D0836964

AVOIDING COMMON
ANESTHESIA ERRORS

CONTRIBUTING EDITORS

RANDAL O. DULL, MD, PhD

Associate Professor of Anesthesiology, Bioengineering, and Pharmaceutical Chemistry
University of Utah School of Medicine
Salt Lake City, Utah

F. JACOB SEAGULL, PhD

Assistant Professor of Anesthesiology
Director of Performance Technology Research
University of Maryland School of Medicine
Baltimore, Maryland

SURJYA SEN, MD

Resident in Anesthesiology
Mayo School of Graduate Medical Education
Mayo Clinic College of Medicine
Rochester, Minnesota

JURAJ SPRUNG, MD, PhD

Consultant, Department of Anesthesiology, Mayo Clinic
Professor of Anesthesiology
Mayo Clinic College of Medicine
Rochester, Minnesota

PETER ROCK, MD, MBA, FCCM

Martin Helrich Professor and Chair
Department of Anesthesiology
The University of Maryland School of Medicine
Anesthesiologist-in-Chief
University of Maryland Medical Center
Baltimore, Maryland

SECTION EDITORS

Michael P. Hutchens, MD, MA – *Intraoperative and Perioperative Management*
Stephen T. Robinson, MD – *Equipment*
Amit Sharma, MD – *Regional Anesthesia, Pain*
Robert D. Valley, MD – *Pediatric Anesthesia*
Laurel E. Moore, MD – *Neuroanesthesia*
Edwin G. Avery, IV, MD – *Cardiac Anesthesia*
Christopher E. Swide, MD – *Obstetric Anesthesia*
F. Jacob Seagull, PhD – *Human Factors*
Kenneth R. Abbey, MD, JD – *Legal Issues*
Norman A. Cohen, MD – *Economic/Practice Issues*

AVOIDING COMMON ANESTHESIA ERRORS

EDITORS

CATHERINE MARCUCCI, MD
Assistant Professor, Department of Anesthesiology
University of Maryland Medical System, Anesthesia Services
Veterans Administration Maryland Health Care System
Baltimore, Maryland

NORMAN A. COHEN, MD
Assistant Professor of Anesthesiology and Perioperative Medicine
Oregon Health and Science University, Portland, Oregon
Chair, Committee on Economics
American Society of Anesthesiologists
Park Ridge, Illinois

DAVID G. METRO, MD
Associate Professor of Anesthesiology
Director, Anesthesiology Residency Program
University of Pittsburgh Physicians
Pittsburgh, Pennsylvania

JEFFREY R. KIRSCH, MD
Professor and Chair of Anesthesiology
Oregon Health and Science University
Portland, Oregon

SERIES EDITOR

LISA MARCUCCI, MD
Assistant Professor of Surgery
Division of Trauma and Critical Care
Department of Surgery
Thomas Jefferson University
Philadelphia, Pennsylvania

The editors acknowledge and thank Lippincott Williams and Wilkins for their generous contribution to the Foundation for Anesthesia Education and Research.

 Wolters Kluwer | Lippincott Williams & Wilkins
Health
Philadelphia · Baltimore · New York · London
Buenos Aires · Hong Kong · Sydney · Tokyo

Acquisitions Editor: Brian Brown
Managing Editor: Nicole Dernoski
Marketing Manager: Angela Panetta
Production Editor: Bridgett Dougherty
Senior Manufacturing Manager: Benjamin Rivera
Design Coordinator: Risa Clow
Compositor: Aptara, Inc.

Copyright © 2008 Lippincott Williams & Wilkins

530 Walnut St.
Philadelphia, PA 19106

All rights reserved. This book is protected by copyright. No part of this book may be reproduced in any form or by any means, including photocopying, or utilized by any information storage and retrieval system without written permission from the copyright owner.

The publisher is not responsible (as a matter of product liability, negligence, or otherwise) for any injury resulting from any material contained herein. This publication contains information relating to general principles of medical care that should not be construed as specific instructions for individual patients. Manufacturers' product information and package inserts should be reviewed for current information, including contraindications, dosages, and precautions.

Printed in the United States of America

Library of Congress Cataloging-in-Publication Data

Avoiding common anesthesia errors / editor, Cathy Marcucci.
    p. ; cm.
  Includes bibliographical references and index.
  ISBN-13: 978-0-7817-8847-2 (case)
  ISBN-10: 0-7817-8847-1 (case)
  1. Anesthesia.   2. Medical errors—Prevention.   I. Marcucci, Cathy.
  [DNLM: 1. Anesthesia—methods.   2. Medical Errors—Prevention & control.
WO 200 A961 2007]
  RD81.A96 2007
  617.9′6—dc22
                                                                2007020749

The publishers have made every effort to trace the copyright holders for borrowed material. If they have inadvertently overlooked any, they will be pleased to make the necessary arrangements at the first opportunity.
    To purchase additional copies of this book, call our customer service department at (800) 638-3030 or fax orders to (301) 824-7390. International customers should call (301) 714- 2324.
    Visit Lippincott Williams & Wilkins on the Internet: http://www.LWW.com. Lippincott Williams & Wilkins customer service representatives are available from 8:30 am to 6:00 pm, EST.

01 02 03 04 05
1 2 3 4 5 6 7 8 9 10

To Charlie and Lisa, my two wonderful children, and heartfelt thanks to my patient spouse. C.M.

Unmeasurable thanks to my wife, Michelle, and my daughter, Allie, who have allowed me the time to pursue my interests. Also, a debt of gratitude to my colleagues at the ASA and AMA for their mentorship and friendship. N.A.C

To my wife Maria, kids (Luke, Nicholas, and Emily) and the anesthesiology residents at the University of Pittsburgh who helped make this possible. D.G.M

To my wife and best friend Robin and my wonderful children, Jodi, Alan, and Ricki for their incredible encouragement and for helping me realize the important priorities in life. J.R.K.

PREFACE

The pressures facing the anesthesiologist or anesthetist are in some ways unique. As always, the patients say it best. Recently, one of the editors of this book was asked the following question, "You mean to tell me that it takes three surgical doctors to take care of just my ear drum, but you and that young fellow over there can take care of all of the rest of me all by yourselves?"

As part and parcel of taking care of "all of the rest" of the patient, the anesthesia provider must fully understand physiology, pathophysiology, and pharmacology; become experts in anesthesia equipment and associated specialized technology; and master skills in airway management and the performance of many procedures. And we must do this in a complex, noisy, and often hostile clinical setting, all while trying as hard as possible to do the right thing and not do the wrong thing! Unfortunately, in spite of everyone's best efforts, mistakes will happen. The editors and authors of this book have had the goal to convey their knowledge from *personally* dealing with and learning from the vast majority of situations in this book, either as a trainee, provider, or a supervisor. We hope that we can impart the knowledge of our pooled experience to the reader who may have limitations due to the nature of their clinical setting or the stage of their career.

It has been suggested facetiously that this book might also be titled "Conversations from the Anesthesiology Break Room," which is exactly what we intended from the outset of this project. There are many excellent standard comprehensive and reference texts available to anesthesia providers and trainees; this book is intended to complement rather than supersede them. Our goal is to provide our collective wisdom in readable, conversational bites, exactly as if you are sitting in the anesthesia office with your supervising faculty or attending and you have about ten minutes before the case starts. Literally, when pondering points for the book, two of our main criteria were "What do we hear the senior staff saying to the junior staff over and over? What was said to us when we were in training that had lasting impact on our practices?" It's also okay with us if the readers laugh a little while reading this book.

In developing the content, we owe a tremendous debt to both our contributing editors and section editors. These individuals contributed expertise, enthusiasm, energy, and ideas and shouldered huge amounts of the work as well. Special thanks to Randal O. Dull, MD, PhD for believing in and "signing onto" the project in its very earliest stages and F. Jacob Seagull,

PhD for helping us with his special expertise in the field of human factors and errors psychology.

We also thank several others for their unique contributions: Katey Millet and Renee Redding for their advice and assistance in preparing the manuscript; the anesthesia residents at the Johns Hopkins Hospital, including Chauncey T. Jones, MD, Andrew M. Gross, MD, and Hassan Ahmad, MD as well as the anesthesia residents at the University of Utah for writing the first chapters and showing us it could be done; Charles W. Emala, MD for his help in finding us authors and editors at Columbia; John L. Cameron, MD for giving us permission to quote him; Sharon Merrick, CCS-P, Coding Manager at ASA's Washington Office, for her technical review of the coding chapters; Michael J. Moritz, MD for his review of the initial chapters of the book; Michael W. Barts, CRNA, for reviewing the topics list and sending us input "from the field;" Deborah Dlugose, CRNA, for her advice, suggestions, and encouragement; and Denis L. Bourke, MD, for his ongoing support.

CATHERINE MARCUCCI, MD
NORMAN A. COHEN, MD
DAVID G. METRO, MD
JEFFREY R. KIRSCH, MD

The authors and editors have unanimously donated their royalties to the Foundation for Anesthesia Education and Research in hopes of further improving the foundation of knowledge in our specialty.

The editors welcome comments and suggestions at sandson. marcucci@comcast.net.

Anesthesiology has evolved to a place in medicine far beyond the traditional provision of intraoperative care, solo or small group practices, and one-office billing processes. The scope of practices in the specialty now encompasses the entire perioperative spectrum, ranging from preoperative assessment and management through postoperative intensive care and acute pain management. Pain medicine also has transitioned from "mom and pop" injection shops to expansive, multidisciplinary practices and hospice care. Even the business processes of anesthesiology, from billing to call responsibilities to exclusive contracting, have become increasingly complex. Thus, medical students, residents, fellows, and other anesthesia students, plus a growing proportion of us older folks who see our practices expanding or who are involved in maintenance of certification, need concise, accurate, and useful information that covers the broad range of topics that we encounter in practice and the business of anesthesiology.

Drs. Cathy Marcucci, Norm Cohen, David Metro, and Jeff Kirsch have provided all anesthesia trainees and many of our practicing anesthesiologists with a book that is terrific. It provides practical advice on many of the most important and often perplexing issues that we see in everyday practice. I am not aware of any other anesthesiology text that is so useful and, to be honest, fun to read. It is not—and was not designed to be—a comprehensive text. Instead, it provides common sense advice for many of our specialty's most important clinical issues in small, easily digestible bites. In addition, many trainees will find the chapters on practice selection and management to be very worthwhile.

The editors have performed a great service for those young men and women who are attracted to our specialty, plus for those of us who have been blessed with the opportunity to care for anesthetized patients, those who are critically ill, and those who require relief from acute or chronic pain. They deserve our thanks for producing such a useful contribution to anesthesia education.

MARK A. WARNER, M.D.
PROFESSOR OF ANESTHESIOLOGY
MAYO CLINIC COLLEGE OF MEDICINE

ACKNOWLEDGMENT

Many thanks to Surjya Sen, MD, who carried full editorial duties for this project, in spite of being a busy resident and fellow, and whose feedback and advice were invaluable. C.M.
I'd like to thank Sharon Merrick, CCS-P, Coding Manager at ASA's Washington Office, for her technical review of the coding chapters. N.A.C.

CONTRIBUTORS

KENNETH R. ABBEY, MD, JD
Assistant Professor
Department of Anesthesiology and
  Perioperative Medicine
Oregon Health and Science University
Anesthesiologist
Department of Anesthesiology and
  Perioperative Medicine
Oregon Health and Science University
Portland, Oregon

HEATHER A. ABERNETHY, MD
Anesthesiologist
Department of Anesthesiology
Meriter Hospital
Madison, Wisconsin

JENNIFER J. ADAMS, MD
Anesthesiologist
Department of Anesthesiology and Critical
  Care Medicine
Johns Hopkins Hospital
Baltimore, Maryland

SHUSHMA AGGARWAL, MD
Associate Professor
Staff Anesthesiologist
Department of Anesthesiology
University of Pittsburgh Medical Centre
Wexford, Pennsylvania

HASSAN M. AHMAD, MD
Resident
Department of Anesthesiology and Critical
  Care Medicine
Johns Hopkins University
House Staff
Department of Anesthesiology and Critical
  Care Medicine
Johns Hopkins Hospital
Baltimore, Maryland

**MOUSTAFA M. AHMED, MD,
MBBCH**
Clinical Assistant Professor
Department of Anesthesiology and Critical
  Care
University of Pennsylvania
Department of Anesthesia Services
Veterans Administration Philadelphia
  Health Care System
Philadelphia, Pennsylvania

**THEODORE A. ALSTON, MD,
PHD**
Assistant Professor
Department of Anesthesia
Harvard Medical School
Anesthesiologist
Department of Anesthesia and Critical Care
Massachusetts General Hospital
Boston, Massachusetts

DOUGLAS W. ANDERSON, DMD
Instructor
Department of Anesthesiology and
  Perioperative Medicine
Oregon Health and Science University
Portland, Oregon

MIRIAM ANIXTER, MD
Visiting Assistant Professor
Department of Anesthesiology
University of Pittsburgh
Staff Attending
Department of Anesthesiology
Children's Hospital of Pittsburgh
Pittsburgh, Pennsylvania

EDWIN G. AVERY, IV, MD
Instructor of Anesthesia
Department of Anesthesia and Critical Care
Harvard Medical School
Chief, Division of Cardiac Anesthesia
Massachusetts General Hospital
Boston, Massachusetts

MICHAEL AXLEY, MD, MS
Resident
Department of Anesthesilogy
Oregon Health and Science University
Portland, Oregon

MICHAEL AZIZ, MD
Assistant Professor
Department of Anesthesiology and
  Perioperative Medicine
Oregon Health and Science University
Portland, Oregon

ANN G. BAILEY, MD
Professor
Departments of Pediatrics and
  Anesthesiology
University of North Carolina
Chapel Hill, North Carolina

PATRICK G. BAKKE, MD
Assistant Professor
Department of Anesthesia and Perioperative
  Medicine
Oregon Health and Science University
Portland, Oregon

RODGER BARNETTE, MD, FCCM
Professor and Chairman
Department of Anesthesiology
Temple University School of Medicine
Chairman
Department of Anesthesiology
Temple University Hospital
Philadelphia, Pennsylvania

STEPHEN R. BARONE, MD
Instructor
Department of Anesthesiology
Weill Cornell Medical College
New York, New York

**MICHAEL W. BARTS, CRNA,
  BSAnesth, AAAPM**
Barts Professional Pain Services, P.C.
Sweet Grass Anesthesia, PLLP
Northern Montana Hospital Anesthesia
  Services
Havre, Montana

SHAWN T. BEAMAN, MD
Visiting Instructor
Department of Anesthesiology
University of Pittsburgh School of Medicine
Montefiore University Hospital
Pittsburgh, Pennsylvania

BRUCE BEN-DAVID, MD
Clinical Associate Professor
Department of Anesthesiology
University of Pittsburgh
Attending Staff/Associate Director
Acute Interventional Postoperative Pain
  Service
Department of Anesthesiology
UPMC-Shadyside Hospital
Pittsburgh, Pennsylvania

ALEXIS BILBO, MD
Resident
Department of Anesthesiology and Critical
  Care Medicine
Johns Hopkins School of Medicine
Baltimore, Maryland

**DANIEL J. BOCHICCHIO, MD,
  FCCP**
Assistant Professor
Department of Anesthesiology
University of Maryland
Colonel, Medical Corps
Deputy Chief Surgeon
National Guard Bureau
Joint Staff
Baltimore, Maryland

CAROL F. BODENHEIMER, MD
Assistant Professor
Department of Physical Medicine and
  Rehabilitation
Baylor College of Medicine
Medical Director
Department of Specialty Rehabilitation
The Institute of Rehabilitation and
  Research
Houston, Texas

KATARINA BOJANIC, MD
Resident
Department of Gynecology and Obstetrics
KB Merkur
Zagreb, Croatia

RYAN J. BORTOLON, MD
Staff Anesthesiologist
Department of Anesthesia
Shriners Hospital for Children-Twin Cities
Minneapolis, Minnesota

RICHARD BOTNEY, MD
Assistant Professor
Department of Anesthesiology and
  Perioperative Medicine
Oregon Health and Science University
Staff Anesthesiologist
Department of Anesthesiology and
  Perioperative Medicine
Oregon Health and Science University
Portland, Oregon

CHARLES D. BOUCEK, MD
Associate Professor
Departments of Anesthesiology and
  Medicine
University of Pittsburgh
Physician
Department of Anesthesiology
Presbyterian University Hospital
Pittsburgh, Pennsylvania

DANIEL R. BROWN, MD, PHD
Chair, Division of Critical Care Medicine
Department of Anesthesiology
Mayo Clinic College of Medicine
Chair, Division of Critical Care Medicine
Department of Anesthesiology
Mayo Clinic
Rochester, Minnesota

JOHN T. BRYANT, IV, MD
Chief Resident
Department of Anesthesiology
University of North Carolina Hospitals
Chapel Hill, North Carolina

ABRAM H. BURGHER, MD
Resident
Department of Anesthesia
Mayo Clinic
Rochester, Minnesota

DAVID A. BURNS, MD
Regional Anesthesiology Fellow
Department of Anesthesiology
University of Pittsburgh
  Presbyterian-Shadyside Hospitals
Pittsburgh, Pennsylvania

STEVEN J. BUSUTTIL, MD, FACS
Assistant Professor
Division of Vascular Surgery
University of Maryland
Chief, Section of Vascular Surgeon
Department of Vascular Surgery
VA Maryland Health Care System
Baltimore, Maryland

MATTHEW CALDWELL, MD
Clinical Assistant Professor
Department of Anesthesiology
University of Michigan Health System
Ann Arbor, Michigan

TAMMILY R. CARPENTER, MD
Instructor
Department of Anesthesiology and
  Perioperative Medicine
Oregon Health and Science University
Anesthesiologist
Department of Anesthesiology and
  Perioperative Medicine
Oregon Health and Science University
Portland, Oregon

THOMAS M. CHALIFOUX, MD
Resident
Department of Anesthesiology
University of Pittsburgh
Pittsburgh, Pennsylvania

JOBY CHANDY, MD
Resident
Department of Anesthesia and Critical Care
Harvard Medical School
Resident
Department of Anesthesia and Critical Care
Massachusetts General Hospital
Boston, Massachusetts

WALTER L. CHANG, MD
Anesthesiologist
Department of Anesthesia
City of Hope Medical Center
Duarte, California

ALAN CHENG, MD
Assistant Professor of Medicine
Department of Medicine
Division of Cardiology
Johns Hopkins University School of
    Medicine
Staff Cardiac Electrophysiologist
Department of Medicine
Division of Cardiology
Johns Hopkins Hospital
Baltimore, Maryland

GRACE L. CHIEN, MD
Chief, Anesthesiology Service
Co–Clinical Director, Operative Care
    Division
Portland Veterans Affairs Medical Center
Associate Professor
Department of Anesthesiology and
    Perioperative Medicine
Oregon Health and Science University
Portland, Oregon

**ROSE CHRISTOPHERSON, MD,
PHD**
Associate Professor
Department of Anesthesiology and
    Perioperative Medicine
Oregon Health and Science University
Staff Anesthesiologist
Department of Operative Care Division
Portland VA Medical Center
Portland, Oregon

MARK CHROSTOWSKI, MD
Resident
Department of Anesthesia and Critical Care
Massachusetts General Hospital
Boston, Massachusetts

NORMAN A. COHEN, MD
Assistant Professor
Department of Anesthesiology and
    Perioperative Medicine
Oregon Health and Science University
Portland, Oregon

IVAN V. COLAIZZI, MD
Resident
Department of Anesthesiology
University of Pittsburgh
Pittsburgh, Pennsylvania

**CHRISTOPHER M. COLVILLE,
MD**
Resident
Department of Anesthesiology and
    Perioperative Medicine
Oregon Health and Science University
Portland, Oregon

THOMAS B. O. COMFERE, MD
Assistant Professor
Department of Anesthesiology, Critical Care
    Division
Mayo Clinic
Senior Associate Consultant
Department of Anesthesiology, Critical Care
    Division
Mayo Clinic
Rochester, Minnesota

ERIK A. COOPER, DO
Resident
Department of Anesthesiology
University of Pittsburgh Medical Center
Pittsburgh, Pennsylvania

ELIZABETH E. COSTELLO, MD
Resident
Department of Anesthesiology
University of Pittsburgh Medical Center
Pittsburgh, Pennsylvania

JENNIFER COZZENS, MD, MPH
Resident
Department of Family Medicine
Oregon Health and Science University
Portland, Oregon

GRANT T. CRAVENS, MD
Resident
Department of Anesthesiology
Mayo Clinic
Rochester, Minnesota

PETER F. CRONHOLM, MD, MSCE
Assistant Professor
Department of Family Medicine and
    Community Health
University of Pennsylvania
Attending
Department of Family Medicine and
    Community Health
Hospital of the University of Pennsylvania
Penn Presbyterian Medical Center
Philadelphia, Pennsylvania

DANIELA DAMIAN, MD
Visiting Instructor
Department of Anesthesiology
University of Pittsburgh School of Medicine
Pittsburgh, Pennsylvania

JAMES F. DANA, MD
Department of Anesthesia and Critical Care
Massachusetts General Hospital
Harvard Medical School
Boston, Massachusetts

RICHARD F. DAVIS, MD, MBA
Professor
Department of Anesthesiology and
    Perioperative Medicine
Oregon Health and Science University
Staff Anesthesiologist
Department of Anesthesiology and
    Perioperative Medicine
OHSU Hospital
Portland, Oregon

M. CONCETTA DECARIA, MD
Resident
Department of Anesthesiology
University of North Carolina
Chapel Hill, North Carolina

MATTHEW V. DECARO, MD, FACC
Clinical Assistant Professor of Medicine
Department of Medicine
Division of Cardiology
Jefferson Medical College
Jefferson Heart Institute
Director Coronary Care Unit
Division of Cardiology
Thomas Jefferson University Hospital
Philadelphia, Pennsylvania

JENNIFER A. DECOU, MD
Resident
Department of Anesthesiology
University of Utah School of Medicine
Salt Lake City, Utah

J. MAURICIO DEL RIO, MD
Resident
Department of Anesthesiology
Pittsburgh, Pennsylvania

JAMES S. DEMEESTER, MD
Clinical Instructor
Department of Anesthesiology and Critical
    Care Medicine
Johns Hopkins Hospital
Baltimore, Maryland

BRANDON C. DIAL, MD
Chief Resident
Department of Anesthesiology
University of Utah
Salt Lake City, Utah

HEATH R. DIEL, MD
Clinical Instructor
Department of Anesthesiology
University of Utah
Salt Lake City, Utah

PEGGY P. DIETRICH, MD
Chief Resident
Department of Anesthesia
University of North Carolina
Chapel Hill, North Carolina

JEFFREY D. DILLON, MD
Instructor
Department of Anesthesiology
University of Utah
Instructor
Department of Anesthesiology
University of Utah Medical Center
Salt Lake City, Utah

RALPH DiRADO, RN
Registered Nurse
Department of Surgical Services
Philadelphia Veterans' Administration
   Medical Center
Philadelphia, Pennsylvania

**DEBORAH DLUGOSE, RN,
   CCRN, CRNA**
Staff CRNA
Anesthesia Services
Veterans Administration Maryland Health
   Care System
Baltimore, Maryland

KAREN B. DOMINO, MD, MPH
Professor
Department of Anesthesiology
University of Washington School of
   Medicine
Seattle, Washington

RANDAL O. DULL, MD, PHD
Associate Professor
Department of Anesthesiology
University of Utah School of Medicine
Salt Lake City, Utah

MUHAMMAD DURRANI, MD
Fellow, Cardiac Anesthesiology
The Johns Hopkins Hospital
Baltimore, Maryland

ERIK S. ECKMAN, MD
Chief Resident
Department of Anesthesiology
University of North Carolina Hospitals
Chapel Hill, North Carolina

JUANITA P. EDWARDS, MD, MS
Resident
Department of Anesthesiology
University of North Carolina
Chapel Hill, North Carolina

JAMEY E. EKLUND, MD
Resident
Department of Anesthesiology
University of Pittsburgh Medical Center
Pittsburgh, Pennsylvania

NABIL M. ELKASSABANY, MD
Clinical Assistant Professor
Department of Anesthesiology and Critical
   Care
University of Pennsylvania
Staff Anesthesiologist
Department of Anesthesiology
Philadelphia VA Medical Center
Philadelphia, Pennsylvania

THOMAS R. ELSASS, MD
Resident
Department of Anesthesiology
University of North Carolina Hospitals
Chapel Hill, North Carolina

WARREN K. ENG, MD
Resident
Department of Anesthesiology
UNC Hospitals Chapel Hill
Chapel Hill, North Carolina

T. MIKO ENOMOTO, MD
Chief Resident
Department of Anesthesiology and
   Perioperative Medicine
Oregon Health and Science University
Portland, Oregon

HEATH A. FALLIN, MD
Resident
Department of Anesthesiology
University of Pittsburgh Medical Center
Pittsburgh, Pennsylvania

HOOMAN RASTEGAR FASSAEI, MD
Resident
Department of Anesthesiology
University of Pittsburgh
Pittsburgh, Pennsylvania

LYNN A. FENTON, MD
Assistant Professor
Department of Anesthesiology and
   Perioperative Medicine
Oregon Health and Science University
Portland, Oregon

BYRON D. FERGERSON, MD
Resident
Department of Anesthesiology
University of Utah School of Medicine
Salt Lake City, Utah

LAURA H. FERGUSON, MD
Resident
Department of Anesthesiology
The University of Pittsburgh Medical
   Center
Pittsburgh, Pennsylvania

MARISA H. FERRERA, MD
Resident
Department of Anesthesiology
University of Pittsburgh
Pittsburgh, Pennsylvania

ALAN C. FINLEY, MD
Resident
Department of Anesthesiology
University of North Carolina Hospitals
Chapel Hill, North Carolina

MICHAEL G. FITZSIMONS, MD
Instructor in Anesthesia
Division of Cardiac Anesthesia
Department of Anesthesia and Critical Care
Massachusetts General Hospital
Boston, Massachusetts

PATRICK J. FORTE, MD
Assistant Professor
Department of Anesthesiology
University of Pittsburgh
Director of Ambulatory Services
Department of Anesthesiology
University of Pittsburgh Medical Center
Pittsburgh, Pennsylvania

BRYAN J. FRITZ, MD
Resident
Department of Anesthesiology
University of Pittsburgh Medical Center
Pittsburgh, Pennsylvania

COSMIN GAURAN, MD
Resident
Department of Anesthesia and Critical Care
Harvard Medical School
Massachusetts General Hospital
Boston, Massachusetts

THERESA A. GELZINIS, MD
Assistant Professor
Department of Anesthesiology
University of Pittsburgh
Staff Anesthesiologist
Department of Anesthesiology
University of Pittsburgh Medical Center
Pittsburgh, Pennsylvania

EDWARD GEORGE, MD, PHD
Lecturer
Department of Anesthesiology
Harvard Medical School
Medical Director, Post Anesthesia Care
   Units
Department of Anesthesia and Critical Care
Massachusetts General Hospital
Boston, Massachusetts

BISWAJIT GHOSH, MD
Clinical Assistant Professor
Department of Anesthesiology
SUNY Downstate Medical Center
Brooklyn, New York

J. SAXON GILBERT, MD
Resident
Department of Anesthesiology and
   Perioperative Medicine
Oregon Health and Science University
Portland, Oregon

**STEPHEN J. GLEICH, BS
(MSIII)**
Medical Student
Mayo Medical School
Mayo Clinic College of Medicine
Rochester, Minnesota

ANDREW M. GROSS, MD
Resident
Department of Anesthesia and Critical Care
   Medicine
Johns Hopkins Hospital
Baltimore, Maryland

KAREN HAND, MD
Assistant Professor
Department of Anesthesiology and
   Perioperative Medicine
Oregon Health and Science University
Anesthesiologist
Department of Anesthesiology and
   Perioperative Medicine
Oregon Health and Science University
Portland, Oregon

**ANNE B. HAUPT, RN, BSN,
CNOR**
Surgical Services
Veterans Administration Maryland Health
   Care System
Baltimore, Maryland

JUSTIN B. HAUSER, MD
Anesthesiologist
Rex Hospital
Raleigh, North Carolina

**ELLIOTT R. HAUT, MD,
FACS**
Assistant Professor
Department of Surgery and Anesthesiology
   and Critical Care Medicine
Johns Hopkins University School of
   Medicine
Attending Surgeon
Department of Surgery and Anesthesiology
   and Critical Care Medicine
Johns Hopkins Hospital
Baltimore, Maryland

NATHAN J. HESS, DO
Resident
Department of Anesthesiology and
   Perioperative Medicine
Oregon Health and Science University
Portland, Oregon

JAMES S. HICKS, MD, MM
Adjunct Associate Professor
Department of Anesthesiology and
   Perioperative Medicine
Oregon Health and Science University
Portland, Oregon

**IBTESAM A. HILMI, MB, CHB,
FRCA**
Assistant Professor
Department of Anesthesiology
University of Pittsburgh Medical Center
Presbyterian Hospital
Pittsburgh, Pennsylvania

J. TODD HOBELMANN, MD
Resident
Department of Anesthesiology and Critical
   Care Medicine
Johns Hopkins Hospital
Baltimore, Maryland

**MICHAEL S. N. HOGAN, MB,
BCH**
Senior Resident
Department of Anesthesiology
Mayo Graduate School of Medicine
Rochester, Minnesota

JEAN-LOUIS HORN, MD
Associate Professor, Director of Regional
    Anesthesia
Department of Anesthesiology and
    Perioperative Medicine
Oregon Health and Science University
Portland, Oregon

**MICHAEL P. HUTCHENS, MD,
    MA**
Assistant Professor
Department of Anesthesiology and
    Perioperative Medicine
Oregon Health and Science University
Attending Anesthesiologist/Intensive
Department of Anesthesiology and
    Perioperative Medicine
Oregon Health and Science University
Portland, Oregon

JAMES W. IBINSON, MD, PhD
Resident
Department of Anesthesiology
University of Pittsburgh Medical Center
Pittsburgh, Pennsylvania

AMY V. ISENBERG, MD
Resident
Department of Anesthesiology
UNC School of Medicine
Chapel Hill, North Carolina

**SERGE JABBOUR, MD, FACP,
    FACE**
Associate Professor of Clinical Medicine
Department of Medicine
Division of Endocrinology, Diabetes and
    Metabolic Diseases
Jefferson Medical College
Thomas Jefferson University
Thomas Jefferson Hospital
Philadelphia, Pennsylvania

MAGGIE JEFFRIES, MD
Clinical Instructor of Anesthesiology
MD Anderson Hospital
Houston, Texas

CHAUNCEY T. JONES, MD
Chief Resident
Department of Anesthesiology and Critical
    Care Medicine
Johns Hopkins University
Baltimore, Maryland

IHAB R. KAMEL, MD
Assistant Professor
Department of Anesthesiology
Temple University School of Medicine
Faculty-Staff Anesthesiologist
Department of Anesthesiology
Temple University Hospital
Philadelphia, Pennsylvania

**SAJEEV S. KATHURIA, MD,
    FACS**
Associate Professor
Department of Ophthalmology
University of Maryland
Baltimore, Maryland

PAUL M. KEMPEN, MD, PhD
Associate Professor
Department of Anesthesiology
University of Pittsburgh
Staff Anesthesiologist
Department of Anesthesiology
Presbyterian University Hospital
Pittsburgh, Pennsylvania

ANGELA KENDRICK, MD
Associate Professor
Department of Anesthesiology and
    Perioperative Medicine
Oregon Health and Science University
Associate Professor
Department of Anesthesiology and
    Perioperative Medicine
Doernbesher Children's Hospital-OHSU
Portland, Oregon

DAVID Y. KIM, MD
Assistant Professor
Department of Anesthesiology
Temple University School of Medicine
Faculty Staff Anesthesiologist
Department of Anesthesiology
Temple University Hospital
Philadelphia, Pennsylvania

JEFFREY R. KIRSCH, MD
Professor and Chair
Department of Anesthesiology and
  Perioperative Medicine
Chief, Chair Quality Executive Committee
Oregon Health and Science University
Portland, Oregon

LAVINIA M. KOLARCZYK, MD
Resident
Department of Anesthesiology
University of Pittsburgh Medical Center
Pittsburgh, Pennsylvania

HILARY KOPROWSKI, II, MD
Resident
Department of Otorhinolaryngology—Head
  and Neck Surgery
University of Maryland
Baltimore, Maryland

ROBERT W. KYLE, DO
Assistant Professor
Department of Anesthesiology
University of North Carolina
Faculty
Department of Anesthesiology
UNC Hospitals
Chapel Hill, North Carolina

KIRK LALWANI, MD, FRCA
Associate Professor of Anesthesiology and
  Pediatrics
Department of Anesthesiology and
  Perioperative Medicine
Oregon Health and Science University
Attending Physician
Department of Anesthesiology and
  Pediatrics
Oregon Health and Science University
Portland, Oregon

**GIORA LANDESBERG, MD,
  DSc, MBA**
Associate Professor
Department of Anesthesia and Critical Care
  Medicine
Hebrew University
Kiryat Hadassah
Chief of Cardiothoracic and Vascular
  Anesthesia
Department of Anesthesia and Critical Care
  Medicine
Hadassah Medical Center
Kiryat Hadassah
Jerusalem, Israel

EUGENE E. LEE, MD
Pediatric Anesthesiology Fellow
Department of Anesthesiology
University of North Carolina
Chapel Hill, North Carolina

LORRI A. LEE, MD
Associate Professor
Department of Anesthesiology
University of Washington
Attending Anesthesiologist
Department of Anesthesiology
Harborview Medical Center
Seattle, Washington

ANNE L. LEMAK, DMD
Resident
Department of Dental Anesthesiology
School of Dental Medicine
University of Pittsburgh
Resident
Department of Anesthesiology
University of Pittsburgh Medical Center
Pittsburgh, Pennsylvania

JAY K. LEVIN, MD
Instructor
Department of Anesthesiology and Critical
  Care Medicine
Johns Hopkins University
Baltimore, Maryland

VINCENT K. LEW, BA (MSII)
Medical Student
School of Medicine
Oregon Health and Science University
Medical Student
Department of Anesthesiology and
    Perioperative Medicine
Oregon Health and Science University
Portland, Oregon

ERICA P. LIN, MD
Resident
Department of Anesthesiology
UNC School of Medicine
Chapel Hill, North Carolina

AMY C. LU, MD, MPH
Fellow
Department of Anesthesia and Critical Care
Harvard Medical School
Resident
Department of Anesthesia and Critical Care
Massachusetts General Hospital
Boston, Massachusetts

EVAN T. LUKOW, DO
Resident
Department of Anesthesiology
University of Pittsburgh
Resident
Department of Anesthesiology
University of Pittsburgh—Presbyterian
    Hospital
Pittsburgh, Pennsylvania

YING WEI LUM, MD
Resident
Department of Surgery
Johns Hopkins Hospital
Baltimore, Maryland

ANNE T. LUNNEY, MD
Resident
Department of Anesthesiology
University of North Carolina
Chapel Hill, North Carolina

CATHERINE MARCUCCI, MD
Assistant Professor
Department of Anesthesiology
University of Maryland Medical System
Anesthesia Services
Veterans Administration Maryland Health
    Care System
Baltimore, Maryland

LISA MARCUCCI, MD
Assistant Professor
Department of Surgery
Thomas Jefferson University
Attending Surgeon
Department of Surgery
Thomas Jefferson University Hospital
Philadelphia, Pennsylvania

JULIE MARSHALL, MD
Resident
Department of Anesthesiology
University of North Carolina
Resident
Department of Anesthesiology
University of North Carolina Hospital
Chapel Hill, North Carolina

JOHN S. MARVEL, DO
Chief Resident
Department of Anesthesiology and Critical
    Care Medicine
Johns Hopkins Hospital
Baltimore, Maryland

GEORGE A. MASHOUR, MD, PHD
Assistant Professor
Department of Anesthesiology
University of Michigan Medical School
Attending Anesthesiologist
Department of Anesthesiology
University of Michigan Health System
Ann Arbor, Michigan

LEENA MATHEW, MD
Assistant Professor
Department of Anesthesiology
Columbia University
New York Presbyterian Hospital
New York, New York

JANEY P. MCGEE, MD
Resident
Department of Anesthesiology
University of North Carolina School of
    Medicine
Resident
Department of Anesthesiology
University of NC Hospitals
Chapel Hill, North Carolina

RYAN C. MCHUGH, MD
Resident
Department of Anesthesiology
Mayo Clinic
Rochester, Minnesota

**VIPIN MEHTA, MBBS, MD,
DARCS, FFARCSI**
Instructor
Department of Cardiac Anesthesia
Harvard Medical School
Staff Anesthesiologist
Department of Cardiac Anesthesia
Massachusetts General Hospital
Boston, Massachusetts

LI MENG, MD, MPH
Assistant Professor
Department of Anesthesiology
University of Pittsburgh
Medical Director of PACU
Department of Anesthesiology
University Pittsburgh Medical Center
Pittsburgh, Pennsylvania

SARAH MERRITT, MD
Fellow
Department of Anesthesiology, Pain
    Division
Johns Hopkins University
Clinical Fellow in Pain Medicine
Department of Anesthesiology, Pain
    Division
Johns Hopkins Medical Institutions
Baltimore, Maryland

RENEE A. METAL, JD
Legal Associate
Rosen Louik and Perry, P.C. Law Firm
Pittsburgh, Pennsylvania

DAVID G. METRO, MD
Associate Professor
Department of Anesthesiology
University of Pittsburgh
Anesthesiologist
Department of Anesthesiology
University of Pittsburgh Medical Center
Pittsburgh, Pennsylvania

LEANDER L. MONCUR, MD
Department of Anesthesia
Loma Linda University Medical Center
Loma Linda, California

LAUREL E. MOORE, MD
Assistant Professor
Department of Anesthesiology
Johns Hopkins University School of
    Medicine
Baltimore, Maryland

MICHAEL J. MORITZ, MD
Professor
Department of Surgery
Penn State College of Medicine
Hershey, Pennsylvania
Chief, Transplant Services
Department of Surgery
Lehigh Valley Hospital
Allentown, Pennsylvania

JEFF T. MUELLER, MD
Instructor
Department of Anesthesiology
Mayo Clinic
Scottsdale, Arizona
Medical Director, Perioperative Services
Mayo Clinic Hospital
Phoenix, Arizona

DANIEL T. MURRAY, CRNA, BSNA, MA
Staff CRNA
Anesthesia Services
Veterans Administration Maryland Health
    Care System
Baltimore, Maryland

PAMELA D. NICHOLS, RN
Surgical Services
Veterans Administration Maryland Health
    Care System
Baltimore, Maryland

ADAM D. NIESEN, MD
Resident
Department of Anesthesiology
Mayo Clinic
Rochester, Minnesota

L. MICHELE NOLES, MD
Assistant Professor
Department of Anesthesiology and
    Perioperative Medicine
Oregon Health and Science University
Portland, Oregon

ALA NOZARI, MD, PhD
Instructor in Anesthesia
Department of Anesthesia and Critical
    Care
Massachusetts General Hospital
Harvard Medical School
Assistant in Anesthesia
Department of Anesthesia and Critical
    Care
Massachusetts General Hospital
Boston Massachusetts

MOHAMMED OJODU, MD
Resident
Department of Anesthesiology
University of Pittsburgh
Pittsburgh, Pennsylvania

JAMES C. OPTON, MD
Resident
Department of Anesthesiology and
    Perioperative Medicine
Oregon Health and Science University
Portland, Oregon

TODD M. ORAVITZ, MD
Assistant Professor
Department of Anesthesiology
University of Pittsburgh
Chief, Hepatic Transplant Anesthesia
VA Pittsburgh Healthcare System
Pittsburgh, Pennsylvania

STEVEN L. OREBAUGH, MD
Associate Professor
Department of Anesthesiology
University of Pittsburgh Medical
    Center-Southside
Staff Anesthesiologist
Department of Anesthesiology
University of Pittsburgh Medical
    Center-Southside
Pittsburgh, Pennsylvania

ANTHONY N. PASSANNANTE, MD
Professor and Vice-Chair
Department of Anesthesiology
UNC Chapel Hill
Chapel Hill, North Carolina

ANGELA M. PENNELL, MD
Resident
Department of Anesthesiology
University of North Carolina
Chief Resident
Department of Anesthesiology
UNC Hospitals-Chapel Hill
Chapel Hill, North Carolina

JORGE PINEDA, JR, MD
Instructor
Department of Anesthesiology and
  Perioperative Medicine
Oregon Health and Science University
Anesthesiologist
Department of Anesthesiology and
  Perioperative Medicine
Oregon Health and Science University
Portland, Oregon

RAYMOND M. PLANINSIC, MD
Associate Professor
Department of Anesthesiology
University of Pittsburgh School of Medicine
Director of Hepatic Transplantation
  Anesthesiology
Department of Anesthesiology
University of Pittsburgh Medical Center
UPMC-Presbyterian
Pittsburgh, Pennsylvania

ANNE E. PTASZYNSKI, MD
Fellow
Department of Anesthesiology
Mayo Graduate School of Medicine
Rochester, Minnesota

JUAN N. PULIDO, MD
Chief Fellow
Division of Critical Care Medicine
Department of Anesthesiology
Mayo Clinic College of Medicine
Rochester, Minnesota

JASON Z. QU, MD
Assistant Professor
Department of Anesthesia
Harvard Medical School
Attending Physician
Department of Anesthesia
Massachusetts General Hospital
Boston, Massachusetts

VIDYA K. RAO, MD
Resident
Department of Anesthesiology
University of Pittsburgh Medical Center
Pittsburgh, Pennsylvania

STEPHEN T. ROBINSON, MD
Associate Professor
Department of Anesthesiology and
  Perioperative Medicine
Oregon Health and Science University
Anesthesiologist
Department of Anesthesiology and
  Perioperative Medicine
Oregon Health and Science University
Portland, Oregon

PETER ROCK, MD, MBA, FCCM
Martin Helrich Professor and Chair
Department of Anesthesiology
The University of Maryland School of
  Medicine
Anesthesiologist-in-Chief
University of Maryland Medical Center
Baltimore, Maryland

RYAN C. ROMEO, MD
Assistant Professor
Department of Anesthesiology
University of Pittsburgh
Staff Anesthesiologist
Department of Anesthesiology
Magee Womens Hospital
Pittsburgh, Pennsylvania

TETSURO SAKAI, MD, PHD
Assistant Professor
Department of Anesthesiology
University of Pittsburgh
Staff Anesthesiologist
Department of Anesthesiology
University of Pittsburgh Medical Center
UPMC Presbyterian/Montefiore
Pittsburgh, Pennsylvania

NEIL B. SANDSON, MD
Director, Residency Training
Sheppard Pratt Health System
Clinical Assistant Professor
University of Maryland Medical School
Department of Psychiatry
Baltimore, Maryland

PRASERT SAWASDIWIPACHAI, MD
Instructor
Department of Anesthesiology
Faculty of Medicine, Mahidol University
Attending Physician
Department of Anesthesiology
Siriraj Hospital
Bangkok, Thailand

SHASHANK SAXENA, MD
Assistant Professor
Department of Anesthesiology
University of Pittsburgh Medical Center
Staff Physician
Department of Anesthesia
VA Pittsburgh Health Care System
Pittsburgh, Pennsylvania

F. JACOB SEAGULL, PHD
Assistant Professor
Director of Education Research
Division of General Surgery
University of Maryland
Baltimore, Maryland

SURJYA SEN, MD
Pain Medicine Fellow
Department of Anesthesiology
Mayo Clinic
Rochester, Minnesota

VALERIE SERA, DDS, MD
Assistant Professor
Division Chief, Adult Cardiac Anesthesia
Department of Anesthesia and Perioperative
   Medicine
Oregon Health and Science University
Portland, Oregon

DAVID A. SHAFF, MD
Instructor
Department of Anesthesiology
Tufts University School of Medicine
Boston, Massachusetts
Senior Staff
Department of Anesthesiology
Lahey Clinic
Burlington, Massachusetts

AMIT SHARMA, MD
Assistant Professor
Department of Anesthesiology
College of Physicians and Surgeons of
   Columbia University
Attending Physician
Department of Anesthesiology
New York Presbyterian Hospital
New York, New York

PHILIP SHIN, MD
Department of Anesthesiology
Columbia University
Housestaff
Department of Anesthesiology
New York Presbyterian Hospital
New York, New York

TODD J. SMAKA, MD
Resident
Department of Anesthesiology and
   Perioperative Medicine
Oregon Health and Science University
Portland, Oregon

KATHLEEN A. SMITH, MD
Resident
Department of Anesthesiology
University of North Carolina
Chapel Hill, North Carolina

JURAJ SPRUNG, MD, PHD
Professor
Department of Anesthesiology
Mayo Clinic College of Medicine
Consultant
Department of Anesthesiology
Mayo Clinic College of Medicine
Rochester, Minnesota

MICHAEL J. STELLA, MD
Assistant Professor
Department of Anesthesiology
University of North Carolina, School of
   Medicine
Assistant Professor
Department of Anesthesiology
North Carolina Children's Hospital
Chapel Hill, North Carolina

MARCUS C. STEPANIAK, CRNA, MS, BSN
Instructor
Department of Anesthesiology and
  Perioperative Medicine
Oregon Health and Science University
CRNA
Department of Anesthesiology and
  Perioperative Medicine
Oregon Health and Science University
Portland, Oregon

JOSEPH B. STRATON, MD, MSCE
Assistant Professor
Department of Family Medicine and
  Community Health
Department of Anesthesiology and
  Critical Care
University of Pennsylvania
Philadelphia, Pennsylvania
Chief Medical Officer
Penn Wissahickon Hospice
University of Pennsylvania Health System
Bala Cynwyd, Pennsylvania

ESTHER SUNG, MD
Resident
Department of Anesthesiology and
  Perioperative Medicine
Oregon Health and Science University
Portland, Oregon

CHRISTOPHER E. SWIDE, MD
Associate Professor
Department of Anesthesiology and
  Perioperative Medicine
Oregon Health and Science University
Staff Anesthesiologist
Department of Anesthesiology and
  Perioperative Medicine
OHSU Hospital
Portland, Oregon

JOSEPH F. TALARICO, DO
Assistant Professor
Department of Anesthesiology
University of Pittsburgh School of Medicine
University of Pittsburgh Medical Center
Pittsburgh, Pennsylvania

ANDREA Y. TAN, MD
Resident
Department of Anesthesiology
University of Pittsburgh
Pittsburgh, Pennsylvania

TERRENCE L. TRENTMAN, MD
Assistant Professor of Anesthesiology
Mayo Clinic
Scottsdale, Arizona

ROBERT D. VALLEY, MD
Professor of Anesthesiology and Pediatrics
Department of Anesthesiology
UNC School of Medicine
Director of Pediatric Anesthesia
Department of Anesthesiology
UNC Hospitals, UNC Children's Hospital
Chapel Hill, North Carolina

JENNIFER VOOKLES, MD, MA
Assistant Professor
Department of Anesthesiology and
  Perioperative Medicine
Oregon Health and Science University
Director, Acute Pain Service
Department of Anesthesiology and
  Perioperative Medicine
Oregon Health and Science University
Portland, Oregon

ANAGH VORA, MD
Resident
Oregon Health and Science University
Portland, Oregon

TOBY N. WEINGARTEN, MD
Assistant Professor
Department of Anesthesia
Mayo Clinic College of Medicine
Rochester, Minnesota

FRANCIS X. WHALEN, JR., MD
Anesthesia Consultant
Department of Anesthesia/Critical Care
  Medicine
Mayo College of Medicine
Rochester, Minnesota

BRADFORD D. WINTERS, MD, PHD
Assistant Professor
Department of Anesthesiology and Critical Care Medicine
Johns Hopkins University School of Medicine
Intensivist
Department of Anesthesiology and Critical Care Medicine
Johns Hopkins Hospital
Baltimore, Maryland

BRIAN WOODCOCK, MB, CHB, MRCP, FRCA, FCCM
Assistant Professor
Director of Medical Student Education
Department of Anesthesiology and Critical Care
University of Michigan
University Hospital
Ann Arbor, Michigan

ANGELA C. WOODITCH, MD
Resident
Department of Anesthesiology
University of Pittsburgh Medical Center
Pittsburgh, Pennsylvania

XIANREN WU, MD
Resident
Department of Anesthesiology
University of Pittsburgh Medical Center
Pittsburgh, Pennsylvania

DENNIS YUN, MD
Fellow in Regional Anesthesia
Department of Anesthesiology
Virginia Mason Medical Center
Seattle, Washington

ANGELA ZIMMERMAN, MD
Assistant Professor
Department of Anesthesiology
Oregon Health and Science University
Portland, Oregon

JOSHUA M. ZIMMERMAN, MD
Clinical Instructor
Department of Anesthesiology
University of Utah
Salt Lake City, Utah

CONTENTS

AIRWAY AND VENTILATION

PEDIATRIC ANESTHESIA   508

OB ANESTHESIA 659

PAIN MEDICINE   711

HUMAN FACTORS   765

LEGAL 795

AVOIDING COMMON ANESTHESIA ERRORS

AIRWAY AND VENTILATION

LINES AND ACCESS

FLUIDS, RESUSCITATION, AND TRANSFUSION

MEDICATIONS

INTRAOPERATIVE AND PERIOPERATIVE

EQUIPMENT

REGIONAL ANESTHESIA

PACU

PEDIATRIC ANESTHESIA

1

NEVER NEGLECT THE BASICS OF
AIRWAY MANAGEMENT

ADAM D. NIESEN, MD AND JURAJ SPRUNG, MD, PHD

Establishing an adequate airway is an important task for every anesthesia provider, as is having a contingency plan in place for a "lost airway." In general, most airway management occurs in the operating room. Before any operation, the anesthesiologist or anesthetist must evaluate the patient's airway and focus on predictors of a difficult airway to minimize the stress and surprise if the airway cannot be secured via the originally planned intervention. Absence of such preparedness could have disastrous consequences.

PATIENT-RELATED CAUSES OF INABILITY TO VENTILATE

The most frequent complications of premature tracheal extubation are hypoventilation, apnea, or obstructive breathing, all frequently associated with hypoxemia and hypercarbia. Immediate postoperative apnea or hypoventilation is most often caused by residual inhaled anesthetic and opioid effects, incomplete reversal of neuromuscular blockade, or the presence of redundant oral tissues. Some patients may have increased sensitivity to anesthetic agents (e.g., elderly, children, patients with obstructive sleep apnea). All this can contribute to loss of airway. Postextubation apnea or hypopnea generally can be resolved with positive-pressure bag-mask ventilation, which may be aided with the placement of an oral or nasopharyngeal airway. However, if ventilation is not achieved, airway patency must be re-established by reintubation or placement of an alternative airway device, such as a laryngeal mask airway (LMA).

Before tracheal extubation, the risk of apnea or hypopnea can be minimized by achieving spontaneous ventilation with adequate tidal volumes and respiratory rate. In addition, anesthetic levels should be low enough to ensure that the patient is able to follow simple commands (e.g., opening eyes, squeezing hands, head lift sustained >5 s). For every patient, the anesthesia provider must check for elegibility for reversal of muscle relaxation by using the twitch monitor, and the reversal agent should be administered well before the end of the surgery to allow enough time for maximal inhibition of pseudocholinesterase. We believe that every patient who has received nondepolarizing muscle relaxants during surgery should receive reversal agents,

© 2006 Mayo Foundation for Medical Education and Research

even if the train-of-four ratio appears visually normal. Exception to that practice should be rare and well considered.

Another possible cause of a lost airway after tracheal extubation is laryngospasm. The highest risk for laryngospasm occurs after induction, just before intubation, or upon emergence from general anesthesia after tracheal extubation as the patient passes through the excitatory phase of anesthesia. Certain patients are at higher risk, such as children and those with a history of smoking, asthma, bronchitis, or bronchiectasis. In addition, certain anesthetic agents, such as desflurane, are more likely to be associated with laryngospasm. If use of bag-mask positive-pressure ventilation with 100% oxygen is unsuccessful in breaking the laryngospasm and maintaining oxygenation, neuromuscular blockade with succinylcholine may be indicated.

MECHANICAL CAUSES OF INABILITY TO VENTILATE

Occlusion of the endotracheal tube by the teeth can occur at virtually any time during anesthesia. It may be due to the patient approximating his or her teeth during emergence or light anesthesia, or to surgical personnel inadvertently applying pressure on the patient's face, causing closure of the teeth. Attempting to breathe spontaneously through an occluded or near-occluded endotracheal tube can cause negative-pressure pulmonary edema, especially in athletic (muscular) patients. In these situations, positive-pressure ventilation could be difficult or impossible. This can be remedied by increasing depth of anesthesia with intravenous agents or administration of muscle relaxants (propofol, lidocaine, or succinylcholine). Typically, after the patient is anesthetized, the endotracheal tube will recoil and airway patency will be re-established. However, when using a wire spiral endotracheal tube, there may be less elastic recoil and the tube may remain partially occluded, requiring emergency tracheal extubation and reintubation with a new tube. This situation is best avoided by placing a "bite block" device, such as an oral airway or other premanufactured hard plastic device, immediately after intubation (especially if muscle relaxants are not used during the operation). Alternatively, a soft bite block may be made from tightly rolled and taped gauze pads placed between the molars.

SURGICAL SITUATIONS CONTRIBUTING TO THE DIFFICULT AIRWAY

Anesthesiologists must exercise special caution when a double-lumen endotracheal tube is changed to a single-lumen tube. The anesthesiologist should critically assess the need for tube exchange because it may be risky in certain patients, such as those who

- Were initially difficult to intubate
- Are morbidly obese

- May be difficult to ventilate via bag-mask device in case reintubation is unsuccessful (beard, obese, facial disfiguration, edentulous)
- Have a compromised airway as a result of the just-performed oral surgery or edema from fluid overload

For these patients it may be safer to keep the double-lumen tracheal tube in place. Alternatively, the anesthesiologist can pull the bronchial lumen into the trachea (after properly deflating both bronchial and tracheal cuffs). After such repositioning, only the tracheal cuff should be reinflated. Another approach is to use a single-lumen tube from the beginning of the case and use a bronchial blocker to perform one-lung ventilation when necessary. However, exchanging the endotracheal tube with "tube exchangers" may not guarantee success.

Although the situation is rare today, special caution should be exercised before tracheal extubation in a patient whose mouth has been wired shut after oral surgery. For these patients, a wire cutter must be readily available at the bedside at all times to facilitate access to the oropharynx in case of emergency. To avoid a potential airway emergency, these patients should be fully awake and responding appropriately to commands before tracheal extubation. All preventive measures should be taken to decrease or eliminate potential postoperative nausea and vomiting, including placing a nasogastric tube and suctioning of gastric contents, administering antiemetic agents, and using a total intravenous anesthetic technique.

PREPARING FOR TRACHEAL EXTUBATION

The scenarios described above clearly illustrate the necessity for always having a backup plan in mind at the time of tracheal extubation. Necessities that always must be available include

1) 100% oxygen source and face mask with bag-mask device
2) Oral suction system
3) Laryngoscope with various blades, endotracheal tube, intubating stylet, and alternative airway device (e.g., LMA)
4) Oral and/or nasopharyngeal airway
5) Induction drugs drawn up and ready, especially succinylcholine

AVOIDING UNEXPECTED LOSS OF THE AIRWAY

After tracheal intubation of every patient, it is crucial to properly secure the endotracheal tube at the appropriate length. In addition, the endotracheal tube should be manually secured (guarded) during any change of the patient's position, as well as during endoscopic procedures. The endotracheal tube should be briefly disconnected from the circuit for transport of the intubated patient from the operating-room bed to the hospital bed. The same caution should be exercised even if simply turning the operating-room table, because tension from the breathing circuit can pull out a previously well-secured endotracheal tube. The endotracheal tube position should also be checked intermittently throughout the operation.

Although the above recommendations may reduce the risk, airway mishaps can still occur. In this emergency situation, members of the surgical team must have clear communication (stop the surgery, prioritize regaining airway access) and the anesthesiologist must take decisive actions. Asking for help from another anesthesia provider may be prudent.

ESTABLISHING AN AIRWAY IN AN EMERGENCY SITUATION

Emergency resuscitation situations can present many difficult airway situations, often in areas not as familiar to the anesthesiologist or not as well equipped as the operating room. This emphasizes the importance of anesthesiologist input when stocking an emergency airway cart. In addition to the traditional tools such as face mask, oral/nasopharyngeal airway, laryngoscope, multiple blade sizes and styles, appropriate-sized endotracheal tubes, and intubating stylet, the cart should also include alternative airway devices (e.g., LMA, intubating LMA, fiber-optic bronchoscope, Bullard scope, light wand, retrograde guidewire intubation, cricothyrotomy kit, and transtracheal jet ventilation). In certain situations, such as a profusely bleeding upper airway, however, a fiber-optic bronchoscope may not be of much help. Well-functioning suction must be immediately at hand. The anesthesia provider should be familiar with alternative devices and be comfortable in using them in an emergency; an emergency airway situation is not a good time to attempt unfamiliar techniques. Consider calling for help early, including from a surgeon in case a surgical airway (emergency tracheotomy, cricothyroidectomy) is needed.

TAKE HOME POINTS

- Lack of airway preparedness can have disastrous consequences when planning extubation of the patient.
- The most frequent complications of premature tracheal extubation are hypoventilation, apnea, or obstructive breathing. Immediate postoperative apnea or hypoventilation is most often caused by residual inhaled anesthetic and opioid effects, incomplete reversal of neuromuscular blockade, or the presence of redundant oral tissues.
- Maintain vigilance for laryngospasm. Be ready to move quickly to positive-pressure ventilation with a mask, or if that fails, succinylcholine.
- Be aware of the special risks involved with changing a double-lumen endotracheal tube to a single-lumen endotracheal tube. Remember that in almost every instance, this maneuver, though advantageous, is optional.
- Do not extubate without being prepared to reintubate if necessary.

SUGGESTED READINGS

Benumof JL. Laryngeal mask airway and the ASA difficult airway algorithm. *Anesthesiology.* 1996;84:686–699.

Gal TJ. Airway management. In: Miller RD, ed. *Miller's Anesthesia.* 6th ed. Vol. 2. Philadelphia: Elsevier Churchill Livingstone; 2005:1617–1652.

Larson CP Jr. Laryngospasm: the best treatment. *Anesthesiology.* 1998;89:1293–1294.

Morgan GE Jr, Mikhail MS, Murray MJ. *Clinical Anesthesiology.* 3rd ed. New York: Lange Medical Books/McGraw-Hill Medical Publishing Division; 2002:59–85.

Practice guidelines for management of the difficult airway: a report by the American Society of Anesthesiologists Task Force on Management of the Difficult Airway. *Anesthesiology.* 1993;78:597–602.

2

BASICS OF AIRWAY MANAGEMENT—PART II (TIPS AND TIDBITS)

CATHERINE MARCUCCI, MD AND
NABIL M. ELKASSABANY, MD

Airway management is both a science and an art, and the wise anesthesia provider will make himself a lifelong student. An informal review of the peer-reviewed anesthesia literature shows that there are at least 25 new manuscripts, case reports, and letters on airway management each month. Similarly, even the "old" drugs in airway management are under ongoing evaluation—the literature for the first months of 2007 contains dozens of reports on the use of succinylcholine, a drug that has been in clinical use for about 60 years. The authors feel strongly that there is also ample opportunity to learn from the spoken tradition as well.

- Try to become expert in each new airway device and technique as it comes out, but remember that the most valuable airway techniques are sometimes the simplest and most basic—a nasal trumpet, a headstrap, or even a jaw thrust. It is best to become proficient with a new airway device on patients with a normal airway before trying to use the new airway device on a complicated patient or in an emergency situation.

- Control your airway situation by controlling your airway drugs. One of the authors saw a case of significant bradycardia probably caused by repeated doses of succinylcholine given to facilitate intubation. The clinical situation then focused on dealing with the bradycardia rather than securing the airway.

- One of the most valuable drugs in airway management is oxygen (the authors had a professor of anesthesia who used to say to put the patient on oxygen first and then think). If difficulty is suspected, have the patient breathe 100% oxygen for 5 minutes. Remember that oxygen utilization by the (nonpregnant) human adult is approximately 3 mL/kg/min. If you have fully denitrogenated the lungs, the chances of having "the oxygen out last the succinylcholine" are increased.

- When you are just learning airway skills, try to do as many mask cases as possible. The successful mask airway is the foundation on which all airway management is based.

- Do not underestimate the amount of airway edema and/or bleeding that can occur with even one or two attempts at laryngoscopy.

© 2006 Mayo Foundation for Medical Education and Research

- Remember that for an intubated patient, the tip of the endotracheal tube (ETT) follows the chin. Flexing the patient's head toward the chest seats the ETT more deeply in the trachea and vice versa.

- Excessive tape on the ETT can be as troublesome as undertaping the ETT. Many senior anesthesia providers have anecdotes involving skin damage to patients' faces or accidentally extubating too soon when "trying to loosen the tape" in advance of being asked to do a planned extubation, such as in a tracheostomy.

- Asking a patient to "squeeze my hand" is not a great pre-extubation test; it really only demonstrates the ability to follow verbal commands. Remember that hand strength is not a standard indication of reversal of neuromuscular blockade. It is best to use standardized methods to assess strength (e.g. head lift, leg lift) before progressing to extubation. It is also suggested that the anesthesia provider ask the patient to do things that are linked functionally to your needs during the first few seconds after extubation: "open your mouth," "take a deep breath," or "try to swallow." This will also increase your confidence that the patient will be able to take a deep enough breath to cough, open their mouth for suction, and be able to control their airway enough to handle secretions.

- A surprising number of serious airway events include the fact that the ETT was actually in the trachea at some point and then was accidentally or purposely removed due to delayed taping, an attempt to change the ETT to a more advantageous size, or the like. A corollary to this is to never feel oversecure when using a tube changer to change the ETT even if the initial airway management was not especially difficult.

- Always be very vigilant when doing airway management in remote locations. The authors feel that the best adjunct intubating aid to take with you is another experienced anesthesia provider. After that, a simple intubating stylet and a laryngeal mask airway are very valuable tools.

- It is surprisingly easy to forget the cricoid pressure and to have working suction when intubating in the intensive care units and other remote locations.

- Always remember to wear your mask and eye protection when intubating in the intensive care units. This is commonly where anesthesia providers incur eye exposures to body fluids (including one of the authors).

- When called to a remote location to do airway management, you, as the expert airway consultant, should expect to assume control of the airway at the time of your arrival.

- One of the most dangerous requests is the call to the intensive care unit to "change the tube," either due to secretions or a ruptured ETT cuff. Exhaust all options before taking out that ETT. Be sure that high airway pressures are not due to a mainstem intubation. Call for a bronchoscope to confirm that there truly are secretions in the ETT. Try a wet throat pack in the supraglottic area if a cuff leak is suspected as the cause of an inability to deliver an appropriate ventilator volume. Do a direct laryngoscopy with the tube in place to make sure that a "leaking ETT cuff" is not just a cuff that has herniated out from the trachea. Be sure "excessive leak" around an ETT isn't due to the combination of the patient requiring high airway pressures (poor pulmonary compliance) and low cuff pressure. When those options are exhausted, call for a colleague.

TAKE HOME POINT

■ Although the authors talk about airway management being an "art," it does not mean that there are not right and wrong ways of doing things. The American Society of Anesthesiologists has developed a difficult airway algorithm that has become a standard that anesthesia providers need to be aware of. The best advice a new practitioner can receive is to always err on the side of caution and to have many possible options in their armamentarium of airway management techniques.

SUGGESTED READING

www.asahq.org/publicationsAndServices/Difficult%20Airway.pdf.

3

CONSIDER PEEP

ANDREA Y. TAN, MD, AND
IBTESAM A. HILMI, MB, CHB, FRCA

Positive end-expiratory pressure (PEEP) is defined as an elevation of alveolar pressure at the conclusion of passive expiration that exceeds atmospheric pressure. PEEP is categorized as applied/extrinsic PEEP or auto/intrinsic PEEP. Extrinsic PEEP is delivered directly through a mechanical ventilator or through a tight-fitting face mask at the end of exhalation. PEEP maintains the patient's airway pressure above atmospheric level by exerting pressure to oppose passive emptying of the lung. Intrinsic PEEP occurs when the lungs fail to deflate fully prior to the next breath, which maintains the alveolar pressure above the atmospheric pressure. If otherwise unspecified, PEEP usually refers to extrinsic PEEP. Both extrinsic PEEP and intrinsic PEEP are covered in this chapter.

EXTRINSIC PEEP

Why Use PEEP? PEEP is used to completely or partially replace the function of the respiratory muscles and therefore correct hypoxemia secondary to alveolar hypoventilation. PEEP is effective in improving arterial oxygenation simply through increasing functional residual capacity (FRC), reducing venous admixture, shifting tidal volume, preventing loss of pulmonary compliance, and decreasing the work of breathing.

Effects of PEEP

Respiratory System. Extrinsic PEEP improves oxygenation by directly affecting alveolar gas exchange and pulmonary mechanics of the respiratory system. Overall, alveolar gas exchange improves through redistribution of fluid within the alveoli. As a result, there is a decrease in intrapulmonary shunting and an improvement in arterial oxygenation. With the addition of PEEP, arterial oxygenation goals may be achieved with a lower fraction of inspired oxygen (FIO_2) and therefore a decreased risk of oxygen toxicity. In terms of lung mechanics, FRC increases and lung compliance improves. PEEP is also responsible for prevention of alveolar collapse, which is of critical importance because the repetitive collapse of lung units at the end of expiration may lead to ventilator-induced lung injury (VILI).

Cardiovascular System. From the cardiovascular standpoint, the addition of PEEP causes a significant increase in intrathoracic pressure. As a result, there is a decrease in venous return and decrease in right and left ventricular

© 2006 Mayo Foundation for Medical Education and Research

preload. This leads to a decline in cardiac output. Biondi et al. showed that at low levels of PEEP the predominant effect is right ventricular (RV) preload reduction. Above 15 cm H_2O PEEP, RV volumes increase and RV ejection fraction (EF) decreases, consistent with increased RV afterload and declines in RV contractility, presumably as a result of increased RV wall stress.

Several possible factors can lead to decrease in cardiac output during application of PEEP. In addition to changes in loading conditions, the leftward septal displacement, systolic and diastolic ventricular interdependence and altered cardiac geometry can all affect cardiac output during the application of PEEP. In any case, the decline in cardiac output may progress toward hypotension and subsequent hypoperfusion of critical organs.

The adverse effects of PEEP on the cardiovascular systems cannot be overlooked. One study has revealed that PEEP may cause tricuspid regurgitation. The combination of increased pulmonary artery pressures, increased vascular resistance, and altered RV geometry may all affect tricuspid valve function. This is critical because the presence of undiagnosed tricuspid regurgitation during mechanical ventilation may invalidate cardiac output values as well as the derived parameters that are determined through thermodilution.

Liver. Effects of PEEP on the hepatic system are also noticeable. The drop in cardiac output causes a decrease in splanchnic blood flow and subsequent decrease in hepatic and portal blood flow. However, an increased in hepatic outflow resistance as a result of impaired venous drainage can lead to the observed liver congestion and hinder the hepatic perfusion. The use of PEEP causes a downward shift of the diaphragm, which further compresses the liver and worsens the hepatic perfusion.

Renal. PEEP causes a decrease in urinary output, sodium excretion, and creatinine clearance. The mechanisms responsible for the decreased urine output are most likely multifactorial, including a decrease in cardiac output, renal blood flow, intravascular volume, and reflex sympathetic nerve activation. There is also an altered release of various hormones including catecholamines, renin–angiotensin–aldosterone, antidiuretic hormone, and atrial natriuretic factor, which contributes to the effects of PEEP on renal function. The patient's volume status and the amount of applied PEEP both contribute to alterations in renal function.

Central Nervous System. The effects of PEEP on cerebral mechanics are numerous. As PEEP is added, there is a notable rise in right atrial pressure. This further translates to an increase in superior vena cava pressure and a decrease in cerebral venous return, resulting in an increase in intracranial pressure (ICP). Other influencing variables include intracranial compliance and body positioning. When the head is elevated above the chest, the transmitted intrathoracic pressure to the intracranial venous sinuses is decreased.

As a result, ICP is minimally affected. In patients with normal ICP, the effect of PEEP can be easily overcome by maintaining normal intravascular volume and systemic blood pressure.

Bronchial Circulation and Thoracic Lymph Drainage. Because it increases the intrathoracic pressure, PEEP affects both bronchial blood flow and thoracic lymph drainage. Lymph drainage from the thoracic duct may be obstructed as a result of PEEP, and edema fluid removal from the lungs may be impaired. Bronchial blood flow may also be affected and interfere with lung repair.

To PEEP or Not to PEEP? Typically, only a small amount of PEEP is needed. About 3 to 5 cm of water is considered the physiologic amount required to overcome the decrease in FRC from bypassing the glottic opening with an endotracheal tube. Use of supraphysiologic PEEP (>5 cm H_2O) may be indicated in certain settings. Specific indications for use of PEEP include acute lung injury, acute respiratory distress syndrome (ARDS), cardiogenic pulmonary edema, diffuse pneumonia requiring mechanical ventilation, and atelectasis associated with severe hypoxemia.

Patients with acute lung injury and ARDS should be managed using lung-protective strategies including (a) low tidal volumes (6 mL/kg), (b) high-frequency ventilation, and (c) PEEP; the main goal is to maintain an acceptable level of PaO_2 but not necessarily a normocarbia (permissive hypercarbia may be allowed). The PEEP may be initiated at 5 cm H_2O and gradually increased to a maximum of 20 cm H_2O. This range allows optimization of arterial oxygenation as well as minimization of adverse effects. These strategies are critical for avoiding ventilator-induced lung injury. Volutrauma, which includes lung overinflation and overstretching of alveoli, barotraumas due to high inflation pressure and high PEEP, and atelectrauma, the repetitive opening and closing of recruitable alveoli, may be avoided. The decrease in VILI will certainly decrease production and release of inflammatory mediators, such as cytokines, $TNF\alpha$, and interleukin-6, which may progress toward systemic inflammatory response and eventual multiple organ dysfunction.

Contraindications to the Use of PEEP. PEEP is not a benign therapy and may be associated with adverse hemodynamic consequences that cannot be overlooked. There are potentially two absolute contraindications to the use of PEEP: hypovolemic shock and undrained high-pressure pneumothorax. Other relative contraindications include hypotension, hypovolemia, intracranial hypertension, unilateral or focal pulmonary disease, pulmonary embolism, and bronchopleural fistula.

Hypotension. Positive-pressure ventilation has been shown to decrease venous return, and this effect is amplified by the addition of PEEP. Furthermore, if the patient is in a hypovolemic state, the hypotension is further accentuated.

Intracranial Hypertension. PEEP should be used cautiously in these cases, because it may decrease the cerebral perfusion pressure (CPP) (the difference between mean arterial pressure and ICP) by either increasing ICP or decreasing mean arterial pressure (MAP). If it is necessary to use PEEP as in the cases listed above, then appropriate monitoring should be obtained to accurately measure both intracranial pressure and MAP. The use of a vasopressor agent may be indicated to maintain the MAP in these circumstances.

Unilateral/Focal Lung Disease. This category includes patients who have severe pneumonia requiring mechanical ventilation. In this case the use of PEEP may worsen hypoxemia, because further ventilation of lung units already under compensatory hypoxic vasoconstriction will only exacerbate ventilation–perfusion mismatch.

Pulmonary Embolism. PEEP may worsen hypoxemia secondary to pulmonary embolism. Increasing the alveolar pressure with PEEP may compress patent pulmonary vessels.

INTRINSIC PEEP

What Is It? Intrinsic PEEP occurs when the alveolar pressure is greater than the atmospheric pressure at the end of normal passive exhalation. It is the end result when there is inadequate time for the lungs to empty secondary to high minute-volume ventilation, restricted expiratory flow, and/or high expiratory resistance.

What Causes It? There are three scenarios in which intrinsic PEEP typically occurs.

1) The first scenario is referred to as high minute-volume ventilation secondary to a high respiratory rate and/or a large tidal volume. An increase in either variable has the same end result, the new breath being initiated before completion of the last exhaled breath, leading to intrinsic PEEP and air trapping.

2) Intrinsic PEEP is also commonly seen when expiratory flow is restricted. This occurs most frequently in patients with chronic lung disease and obstructive airway disease. The airways are constricted from limited expiratory flow as in bronchospasm, inflammation, or severely decreased pulmonary compliance such as occurs in ARDS.

3) The third type of intrinsic PEEP is seen with expiratory resistance. This may occur because of a kinked endotracheal tube or one with a narrowed diameter, secondary to accumulation of secretions. It may also present in cases in which the patient is agitated and/or in pain.

Complications of Intrinsic PEEP. It is important for the clinician to determine the underlying cause of intrinsic PEEP because there are potentially devastating sequelae. Intrinsic PEEP may result in a significantly increased work of breathing, which may make it more difficult to wean a patient off a ventilator. Alveolar gas exchange may decrease, resulting in a lower arterial oxygen tension. This may be explained by an uneven distribution of intrinsic PEEP among lung units compared to when extrinsic PEEP is used. Finally, hemodynamic instability may occur. Intrinsic PEEP creates an increase in intrathoracic pressure, which decreases preload of both ventricles and decreases left ventricular compliance. Once this occurs, there is a resultant increase in right ventricular afterload and pulmonary vascular resistance, which leads to a decrease in cardiac output.

Management of Intrinsic PEEP. Various techniques may be utilized to minimize intrinsic PEEP. These include aggressive bronchodilator therapy, adequate pain control and/or sedation, and minimization of the inspiratory-to-expiratory ratio. In patients who are actively breathing, continuous positive airway pressure (CPAP) or extrinsic PEEP may be used to counter intrinsic PEEP. However extrinsic PEEP should be used with caution in this setting, as it may potentially worsen hyperinflation and compromise the patient's hemodynamic status.

TAKE HOME POINTS

- PEEP comes in two varieties: applied/extrinsic PEEP and auto/intrinsic PEEP.
- Positive pulmonary effects associated with PEEP include improvements in arterial oxygenation (PaO_2), recruitment of lung units, lung compliance, and increased functional residual capacity.
- The hemodynamic effects of PEEP include decreased venous return and biventricular preload, and subsequent decreased cardiac output.
- PEEP also has widespread multiorgan effects, including:
  - Liver: decreased splanchnic blood flow, resulting in liver congestion and hypoperfusion
  - Kidneys: decreased renal blood flow, resulting in decreased urine output, decreased sodium excretion, decreased creatinine clearance, and altered hormonal release
  - Brain: decreased cerebral venous return, resulting in increased ICP
  - Bronchial circulation: decreased bronchial blood flow, resulting in impaired lung repair
  - Thoracic lymph drainage: thoracic duct obstruction, resulting in impaired removal of edema from the lungs
- Key indications for use of PEEP include treatment of acute lung injury, acute respiratory distress syndrome (ARDS), cardiogenic pulmonary edema, diffuse pneumonia, and atelectasis with associated severe hypoxemia.

- Relative contraindications to use of PEEP include hypotension, hypovolemia, intracranial hypertension, unilateral or focal pulmonary disease, pulmonary embolism, and bronchopleural fistula.
- Intrinsic PEEP occurs when there is inadequate time for the lungs to empty secondary to high minute-volume ventilation, restricted expiratory flow, and/or expiratory resistance.
- Negative sequelae associated with intrinsic PEEP include difficulty weaning patient from the ventilator, decreased alveolar gas exchange, and hemodynamic instability.
- Techniques to minimize intrinsic PEEP include bronchodilator therapy, administration of analgesics and sedatives, and addition of CPAP or extrinsic PEEP.

SUGGESTED READINGS

Acute Respiratory Distress Syndrome Network. Ventilation with lower tidal volumes as compared with traditional tidal volumes for acute lung injury and the acute respiratory distress syndrome. *N Engl J Med.* 2000;342:1301–1308.

Artucio H, Hurtado J, Zimet L, et al. PEEP-induced tricuspid regurgitation. *Intensive Care Med.* 1997;23:836–840.

Biondi J, Schulman D, Soufer R, et al. The effect of incremental positive end-expiratory pressure on right ventricular hemodynamics and ejection fraction. *Anesth Analg.* 1988;67:144–151.

Brinker JA, Weiss JL, Lappe DL, et al. Leftward septal displacement during right ventricular loading in man: demonstration by two-dimensional ECHO. *Circulation.* 1980;63:87–95.

Mughal M, Minai O, Culver D, et al. Auto-positive end-expiratory pressure: mechanisms and treatment. *Cleveland Clin J Med.* 2005;72(9):801–809.

The National Heart, Lung, and Blood Institute ARDS Clinical Trials Network. Higher versus lower positive end-expiratory pressures in patients with the acute respiratory distress syndrome. *N Engl J Med.* 2004;351:327–336.

Robotham JL, Bell RC, Badke FR, et al. Left ventricular geometry during positive end-expiratory pressure in dogs. *Crit Care Med.* 1985;13:617–624.

Santamore WP, Lunch PR, Meier G, et al. Myocardial interaction between the ventricles. *J Appl Physiol.* 1976;41(3):362–368.

Tobin M. *Principles and Practice of Mechanical Ventilation.* 2nd ed. New York: McGraw Hill; 2006:273–325.

4

A VARIETY OF TECHNIQUES PROVIDE ACCEPTABLE ANESTHESIA FOR AWAKE INTUBATION OF THE AIRWAY; ULTIMATELY, THE MOST IMPORTANT FACTORS ARE OPERATOR EXPERIENCE AND ADEQUATE TIME

CHAUNCEY T. JONES, MD

Awake fiber-optic intubations are an integral component of known difficult airway management. Operator experience in managing these airways is the most important variable. However, preparation of the patient and the airway weigh heavily in achieving a successful awake intubation.

Preparation of the patient involves discussion of what to expect and how the patient can help the process go smoothly, and then mild sedation, as respiratory status permits. However, sedation should not be to the point of airway obstruction or disinhibition of the patient.

Preparation of the airway involves administering an antisialagogue (such as 0.2 to 0.4 mg glycopyrrolate) to block the secretory reflex and anesthetizing the entire route that the intubation will take, whether nasal or oral. This course can be divided into nasal and oral cavies; nasopharyngeal, oropharyngeal, and hypopharyngeal regions of the pharynx; or subglottic regions, which include the larynx and trachea. The innervation of these regions must be blocked for successful awake intubation.

INNERVATION

Nasal cavity innervation is derived from two branches of the trigeminal nerve (V), the ophthalmic (V1) and the maxillary (V2). The anterior ethmoid nerve (from V1) innervates the anterior aspects of the nasal cavity and septum. The posterior nasal cavity and septum are innervated primarily by the lateral posterior superior, lateral inferior posterior, and nasopalatine nerves of V2.

The sensory innervation of the oral cavity and muscles of mastication derive from the mandibular branch of the trigeminal nerve (V3). Muscles of the tongue are supplied primarily by the hypoglossal, CN XII. Its general sensory path is from the lingual nerve, a branch of V3, for the anterior two thirds, and by the glossopharyngeal nerve, CN IX, for the posterior one third. The hard and soft palate are innervated by the greater and lesser palatine nerves, respectively, which are branches from V2.

Sensory innervation of the entire pharynx and epiglottis is supplied primarily by the glossopharyngeal nerve, CN IX, and motor nerve supply is

ⓒ 2006 Mayo Foundation for Medical Education and Research

from the vegas nerve, CN X. The superior laryngeal nerve, derived from the vegas nerve, CN X, supplies sensory to the larynx above the true vocal cords as well as to the cricothyroid muscle. The recurrent laryngeal nerve, also from the vegas, CN X, supplies all other muscles of the larynx and sensation at the level of vocal cords and below. Recurrent laryngeal nerve also supplies sensory and motor components to the trachea.

Several protective reflexes can be elicited with airway manipulation, including gag, glottic closure (laryngospasm), and cough. These reflexes can be blocked by either their afferent (sensory) and/or efferent (motor) components. Input for the gag reflex is the glossopharyngeal nerve, CN IX, and output is the vegas, CN X. Fibers for glottic closure reflex are superior laryngeal for afferent and both superior and recurrent laryngeal for efferent. Other reflexes that may also be encountered are bronchospasm reflex, secretory reflex, vomiting reflex, and cardiovascular reflex.

ANESTHETIZATION OF THE AIRWAY

Anesthetization of the airway for awake fiber-optic intubation can be achieved by a number of techniques and can be adjusted to the patient, the operator preference, and availability of supplies (Table 4.1). These often include a mixture of topicalization and nerve blocks. Topicalization methods include direct application of lidocaine or viscous lidocaine, aerosol spray, atomization, or nebulization (Table 4.2). Common nerve blocks include glossopharyngeal, superior laryngeal, and translaryngeal. Other blocks may be performed, such as maxillary and mandibular nerve blocks. However, these are more invasive with a lower risk/benefit ratio, and their relevant terminal nerves can easily be blocked topically.

TABLE 4.1	COMMONLY USED TOPICAL METHODS FOR AIRWAY BLOCKS	
METHOD	LOCAL ANESTHETIC	NOTES
Nasal topical	1. 4% cocaine 2. 2% to 4% lidocaine or viscous lidocaine with 1% phenylephrine	Cocaine and phenylephrine cause vasoconstriction and decrease chance of epistaxis
Aerosol spray	Benzocaine	Risk of methemoglobinemia if maximum dose exceeded
Atomizer	4% lidocaine	Usually takes longer to work than direct topicalization
Nebulizer	4% lidocaine	Usually takes longer to work than direct topicalization
Syringe	2% to 4% lidocaine	Can be injected through nasal trumpet or slowly deposited onto the posterior tongue and run inferiorly to reach the hypopharynx

TABLE 4.2	COMMONLY USED LOCAL ANESTHETICS FOR AIRWAY BLOCKS			
DRUG	**CLINICAL USE**	**ONSET**	**DURATION (MIN)**	**MAXIMUM DOSE**
Cocaine	Topical (nasal)	Slow	30–60	1.5 mg/kg
Benzocaine	Topical	Fast	5–10	200 mg
Lidocaine	Topical/nerve blocks	Medium/fast	30–60/60–180	4 mg/kg no epi; 7 mg/kg with epi

Nasal Cavity/Nasopharynx. Anesthetization of the V1 and V2 branches of the nasal cavity can be achieved with cocaine or lidocaine. Cocaine also provides vasoconstriction to decrease the incidence of epistaxis. Phenylephrine can be added to lidocaine to provide the same result. A 3:1 combination of 4% lidocaine with 1% phenylephrine will yield a 3%/0.25% solution that can be applied by inserting a cotton-tipped applicator. Alternatively, 2% viscous lidocaine can be mixed with phenylephrine to make a similar suspension and applied with a cotton-tipped applicator as well as serially increasing sizes of nasal airways. This technique not only anesthetizes and vasoconstricts the nasal cavity, it also lubricates and dilates it to the desired-sized endotracheal tube, usually 7.0. A nasal trumpet usually extends farther into the nasopharynx and provides better nasopharyngeal block than a cotton-tipped applicator. In addition, a slip-tip syringe can be used to inject several milliliters of 2% to 4% lidocaine through the nasal trumpet to further anesthetize the nasopharynx, oropharynx, and hypopharynx as the solution travels down the pharynx.

A contraindication to this technique is trauma to the nasal cavity. Relative contraindications include uncontrolled hypertension and coagulopathy.

Oral Cavity/Oropharynx. The oral cavity (mandibular nerve V3) is not usually affected by pain during oral awake fiber-optic intubation and thus does not have to be blocked, but usually it is at least partially blocked by several of the methods utilized for blocking the oropharynx. The oropharynx (glossopharyngeal nerve, CN IX) does need to be blocked. This can be achieved with any number of procedures: gargling several milliliters of 2% to 4% lidocaine and then expectorating the solution; using an aerosol spray such as benzocaine spray; atomization; nebulization; or applying lidocaine-soaked pledgets directly to the oropharynx. If oral awake intubation is planned, prevention of the patient biting the endotracheal tube or scope is needed. The muscles of mastication usually are not blocked, but rather, a bite block or oral airway is inserted.

A direct glossopharyngeal nerve block can be performed by either an intraoral or peristyloid approach. For the intraoral approach, adequate mouth opening and topicalization for the patient to tolerate the block are needed. The tongue is distracted in an anteroinferior direction, which can be done with a laryngoscope blade or tongue depressor. The base of the tonsillar pillar is identified and a 25-gauge spinal needle is advanced submucosally at the caudal-most portion of the pillar. Aspiration before injection to rule out intravascular location is important, given the close proximity of the internal carotid artery. Then 5 mL of local anesthetic can be injected. The same process is repeated on the other side. The glossopharyngeal block is sometimes avoided by junior practitioners, however, there are clinicians who have used it routinely for many years with great success.

The peristyloid approach requires access to the lateral neck and ability to identify bony landmarks. The midpoint of a line between the mastoid process and the angle of the mandible is identified. Deep to this should be the styloid process, which can sometimes be felt with deep palpation. The overlying skin is injected with a wheel of local anesthetic and a 22-guage needle is inserted perpendicular to the skin. This is advanced until the styloid process is contacted, usually in 1 to 2 cm. The tip of the needle is then walked off the process posteriorly. Once contact is lost, and after negative aspiration for blood, 5 to 7 mL of local anesthetic is injected. The process is repeated on the contralateral side.

Contraindications for glossopharyngeal nerve block include overlying infection and coagulopathy.

Hypopharynx. The hypopharynx is usually anesthetized by the methods used for the oropharynx as the local anesthetic migrates inferiorly. In addition, a syringe can be used to trickle anesthetic down the posterior tongue and onto the hypopharynx. If an oral airway is in place, it can be used as a conduit to direct local anesthetic to the hypopharynx. Local anesthetic can also be injected under direct visualization through the port of the fiber-optic scope.

Larynx. The larynx may be reached with local anesthetic using the same methods as for anesthetizing the oropharynx and hypopharynx, such as an atomizer, a nebulizer, or by trickling anesthetic down the posterior tongue. Local anesthetic can be deposited on the larynx through the fiber-optic scope as well.

A superior laryngeal nerve block can be used to block the nerve directly. The patient is placed in a supine position and the neck fully extended. The hyoid bone is identified by careful palpation. Once identified, it is displaced toward the ipsilateral side of injection and a 25-gauge needle is advanced until it makes contact with the greater cornu of the hyoid bone. The needle is then walked off inferiorly and advanced 2 to 3 mm to place the tip between the thyrohyoid membrane laterally and the laryngeal mucosa medially. After negative aspiration for air and blood, 2 to 3 mL of local anesthetic is injected.

The process is repeated on the contralateral side. Alternatively, the superior laryngeal nerve can be blocked topically by applying 4% lidocaine on a pledget to the bilateral piriform fossa for several minutes.

Contraindications include coagulopathy and an inability to extend the neck.

Vocal Cords and Trachea. The vocal cords and trachea may be anesthetized by several of the procedures mentioned previously as anesthetic is aspirated or inhaled. However, they are more reliable and completely blocked by direct injection of local anesthetic through a fiber-optic scope or translaryngeal block.

A translaryngeal or transtracheal nerve block is used to anesthetize the true vocal cords and the trachea. It can also block some supraglottic structures as it is coughed out through the vocal cords. The patient is placed in a supine position and the neck extended. The cricothryoid membrane is identified in its midline location. The overlying skin is injected with local anesthetic. A 22-gauge needle on a 10-mL syringe with 3 mL of 4% lidocaine is introduced perpendicular to the skin and advanced while continuously aspirating for air. Positive air aspiration indicates that the needle tip is in the trachea. Care must be taken not to advance into the posterior wall of the trachea. Once correct position is confirmed, the local anesthetic is injected as the patient inhales and the needle is quickly removed, as injection will elicit a cough. Some operators prefer to use a catheter-over-needle technique, with only the catheter left in place while injecting.

Performing a series of topical and/or regional nerve blocks to anesthetize the involved branches of the V1, V2, V3, glossopharyngeal, and vegas nerves as described above will make the experience of awake fiber-optic intubation more tolerable for the patient and significantly increase the chance of a successful procedure.

TAKE HOME POINTS

- Watch as many of these awake airway procedures as possible—operator experience is one of the most important variables in providing anesthesia for the airway smoothly and efficiency, and every experienced anesthesia provider has his or her own favorite techniques.
- Always extend as much empathy and patience to the patient as possible, remember that even when everything goes smoothly, this is not the easiest thing in the world for anybody, most of all the patient. If he asks to stop a minute to catch his breath, stop a minute.
- A variety of sedation techniques will work, but don't try to substitute heavy sedation for inadequate topical anesthesia. Be aware that droperidol will make the patient appear sedated and compliant, but the anesthesia

provider has to be prepared for the patient to later describe feeling like a zombie that couldn't run away.

- Most anesthesia providers use a lidocaine nebulizer as well as blocks.
- The other important "ingredient" in providing anesthesia to the airway is *time*!
- Check with the surgeons (particularly the ENT surgeons) before doing a transtracheal block; they will sometimes ask you not to broach the trachea with a needle in advance of their procedure.

SUGGESTED READINGS

Fulling PD, Roberts JT. Fiberoptic intubation. *Int Anesthesiol Clin.* 2000;38(3):189–217.

Miller RD, ed. *Miller's Anesthesia.* 6th ed. Philadelphia: Elsevier Churchill Livingstone; 2005:1641–1646, 1708–1709.

Simmons ST, Schleich AR. Airway regional anesthesia for awake fiberoptic intubation. *Reg Anesth Pain Med.* 2002;27(2):180–192.

5

An Awake Intubation Should Not Be a Traumatic Experience for the Patient

Chauncey T. Jones, MD

To some, the phrase "awake intubation" may conjure up thoughts of medieval torture tactics. Indeed, intubations are commonly performed without sedation during code situations on semiconscious patients. However, in the operating room and in other controlled situations, awake intubations should not be a traumatic experience for the patient.

Anesthesiologists must possess sound management skills with difficult airways. Most American Society of Anesthesiologists (ASA) closed claims studies are related to inadequate oxygenation or ventilation. Part of the preoperative evaluation by the anesthesiologist is to determine how endotracheal intubation can be safely executed. In most instances, induction of anesthesia followed by asleep intubation is reasonable. In certain patients, however, awake intubation may be safest. Indeed, awake intubation is part of the ASA Difficult Airway Algorithm.

Indications for Awake Intubation

The decision for an awake intubation may be based on a history of difficult ventilation and/or intubation during prior anesthesia. The indication for surgery may require awake intubation. For example, you may be asked to anesthetize a patient with severe cervical spine instability, requiring awake intubation and awake positioning; or a patient might have a head and neck mass that is partially obstructing the airway or compressing the trachea. Information obtained from history and physical examination is also useful and may reveal congenital syndromes, abnormal facial structure such as micrognathia, morbid obesity, obstructive sleep apnea with poor respiratory reserve, severe aspiration risk, or significant hemodynamic instability.

Nasal Versus Oral

Most intubations are performed orally, unless there is a contraindication. Nasal intubations are used for oral surgeries in which an endotracheal tube would hinder the operation, or if the mandible is to be wired closed. Nasal intubation can be performed on patients with poor mouth opening and to aid patient comfort and oral hygiene if immediate postoperative extubation is not planned. Fiber-optic nasal intubation is often technically easier

---

© 2006 Mayo Foundation for Medical Education and Research

than oral fiber-optic intubation, and a blind nasal intubation can also be employed.

Contraindications to nasal intubation include coagulopathy, abnormal nasal anatomy, sinusitis, and facial trauma where there may be a basilar skull fracture. Complications of nasal intubation include epistaxis, trauma to nasal structures, sinusitis with possible bacteremia, and cribriform plate perforation resulting in cerebral injury/death.

TECHNIQUES

There are multiple ways to perform an awake intubation. Common to all awake techniques is preparation of the patient and the airway. Letting the patient know what to expect is a key component to success. Mild sedation, as respiratory status permits, is also helpful. Preparation of the airway includes administration of antisialagogues and anesthetization of the airway with topical and regional techniques (see Chapter 4).

Currently, the most commonly employed technique is oral or nasal fiber-optic intubation. Keep in mind that fiber-optic scopes are not always available and are not a requirement for awake intubation. Other options include blind nasal intubation, laryngoscopy, or some combination of techniques. Keep in mind that an ultimate option may be a surgical airway.

FIBER-OPTIC INTUBATION

First, become familiar with and test the equipment. Verify adequate light source, focus, and white balance if applicable. Scope manipulation is most efficient when the shaft is devoid of slack and held taught. All scope maneuvers are controlled by the dominant hand with the up/down lever, by rotating the wrist, and scope advancement or withdrawal. Obtain suction for the scope. Test the cuff on the endotracheal tube (ETT), usually 7.0 or smaller, and soften it in warm solution. Lightly lubricate the shaft of the scope to facilitate easy passage of the ETT. To prevent fogging, antifog solution can be applied to the scope tip, or the tip can simply be placed in warm saline. Patient position can be sitting, semirecumbent, or supine with the head in neutral position.

For nasal intubation, insert the endotracheal tube into the previously anesthetized, dilated, and vasoconstricted nasal passage (see Chapter 4) until the tip is in the oropharynx. This serves as a conduit to introduce the fiber-optic scope and guide it toward its destination. Alternatively, some anesthesiologists prefer to have the scope tip threaded through the ETT, but introduce the scope tip first and let it serve as a guide for the ETT—similar to the Seldinger technique for inserting central venous catheters.

Once the scope tip is in the oropharynx, the key is to stay midline, maneuver the scope anteriorly, and identify relevant structures. Anterior displacement of the tongue is helpful. This can be done by having an assistant grasp the tongue with gauze. Ideally, with advancement of the scope, one should see posterior tongue, epiglottis, arytenoids, vocal cords, trachea, and carina. Ask the patient to take a deep breath or pant just before traversing the vocal cords. The ETT can then be advanced into the trachea over the scope while maintaining visualization of the carina. The ETT may sometimes meet resistance as it contacts the arytenoids. If this is encountered, rotate the ETT 90 degrees. Distal ETT location can be confirmed with the scope. With the scope tip at the carina, use the nondominant hand to hold the scope at the proximal end of the ETT. Withdraw the scope until the distal end of the ETT can just be seen through the scope and stop. The distance from the nondominant hand to the proximal end of the ETT is the height of the ETT tip above the carina.

Oral fiber-optic intubations are similar to nasal fiberoptic bronchoscopy (FOB) except that an oral airway or bite block should be used to prevent operator injury or scope damage. The technique is often more technically difficult because a more acute angle must be managed. A jaw thrust may help.

BLIND NASAL

The blind nasal technique can be used when blood or secretions impede visualization with the fiber-optic scope. Prepare the airway as described in Chapter 4. During the procedure, have the patient pant. Using a 7.0 ETT, introduce it through the nasal passage and slowly advance. Patient respirations can be heard through the ETT. Advance toward the respirations as a guide. If respiratory sounds through the ETT disappear, advancement into the esophagus is likely and the ETT should be withdrawn and redirected. The ETT can be rotated to maintain a midline position. If there is no a concern for cervical spine instability, the neck can be extended or flexed to help facilitate intubation. Special endotracheal tubes are available that have a drawstring to help manipulate the tip of the endotracheal tube.

If blind nasal intubation is unsuccessful and there is no contraindication to oral instrumentation, the technique can be converted from blind to oral by using laryngoscopy and Magill forceps to help aid the nasal intubation.

AWAKE LARYNGOSCOPY

Awake direct laryngoscopy and intubation can be performed on patients after anesthetization of the airway, which will also attenuate gag and cough reflexes (see Chapter 4). Once the vocal cords are identified, intubate as the patient inhales. Awake indirect laryngoscopy and intubation can be done in a similar manner with the Bullard scope. The Bullard scope can be helpful for patients with a small mouth opening and anterior airways.

- Awake intubation is part of the ASA Difficult Airway Algorithm.
- Indications for awake intubation include cervical spine instability, head and neck mass, congenital syndromes, morbid obesity, or severe aspiration risk.
- Proper preparation of the patient and airway is paramount.
- Remember that awake intubations do not have to be via fiber-optic scope— other techniques include blind nasal placement of the ETT and direct laryngoscopy.
- Do *not* "torture" the patient—if he or she is crying or asking for you to stop, *stop* and reassess your technique and airway preparation.

SUGGESTED READINGS

American Society of Anesthesiologists Task Force on Management of the Difficult Airway. Practice Guidelines for the Management of the Difficult Airway. *Anesthesiology*. 1993;78:579.

Caplan RA, Posner KL, Ward RJ, et al. Adverse respiratory events in anesthesia: a closed claims analysis. *Anesthesiology*. 1990;72:828–833.

Fulling PD, Roberts JT. Fiber-optic intubation. *Int Anesthesiol Clin*. 2000;38(3):189–217.

Miller RD, ed. *Miller's Anesthesia*. 6th ed. Philadelphia: Elservier Churchill Livingstone; 2005:1641–1646, 1708–1709.

6

A HIGH INSPIRED CONCENTRATION OF OXYGEN IS CONTRAINDICATED IN CERTAIN CIRCUMSTANCES

XIANREN WU, MD AND DAVID G. METRO, MD

The concept of oxygen toxicity in certain circumstances is well known among medical professionals. To anesthesia providers, however, the most common errors concerning oxygen toxicity are in the following assumptions: (a) the benefits of oxygenation will outweigh its potential toxic effects; (b) it is irrelevant in the emergency department (ED) or the operating room (OR), where long-term exposure to high concentration oxygen is rare; and (c) damage from high-concentration oxygen is mild to moderate.

Indeed, the importance of oxygenation cannot be exaggerated, and the most well-known toxicities take days to develop clinical signs after exposure to high-concentration oxygen (hyperbaric oxygen is not discussed in this chapter). Certainly, a high inspired concentration of oxygen is warranted in some situations—for instance, if a patient who is being turned prone and placed in pins becomes extubated, the anesthesia providers have several minutes longer to turn him back over and get him reintubated if he is being ventilated with 100% oxygen as opposed to an intentionally lowered FiO_2. In the past decades, however, we have come to realize that oxygen toxicity can have very acute and significant effects in multiple clinical scenarios such as cardiopulmonary resuscitation (CPR), cardiopulmonary bypass (CPB), and organ transplantation. It is clearly an inevitable issue confronting every anesthesia provider in the intensive care unit (ICU), the OR, or the ED. Avoiding oxygen toxicity may not only avoid tissue damage, it may also reduce mortality.

We will briefly discuss several clinical scenarios of oxygen toxicities. Among them, pulmonary injuries secondary to prolonged exposure and retinopathy of prematurity might be viewed as "chronic" toxicity of high concentration oxygen, whereas the others represent acute detrimental effects, happening minutes to hours after exposure to high oxygen concentrations.

PROLONGED EXPOSURE (ICU VENTILATION)

The damage resulting from prolonged exposure to high oxygen concentrations involves several organ systems, including the lungs (fibrosis, hemorrhage, atelectasis, edema, and hyaline membrane damage), the central nervous system (CNS) (convulsion, paralysis, and death), the testes, and blood

© 2006 Mayo Foundation for Medical Education and Research

cells (hemolysis). Pulmonary injuries are the most common sequelae in human beings. The mechanisms are still not fully understood. It is generally held that oxygen toxicity in human beings can be avoided if 100% O_2 is taken for less than 12 hours, or 80% for less than 24 hours, or 60% for less than 36 hours. This is relevant to patients with respiratory failure who need prolonged respiratory support. As a general rule, oxygen concentration should be reduced to the lowest possible level. Unfortunately, this often is a challenging task when patients need a higher FiO_2 for oxygenation. It is important to optimize other factors, such as positive end-expiratory pressure (PEEP) and ventilation modes before increasing oxygen concentration is considered.

RETINOPATHY OF PREMATURITY
High oxygen concentration was associated with increased incidences of retinopathy of prematurity (ROP) in the 1940s. During the 1950s and 1960s, the oxygen tension of incubators was decreased. The incidence of ROP decreased as expected, but mortality seemed to increase. Based on recent studies, the 2002 American Association for Respiratory Care (AARC) guideline recommended that for infants less than 37 weeks' gestation, PaO_2 should be kept lower than 80 mm Hg.

CONGENITAL HEART DISEASES
Inhalation of oxygen may substantially reduce pulmonary vascular resistance in infants with pulmonary hypertension. If there is an intracardiac shunt, such as in hypoplastic left heart or a single ventricle, the balance between pulmonary and systemic circulations may be disrupted, causing left-to-right shunting and potentially devastating consequences within minutes. This is extremely important in the induction of anesthesia when denitrogenation with 100% oxygen would otherwise be routine.

ACCENTUATION OF HYPERCAPNIA
Giving oxygen to patients with compensated respiratory failure should be done cautiously, as the treatment may worsen hypercapnia. This rapid consequence is more a "physiologic" than a "toxic" effect of high-concentration oxygen. Its mechanisms include decreased stimuli on the peripheral chemoceptors, worsened V/Q mismatch, and increased CO_2–hemoglobin dissociation.

ABSORPTION ATELECTASIS
In patients with a low regional V/Q ratio in the lungs, the involved alveoli are kept open mainly by nitrogen. Inhalation of high-concentration oxygen maximizes the nitrogen partial pressure gradients between alveoli and palmary capillaries, enhances absorption of nitrogen in the alveoli, and completely

collapses the poorly ventilated alveoli. Most often in the elderly, the resultant increased shunting may be as high as 11% and take place as rapidly as 30 min after inhalation of pure oxygen.

CARDIOPULMONARY RESUSCITATION

Numerous animal experiments and clinical studies suggest that 100% oxygen used during CPR may be detrimental, especially in neonates. Davis et al. analyzed the outcomes in five separate clinical trials (1,302 cases total) that compared resuscitations with either 100% oxygen or room air in neonates with asphyxia. Although no original study found any difference in mortality rates between groups, the pooled data revealed a significant benefit of room air resuscitation for infants (relative risk of 0.71). It is estimated that one death would be prevented for 20 patients if air, instead of 100% oxygen, were used for resuscitation. During the 2005 International Consensus Conference on Cardiopulmonary Resuscitation, it was acknowledged that excessive oxygen given during resuscitation may cause oxidant injury and should be avoided, especially in premature infants. However, the current evidence was weighed as insufficient to specify the concentration of oxygen to be used initially, or to indicate a change in the oxygen concentration afterward. In the 2005 American Heart Association (AHA) guidelines, the standard approach to resuscitation is still to use 100% oxygen. However, it accepts use of an oxygen concentration of less than 100% (or room air) for neonatal resuscitation.

In contrast, the existing evidence of oxygen toxicity in adult CPR is much less compelling. The major concern is still focusing on airway, breathing, and circulation (ABC), and giving 100% oxygen during resuscitation remains preferred.

CARDIOPULMONARY BYPASS

High oxygen concentration may be toxic during CPB. Pizov et al. reported in a clinical study that ventilation with 100% oxygen during surgery and insuflation of the lungs with 100% oxygen during CPB was associated with a lower PaO_2/FiO_2 ratio and a higher TNF level in bronchoalveolar lavage, as compared to the control group that was treated with air instead of 100% oxygen. Patients with pre-existing hypoxia/cyanosis may be even more vulnerable to oxygen damage. In animal models, Morita et al. demonstrated that CPB primed and run with the conventional hyperoxic perfusate was associated with more reperfusion injuries and poorer myocardial functions compared with those with hypoxic or normoxic perfusate. However, there are no further studies exploring whether avoiding hyperoxic ventilation and lung insuflation has any significant effects on clinical outcome. A consensus on this issue has not been reached in clinical practice.

ORGAN TRANSPLANTATION

Research data supports the thought that hyperoxic reperfusion may exacerbate ischemia/reperfusion injury in organ transplantation. Here are a couple of examples. Detterbeck et al. demonstrated that hyperoxic reperfusion in lung transplantation in animals decreased PO_2 and shortened survival time. In another animal experiment, hyperoxic reperfusion after 30 minutes of complete renal ischemia was associated with sustained elevation of creatinine and blood urea nitrogen (BUN), while normoxic reperfusion caused only transient elevation. However, so far there is no established guideline that defines an optimal oxygen tension for initiation of reperfusion in organ transplantation.

OTHER ISSUES

It has been reported that inhalation of high-concentration oxygen causes vasoconstriction of coronary and retinal arteries. In patients who have received bleomycin, the risks for oxygen toxicity are significantly elevated.

The mechanisms for oxygen toxicity are associated with excessive production of free oxygen radicals. Many antioxidants have been shown to have promising effects in the laboratory, but none has been used successfully in the clinical realm to attenuate oxygen toxicity from prolonged exposure or during ischemia/reperfusion.

TAKE HOME POINTS

- Prolonged exposure to high-concentration oxygen may cause significant tissue injuries, such as pulmonary fibrosis, hemorrhage, edema, hyaline membrane, and ROP.
- Acute and devastating oxygen toxicity should be anticipated in the following situations: (a) patients with chronic obstructive pulmonary disease (COPD), (b) patients with regional decreased V/Q ratio in the lungs, (c) patients with pulmonary hypertension and congenital heart diseases, and (d) neonatal CPR patients.
- High oxygen concentration may be toxic in the following situations: adult CPR, lung injuries in CPB, aortic cross-clamping/declamping, and organ transplantation.
- Antioxidant treatments are still experimental. Therefore, identifying patients with increased risks and avoiding oxygen toxicity is important.

SUGGESTED READINGS

American Heart Association. 2005 American Heart Association (AHA) guidelines for cardiopulmonary resuscitation (CPR) and emergency cardiovascular care (ECC) of pediatric and neonatal patients: pediatric basic life support. *Pediatrics*. 2006;117:e989–e1004.

Benumof JL. Respiratory physiology and respiratory function during anesthesia. In: Miller RD, ed. *Miller's Anesthesia*. Philadelphia: Churchill Livingstone; 2000:578–618.

Day RW, Barton AJ, Pysher TJ, et al. Pulmonary vascular resistance of children treated with nitrogen during early infancy. *Ann Thorac Surg.* 1998;65(5):1400–1404.

El-Lessy HN. Pulmonary vascular control in hypoplastic left-heart syndrome: hypoxic- and hypercarbic-gas therapy. *Respir Care.* 1995;40(7):737–742.

Frank L, Massaro D. The lung and oxygen toxicity. *Arch Intern Med.* 1979;139:347–350.

Morita K, Ihnken K, Buckberg GD, et al. Role of controlled cardiac reoxygenation in reducing nitric oxide production and cardiac oxidant damage in cyanotic infantile hearts. *J Clin Invest.* 1994;93:2658–2666.

Myers TR, American Association for Respiratory Care (AARC). AARC clinical practice guideline: selection of an oxygen delivery device for neonatal and pediatric patients—2002 revision & update. *Respir Care.* 2002;47:707–716.

Riordan CJ, Randsbeck F, Storey JH, et al. Effects of oxygen, positive end-expiratory pressure, and carbon dioxide on oxygen delivery in an animal model of the univentricular heart. *J Thorac Cardiovasc Surg.* 1996;112(3):644–654.

Zwemer CF, Whitesall SE, D'Alecy LG. Cardiopulmonary-cerebral resuscitation with 100% oxygen exacerbates neurological dysfunction following nine minutes of normothermic cardiac arrest in dogs. *Resuscitation.* 1994;27:159–170.

7

UNDERSTAND AND TAKE ADVANTAGE OF THE UNIQUE PROPERTIES OF HELIUM FOR THE MANAGEMENT OF THE COMPROMISED AIRWAY

J. MAURICIO DEL RIO, MD AND THERESA A. GELZINIS, MD

A 22-month-old girl began coughing while eating some sunflower seeds. Shortly thereafter, she appeared to be gasping for air. Her mother performed back blows and called for an ambulance. In the emergency department she was awake, alert, and sitting forward with obvious stridor, increased work of breathing, frequent coughing, and drooling. The patient was transported emergently to the operating room for airway management. When you arrive, her vital signs are blood pressure 119/76 mm Hg, respiratory rate 66 breaths/min, heart rate 160 beats/min, and pulse oximetry 90% with some blow-by oxygen. Examination of the chest reveals mild retractions and faint bilateral wheezing. While awaiting the arrival of the ENT surgeon, the patient has intermittent episodes of perioral cyanosis, repetitive coughing, and worsening stridor.
How would you manage this patient?

Since 1934, when helium was first described as therapy for upper-airway obstruction and asthma exacerbation, it has been advocated for the treatment of a wide variety of respiratory conditions. However, the optimal application and effectiveness of the helium–oxygen mixture (heliox) for managing air flow obstructive disorders has not been clearly supported by the evidence. It is important to understand the mechanism of action and the scenarios in which this therapy is and is not warranted.

PHYSICAL PROPERTIES OF HELIUM

Helium is a colorless, odorless, tasteless, monatomic element. It is the first noble gas in the periodic table, with an atomic number of 2 and an atomic weight of 4 g/mol. Helium is the second most abundant element in the universe but relatively rare on earth, representing 0.000524% of the atmosphere. With the lowest boiling and melting points of the elements, helium exists as a gas except in extreme conditions. In natural conditions, most helium is created by the radioactive decay of heavier elements and is trapped within natural gas in concentrations up to 7%. Helium is extracted from natural gas by fractional distillation. At a temperature near absolute zero the liquid helium has virtually no viscosity, a property called superfluidity.

© 2006 Mayo Foundation for Medical Education and Research

As a consequence of its low atomic weight, the density of helium is the lowest of any gas except hydrogen; unlike hydrogen, it is nonflammable. Helium's low density allows CO_2 to diffuse five times more rapidly through a helium–oxygen mixture than through air or oxygen. Being biologically inert, helium has no direct pharmacologic effects and has no intrinsic bronchodilatory or anti-inflammatory properties. For the same reasons, it has no known toxic effects, even when used for extended periods of time.

HELIOX

Heliox is a mixture of helium and oxygen gases. Standard heliox cylinders contain 80:20 heliox, though heliox also is also available in 70:30 and 60:40 mixtures. Commercial-grade heliox is available in H-size cylinders, which contain approximately 1,200 L of gas, at approximately 2,200 psi. If the patient requires supplemental oxygen, this limits the helium concentration that can be administered.

HISTORICAL USES OF HELIOX

Helium was discovered in 1868 by a French astronomer, Janssen, as a bright yellow line in the spectrum of the sun during a solar eclipse. The new element was first isolated on Earth in 1895 by a British chemist, Ramsay. At the time of its discovery, helium had no practical use. Heliox was first used physiologically to create breathing environments for diving. It reduced the formation of nitrogen bubbles responsible for decompression illness in divers and allowed them to work at depth for extended periods of time. In 1934, Barach noted the biologic inertness of heliox; he found no ill effects in mice exposed to a high helium concentration for 2 months. Those experiments were followed by clinical investigations of its potential benefits for various disorders, including asthma and infant airway obstruction. Barach noted evidence of relief within 6 to 10 breaths, with dyspnea returning in as little as 3 to 4 breaths after discontinuation of heliox. After the late 1930s, little was reported about clinical applications of heliox until 1979. Since then, there has been a resurgence in the investigation of its potential uses.

PHYSICS OF FLUID FLOW WITH HELIOX

The behavior of a fluid in flow is related to two intrinsic properties of the fluid: density and viscosity. The density of a substance is its mass per unit volume. Because 1 gram molecular weight of a gas occupies a volume of 22.4 L under standard conditions, gas density is its gram molecular weight divided by 22.4 L. The density of helium is thus 0.179 g/L. Oxygen's molecular weight is 32 g, so its density is 1.43 g/L. Viscosity is an internal property of a fluid. Viscosity causes resistance to flow. A fluid with a high viscosity strongly resists flow.

Gas flow can vary from laminar at one end of the spectrum to turbulent at the other. Under normal circumstances, gas flow in many parts of the respiratory tract is largely laminar and follows the Hagen–Poiseuille law. This law states that the fluid flow rate (Q) through a straight tube of uniform bore is proportional to the pressure gradient (ΔP) and the fourth power of the radius (r), and is related inversely to the viscosity of the gas (μ), and the length (l) of the tube:

$$\dot{Q} = \frac{\Delta P \pi r^4}{8\mu l}$$

Flow varies directly with pressure, so quadrupling the pressure will quadruple the flow; it also varies as the fourth power of the radius, so doubling the radius will increase flow by a factor of 16. Note that laminar flow is viscosity-dependent and density-independent. Because the viscosity of helium, oxygen, and air is similar and laminar flow velocity is independent of density, heliox has no effect on areas of laminar flow.

Turbulent flow occurs in constricted passages and follows a different law:

$$\dot{Q} = k\sqrt{\frac{\Delta P}{\rho}}$$

Compared with laminar flow, turbulent flow is less efficient. Flow increases with the square root of the pressure gradient, so quadrupling the pressure gradient merely doubles the flow. Decreasing the density will also increase the flow. As flow velocity decreases and/or airway resistance increases, there is a critical level at which the flow pattern changes from laminar to turbulent. This transitional zone is defined by Reynolds number (Re):

$$Re = \frac{V D \rho}{\mu}$$

where V represents the mean velocity of the gas, D represents airway diameter, ρ represents the gas density, and μ is the viscosity of the gas. The Reynolds number is the ratio of inertial forces (density-dependent, viscosity-independent) to viscous forces (viscosity-dependent, density-independent). Laminar flow occurs at low Reynolds number (Re $<$2,100) when viscous forces are dominant and is characterized by smooth, constant fluid motion. Turbulent flow occurs at high Reynolds number (Re $>$4,000) and is dominated by inertial forces, producing random eddies, vortices, and other flow fluctuations. Transitional flow lies between these values and displays qualities of both types of flow.

While breathing air, there is an insignificant difference in relative gas density at various oxygen concentrations. However, by replacing nitrogen

with helium, there is a wide variability in the density between the different oxygen concentrations. As a result, the Reynolds number is decreased,
making flow more likely to be laminar. With extremely turbulent flow patterns, flow rate becomes dependent on gas density according to the Bernoulli
equation:

$$Q = (2\,\Delta P/\rho)^{1/2}$$

Therefore, by using helium as the carrier gas, heliox will reduce the density
of the inspired gas and will provide a higher flow rate even if the flow remains
turbulent. This results in a lower resistance to gas flow, allowing for increased
bulk flow through high-resistance airways and converting some or all of the
turbulent flow to laminar flow. In the end, there is increased oxygen flow and
decreased work of breathing.

CLINICAL USE OF HELIOX

Air flow patterns in the pulmonary system are products of the physical
conditions in the airway (e.g., diameter, anatomic shape, branching, and
smoothness of airway lining) and the composition of the inhaled gas. Air
flow in the lung periphery is primarily laminar because of the large cross-
sectional surface area through which the gas flows. Conversely, air flow in
the larger upper airways is turbulent, with relatively high flow and relatively
small cross-sectional surface area. The flow characteristics in the airways
may also vary depending on the inspiratory and expiratory flow rates. During normal breathing, a transition from turbulent to laminar flow occurs
from the trachea to around the second generation of bronchi. However, in
patients with airway obstruction, turbulent flow occurs randomly and more
frequently, even at low respiratory and flow rates. This leads to increased
work of breathing. In patients with increased airway resistance, heliox administration will reduce resistance to flow, which will lead to decreased work of
breathing.

ADMINISTRATION

Helium has a very high diffusion coefficient, which requires it to be stored
in special, tightly sealed containers. In order to achieve a sufficient helium
concentration ($>50\%$) to gain maximal advantage from the helium, the administration system needs to be "helium-tight". Therefore, the most effective heliox systems are closed systems. The system should be also high-flow,
with sufficient flow to meet or exceed the patient's minute volume and peak
inspiratory flow, and to minimize dilution with ambient air. Flushing a high
flow of heliox into the patient's airway is expensive and can be wasteful.
Hence, the delivery method should include a reservoir and an on-demand
delivery system that minimize total flow and helium requirements.

Heliox can be used in patients who are breathing spontaneously, but also in the settings of both invasive mechanical ventilation (e.g., with tracheal intubation) and noninvasive mechanical ventilation.

BENEFICIAL RESPIRATORY EFFECTS
- Reduces transpulmonary pressure requirement
- Increases tidal volume
- Improves homogeneity of gas distribution
- Improves elimination of CO_2
- Improves delivery of aerosolized medications

POSSIBLE CLINICAL APPLICATIONS
- Upper-airway obstruction
- Postextubation stridor
- Croup
- Bronchiolitis
- Asthma exacerbation
- Chronic obstructive pulmonary disease (COPD) exacerbation
- Pulmonary function testing

Being used for these purposes, in different clinical trials, heliox therapy has been shown to:
- Relieve stridor, reduce work of breathing, and reduce respiratory distress
- Allow time to assess patient's airway and clinical status
- Allow time to prepare for further interventions
- Act as a therapeutic bridge to allow time for definitive treatments to become effective
- Act as an alternative to effective treatments when they are contraindicated
- Prevent intubation in patients with impending respiratory failure
- Decrease the need for intubation or reintubation in perioperative settings
- Be clearly useful for upper-airway obstruction
- Provide greater benefit in patients with a greater degree of respiratory distress
- Shorten the length of perinatal ICU stay in infants with bronchiolitis
- In croup, improves respiratory distress, though not better than conventional therapies

FOR ASTHMA EXACERBATION
- Conventional treatment is sufficient for the majority of patients.
- First-line use of heliox is not warranted for most patients.
- Heliox is more effective for patients with the most severe exacerbations and air flow obstruction.
- The beneficial effects seem to be most efficacious when heliox is used early (before 24 h).

- Early use may decrease dyspnea and improve gas exchange, especially when implementing conventional therapies that require hours for full effect (e.g., steroids).
- Heliox can be used as a temporizing measure to prevent intubation.
- Heliox has a relatively safe treatment profile, and clinical benefits should be rapid.

FOR SEVERE COPD

- Heliox may improve alveolar ventilation and gas transfer (decreasing $PaCO_2$).
- Heliox may reduce the need for intubation.
- Heliox should be considered in individual cases when intubation is required but would be undesirable.
- Wide-scale use of heliox cannot be recommended based on clinical evidence.

RISKS OF HELIOX USE

Hypoxemia/Anoxia. There is a possibility of delivering a gas mixture that contains <21% oxygen. This risk is reduced by administering only heliox that contains at least 20% oxygen. The cylinder should be mixed and tested before use. The use of an oxygen analyzer in line with the gas output provides monitoring to prevent hypoxemia. There have been reports of hypoxia during heliox administration in preterm infants who have a history of bronchopulmonary dysplasia and subglottic stenosis. This could be related to the reduction of lung volume and the increased intrapulmonary shunt.

Volutrauma/Barotrauma. Heliox's flow is faster than that of air or oxygen. Consequently, when using a flow meter calibrated for oxygen or air, a correction factor (based on the helium concentration) must be applied to correct for the difference in flow rate. The heliox correction factors are generally rounded off to 1.4 for 60:40, 1.6 for 70:30, and 1.8 for 80:20. Thus, when an oxygen flow meter delivering 80:20 heliox reads 10 L/min, it is actually delivering 18 L/min. If a system delivers more than the set volume, there is a risk of volume-induced injury, pressure-induced injury, or hypocarbia. This is of particular concern with closed systems that are not designed for heliox administration.

Inadequate Delivery of Aerosolized Medications. Poorly adjusted flow of heliox in a nebulizer can result in a subtherapeutic dose or can increase the dose delivered to the lungs above the intended levels.

Hypothermia. Hypothermia has been associated with hood administration of heliox to infants. Heliox has a high thermal conductivity with consequent risk of hypothermia when the gas temperature is <36°C, especially when it is administered for long periods. The risk of hypothermia can be avoided with adequate warming and humidification of the inhaled gas.

- Heliox is clearly useful in patients with upper-airway obstruction.
- It can relieve stridor, reduce work of breathing, and reduce respiratory distress.
- It may decrease the need for intubation or reintubation in perioperative settings.
- It can allow time for other interventions or therapies to become effective.
- Heliox must be administered with devices designed for that purpose.
- Definitive clinical evidence is needed to elucidate its role.

SUGGESTED READINGS

Andrews L, Lynch M. Heliox in the treatment of chronic obstructive pulmonary disease. *Emerg Med J*. 2004;21(6):670–675.

Brown L, Sherwin T, Perez JE, et al. Heliox as a temporizing measure for pediatric foreign body aspiration. *Acad Emerg Med*. 2002;9:346–347.

Chevrolet JC. Helium oxygen mixtures in the intensive care unit. *Crit Care*. 2001;5(4):179–181.

Fink JB. Opportunities and risks of using heliox in your clinical practice. *Respir Care*. 2006;51(6): 651–660.

Gupta VK, Cheifetz IM. Heliox administration in the pediatric intensive care unit: an evidence-based review. *Pediatr Crit Care Med*. 2005;6(2):204–211.

Hess DR. Heliox and noninvasive positive-pressure ventilation: a role for heliox in exacerbations of chronic obstructive pulmonary disease? *Respir Care*. 2006; 51(6):640–650.

Hess DR, Fink JB, Venkataraman ST, et al. The history and physics of heliox. *Respir Care*. 2006;51(6):608–612.

Myers TR. Use of heliox in children. *Respir Care*. 2006;51(6):619–631.

Venkataraman ST. Heliox during mechanical ventilation. *Respir Care*. 2006;51(6):632–639.

8

Remember That There Are Special Considerations Involved With Both Intubation And Chronic Airway Management Of Burn Patients

MARISA H. FERRERA, MD AND SHUSHMA AGGARWAL, MD

Burns can result from thermal, chemical, electrical, or radiation injury. Thermal injury is most common, accounting for up to 90% of all burn insults. Carbon monoxide poisoning is the most frequent cause of death during and immediately after a fire. If the patient survives the first few hours, morbidity and mortality are related to the total body surface area involved, the depth of the burn, and the patient's age. The likelihood of airway compromise increases with more serious burns.

Characteristics of major burns include:

1) Partial-thickness burns involving >25% of total body surface area (TBSA) in adults
2) Full-thickness burns involving >10% of TBSA
3) Presence of inhalational injury
4) Involvement of the face, eyes, ears, hands, feet, or perineum causing impairment
5) Caustic chemical burn etiology
6) High-voltage electrical burns
7) Burns in patients with coexisting debilitating disease

Characteristics of moderate burns include:

1) Partial-thickness burns involving 15% to 25% of TBSA in adults
2) Full-thickness burns involving 2% to 10% TBSA

Burns range from first- to fourth-degree, depending on the depth of the destroyed skin. First-degree burns are limited to the epidermis. Second-degree burns extend into the dermis and are divided into superficial and deep partial-thickness burns based on upper or lower dermis involvement, respectively. Third-degree burns include the entire epidermis and dermis, and fourth-degree burns extend into muscle, fascia, or bone.

Total body surface area of burned skin is estimated using the "rule of nines." Body parts are divided into allotments or multiples of 9% (*Table 8.1*).

ACUTE MANAGEMENT

Burn patients with inhalational injury may require endotracheal intubation and ventilatory support at the site of the fire. If the patient has an endotracheal

© 2006 Mayo Foundation for Medical Education and Research

TABLE 8.1	RULE OF NINES	
Entire head and neck		9%
Each arm		9%
Anterior upper/lower trunk		18%
Posterior upper/lower trunk		18%
Each lower extremity		18%
Genitals and perineum		1%
Each hand		1%

tube (ETT) on arrival to the hospital, do not change the tube; it may be difficult to get another one in place. It is not unusual that burn patients present asymptomatically. These patients have the potential to become problematic because of subsequent sequelae of burn injury that lead to a challenging airway. Burn patients develop excessive amounts of upper- and lower-airway edema as a result of mucosal destruction and capillary leakage that is further exacerbated by fluid resuscitation. Airway edema and narrowing continues for 12 to 24 hours after the initial burn insult. A thorough history and physical are helpful in determining which patients are candidates for early intubation. While assessing the patient, administer oxygen by face mask and monitor oxygen saturation with pulse oximetry.

History. A burn injury that occurs in an enclosed space with highly combustible material is very suspicious for inhalation injury. Patients who report coughing, drooling, hoarseness, dysphonia, and dysphagia are at risk of airway swelling.

Physical Exam. Facial burns and the presence of oral soot correlate highly with airway edema and impending airway compromise. Other signs include singed facial hair, soot in the nose, stridor, and respiratory distress.

Diagnosis. The diagnosis of inhalation injury is made primarily by history and physical examination. Patients who demonstrate the above signs and symptoms should undergo endotracheal intubation. In addition, patients with a partial pressure of arterial oxygen (PaO_2) < 60 mm Hg, $PaCO_2$ >50 mm Hg (acutely) on room air, or a PaO_2 <200 mm Hg on 100% oxygen also require intubation. Computed tomography (CT) scan and radiographs of the chest are not helpful in the acute setting. Some facilities advise using fiberoptic bronchoscopy every 3 to 4 hours to diagnose impending airway obstruction; however, this recommendation may not be clinically practical.

Management. Initial management includes securing the airway, breathing, and circulation (ABC) as in any other form of injury. If the patient's history and physical are indicative of airway compromise, perform endotracheal intubation early, before it becomes a technical challenge. Inform the entire team of physicians of the primary approach and alternative plans for managing the airway. Difficult-airway equipment should be readily available.

As per the American Society of Anesthesiologists (ASA) Difficult Airway Algorithm, elective measures are appropriate when the physician is able to ventilate the patient (www.asahq.org/Newsletters/2005/11-05/2003TraumaAlgorithm.html).

If a "can't ventilate, can't intubate" situation arises, the physician should approach the airway based on the Difficult Airway Algorithm.

The most suitable elective methods of securing the airway in a burn patient are discussed below.

1) Direct vision laryngoscopy is the most commonly used technique for endotracheal intubation. However, if the patient has inadequate mouth opening, limited range of neck motion, and distorted postburn airway anatomy, consider alternate routes of intubation.

2) Flexible fiberoptic laryngoscopy is the alternative method of choice because it can overcome the problems of direct-vision laryngoscopy.

3) Retrograde wire technique is useful when bleeding prevents adequate visualization of the airway. This is best performed by a provider with experience.

4) Tracheostomy is done electively in a sterile environment, usually by a surgeon. Avoid surgical tracheostomy if possible because of the high incidence of pulmonary sepsis, subglottic stenosis, fistula formation, and subsequent death.

Succinylcholine, a depolarizing muscle relaxant, should be avoided when intubating burn patients. Succinylcholine can produce dangerous levels of hyperkalemia, leading to cardiac arrest. The greatest risk of hyperkalemia occurs within 2 weeks to 6 months after the burn injury.

Be careful when using non-depolarizing muscle relaxants initially. Because there is a possibility of failed intubation, the patient may need to have spontaneous ventilation reestablished. Interestingly, patients are generally resistant to the effects of non-depolarizing muscle relaxants. This desensitization appears by post-injury day 7 and may last up to 70 days.

Nasotracheal intubation is suggested if facial trauma or burns do not preclude its use. Patients tolerate this method better, especially those who need intubation for an extended period of time. The risk of sinusitis increases after 4 days of nasotracheal intubation. Do not extubate patients who require multiple repeat surgeries until the planned surgical course of treatment is completed. If extubation occurs, the provider may run into the same problems faced acutely as well as complications that occur in the chronic setting.

Dressing changes and irrigation and débridement of the wound are common procedures done in the early days after burn injury. If the patient does not require airway support with intubation, these procedures are done under monitored anesthesia care with mask ventilation. Short-acting medications such as midazolam, propofol, and ketamine are the anesthetic agents of choice.

High-frequency positive-pressure ventilation (HFPV) is beneficial in preventing barotrauma and pneumonia in patients with inhalational injury. Tidal volumes of 1 to 3 mL/kg are given at frequencies of 100 to 3,000 cycles per minute. This method of ventilation allows adequate recruitment of collapsed alveoli while avoiding high peak airway pressures. Proper gas humidification is required to avoid severe necrotizing tracheobronchitis.

CHRONIC MANAGEMENT

Chronic complications in burn patients include wound contracture and tracheal stenosis, which make late or subsequent attempts at intubation difficult.

History. Patients with third- and fourth-degree burns are likely to develop scar contracture. Face and neck contractures make intubation challenging by preventing adequate oral opening, neck flexion, and head extension. Contractures in patients with circumferential full-thickness chest wall burns have problems with chest wall motion, decreasing the ability to ventilate the lungs adequately.

Direct inhalational injury, scar contracture, and/or mechanical damage from the endotracheal tube, tracheostomy tube, or their respective cuffs put burn patients at risk for tracheal stenosis. Stenosis is caused by pressure necrosis with subsequent healing and scar formation. Prolonged intubation and repeated intubation are additional factors that play a role in stenosis formation. Patients may report dyspnea or may have a history of requiring smaller endotracheal tubes for repeated intubations.

Physical. Findings of stenosis are made by fiberoptic bronchoscopy. Most stenoses occur in the subglottic region, but they can also involve the upper and lower trachea or a combination of these. Stridor is indicative of stenosis.

Management. Tracheal stenosis is difficult to treat once it occurs. Prevention is the key to management. Although inhalational injury causes tracheal stenoses in and of itself, the risk can be decreased by using low-pressure cuffs (<20 cm H_2O), ensuring tube stability, and minimizing the number and length of intubations. Early tracheal resection should be avoided because of high restenosis rates.

The approach to airway management in the chronic setting is similar to that in the acute setting. However, there are key differences. In the nonemergency pathway, successful intubation is more likely with fiberoptic bronchoscopy because it allows the provider to detect the presence of subglottic and tracheal stenoses. As stated previously, maintain open communication with the surgical team. When endotracheal intubation is needed emergently, their surgical skills will be required to release wound contractures to make head and neck manipulation less difficult, or they may be needed to secure a surgical airway.

TAKE HOME POINTS

- A detailed history and physical examination are essential in predicting airway compromise.
- It is safer to intubate sooner rather than later.
- Avoid succinylcholine.
- Elective tracheostomy in burn patients is associated with a high incidence of complications.
- Utilize a team approach. Maintain open communication with the surgical team.
- Have the appropriate equipment and personnel to manage a difficult airway readily available.

SUGGESTED READINGS

American Society of Anesthesiologists. Difficult Airway Algorithm. www.asahq.org/Newsletters/2005/11-05/2003TraumaAlgorithm.html.

Herndon D, ed. *Total Burn Care*. 2nd ed. London: WB Saunders; 2002:224, 233–240, 247, 251.

Madnani DD, Steele NP, de Vries E. Factors that predict the need for intubation in patients with smoke inhalation injury. *Ear Nose Throat J*. 2006;85(4):278–280.

Saffle JR, Morris SE, Edelman L. Early tracheostomy does not improve outcome in burn patients. *J Burn Care Rehab*. 2002;23(6):431–438.

Yang J, Yang W, Chang L, et al. Symptomatic tracheal stenosis in burns. *Burns*. 1999;25:72–90.

9

CONSIDER THE USE OF LIDOCAINE IN THE CUFF OF THE ENDOTRACHEAL TUBE, BUT BE AWARE OF THE RISKS AND ALTERNATIVES

JAMEY E. EKLUND, MD AND PAUL M. KEMPEN, MD, PhD

Anesthesia providers must mitigate the undesired hemodynamic and neuromuscular responses to intubation. Usually (but of course, not always!), large doses of induction drugs and neuromuscular blockade smooth the way during intubation. Intraoperatively, an adequate level of inhalational anesthetic plus opioids will help the patient tolerate the endotracheal tube (ETT). On extubation, however, the dissipating anesthetic effects and re-emerging pharyngotracheal reflexes may lead to coughing and adverse symptoms, including tachyarrhythmias and increased intracranial, intraocular, or intravascular pressures, via the airway-circulatory reflex.

The incidence of coughing at extubation varies between 6.6% and 96%. Mitigating circulatory-airway reflex symptoms is especially important in patients with cardiovascular and reactive airway disease, neurosurgery, and certain head, neck, or ophthalmologic conditions. Multiple anesthetic strategies to prevent ETT-stimulated coughing have been described, including:

1) Elimination of the ETT completely during general anesthesia (i.e., mask anesthetics) or extubation during profound anesthesia when the ETT is no longer necessary (known universally as a "deep extubation")
2) Use of local anesthetic via systemic intravenous (IV) or topical endotracheal administration

Anesthesia providers must consider patient history, co-morbidities, and surgical needs to select appropriate strategies.

INTRACUFF LIDOCAINE (ICL)

Nonionized lidocaine has been shown to diffuse readily along a concentration gradient through the lipophilic plastic of an ETT cuff sufficiently to anesthetize adjacent mucosa, typically sparing the vocal cords (which are not in contact with the cuff). The cuff serves as a reservoir of local anesthetic. Comparing equal volumes of intracuff saline versus lidocaine, the incidence of postextubation coughing has been shown to be 59% versus 38%, respectively. Saline-filled cuffs functioned as the control and were shown to have comparable efficacy to air-filled cuffs. Estebe et al. extensively studied various concentrations of lidocaine (2% to 10%), as well as alkalinization of the lidocaine solution. Higher lidocaine concentrations and alkaline solution

© 2006 Mayo Foundation for Medical Education and Research

pH effectively increase the available nonionized, lipophilic, and diffusible lidocaine. Alkalinization increases the available nonionized and diffusible lidocaine at any given concentration.

Risks. Although the use of lidocaine in the ETT cuff is appealing, serious potential risks deserve consideration. Plain or alkalinized lidocaine solutions (2% to 4%) are clinically effective while limiting exposure to potentially toxic (gram) amounts of intratracheal lidocaine from 10% solutions, should the approximately 10-mL-volume cuff rupture. Filling and deflating the cuff with noncompressible aqueous solutions typically occur much more slowly than with air, whereas similarly, complete elimination of intracuff air and the pressure–volume effects from N_2O can be difficult. Many studies of intracuff lidocaine employed direct manometry to avoid excessive pressure; others inflated cuffs until positive-pressure ventilation at 20 cm H_2O was confirmed without air leak. Prolonged cuff pressure >20 cm H_2O can tamponade mucosal perfusion and result in tissue necrosis. Fluid-filled intracuff pressures may be difficult to assess, with slow fluid flow between pilot and tracheal balloons. Anesthesia providers who are unfamiliar with or unaware of fluid-filled cuffs may not completely empty them at extubation during the 1- to 2-second deflation attempt that is typical for air. Thus, the noncompressible fluid-filled ETT balloon may lead to vocal cord trauma when it is inadvertently pulled through the glottic opening. Although extubation with air-filled balloons was not found to cause arytenoid subluxation in several cadavers, the effect of fluid-filled balloons is unknown.

Albeit rare, cuff rupture has been reported, and lidocaine can be rapidly absorbed through the lung. Although diffusion from 10% lidocaine via intact ETT cuffs did not reach toxic plasma levels, systemic toxicity could occur if the cuff ruptures and releases >1 gram of lidocaine into circulation. Cuffs with pinhole-sized defects filled at minimal pressure typically leak slowly, thus limiting peak and rapid uptake and potential lidocaine toxicity. Knight et al. studied high-dose administration of lidocaine in a patient population to assess systemic toxicity. After induction with 6 mg/kg of lidocaine and maintenance anesthesia of 0.6 mg/kg diazepam and 50% N_2O, a total of 21 mg/kg lidocaine via controlled intravenous infusion was administered up to the point of cardiac bypass without toxicity. Peak plasma concentrations of 9.5 mcg/mL were noted at sternotomy. Indeed, rapid parenteral injections carry a higher risk of toxicity; but based on this study, systemic toxicity should not be clinically evident in adults with doses smaller than 100 mg intravenous push or 160 mg via tracheal instillation.

Time-dependent diffusion of lidocaine from the cuff effectively limits toxicity, as hepatic metabolism occurs with a $T_{1/2}$ of 90 minutes. With excessive pressure and resulting tracheal mucosa ischemia, systemic absorption may be further curtailed. In vitro studies demonstrated that higher concentrations of lidocaine (4% vs. 2%), prolonged duration for diffusion (360 minutes vs. 60 minutes), and "priming" cuff membranes (by prefilling them) resulted in a maximum diffusion of only 17.49 mcg lidocaine. A similar independent study noted as much as 1% of a 4% lidocaine solution diffusing after 6 hours, whereas alkalinized lidocaine resulted in 65% diffusion of the stock solution (2 mL of 2% lidocaine) after 6 hours. Sufficient time must elapse for an effective topical accumulation of mucosal lidocaine, making intracuff lidocaine questionably effective in surgeries lasting <1 hour. Typically, cuffs are also prefilled significantly in advance to saturate the cuff membrane and to eliminate air, which may limit clinical utility in high-volume and rapid-turnover practices. Two separate in vivo studies comparing control to lidocaine-filled cuffs showed very significant cough suppression (5% vs. 70% and 16% vs. 38% to 44%, respectively). The primary goal of intracuff lidocaine is to prevent adverse hemodynamic and oxygenation changes. Unfortunately, this occurred with limited success: "The emergent hemodynamic and oxygenation saturation data were similar for all three groups [air, saline, lidocaine]"—Fagan et al.

ALTERNATIVES

The minimal anesthetic concentration for suppression of the airway-circulatory reflex from the ETT at extubation (MAC extubation on MAC_{ex}) is comparable to the stimulus of skin incision and is effectively managed at 1.2 MAC. Extubation at MAC_{ex} can effectively mitigate hemodynamic and hyperreactive airway responses from tracheal stimulation once the ETT is no longer required. "Deep extubation" involves removing the ETT while the patient is in a surgical plane of anesthesia. Removing the endotracheal tube can subsequently reduce anesthetic depth requirements, as surgical stimulation abates and dressings are applied, and can thus expedite emergence and transfer to the postoperative acute care unit. The anesthesia provider must, however, demonstrate airway skills to ensure adequate ventilation throughout emergence. Deep extubation is best performed after spontaneous respiration becomes evident. Removing an unnecessary ETT results in a situation equivalent to anesthesia via mask ventilation and with similar contraindications (i.e., high aspiration risk, difficult airway/high ventilation pressure requirements). Daley et al. showed that most anesthesia providers are hesitant to extubate in a deep plane of anesthesia because of aspiration risk. Thus, placement of a Salem sump (naso-gastric tube) after intubation (with removal immediately before extubation) maximizes stomach decompression and helps identify particulate stomach content.

Lidocaine, 1 to 2 mg/kg intravenous push 1 minute before extubation, effectively suppresses cough. Other intravenous medications that can also reduce coughing at extubation include opiates, propofol, succinylcholine, beta-adrenergic blockers, and dexmedetomidine. However, most systemi-cally administered medications, including lidocaine, also increase anesthetic depth, increase sedation, and/or decrease respiratory drive, and thereby unnecessarily prolong emergence from inhalation anesthetics. Lidocaine plasma concentrations of 3 mcg/mL are required to suppress the cough reflex, while contributing 0.15 MAC of anesthetic effects. Animal studies also confirm that as little as 1 mcg/mL of lidocaine contributes significantly to inhalational anesthetic effects. Because many IV medications have anti-tussive properties, it is clinically difficult to attribute specific mitigation of cough alone to acutely injected lidocaine, without invoking general anesthetic effects per se.

Topical tracheal lidocaine has been effectively demonstrated to reduce the incidence of coughing. Patients undergoing awake fiber-optic intubation are routinely anesthetized topically and are without reaction upon tracheal contact. ETT lubrication with nonaqueous lidocaine jelly may be irritating to the mucosa and is therefore discouraged. Available instillation methods of aqueous solutions include LTA (Hospira, Chicago, IL) at intubation, spray-ing lidocaine down the ETT tube lumen, or via the LITA tube (Sheridan Catheter Corp., Argyle, NY). The LITA tube has an integrated injection port to allow simultaneous injection above and below the cuff via a separate injection port. Although Gonzalez et al. demonstrated the LITA's effective in decreasing cough, LITAs are twice as expensive as regular ETTs, can fail when fenestrations become plugged, and must be inserted at induction for routine use at extubation. An inflated cuff may limit lidocaine from quickly reaching underlying mucosa, while mucosal innervation may be interrupted from above and below the cuff. Likewise, lidocaine may flow beneath the cuff via the film of tracheal secretions. Complete topical effects may require time, whereas systemic transpulmonary effects develop rapidly.

Spraying lidocaine solution down the ETT is a practical and effective alternative to intracuff application. Patients often cough briefly, thus dis-tributing lidocaine throughout the airway and facilitating systemic effects via lung absorption. More effectively, the lidocaine can be trickled in over 10 to 20 seconds via a Luer-Lok port on the airway elbow. With the cuff completely deflated, a sustained insufflation/Valsalva maneuver directs the lidocaine upward to the vocal cords and mucosa adjacent the cuff. This is best performed under anesthesia as ventilatory drive returns in response to normalization of the CO_2 levels and before complete reversal of neuro-muscular blockade, thus facilitating air and lidocaine "bubbling up" through relaxed vocal cords. Upon completion of the injection, neuromuscular block-ade is reversed. After typically 20 to 30 seconds, maximal topicalization and a return of regular spontaneous respiration develops. At this point, a rapid deflation of the cuff resulting in no reaction or change in respiration (i.e., as evidenced on $ETCO_2$ tracing) tests to identify adequate topical anesthesia to allow uneventful extubation. This topical effect lasts about 15 to 20 minutes and allows removal of the ETT without significant hemodynamic or respiratory changes. Topically eliminating tracheal stimulus appears to be protective against laryngospasm at all depths of extubation. Although Burton at al. original description recommends 4 mL of 4% lidocaine solution, 5 mL of 2% lidocaine solution is equally effective in our practice. The airway-circulatory reflex is effectively suppressed with 2% lidocaine dosed at 1 mg/kg via intratracheal instillation. The lowest effective dose via intratracheal instillation that effectively mitigates hemodynamic changes immediately before extubation and that has consistent duration of such effects remains to be shown definitively.

TAKE HOME POINTS

- Intracuff lidocaine is effective for cases >1 hour in duration but may carry significant risks and requires significant preparation.
- Lower concentrations of lidocaine are more effective when alkalinized and are less likely to result in systemic toxicity should the cuff rupture.
- Use of manometry is useful to prevent mucosal ischemia but is underutilized.
- Endotracheal instillation appears to be a safe, easy, effective, and widely available technique.
- Clinical skill and experience are required to safely match available techniques to appropriate patients, and the use of intratracheal local anesthetics to remove the ETT is typically contraindicated in patients "at risk" for aspiration.

SUGGESTED READINGS

Altinas F, Bozkurt P, Kaya G, et al. Lidocaine 10% in the endotracheal tube cuff: blood concentrations, haemodynamic and clinical effects. *Eur J Anaesthesiol.* 2000;17(7):436–442.

Asai T, Koga K, Vaughan RS. Respiratory complications associated with tracheal intubation and extubation. *Br J Anaesth.* 1998;80(6):767–775.

Bidwai AV, Bidwai VA, Rogers CR, et al. Blood pressure and pulse-rate responses to endotracheal extubation with and without prior injection of lidocaine. *Anesthesiology.* 1979;51(2):171–173.

Burton AW, Zornow MH. Laryngotracheal lidocaine administration. *Anesthesiology.* 1997;87(1):185–186.

Daley MD, Norman PH, Coveler LA. Tracheal extubation of adult surgical patients while deeply anesthetized: a survey of United States anesthesiologists. *J Clin Anesth.* 1999;11(6):445–452.

Diachun CA, Tunink BP, Brock-Utne JG. Suppression of cough during emergence from general anesthesia: laryngotracheal lidocaine through a modified endotracheal tube. *J Clin Anesth.* 2001;13(6):447–451.

Difazio C, Neiderlehner J, Burney RG. The anesthetic potency of lidocaine in the rat. *Anesth Analg.* 1976;55(6):818–821.

Dollo G, Estebe JP, Le Corre P, et al. Endotracheal tube cuffs filled with lidocaine as a drug delivery system: in vitro and in vivo investigations. *Eur J Pharm Sci.* 2001;13(3):319–323.

Estebe JP, Dollo G, Le Corre P, et al. Alkalinization of intracuff lidocaine improves endotracheal tube-induced emergence phenomena. *Anesth Analg.* 2002;94(1):227–230.

Estebe JP, Gentili M, Le Corre P, et al. Alkalinization of intracuff lidocaine: efficacy and safety. *Anesth Analg.* 2005;101(5):1536–1541.

Fagan C, Frizelle HP, Laffey J, et al. The effects of intracuff lidocaine on endotracheal-tube induced emergence phenomena after general anesthesia. *Anesth Analg.* 2000;91(1):201–205.

Gefke K, Andersen LW, Freisel E. Lidocaine given intravenously as a suppressant of cough and laryngospasm in connection with extubation after tonsillectomy. *Acta Anaesthesiol Scand.* 1983;27(2):111–112.

Gonzalez RM, Bjerke RJ, Drobycki T, et al. Prevention of endotracheal tube-induced coughing during emergence from general anesthesia. *Anesth Analg.* 1994;79(4):792–795.

Himes RS, DiFazio CA, Burney RG. Effects of lidocaine on the anesthetic requirements for nitrous oxide and halothane. *Anesthesiology.* 1997;47(5):437–440.

Huang CJ, Tsai MC. In vitro diffusion of lidocaine across endotracheal tube cuffs. *Can J Anaesth.* 1999;46(1):82–86.

Jee D, Park SY. Lidocaine sprayed down the endotracheal tube attenuates the airway-circulatory reflexes by local anesthesia during emergence and extubation. *Anesth Analg.* 2003;96(1):293–297.

Kempen PM. Extubation in adult patients: who, what, when, where, how and why? *J Clin Anesth.* 1999;11(6):441–444.

Kempen PM. Reply: laryngotracheal lidocaine administration. *Anesthesiology.* 1997;87(1):186.

Knight PR, Droll DA, Nahrwold ML, et al. Comparison of cardiovascular responses to anes-thesia and operation when intravenous lidocaine or morphine sulfate is used as adjunct to diazepam-nitrous oxide anesthesia for cardiac surgery. *Anesth Analg.* 1980;59(2):130–139.

Leech P, Barker J, Fitch W. Proceedings: Changes in intracranial pressure and systemic arterial pressure during the termination of anaesthesia. *Br J Anaesth.* 1974;46(4):315–316.

Miller RD, ed. *Miller's Anesthesia.* 6th ed. New York: Elsevier; 2005.

Navarro RM, Baughman VL. Lidocaine in the endotracheal tube cuff reduces postoperative sore throat. *J Clin Anesth.* 1997;9(5):394–397.

Paulsen FP, Rudert HH, Tillmann BN. New insights into the pathomechanism of postintubation arytenoids subluxation. *Anesthesiology.* 1999;91(3):659–666.

Sant 'ambrogio G, Remmers JE, deGroot WJ, et al. Localization of rapidly adapting receptors in the trachea and main stem bronchus of the dog. *Respir Physiol.* 1978;33(3):359–366.

Sconzo JM, Moscicki JC, DiFazio CA. In vitro diffusion of lidocaine across endotracheal tube cuffs. *Reg Anesth.* 1990;15(1):37–40.

Soltani HA. Letter to the editor. *J Clin Anesth.* 2004;16(1):80.

Steinhaus JE, Gaskin I. A study of intravenous lidocaine as a suppressant of cough reflex. *Anesthesiology.* 1963;24:285–290.

Sumpelmann R, Krohn S, Strauss JM. Laryngotracheal administration of local anesthetics—is the effect mediated by systemic absorption? *Anesth Analg.* 1995;80(2):430–431.

Yukioka H, Yoshimoto N, Nishimura K, Fujimori M. Intravenous lidocaine as a suppressant of coughing during tracheal intubation. *Anesth Analg.* 1985;64(12):1189–2292.

10

ALWAYS TROUBLESHOOT AN INCREASE IN PEAK AIRWAY PRESSURE

ADAM D. NIESEN, MD AND JURAJ SPRUNG, MD, PhD

Occasionally, the anesthesiologist needs to troubleshoot elevated peak airway pressure in an intubated patient. Although each patient has a different baseline peak airway pressure, the anesthesiologist must investigate possible causes of a sudden increase in ventilating pressure. For the most part, these pressure increases can be attributed to problems related to the patient, to airway/ventilation equipment, or even to positioning of surgical staff and equipment.

CONSEQUENCES OF ELEVATED VENTILATORY PRESSURE

Any sudden increase in peak airway pressures requires immediate attention. Barotrauma (trauma resulting from high peak pressure) or volutrauma (trauma to the lungs resulting from overstretched alveoli caused by increased tidal volume) can result from prolonged positive-pressure ventilation at high pressures and/or unrestricted lung expansions. Overstretch of alveoli may cause disruption of the alveolar–capillary membrane, thereby causing an increase in pulmonary vascular permeability and pulmonary edema. High peak inspiratory pressure (PIP) may also cause pneumothorax and pneumomediastinum. As a consequence, an acute respiratory distress syndrome–like picture, referred to as ventilator-induced lung injury, may develop. To prevent ventilator-induced lung injury, excessive PIP should be avoided and alveolar plateau pressures should be maintained below 30 cm H_2O.

In addition to injuring lungs, high airway pressures may also affect hemodynamics. If excessive positive end-expiratory pressure (PEEP) is used, or if auto-PEEP is generated by breath stacking, cardiac output may be adversely affected through increase in intrathoracic pressure, which can impede venous return to the right ventricle. In addition, compression of pulmonary vessels may increase right ventricular afterload, which in turn decreases right ventricular stroke volume and causes right ventricular dilatation. This subsequently shifts the interventricular septum toward the left ventricle, further reducing left ventricular preload and stroke volume. If breath stacking is prolonged and severe, cardiovascular collapse may ensue, appearing as pulseless electrical activity.

Airway/Ventilation Equipment Problems

One of the most important strategies in preventing high airway pressure–induced lung injury is to thoroughly check the anesthesia machine and breathing circuit system (including inspiratory and expiratory valves) before each use. In this way, mechanical problems can be remedied early. However, the fact that the machine was checked does not rule it out as the source of a sudden problem. Some examples include a suddenly stuck manual PEEP valve, a PEEP valve placed incorrectly into the inspiratory limb of the breathing circuit (this rarely happens because contemporary anesthesia machines have a built-in PEEP valve), a stuck expiratory valve causing breath stacking, or a faulty pressure-relief (pop-off) valve during spontaneous breathing. Other causes of high circuit pressures have been described, such as malfunctioning of ventilator relief and control valves, scavenger system blockage, or occlusion of the muffler on the ventilator. Any of these can result in elevated peak airway pressures and should be considered in determining the underlying cause of elevated pressures in the breathing circuit.

After initiation of mechanical ventilation, the pop-off valve should be set to the "open" position. With resumption of spontaneous breathing at the end of the case, if this valve were closed and this remained unnoticed, high pressure (50 to 60 mm Hg) could develop in the breathing circuit and in the patient's lungs. This high pressure can be further aggravated by flushing bypass oxygen into the system. The same applies when, after the circuit has been disconnected and then reconnected to a tracheal tube, in order to fill the ventilator bellows, an anesthesiologist pushes the oxygen bypass button simultaneously with mechanical inspiration. During this maneuver, all gas delivered to the circuit is directed toward the patient's lungs, potentially causing barotrauma.

Patient-Related Problems

One of the most clinically apparent causes of increased peak airway pressures in the practice of anesthesia is the patient coughing or bucking during light anesthesia. This is often resolved simply by increasing the depth of anesthesia by increasing inspiratory concentration of inhaled anesthetic, or administration of intravenous (IV) anesthetic (e.g., propofol, lidocaine) or IV opioid.

Bronchospasm is a frequent cause of increased PIP. Auscultation of the lung fields can confirm this diagnosis if expiratory wheezes are present. Extreme cases of bronchospasm may be associated with no wheezing because air may not be moving. Bronchospasm can also be a part of intraoperative allergic reactions (anaphylactic or anaphylactoid reactions), but rash, tachycardia, and hypotension frequently will be associated. Treatment with albuterol, epinephrine, or diphenhydramine, deepening of inhalational anesthesia, and discontinuing or avoiding the offending agent can help relieve this type of bronchospasm. Reviewing the patient's allergies and avoiding those drugs and other similar compounds is the easiest way to prevent such anaphylactic reactions.

Wheezing. Intraoperative wheezing with high PIP can also be caused by endotracheal tube narrowing (tube kinking, the patient biting the tube, over-inflation of the tube cuff causing occlusion of the lumen) or increased airway secretions. Even a dislodged nasal turbinate has been described to occlude the endotracheal tube, causing inability to ventilate the lungs. Passing a flexible suction catheter through the endotracheal tube can help confirm patency and, in the case of secretions, can help remedy the problem. However, direct visualization with a fiber-optic bronchoscope is the "gold standard" for determining the definitive cause of endotracheal tube obstruction. Secretions distal in the tracheobronchial tree or foreign-body aspiration can produce similar signs and are unlikely to be identified by the suction catheter test, requiring further exploration with fiber-optic bronchoscopy or possibly chest radiography in the case of a foreign body. External compression of the airway by surgical equipment or personnel also can cause an acute increase in PIP, and if recognized, can be easily remedied by communicating the problem and possible solutions to the surgical staff.

Positioning. When a patient is placed in a steep Trendelenburg position, increased peak airway pressures may be encountered, especially if the patient is morbidly obese. This position causes the abdominal contents and overlying chest structures (large breast) to shift in the cranial direction. In that case, an endotracheal tube placed in the distal part of the trachea may move farther toward the carina tracheae and may even result in endobronchial intubation. This may result in increased peak airway pressure; however, a sudden decrease in end-tidal CO_2 concentration on capnography may be suggestive of endobronchial migration of the tracheal tube. Furthermore, endobronchial intubation can be detected by auscultation for bilateral breath sounds—if they are absent, withdrawing the endotracheal tube is mandatory. The anesthesiologist should always observe the tracheal tube depth markings (labeled in centimeters) to prevent accidental tracheal extubation, which in a patient with a difficult airway can be particularly catastrophic.

Decreased Pulmonary and Chest Wall Compliance. A gradual decrease in pulmonary compliance with an increase in PIP during massive fluid administrations may be indicative of pulmonary edema. Furthermore, continuous monotonous ventilation without PEEP may result in gradual atelectasis, which will increase overall stiffness of the lungs. Occasional intraoperative performance of the vital capacity (recruitment) maneuver may be therapeutic. Rarely, decreased chest wall compliance can be encountered with use of opioids. Centrally mediated muscle contraction can be seen usually after quick and large boluses of opioids, particularly fentanyl, sufentanil, and alfentanil. Chest wall rigidity caused by opioids can be severe enough to impede ventilation. Fortunately, treatment with neuromuscular blockade is an effective method for reversing chest wall rigidity and allowing adequate ventilation. A similar situation with decreased chest wall compliance may occur if additional force is applied to the chest (e.g., surgical equipment, surgical staff leaning on chest).

Acute Decreases in Lung Parenchymal Volume. Anything that increases the intraabdominal volume (e.g., insufflation of the abdomen for laparoscopic surgery, ascites, abdominal packing) may also elevate PIP. Similarly, compression of the lung parenchyma by pleural effusion or tension pneumothorax can affect airway pressures. Evacuation of pleural fluid by needle aspiration is helpful but should be done before anesthesia and mechanical ventilation; even then, signs of pneumothorax must be excluded before mechanical ventilation is initiated. In the case of pneumothorax, even a simple pneumothorax can become a tension pneumothorax when positive-pressure ventilation is used. If a tension pneumothorax is suspected intraoperatively, immediate needle decompression is indicated. This is performed by inserting a 14-gauge over-the-needle catheter into the second intercostal space at the midclavicular line on the affected side. This will convert a tension pneumothorax to an open pneumothorax, buying time until a chest tube can be placed.

CONCLUSION

Every anesthesiologist must be able to quickly troubleshoot increased ventilatory pressure during anesthesia. Ignoring it may result in severe consequences and induce serious injury to the patient's lungs.

TAKE HOME POINTS

- A sudden increase in peak airway pressure requires immediate investigation.
- Barotrauma or volutrauma can lead to ventilator-induced lung injury.
- High airway pressures can also affect hemodynamics, including increases in thoracic pressures, compression of pulmonary vasculature, and a decrease in biventricular output.
- A thorough machine check-out does not eliminate the possibility of an intraoperative machine failure as the cause of high airway pressures.
- Consider patient-related problems as well, including bronchospasm, decreases in lung compliance, and acute decreases in lung volume.
- Fiber-optic bronchoscopy is the gold standard to rule out an obstruction of the endotracheal tube as a source of increased airway pressures.

SUGGESTED READINGS

Moon RE, Camporesi EM. Respiratory monitoring. In: Miller RD. *Miller's Anesthesia*. 6th ed. Vol 1. Philadelphia: Elsevier Churchill Livingstone; 2005;1437–1481.

Morgan GE Jr, Mikhail MS, Murray MJ. *Clinical Anesthesiology*. 3rd ed. New York: Lange Medical Books/McGraw-Hill Medical Publishing Division; 2002;40–58, 951–954.

Myles PS, Madder H, Morgan EB. Intraoperative cardiac arrest after unrecognized dynamic hyperinflation. *Br J Anaesth*. 1995;74:340–342.

Sethi JM, Siegel MD. Mechanical ventilation in chronic obstructive lung disease. *Clin Chest Med*. 2000;21:799–818.

11

AVOID COMMON AIRWAY AND VENTILATION ERRORS IN MORBIDLY OBESE PATIENTS

FRANCIS X. WHALEN, JR, MD AND
JURAJ SPRUNG, MD, PHD

Over the past 20 years, the incidence of obesity has increased significantly in both adults and children. Obesity is defined as a body mass index (BMI) of 30 kg/m^2 or greater. The latest data from the U.S. National Center for Health Statistics show that 32% of adults aged 20 years and older—more than 60 million people—are obese, up from 22% in the 1988–1994 data. This increase is not limited to adults; the percentage of young people who are overweight has more than tripled since 1980.

For the anesthesiologist, this means that greater numbers of morbidly obese patients will require care. Concerns with regard to morbid obesity include:

- Airway and ventilatory management
- Drug dosing
- Injuries related to positioning
- Coronary artery disease, hypertension, pulmonary hypertension, and cor pulmonale
- Glucose control, hyperlipidemia
- Increased incidence of various postoperative complications
- Sleep-disordered breathing (central or obstructive sleep apnea).

This chapter focuses on airway management and ventilatory issues in morbidly obese patients, although morbid obesity affects virtually every organ system.

Several studies have compared the difficulties in intubating the trachea in morbidly obese and normal-weight patients. Intubation is more difficult in morbidly obese persons, although BMI alone has not been shown to be an independent predictor of difficult intubation. Neck circumference and Mallampati score have been shown to be more accurate indicators of a difficult airway: neck circumference of 40 cm was associated with a 5% incidence of a difficult airway, and a 60-cm circumference was associated with a 35% incidence of difficulty.

Morbidly obese patients have a lower functional residual capacity, larger alveolar-to-arterial oxygen gradient, and a higher tendency for hypoventilation during sedation; all these factors make them more prone to oxyhemoglobin desaturation during tracheal intubation. Positioning of morbidly obese patients in the reverse Trendelenburg position has been shown to allow a longer period of apnea without oxyhemoglobin desaturation, as well as lower respiratory system compliance once mechanical ventilation has resumed. Therefore, the reverse Trendelenburg position may give the operator more time for airway management and also may reduce the incidence of pulmonary aspiration.

ESTABLISHING THE AIRWAY

In morbidly obese patients with a high Mallampati score or large neck circumference, awake fiber-optic intubation should be considered a first-choice technique for tracheal intubation. Other possibilities include performing the tracheal intubation with rigid intubating devices designed for a "difficult airway," such as a Glidescope, Bullard laryngoscope, or Wuscope. After being sedated, morbidly obese patients, especially those with sleep apnea, are prone to upper-airway collapse, which thus contributes to increased resistance and obstructive apnea. This situation may convert an elective airway to an emergency procedure. Spontaneous breathing will provide oxygenation and the airway will open to a greater degree, thus providing a better view. Therefore, all attempts should be made to preserve spontaneous ventilation during management of a difficult airway. Alternative airway management, such as translaryngeal illumination with a lighted stylette (e.g., Lightwand), may not be effective in these patients because of increased soft tissue over the anterior neck or redundant tissue in the posterior pharynx.

If endotracheal intubation is difficult and/or mask ventilation is suboptimal, alternative strategies must be available. A laryngeal mask airway (LMA), intubating LMA, or Combitube can be used to establish ventilation and maintain oxygenation. Cricothyroidotomy or tracheostomy are the last options, although these can be difficult in obese patients because of lack of recognizable landmarks and excessive tissue. Some reports have noted using ultrasonography-guided placement of a tracheostomy in morbidly obese patients.

Use of the LMA in morbidly obese patients is plagued by the fear of gastric aspiration. However, no reports have noted increased pulmonary aspiration of gastric contents in obese patients, and contrary to popular belief, retrieval of gastric contents in these patients revealed low residuals. When placed electively after induction of anesthesia in morbidly obese patients, the LMA is an effective airway tool. The intubating LMA has been used effectively in obese patients with a difficult airway. This device provides adequate ventilation, creates additional time for airway management, and assists in placement of an endotracheal tube.

ASSOCIATED PROBLEMS

Sleep-disordered breathing is associated with morbid obesity; however, the vast majority of these patients are not diagnosed before the perioperative period. Additional predictors for obstructive sleep apnea include neck circumference in men and BMI in women. Patients with obstructive sleep apnea are more sensitive to respiratory depression from anesthetics and sedatives. They are at increased risk of airway obstruction or apnea postoperatively, which may precipitate a situation that requires urgent establishment of an airway. Timely intervention with noninvasive ventilation in these patients in a monitored setting may be life-saving. Specifically, if the patient has a prescribed level of continuous or biphasic positive airway pressure preoperatively, these treatments should be initiated immediately postoperatively.

VENTILATION AFTER THE AIRWAY IS ESTABLISHED

Morbidly obese patients have lower functional residual capacity when supine, which leads to an increased alveolar-to-arterial oxygen gradient and may contribute to faster development of hypoxemia. A ventilation strategy that uses a larger tidal volume will not improve oxygenation, and data are emerging that high tidal volumes may actually worsen postoperative outcome as a result of lung injury. Isolated effects of positive end-expiratory pressure (PEEP) of 10 cm H_2O used intraoperatively only modestly improve oxygenation in morbidly obese anesthetized patients. During induction of anesthesia, the application of 10 cm PEEP has been shown to decrease atelectasis and improve PaO_2 in morbidly obese patients. Preoxygenation with an FIO_2 of 60% versus 100% may be advantageous because it does not contribute to the development of postinduction (absorption) atelectasis.

TAKE HOME POINTS

- Tracheal intubation may be more difficult in morbidly obese patients. Therefore, careful assessment of the airway, precise management, and development of alternative intubating strategies are mandatory.
- These patients are at higher risk for airway compromise because of obstructive sleep apnea; therefore, sedation should be gradual, and spontaneous breathing must be maintained.
- When establishing a difficult airway in a morbidly obese patient, awake fiber-optic intubation is the technique of choice because it decreases the risk of a "lost airway."
- Appropriate positioning in the reverse Trendelenburg position with a wedge placed below the shoulders and maximal "sniffing position" will facilitate control of the airway.
- Finally, full readiness with alternative intubating devices will help in avoiding potential disasters.

SUGGESTED READINGS

Boyce JR, Ness T, Castroman P, et al. A preliminary study of the optimal anesthesia positioning for the morbidly obese patient. *Obes Surg.* 2003;13:4–9.

Brodsky JB, Lemmens HJ, Brock-Utne JG, et al. Morbid obesity and tracheal intubation. *Anesth Analg.* 2002;94:732–736.

Centers for Disease Control and Prevention [homepage on the Internet]. Overweight and obesity: home [updated 2006 March 22, cited 2006 May 9]. Available from: www.cdc.gov/nccdphp/dnpa/obesity.

Coussa M, Proietti S, Schnyder P, et al. Prevention of atelectasis formation during the induction of general anesthesia in morbidly obese patients. *Anesth Analg.* 2004;98:1491–1495.

Frappier J, Guenoun T, Journois D, et al. Airway management using the intubating laryngeal mask airway for the morbidly obese patient. *Anesth Analg.* 2003;96:1510–1515.

Juvin P, Lavaut E, Dupont H, et al. Difficult tracheal intubation is more common in obese than in lean patients. *Anesth Analg.* 2003;97:595–600.

Keller C, Brimacombe J, Kleinsasser A, et al. The Laryngeal Mask Airway ProSeal[TM] as a temporary ventilatory device in grossly and morbidly obese patients before laryngoscope-guided tracheal intubation. *Anesth Analg.* 2002;94:737–740.

Pelosi P, Ravagnan I, Giurati G, et al. Positive end-expiratory pressure improves respiratory function in obese but not in normal subjects during anesthesia and paralysis. *Anesthesiology.* 1999;91:1221–1231.

Sprung J, Whalley DG, Falcone T, et al. The effects of tidal volume and respiratory rate on oxygenation and respiratory mechanics during laparoscopy in morbidly obese patients. *Anesth Analg.* 2003;97:268–274.

Sustic A, Zupan Z, Antoncic I. Ultrasound-guided percutaneous dilatational tracheostomy with laryngeal mask airway control in a morbidly obese patient. *J Clin Anesth.* 2004;16:121–123.

12

PLAN FOR AN AIRWAY FIRE WITH EVERY HEAD AND NECK CASE

JULIE MARSHALL, MD

A 67-year-old woman with a history of chronic obstructive pulmonary disease (COPD) with a home oxygen requirement of 3 L/min by nasal cannula and coronary artery disease was admitted to the burn unit. She had been involved in a house fire after falling asleep while smoking and dropping her cigarette. She sustained an inhalation injury and was intubated in the intensive care unit (ICU) for 2 weeks before coming to the operating room (OR) for a tracheostomy. The procedure was done using the in situ *polyvinyl chloride endotracheal tube. During the procedure, you had trouble maintaining her blood pressure under anesthesia and were reluctant to use pressors due to recent skin grafts. Because she was tolerating only about 0.6% isoflurane and not much midazolam, you added 20% nitrous oxide to her inspired oxygen. Unfortunately, she suffered desaturation of her SpO₂ and ST segment changes with attempts to further lower the FiO₂. As the airway was entered with electrocautery at the tracheostomy site, a flame was noted that flashed from the tracheostomy. What might have been done to decrease this risk? Now that a fire has occurred, what should be done?*

One of the primary responsibilities of the anesthesia provider is the management of the airway, including anticipating the airway problems that may arise during surgery. Airway fires are complications that are both dramatic and critical when they occur. Selecting an anesthetic plan that decreases the risk of fire is one of the first priorities in airway management. If an airway fire does occur, an anesthesia provider must know what to do to minimize harm to the patient.

The risk of fire occurs whenever the fire triad is present. The fire triad consists of an ignition source, fuel, and oxidizer. It must be recognized that these elements are nearly always present in the OR! During head and neck surgery, these elements are not only present but in close proximity. The oxidizer, oxygen or nitrous oxide, is provided by the anesthesiologist through the endotracheal tube into the surgical site. The ignition source is provided by the surgeon, usually in the form of an electrocautery device or laser. The fuel in airway fires may be the endotracheal tube, packing in the airway, and necrotic or charred tissue. If an endotracheal tube is ignited in a patient,

---

© 2006 Mayo Foundation for Medical Education and Research

the flow of gas through the tube can create a "blowtorch"-type flame that can injure more distal structures. Fires that occur at tracheostomy sites as the airway is entered have been reported to cause more local injury and flames that enter the OR environment instead of the distal lungs. Oral and pharyngeal procedures performed in children with uncuffed tubes may result in airway fire because of the leak of oxygen-rich gas into the site on surgery.

The endotracheal tube is the fuel source that is most consistently present in the airway. It has been shown that red rubber, polyvinyl chloride, and silicone endotracheal tubes are all flammable at <26% oxygen. To decrease the risk of combustion, anesthesiologists historically wrapped the endotracheal tubes in metal tape. This practice is not often used today because the tape may loosen, thereby exposing areas of the tubing, it does not cover the cuff, and the tubes may kink easily. Commercially available "laser-resistant" tubes are flexible metal tubes that are more resistant to combustion and may be a better choice for airway surgery. However, these tubes are more bulky and may be more difficult to place. The cuff of the endotracheal tube may be filled with methylene blue; in the event of a cuff perforation, the color change will notify the surgeon. The necessity for an endotracheal tube should be discussed with the surgeon as well. Some procedures may be done with intermittent apnea, although this may require a higher FiO_2 during episodes of ventilation.

Common procedures that carry a high risk of airway fire include tracheostomy, tonsillectomy, adenoidectomy, airway tumor debulking, oral surgery, and tracheal reconstructions. Because it is inevitable that the fire triad will be present and in close proximity during ENT procedures, steps must be taken to minimize the risk.

The surgeon must be in communication with the anesthesiologist about the surgical plan including any planned airway or intraoral procedures. If there is a portion of the surgery that precedes the high-risk portion of the case, the anesthesia provider should be notified as the airway portion approaches so that adjustment may be made to lower the FiO_2 if needed.

Minimizing the FiO_2 is one of the trickiest aspects of managing the fire triad, even for experienced anesthesia providers. It is especially difficult in patients who have poor lung function or tenuous cardiovascular status. The risk of using a higher FiO_2 must always be weighed against the risk of fire and the alternative options available to the surgeon. Remember that both oxygen and nitrous oxide are flammable to equal degrees, so a mixture of a low oxygen flow with air may be a safer option. If there is difficulty in maintaining the patient at a low FiO_2, the surgeon must be notified so that he or she can use non–heat-generating surgical tools (scalpel instead of electrocautery) or modify the surgical plan. Also, during intraoral or pharyngeal procedures, wet packing may be placed to decrease the leakage of oxygen-rich gas into the surgical site. Care must be taken that these stay moist, because dry packing will act as an additional source for ignition.

If an airway fire occurs, because of poor planning or in spite of good planning, care must be taken to prevent further harm. The oxidizer should be removed by stopping ventilation. The endotracheal tube is removed to remove the source of fuel and prevent further thermal burns. The patient should be ventilated and reintubated. After the patient has stabilized, the extent of damage should be determined with bronchoscopy and any additional relevant workup or treatment (arterial blood gas (ABG), steroids, tracheotomy) considered immediately. The management should be tailored to the specific clinical situation.

So what could have been done differently for the patient above, who sustained an airway fire during tracheostomy? Changing the polyvinyl tube to a metal tube would not be warranted for this procedure. Using a gas mixture of oxygen and air, instead of oxygen and nitrous oxide, would have decreased the amount of oxidizer present and should have been done. The surgeons should have been notified of the difficulty in decreasing the FiO_2 so an alternative method of entering the airway could be utilized, such as a scalpel. (*Actually*, the surgeons should have known not to use electrocautery to enter the airway in the first place, and should have been reminded by the anesthesia provider, who should have been on his or her feet, hanging over the drapes and watching every move). Once the fire occurred, the steps of disconnecting from the circuit, extubation, extinguishing the flame, ventilation, and reintubation would have been appropriate.

Finally, there have been some reports of keeping patients intubated after airway fires during tracheotomy if the fire has been extinguished. This is because of the risk of extubating patients who usually have prior lung disease, as does the patient in our example. Following stabilization, appropriate measures include bronchoscopy, ABG, chest radiography, and continuing with the tracheotomy.

TAKE HOME POINTS

- The fire triad is both present and in close proximity in the airway—develop a method to remind yourself of that for every case.
- Minimize oxidizer FiO_2 and nitrous oxide concentration.
- Minimize ignition generators—electrocautery or laser time.
- Metal tubes are harder to ignite, but all tubes can combust.
- If a fire occurs, disconnect from the circuit, extubate, extinguish the flame, ventilate, reintubate, then do diagnostic tests and treatment.

Suggested Readings

Chee WK, Benumof JL. Airway fire during tracheostomy: extubation may be contraindicated. *Anesthesiology*. 1998;89(6):1576–1578.

Ehrenwerth J, Seifert H. Electrical and fire safety. In: Barash PG, Cullen BF, Stoelting RK, eds. *Clinical Anesthesia*. 5th ed. Philadelphia: Lippincott Williams & Wilkins; 2006: 149–207.

Mattucci KF, Militana CJ. The prevention of fire during oropharyngeal electrosurgery. *Ear Nose Throat Journal*. 2003;82(2):107–109.

Rampil IJ. Anesthesia for laser surgery. In: Miller RD, ed. *Miller's Anesthesia*. 6th ed. Philadelphia: Elsevier Churchhill Livingstone; 2005:2573–2587.

13

KNOW HOW TO PERFORM A CRICOTHYROIDOTOMY

LISA MARCUCCI, MD AND HILARY KOPROWSKI, II, MD

Although instances when management of an airway has progressed down the algorithm to the need for an emergency surgical airway are fortunately rare, it is sometimes necessary to perform this procedure to gain control of the airway. In the past, there was most likely "a surgeon within earshot," but with the advent of more restricted residency work hours and the need to do more cases to generate the same billing income, surgeons are "spread more thinly" than in the past.

A cricothyroidotomy is a variant approach to tracheostomy and is considered by surgeons to be the preferred technique for initial emergent surgical airway management. The cricothyroid membrane is generally easy to locate and is fairly avascular. Because cricoid cartilage chondritis with the unfortunate sequelae of subglottic stenosis can develop after cricothyroidotomy, revision to a conventional tracheostomy, usually at the second or third tracheal ring (which involves exposing and separating the strap muscles and dividing the thyroid isthmus) is generally performed within 24 hours.

The most important step in performing a cricothyroidotomy successfully is making the decision to do one. The second most important step is remaining calm; it is the authors' opinion that most anesthesiologists have the technical skills necessary to facilitate an "emergency surgical airway" via cricothyroidotomy.

The steps used by general surgeons in performing emergent cricothyroidotomy are as follows.

1) Position yourself on the side of the bed where your dominant hand is cephalad (i.e., if you are right-handed you will be standing by the patient's left shoulder).

2) Do not prep the neck—this is an emergency procedure and seconds count.

3) Palpate the cricoid membrane—this lies above the cricoid cartilage and below the thyroid cartilage. It is the exact location where transtracheal lidocaine is injected for anesthesia for an awake airway technique.

4) Ask for a no. 10 blade.

5) With your dominant hand moving from *foot to head*, use the belly of the blade to make a *longitudinal* incision in the midline 4 cm long superficial to the cricoid membrane.

© 2006 Mayo Foundation for Medical Education and Research

6) Take care to stay in the midline. Large anterior thyroid veins run on either side of the midline and can cause bleeding sufficient to completely obscure the field.

7) Do not be stingy on the length of the incision. A long incision allows the tissues to "gap open" and will make visualization of the trachea easier.

8) Apply enough pressure to the blade to reach the level of the cricoid membrane with two passes.

9) If the person is obese, ask for instruments to retract the tissue. You will need two (one for each side). Army–Navy, thyroid rectors, or vein retractors are all acceptable choices.

10) Once at the cartilage level, palpate again for the cricoid membrane.

11) When the cricoid membrane is located, use the no. 10 blade to "poke through" the cricoid cartilage.

12) You will know you are in the airway when there is "sputtering and splashing." Take care not to have your face too close to the operative field when performing this step so as not to have a splash exposure.

13) Without removing the blade, turn it 180 degrees several times to widen the opening.

14) Still without removing the blade, move it from your dominant hand to your nondominant hand and retract the lower edge of the incision you have just made toward the feet with the side of the blade. Do not take the blade out of the airway at any time before the endotracheal tube is placed. The incision will "close shut" and you will have difficulty relocating the site where you entered the airway.

15) With your now free dominant hand, take a 6.0 cuffed styletted endotracheal tube; have an assistant bend the tip to an approximate angle of 75 to 90 degrees.

16) Insert the tube with a curving motion.

17) Remove the stylet and check for good air flow and return of CO_2 per standard anesthesia protocol.

18) Do not let go of the tube until it has been sewn into place. Securing the tube and closing the incision is probably best done by your hopefully soon to be arriving surgical colleagues.

19) If at any stage bleeding is experienced, do not use cautery. This risks igniting the surrounding oxygen and putting the patient and staff at extreme risk.

20) Do not be concerned about the esthetics of the incision or where the tube actually entered the airway or the comments of colleagues. Remember, there is almost no incision that a plastic surgeon cannot revise and almost no tracheal or laryngeal injury that an otolaryngologist cannot repair. Your colleagues will undoubtedly be polite as they know that an anesthesiologist performing a cricothyroidotomy is the very definition of an emergency situation.

14

DO NOT OVERINFLATE THE CUFF OF THE ENDOTRACHEAL TUBE

J. TODD HOBELMANN, MD

You are supervising a junior resident for the first time and are proceeding nicely through the start of a femoral-dorsal pedis bypass. You are helping your CA-1 place an arterial line when two senior anesthesiologists make a surprise visit to your room. You have a slight sinking feeling when you notice that one of them is holding a small manometer. He applies it to the balloon of the endotracheal tube (ETT) and you find that the measured pressure in the cuff of the ETT is 65 cm H_2O. This particular colleague happens to have a PhD in biomedical engineering (and the other person has an interest in tracheal injuries), so you know that there is not even a chance of arguing about it. You have been busted by the cuff police.

The cuff of an endotracheal tube is an essential piece of modern anesthesia. It serves as a seal of the airway—decreasing the likelihood of aspirating pharyngeal secretions into the trachea and lungs (debatable) and allowing adequate positive-pressure ventilation. It also serves to anchor the ETT in place, thus allowing position changes during surgery with less risk of mainstem intubation or inadvertent extubation. Traditionally, we learn in anesthesiology that the cuff pressures of the ETT should be within the range of 20 to 30 cm H_2O. Although these numbers are very strict in pediatric anesthesia (and a component of every pediatric anesthesiology text), cuff pressure in adults is of key importance as well.

The pediatric airway differs in many ways from that of an adult. One of the key differences is the location of the narrowest portion of the airway. Remember that the adult airway is cylindrical-shaped, with the tightest area being between the vocal cords or glottis. However, in neonates, infants, and young children, the airway is more funnel-shaped and becomes tightest at the level just below the glottic aperture (the subglottis). Because the pediatric subglottic region can be very narrow, anesthesiologists often do not use cuffed ETTs unless the patient is around age 8 to 10 years or older. In many circumstances, without a cuff, the diameter of the ETT itself may often be too wide for the airway, even when it passes easily beyond the cords. It is not uncommon in pediatric cases that the anesthesiologist changes to a smaller ETT for this reason. Above 30 cm H_2O, the pressure exerted by the tube on the subglottis for a prolonged operation may cause mucosal ischemia,

© 2006 Mayo Foundation for Medical Education and Research

resulting in sloughing of the mucosal lining and potentially resulting in subglottic stenosis or worse.

With modern single-lumen ETTs (those that are low-pressure, high-volume), catastrophic consequences are relatively rare in the operating room, especially for adult cases. With older ETTs (high-pressure, low-volume), overinflation of the cuff could result in severe morbidity such as rupture of the trachea, tracheal–innominate artery fistulas, and tracheo–carotid artery erosions. Luckily, the biggest complication of having an ETT inflated in the airway during modern anesthesia is postoperative sore throat. Nonetheless, animal data imply that overinflation of modern ETT cuffs may result in serious ciliary damage and reduced tracheal blood flow (more severe in hypotensive states).

Of note, another operating room population of concern with respect to ETT cuff pressure is patients undergoing thoracic cases involving lung isolation with a double-lumen ETT. The cuff on the bronchial lumen can easily be overinflated and result in bronchial edema and stenosis (as this cuff is often of lower volume and higher pressure than the standard tracheal cuff). Proper practice requires the provider inflate this cuff with only the minimal pressure required to offer adequate lung isolation. Once isolation is no longer required, the cuff should be deflated.

It has long been known that there are limited ways of detecting true cuff pressure in the operating room during adult cases. Previous studies have demonstrated that manual palpation of the cuff generally underestimated cuff pressure. A well-performed study from 2004 suggested the use of manometry in gathering accurate data regarding ETT cuff pressure. This suggestion may be taken under stronger consideration in the intensive care unit (ICU) setting, where patients remain intubated for prolonged periods of time. However, utilization of manometry could well be warranted for longer cases, such as transplants, and cardiac and neurosurgery. This has not gained wide acceptance in clinical practice at this time.

TAKE HOME POINTS

- ETT cuff pressure has implications in anesthesia.
- ETT cuff pressure is of vital importance in the pediatric population to avoid serious airway consequences.
- Maximum cuff pressure should not exceed 20 to 30 cm H_2O.
- Be especially careful not to overinflate the blue cuff on the bronchial side of a double-lumen tube.
- After intubation, inflate the cuff just enough to prevent an air leak.
- Manual palpation of the balloon is not reliable in determining cuff pressures.

SUGGESTED READINGS

Braz JR, Navarro LH, Takata IH, et al. Endotracheal tube cuff pressure: need for precise measurement. *Sao Paulo Med J.* 1999;117:243–247.

Curiel Garcia JA, Guerrero-Romero F, Rodriguez-Moran M l. Cuff pressure in endotracheal intubation: should it be routinely measured? *Gac Med Mex.* 2001;137:179–182.

Fernandez R, Blanch L, Mancebo J, et al. Endotracheal tube cuff pressure assessment: pitfalls of finger estimation and need for objective measurement. *Crit Care Med.* 1990;18:1423–1426.

Gottschalk A, Burmeister MA, Blanc I, et al. Rupture of the trachea after emergency endotracheal intubation. *Anasthesiol Intensivmed Notfallmed Schmerzther.* 2003;38:59–61.

Sengupta P, Sessler DI, Maglinger P, et al. Endotracheal tube cuff pressure in three hospitals, and the volume required to produce appropriate cuff pressure. *BMC Anesthesiology.* 2004;4:8.

15

DON'T UNDERREPRESENT THE RISKS ASSOCIATED WITH THE USE OF A LARYNGEAL MASK AIRWAY

SURJYA SEN, MD

A 57-year-old, otherwise healthy professional concert singer presents for an elective outpatient prostate biopsy for suspected adenocarcinoma. He has a healthy body mass index (BMI), and physical exam indicates that he would be a grade 1 intubation. He reports that 10 years ago he experienced hoarseness and prolonged throat and mouth pain after intubation for an emergency appendectomy. He concludes this bit of history by volunteering, "I almost sued the guy that jammed that tube down my throat; I couldn't do my concert dates for two months." He had surgery for a meningomyocele as an infant (wouldn't you just know), so a spinal is out. He inquires whether there are any other options. When you suggest a laryngeal mask airway, he replies, "Well, that sounds great, Doc, but are there any drawbacks to having anesthesia with this 'ellemae' thing?"

In 1983, Dr. Archie Brain introduced the laryngeal mask airway (LMA) as a device to secure the airway without the use of direct laryngoscopy. By 1988 the LMA became commercially available worldwide, and by 1991 the U.S. Food and Drug Administration had approved its use in the United States. Soon thereafter, the device gained rapid popularity because of its advantages over other options for airway control—namely, direct laryngoscopy with endotracheal intubation or bag-mask ventilation (*Table 15.1*). These days, the LMA is an essential piece of equipment on every emergency airway cart and has become nearly ubiquitous in outpatient anesthesia. Despite its many advantages, however, the use of an LMA does carry a small but significant set of risks. Every anesthesia provider should be familiar with these risks—not only to recognize potential complications if they occur, but also to counsel patients properly when requesting informed consent.

DISADVANTAGES AND COMPLICATIONS

LMA Misplacement. The first requirement to placing an LMA successfully is proper positioning. Problems such as a folded tip, supraglottal placement, and an improper seal over the upper esophagus can usually all be resolved with repositioning. Just as with endotracheal intubation, verification of proper LMA placement immediately after insertion is imperative.

ⓒ 2006 Mayo Foundation for Medical Education and Research

TABLE 15.1 SOME ADVANTAGES OF THE LMA

- Use in an ACLS algorithm for difficult airway.
- Use in the absence of trained personnel to perform tracheal intubation or surgical airway.
- Use when direct laryngoscopy equipment malfunctions.
- Use in reactive airway disease when endotracheal intubation may be overstimulating.
- Less intraocular pressure increases when compared to endotracheal intubation.
- Less local trauma and better hemodynamic stability during insertion than with direct laryngoscopy and endotracheal intubation.
- Less incidence of "sore throat" and "hoarse voice" when compared to endotracheal intubation.
- Less gastric insufflation when compared to face-mask ventilation.
- Better air-tight seal, less hand fatigue, and more stability than a face mask.
- Less manipulation of the patient's head, neck, and jaw.

End-tidal capnography, bilateral breath sounds, and auscultating over the laryngopharynx for evidence of leaks should be essential parts of a preliminary check after initial positioning. The placement should be periodically verified throughout the case and after any repositioning of the patient.

Mucosal Injury and Sore Throat. With a mean incidence of approximately 10%, mucosal injury is usually recognized by blood on the LMA after removal. The main causes are usually cuff pressure on the pharyngeal mucosa (though cuff pressures are typically less than that required for mucosal perfusion) and manipulation during insertion. Sore throats are more common, with a mean incidence of 18%, but are still less common than are typically seen with endotracheal intubation.

Gastric Inflation. Though certainly not as effective as an endotracheal tube in preventing gastric inflation, the LMA is superior to mask ventilation. The risk of gastric inflation is usually present because most patients may require some assisted ventilations during the anesthetic. Adherence to strict nothing-by-mouth (NPO) guidelines and careful patient selection (i.e., not using an LMA electively in patients with severe reflux or in patients who are obese) can help minimize the risks of regurgitation and aspiration that can come with overinflation of the stomach. It is worthwhile noting that the Proseal brand of LMA has a separate esophageal drainage tube that can help reduce the risk of gastric inflation and subsequent regurgitation.

Regurgitation and Aspiration. In an elective situation, if there is any definable preoperative risk of regurgitation or aspiration in a patient, the anesthesia provider should not chose an LMA. Endotracheal tubes are reliably better at minimizing this risk. In cases when aspiration does occur with an LMA (incidence rates are reported at approximately 0.02%), malposition and/or gastric inflation are often the cause. In a review of the literature, Keller et al.

found several other factors that may increase the risk: *inadequate depth of anesthesia, intra-abdominal surgery, upper gastrointestinal disease, lithotomy position, patient movement, exchanging the LMA for an endotracheal tube, multiple insertion attempts, opioids, diabetes with gastroparesis, obesity, and cuff deflation.* Catastrophic outcomes including brain injury and death have also been reported.

Hyperinflation of Cuff. Multiple studies have demonstrated that LMA cuff pressures increase over the course of an operation when nitrous oxide is used. The increase in cuff pressures correlated directly with the length of the procedures (as high as 42 mm Hg in procedures that lasted from 2 to 5 hours). Cuffs that were constructed from polyvinyl chloride (PVC) seemed less susceptible to hyperinflation. The clinical correlate to these increased pressures is not clear (though some authors have reported cases of nerve injuries thought to be related to high pressures), but anesthesia providers will be well advised to check the inflation pressures of the LMA cuff periodically over the course of a long procedure when nitrous oxide is being used.

Nerve Injury. Various nerve injuries have been reported with the use of an LMA. Injuries to the recurrent laryngeal, superior laryngeal, hypoglossal, and lingual nerves have all been reported. Implicated causes have ranged from high cuff pressures to malpositioning. Most are reported to have resolved within 6 months.

Mediastinitis and Retropharyngeal Abscess Formation. In a recent "case and commentary" discussion of laryngeal mask airways posted on Agency for Healthcare Research and Quality (ahrq.gov), the occurrence of mediastinitis and retropharyngeal abscess formation was reported. This complication is worth noting because systemic manifestations such as fevers and myalgias combined with "a fullness in the neck" may warrant an emergency evaluation of possible retropharyngeal perforation, abscess formation, and mediastinal involvement. Definitive therapy with antibiotics and surgical drainage were reported to be effective for the complication.

TAKE HOME POINTS

- LMAs may offer an advantage over endotracheal intubation or prolonged mask anesthesia in certain well-selected cases.
- Despite certain advantages, however, patients should be appropriately counseled regarding the associated complications that may occur.
- Never compromise the aspiration risk of a patient when selecting an LMA; endotracheal anesthesia is decidedly better.
- Beware of high cuff inflation pressures with prolonged nitrous anesthesia—nerve injuries may occur.

SUGGESTED READINGS

Brain AIJ. The laryngeal mask airway—a new concept in airway management. *Br J Anesth.* 1983;55:801–805.

Bruce IA, Ellis R, Kay NJ. Nerve injury and the laryngeal mask airway. *J Laryngol Otol.* 2004;118(11):899–901.

Cook TM, Lee G, Nolan JP. The Proseal™ laryngeal mask airway: a review of the literature. *Can J Anesth.* 2005;52(7):739–760.

Danks RR, Danks B. Laryngeal mask airway: review of indications and use. *J Emer Nursing.* 2004;30(1):30–35.

Jahr JS, Hosseini P. Web morbidity and mortality case discussion. Agency for Healthcare Research and Quality. www.webmm.ahrq.gov/case.aspx?caseID=139, November 2006.

Keller C, Brimacombe J, Bittersohl J, et al. Aspiration and the laryngeal mask airway: three cases and a review of the literature. *Br J Anaesth.* 2004;93(4):579–582.

Maino P, Dullenkopf A, Bernet V, Weiss M. Nitrous oxide diffusion into the cuffs of disposable laryngeal mask airways. *Aneasthiology.* 2005;60(3):278–282.

Ouellette RG. The effect of nitrous oxide on laryngeal mask cuff pressure. *AANA J.* 2000;68(5): 411–414.

Trevisanuto D, Micaglio M, Ferrarese P, Zanardo V. The laryngeal mask airway: potential applications in neonates. *Arch Dis Child Fetal Neonat Ed.* 2004;89(6):F485–F489.

16

DO NOT BE INTIMIDATED BY THE PLACEMENT AND USE OF DOUBLE-LUMEN ENDOTRACHEAL TUBES

JAY K. LEVIN, MD

The use of double-lumen endotracheal tubes (DLTs) is standard practice for thoracic and other surgical procedures requiring one-lung ventilation, as well as in life-threatening conditions requiring lung isolation, such as hemoptysis. Although the techniques for accurate placement and ventilation with DLTs are more complex than for placement of a standard endotracheal tube, practitioners should be no more intimidated by them than by any other (slightly advanced) airway procedure. The trick to the placement and use of a DLT is to take it step by step. Remember that appropriate caution in placing DLTs is always warranted (never force "the square peg in a round hole"), but no more than in any other area of anesthetic practice.

DLTs are designed to ventilate one lung while isolating the contralateral side. There are design differences depending on the manufacturer, but all DLTs consist of a tracheal lumen and endobronchial lumen. Sizes of DLTs vary from 26 to 41 French (one French equals 1/3 mm and is a measurement of diameter). A 39 F DLT is equivalent to a 9.5-mm-internal-diameter endotracheal tube. Choosing the "proper size" has been a topic of many investigations, including the use of chest radiographs and computerized tomography (CT) scans to measure tracheal and bronchial diameter. No one method has proven an absolute predictor of the "optimal" size of DLT or, in other words, the size DLT that results in the fewest minor and major complications for any given patient but that still functions reliably in the intraoperative period. Traumatic airway injuries are common with double-lumen endotracheal tubes, with a high incidence of hoarseness and sore throat, and presumably an oversized tube will contribute to this unnecessarily. However, undersizing a DLT could lead to distal migration and possible pneumothorax.

The typical method of placing a left DLT is to use direct laryngoscopy to pass the bronchial tip through the vocal cords, remove the stylet, and then advance the tube until the "double" portion passes through the larynx. At this point, for proper placement in the left bronchus, a "blind" or fiberoptic technique may be used. In the "blind" technique, the tracheal cuff is placed past the vocal cords, the tube is rotated counterclockwise, and the

© 2006 Mayo Foundation for Medical Education and Research

tube is advanced until it meets resistance (approximately 28 to 30 cm at the teeth). Using the fiber-optic method, the bronchial tip is placed past the vocal cords, the scope is placed through the bronchial lumen and driven into the left mainstem bronchus, and the tube is advanced over the scope into the left side.

There are advantages and disadvantages to each technique for initial placement of DLTs. The fiber-optic scope technique is favored by some senior practitioners and is often described as the technique of choice. However, a fiber-optic scope may not be available or may not be helpful in situations of significant hemorrhage or secretions, and one must rely on clinical skills for proper positioning.

The "blind" technique allows for rapid placement without the need for excess equipment other than a stethoscope for auscultation to confirm correct placement. Unfortunately, malposition requiring further manipulation has been reported as from 30% to 78%. Leaving the stylet in place for the entire "blind" placement has demonstrated improved success, although the potential risk for airway trauma may outweigh this benefit. An additional technique reported increased success by insufflating 2 mL of air into the bronchial cuff after placement, withdrawing while holding the pilot balloon until it collapsed, deflating the bronchial cuff, and advancing 1.5 cm. Proper placement occurred in 26 of 29 left-sided DLT attempts. One major disadvantage with the "blind" method beyond lower success rates is the inability to visualize anatomic problems. An example is thoracic aortic aneurysms, which can compress the left main bronchus, impairing placement and potentially leading to aneurysm rupture by "blind" DLT placement.

Left-sided double-lumen placement can be confirmed by auscultation or by fiber-optic visualization. With proper technique, clinical confirmation can be performed successfully with a stethoscope. First, inflate the tracheal cuff and listen for bilateral breath sounds. Clamp the tracheal side, open the tracheal vent, and listen for a leak on the tracheal side. Inflate the bronchial cuff until the leak disappears, usually less than 2 mL and never more than 3 mL. Isolation is confirmed by the loss of breath sounds on the tracheal side and preserved sounds on the bronchial side. Bilateral breath sounds should return after the clamp is removed and the vent is closed.

If the auscultation technique does not confirm placement, fiber-optic confirmation is warranted, if available. One should always find the right upper-lobe bronchus to confirm accurate placement in the left side. The bronchial cuff should be barely seen or, with BronchCath Mallinckrodt DLTs, a black line marks 4 cm from the distal tip of the bronchial lumen. Because the left main bronchus is longer than 5 cm in both men and women, this should provide ideal placement.

Insufflation of the bronchial cuff is an important part of final placement of the DLT. If the patient is to be placed in the lateral decubitus position, it may be best to insufflate the bronchial cuff after final positioning to prevent the DLT from being displaced as well as to avoid overinflating the cuff. There are alternative methods to auscultation to determine the minimal amount of air needed for lung isolation to prevent mucosal ischemia. While ventilating, 0.5 mL of air at a time (not to exceed 3 mL) is injected into the bronchial cuff, a bare hand or arm is placed over the bronchial vent, and the bronchial side is clamped. The leak will disappear when isolation is achieved. Another technique involves placing a nasogastric tube tip in the bronchial lumen and the other end in a bottle of saline while slowly injecting air into the cuff until bubbles are no longer apparent. *Always remember to deflate the bronchial cuff when lung isolation is no longer necessary.*

The choice of the appropriate tidal volume for one-lung ventilation (OLV) is an important area of evolving practice. Recent evidence suggests that lower lung volumes during OLV (5 mL/kg) with positive end-expiratory pressure (PEEP) during esophagectomy, a "protective ventilation strategy" similar to that used in acute lung injury (ALI) patients, resulted in decreased inflammatory response, improved lung function, and earlier extubation. In patients with obstructive lung disease, there is the possibility for auto-PEEP with larger tidal volumes (TVs) if adequate time is not allowed for exhalation. Maintaining peak pressures >40 cm H_2O and higher tidal volumes led to a higher incidence of postpneumonectomy ALI and respiratory failure. These considerations suggest that the higher traditional TVs of 9 to 12 mL/kg should be reduced during OLV.

The use of PEEP is sometimes considered controversial because of concern that capillary compression will cause shunting of blood flow away from the ventilated lung. However, given the prevalence of atelectasis contributing to hypoxemia and the body of data showing the protective role of PEEP in reducing ventilator-associated lung injury, the use of moderate PEEP (4 to 8 cm H_2O) is recommended. In general, if a manual recruitment maneuver improves oxygenation, then PEEP will help maintain that effect.

TAKE HOME POINTS

- Double-lumen endotracheal tubes provide a simple means for one-lung ventilation and lung isolation.
- The ability to properly place and confirm DLT position needs to be part of every anesthesia practitioner's repertoire.
- Seek out these cases and take the airway management one step at a time: "Number one, have we intubated the trachea? Number two, what

information do we have that the bronchial lumen is where we want it?" and then proceed down the algorithm.

- The editor recommends that junior practitioners take a try at confirming placement by auscultation before using the fiber-optic method. It is a great way to really get a sense of how the DLT will function later in the case.

- If the DLT is "not working," remember that unless you have turned the whole thing 180 degrees, it is either in too far or not in far enough. If you can't figure out which is the case, consider withdrawing the bronchial lumen into the trachea and starting over.

- Once placement has been confirmed, avoid taping it to what will be the dependent side of the face, and don't "overtape" it. Occasionally, the DLT will have to be moved several millimeters during the case, and many practitioners have had to struggle with peeling a wad of tape off the side of the patient's face that has been positioned in the foam head ring.

- With careful placement and a lung-protective strategy with lower TVs, and the use of PEEP, proper use of DLTs may provide postoperative benefits and better surgical outcomes.

SUGGESTED READINGS

Alliaume BA, Coddens J, Deloof T. Reliability of auscultation in positioning of double-lumen endobronchial tubes. *Can J Anesth*. 1992;39:687–690.

Bahk JH, Lim YJ, Kim CS. Positioning of double-lumen endobronchial tube without the aid of any instruments: an implication for emergency management. *J Trauma*. 2000;49:899–902.

Brodsky JD, Macario A, Mark JBD. Tracheal diameter predicts double lumen tube size: a method for selecting left double-lumen tubes. *Anesth Analg*. 1996;82:861–865.

Chow MYH, Liam BL, Lew TWK, et al. Predicting the size of double lumen endobronchial tube based on tracheal diameter. *Anesth Analg*. 1998;87:158–163.

Fernandez-Perez ER, Keegan MT, Brown DR, et al. Intraoperative tidal volume as a risk factor for respiratory failure after pneumonectomy. *Anesthesiology*. 2006;105:14–18.

Hannalah M, Benumof JL, Silverman PM, et al. Evaluation of an approach to choosing a left double lumen tube size based on chest computed tomographic scan measurement of left mainstem bronchial diameter. *J Cardiothoracic Vasc Anesth*. 1997;11:168–174.

Huang CC, Chou AH, Liu HP, et al. Tension pneumothorax complicated by double lumen endotracheal tube intubation. *Chang Gund Med J*. 2005;28:503–507.

Kaplan JA, Slingler PD, ed. *Thoracic Anesthesia*. 3rd ed. Elsevier; Philadelphia, PA, 2003.

Klein U, Karzai W, Bloos F, et al. Role of fiberoptic bronchoscopy in conjunction with the use of double-lumen tubes for thoracic anesthesia. *Anesthesiology*. 1998;88:346–350.

Knoll H, Ziegler S, Schreiber JU, et al. Airway injuries after one-lung ventilation: a comparison between double-lumen tube and endobronchial blocker: a randomized, prospective, controlled trial. *Anesthesiology*. 2006;105:471–477.

Lieberman, Littleford J, Horan T, et al. Placement of left double-lumen endobronchial tubes with or without a stylet. *Can J Anesth*. 1996;43:238–242.

Michelet P, D'Journo XB, Roch A, et al. Protective ventilation influences systemic inflammation after esophagectomy: a randomized controlled study. *Anesthesiology*. 2006;105:911–919.

Slinger P. Pro: low tidal volume is indicated during one-lung ventilation. *Anesth Analg*. 2006;103:268–270.

17

DO NOT UNDERESTIMATE THE DIFFICULTY OF REINTUBATING A PATIENT WHO HAS UNDERGONE CAROTID ENDARTERECTOMY OR CERVICAL SPINE SURGERY

HEATH R. DIEL, MD AND RANDAL O. DULL, MD, PhD

Anesthesia providers do not always appreciate the potential difficulties in reintubating patients who have undergone carotid endarterectomy and cervical spine surgery. Because these patients do not have tumors and usually do not initially present with stridor or signs of vocal cord paralysis (unless there has been a previous stroke), the initial intubation often is uncomplicated. During the operative phase there are many important physiologic issues, such as management of hemodynamics and maintenance of organ perfusion, that compete with the anesthesia provider's attention to airway issues. Prompt emergence and extubation is desired to facilitate postoperative neurologic checks and to avoid hypertension and coughing at the time of emergence. However, at all times, anesthesia providers must be alert for postextubation airway issues. It can be extremely difficult to get the airway secured after failed extubation even if the initial intubation was uncomplicated. This is a situation to consider very carefully before planning a "trial of extubation" or a "let's see how he does without the tube" maneuver.

The causes of postoperative respiratory dysfunction after carotid endarterectomy or cervical spine fusion include laryngeal or pharyngeal edema, hematoma, cerebrospinal fluid (CSF) leak, recurrent laryngeal nerve dysfunction, carotid body dysfunction, cervical fusion, malalignment, and improperly applied bandages.

EDEMA/HEMATOMA

Postoperative cervical edema is present in every anterior neck procedure to some degree and occurs in cervical laminectomy because of prone positioning. In carotid endarterectomy patients, computed tomographic studies have shown a 25% to 60% reduction in airway volume and a 200% to 250% increase in retropharyngeal mass as a result of edema alone. Edema of the larynx and pharynx is thought to be caused by venous and lymphatic disruption, as well as direct tissue trauma with increased capillary permeability secondary to release of local inflammatory mediators. Tissue edema can be difficult to gauge clinically if the patient has remained in the supine position. There can be significant internal compression of airway structure with little

© 2006 Mayo Foundation for Medical Education and Research

or no change in neck circumference, and stridor may not be heard until the airway has narrowed to 4 mm. Also, unilateral tissue disruption can cause bilateral edema. Edema is rarely the sole cause of respiratory distress leading to reintubation, but it compounds the effects of other problems that might arise (such as hematoma) and can make visualization of the vocal cords for reintubation extremely difficult. If the edema has occurred because of prone positioning, elevating the head of the bed to 30 degrees during emergence can reduce soft tissue edema.

Significant hematoma occurs in about 1.4% to 10.0% of carotid endarterectomy patients, with higher frequency in cases involving coagulopathies and heparin use without reversal. Frequently, hematomas do not develop until several hours into the postoperative phase, and the "carotid take-back" patient is often hypertensive, hypercarbic, and partially obtunded as well. Reintubation in this situation can be one of the most difficult airway situations to manage, and the airway can quickly become a truly emergency situation. Surgical evacuation of the hematoma without regard for aseptic technique may be sufficient to relieve the obstruction until oral direct laryngoscopy can be performed. The authors recommend that anesthesia providers have available maximum airway support in terms of personnel and equipment when reintubating any patient who has developed significant hematoma after carotid or cervical neck surgery.

Cerebrospinal Fluid Leak

Cerebrospinal fluid leak is a possible complication of anterior cervical vertebral fusion and occurs when the integrity of the dura mater and arachnoid tissue is disrupted. Collection of CSF can cause impaired ventilation as a result of mass effect, very similar to hematoma formation.

Recurrent Laryngeal Nerve Injury

Recurrent laryngeal nerve injury happens most often after thyroid surgery but is a recognized complication of carotid endarterectomy and anterior cervical spine surgery as well. Acute dysfunctions of the recurrent laryngeal nerve occur in about 0.2% to 10.0% of carotid surgery cases, but, fortunately, less than 1.0% involve permanent injuries.

The recurrent laryngeal nerve runs in the groove between the trachea and esophagus and innervates all the muscles of the larynx except the cricothyroid muscle. Injury is usually the result of ischemia, surgical manipulation, dissection, stretching, or compression. Unilateral dysfunction results in unilateral vocal cord adduction and hoarse voice. Bilateral dysfunction causes airway obstruction from bilateral cord adduction. The anesthesiologist should be aware of the preoperative function of the recurrent laryngeal nerves and patients with hoarse voice related to stroke or prior surgery. These patients may benefit from preoperative evaluation. Upon emergence and extubation, bilateral laryngeal nerve dysfunction presents as immediate airway obstruction requiring intervention.

CAROTID BODY DYSFUNCTION

The carotid body functions primarily as a chemoreceptor for blood oxygen and carbon dioxide content. Surgical denervation secondary to carotid endarterectomy impairs the patient's physiologic response to hypoxia. Patients treated with respiratory depressants such as opiates are at greater risk for postoperative hypoxia

CERVICAL MISALIGNMENT

Cervical misalignment is an unusual but possible complication of cervical spinal fusion. Misalignment can cause structural impingement of the airway, which, coupled with edema, can lead to ventilation deficiencies. Also, cervical fusion limits neck extension, and this could contribute to difficult postoperative reintubation.

SURGICAL DRESSINGS

Supportive dressings after neck surgery can cause airway obstruction by impeding venous and lymphatic drainage and worsening edema. Large dressings also obscure visualization of the operative site and may cover signs of bleeding that would alert the anesthesia and postoperative acute-care staff to a developing hematoma. Cervical collars should be sized appropriately and allow for some postoperative expansion due to edema. It should be obvious but bears stating that excessively tight or circumferential neck bandages should never be used. The authors are aware of several cases of apparent airway obstruction after carotid endarectomy that were relieved when the neck dressing was removed.

SUGGESTED READINGS

Allain R, Marone L, Meltzer L, et al. Carotid endarterectomy. *Int Anesthesiol Clin*. 2005;43(1): 15–38.

American Society of Anesthesiologists Task Force. A management of the difficult airway. Practice guidelines for management of the difficult airway. An updated report. *Anesthesiology*. 2003;95:1269–1277.

Ballotta E, Da Giau G, Renon L, et al. Cranial and cervical nerve injuries after carotid endarterectomy: a prospective study. *Surgery*. 1999;125:85–91.

Bukht D, Langford RM. Airway obstruction after surgery in the neck. *Anesthesia*. 1983;38: 389–390.

Carmichael EJ, McGuire G, Wang D, et al. Computed tomographic analysis of airway dimensions after carotid endarterectomy. *Anesth Analg*. 1996;83:12–17.

Curran AJ, Smyth D, Sheehan SJ, et al. Recurrent laryngeal nerve dysfunction following carotid endarterectomy. *J R Coll Surg Edinb*. 1997;42(3):168–170.

Hughes R, McGuire G, Montanera W, et al. Upper airway edema after carotid endarterectomy: the effect of steroid administration. *Anesth Analg*. 1997;84:475–478.

Ichinose K, Kozuma S, Fukuyama S, et al. A case of airway obstruction after posterior occipito-cervical fusion. *Masui*. 2002;51(5): 513–515.

Joseph MM, Kaufman W, Shindo M, et al. Complications of anesthesia for head-neck and reconstructive surgery. *Semin Anesth.* 1996;15:203–211.

Jung A, Schram J, Lehnerdt K, et al. Recurrent laryngeal nerve palsy during anterior cervical spine surgery: a prospective study. *J Neurosurg Spine.* 2005;2(2):123–127.

Kreisler NS, Durieux M, Spickermann BF, et al. Airway obstruction due to a rigid cervical collar. *J Neurosur Anesthesiol.* 2000;2:118–119.

McRae K. Anesthesia for airway surgery. *Anesthesiol Clin North Am.* 2001;19(3):497–541.

Penberthy A, Roberts N. Recurrent acute upper airway obstruction after anterior cervical fusion. *Anaesth Intensive Care.* 1998;26(3):305–307.

18

DO NOT START THE AIRWAY MANAGEMENT OF A LUDWIG ANGINA PATIENT UNTIL PERSONNEL AND EQUIPMENT FOR A DEFINITIVE (SURGICAL) AIRWAY ARE ASSEMBLED

ANNE L. LEMAK, DMD AND TODD M. ORAVITZ, MD

Ludwig angina is more formally known as septic cellulitis of the submandibular, submental, or sublingual spaces. Ludwig angina is most often the result of a dental abscess of the second or third mandibular molar, before or after tooth extraction, and presents as diffuse swelling of the floor of the mouth and airway. Symptoms can arise quickly and may consist of neck swelling, redness and pain, fever, chills, fatigue, earache, drooling, confusion, and eventually, airway collapse. Prompt treatment is compulsory to prevent the spread of infection and asphyxiation associated with subsequent airway edema.

Ludwig angina is typically caused by hemolytic streptococci from normal oral flora, but it may be caused by a combination of both aerobic and anaerobic bacteria resulting in the infectious process. The swelling in the floor of the mouth may be so extensive that the tongue is displaced upward and posterior, occluding the mouth and oropharynx, and if left untreated, the infection may spread caudally into the thoracic cavity and result in an abscess of the pericardium and lungs or throughout the body as septic shock. Patients may present with extreme lethargy, dehydration, and shortness of breath, and require immediate medical attention.

Treatment of the Ludwig angina patient depends on the extent of airway involvement. A less extensive case may simply require incision and drainage, surgical decompression, and a full course of broad-spectrum antibiotics. However, to determine the degree of inflammation, a computerized tomographic (CT) scan of the head and neck may be warranted as the first step to treatment. A thorough history and physical should also be obtained, and the patient's anesthesia team should work in conjunction with the surgeons to devise a comprehensive treatment plan. Managing the Ludwig patient may be complex, as he or she may be unable to talk or open his or her mouth adequately for incision and drainage of the affected area. Difficulty opening the mouth in combination with airway edema and displacement of the tongue presents the potential for serious anesthetic risk and complication. A definitive anesthetic strategy, along with backup preparations, is highly recommended for any Ludwig patient.

© 2006 Mayo Foundation for Medical Education and Research

The anesthesia provider(s) should carefully examine the airway, evalu-ating all the usual components including Mallampati class, oral opening, cer-vical range of motion, thyromental distance, and presence/absence of teeth. Additionally, in the Ludwig angina patient, the degree of airway edema, both clinically and radiographically, ability to swallow, amount of secretions, and mobility of the tongue need to be assessed. Tongue mobility is a fairly unique consideration in the Ludwig patient, as the disease process itself involves the submandibular space, which may become edematous and hardened. This is important with respect to airway management because during routine laryn-goscopy the tongue is displaced into the submandibular space. In the Ludwig patient, if that space is diminished or unavailable, it can make visualization of the vocal cords and subsequent intubation quite difficult. The anesthesi-ologist and surgeon may proceed only after this checklist has been carefully evaluated and a clear plan has been devised.

The airway of a Ludwig patient may be deceiving in that it may appear to be unobstructed when the patient is awake and breathing spontaneously, but that may change dramatically after induction and paralyzation. Topically anesthetizing a patient's larynx and trachea in order to take an "awake look" may not be beneficial, as visualization of laryngeal anatomy postinduction may be greatly reduced compared to that of the awake patient, because of decreased laryngeal muscle tone. Muscle relaxants may allow the edematous tissues adjacent to the trachea to relax after induction and occlude an airway that was patent in an awake Ludwig patient, possibly resulting in difficult, if not impossible, ventilation and/or intubation. Multiple intubation attempts or manipulations of a Ludwig patient's airway can be especially harmful, as it may cause the accumulation of blood and secretions in the pharynx and can potentiate further complications in already dire circumstances. For these reasons, direct laryngoscopy after topicalization of the airway is not advised in the Ludwig angina patient.

For the mildest cases of Ludwig angina, traditional direct laryngoscopy after routine induction may be sufficient. If this route is undertaken, it is advisable to have emergency airway equipment in the operating room should either ventilation or intubation prove more difficult than anticipated. For example, a laryngeal mask airway (LMA) may prove more effective than bag-mask ventilation if soft tissue collapse is a problem. Even more important than emergency airway equipment, however, is the presence in the operating room during induction of an experienced surgeon ready to provide a surgical airway should ventilation and intubation prove impossible.

For moderate Ludwig angina patients, a safer means of obtaining a se-cure airway is to carry out an awake intubation, in which the patient retains consciousness and spontaneous respirations until the endotracheal tube is in place. Before beginning an awake intubation, the patient must be fully informed of what he or she is about to experience, and he or she must be willing and able to cooperate with the anesthesiologist in attaining adequate airway anesthesia. To overcome the laryngeal reflexes and anesthetize the airway, a variety of methods may be used. Supraglottic anesthesia can be obtained via nebulized topical anesthetic followed by lidocaine-soaked pledgets, gargles, or sprays. Bilateral superior laryngeal nerve blocks may also be performed to anesthetize the cricothyroid muscle and to ameliorate sensation from the base of the tongue to the vocal cords. Patients with a full stomach, evidence of a tumor at the site of block, and those with an active infection at the site of injection are contraindications to the use of this nerve block. Because tracheal nerve blocks can be somewhat uncomfortable, benzodiazepines and/or opioids may be used to offset the stress associated with this procedure. Caution must be taken to ensure that the patient maintains spontaneous respirations and does not become oversedated. Infraglottic anesthesia may also be warranted and can be achieved via a transtracheal nerve block by injecting via the cricothyroid membrane with 2% lidocaine. Once full airway anesthesia is accomplished, the anesthesiologist can proceed with intubation. The endotracheal tube can be passed by means of a flexible fiber-optic bronchoscope, a direct-vision, lighted stylet (Shikani optical stylet or retromolar scope), or via an intubating laryngeal mask airway (Fastrach LMA). Care must be taken to avoid contacting abscessed areas in the mouth and oropharynx with airway instruments to prevent purulent discharge from migrating into the lungs. Once the trachea has been successfully intubated and endotracheal tube (ETT) position confirmed with positive end-tidal CO_2 and auscultation, the anesthesiologist can induce general anesthesia and the surgical procedure may begin. An experienced surgeon should be present in the operating room, ready to do an emergency tracheostomy, during any awake intubation attempt.

One important point to remember when considering awake intubation in a patient with Ludwig angina is that airway topical anesthetization itself may be difficult. The infected laryngeal tissues will likely be acidotic, which means that a greater percentage than normal of the local anesthetic will remain in its ionized form. Because the nonionized form traverses the neuronal membrane, the effectiveness of the local anesthetic may be reduced and the degree of airway anesthesia may be suboptimal.

Ludwig angina patients who present with advanced disease, evidenced by labored respirations, drooling, or limited mouth opening, are candidates for awake tracheostomy. An experienced surgeon should always be present in the operating room, ready to perform an emergency tracheostomy, regardless of the apparent level of airway involvement.

The decision to extubate the patient upon conclusion of the surgical procedure is based on the extent of the infection and the level of edema present. For more serious infections, a timely course of antibiotics may be necessary to alleviate the swelling and allow for an unimpeded airway before extubation. For patients of this type, who were preoperatively classified as having a "difficult" airway, a decision to remain intubated should be made, along with arrangements for postoperative sedation. All patients with considerable edema of the pharynx, submandibular space, and tongue should remain intubated indefinitely, until it is certain that a natural airway can be maintained. It is not uncommon for a Ludwig patient to remain intubated and mechanically ventilated for several days postoperatively, until extubation criteria have been met. It is mandatory that any patient with Ludwig angina who was intubated orally be able to breathe around the endotracheal tube with the cuff deflated before extubation. This helps to ensure that the edema has subsided and a patent airway is present without the endotracheal tube in place. In patients who have required a tracheostomy, maintaining the tracheostomy site is inevitable; however, whether the patient is kept on mechanical ventilation or allowed to breathe spontaneously depends on the patient's prior medical history (presence or absence of lung disease, localized versus systemic infection, etc).

In any Ludwig angina case, meticulous attention must be paid to devising and executing the safest and most thorough anesthetic and surgical plan. A thorough understanding of the "difficult" airway algorithm is paramount, as well as a close collaboration among all involved parties on the surgical and anesthesia teams. A prompt and comprehensive strategy is the key to enduring the most serious of circumstances challenging a Ludwig angina patient.

TAKE HOME POINTS

- Ludwig angina is most commonly seen after dental work. A typical scenario is for the patient to present in the evening or on a weekend after an urgent call to the dentist or endodontist that resulted in referral to the emergency department.
- Airway assessment for these patients incorporates all the basics, plus an assessment of tongue mobility, drooling and/or pooling of secretions, and ability to swallow.
- *Do not "spray the patient up for a quick look" while you are waiting for the surgeons to arrive.* This can and has resulted in patient mortality.
- Depending on the severity of the airway obstruction, either very careful awake or anesthetized techniques are appropriate. Err on the side of conservative treatment.

■ Do not attempt an airway maneuver unless you can rapidly progress to a definitive, surgically secured airway. This mandates the presence of an experienced surgeon, ready to do a surgical airway.

SUGGESTED READINGS

Barash PG, Cullen BF, Stoelting RK. *Clinical Anesthesia.* 4th ed. Philadelphia: Lippincott Williams & Wilkins; 2001:1000–1001.

Stoelting RK, Dierdorf SF. *Anesthesia and Co-existing Disease.* 4th ed. Philadelphia: Churchill Livingstone; 2002:579. www.nlm.nih.gov/medlineplus/ency/article/001047.htm

19

REMEMBER THAT THE IV START IS YOUR FIRST CHANCE TO MAKE A FAVORABLE IMPRESSION ON THE PATIENT

HASSAN M. AHMAD, MD AND CATHERINE MARCUCCI, MD

Intravenous access is a crucial part of anesthesia care, and placement and management of lines are important skills for an anesthesiologist. Virtually all anesthetics require some degree of intravenous (IV) access, whether it is for induction of general anesthesia, administration of medications, fluid resuscitation, or blood sampling.

The majority of adult surgical cases start with a peripheral IV for induction of general anesthesia, initiation of conduction blockade, or conscious sedation (for pediatric cases, it is usually appropriate to induce via an inhalational agent; however, endotracheal intubation should not be attempted until IV access is obtained). When performing regional anesthesia, it is also important to have an IV, not only for the administration of sedative and anxiolytic medications, but also to respond to potential hemodynamic changes related to neuraxial or peripheral blocks.

Peripheral IV placement can be one of the most challenging procedures in anesthesia, especially for beginners. When placing a peripheral IV, always make sure to:

- The initial needle stick can be very unpleasant for some people and a startled patient may move suddenly, making the procedure more difficult.
- If your operating room has a practice that allows IVs to be started in seated patients, always ask about and watch for vasovagal reactions. It seems counterintuitive, but often the patients who have the worst vasovagal reactions are the youngest and healthiest. One of the authors once saw a strapping young ex-marine slide right out of his chair onto the ground. Of course, there was a huge ruckus in the preoperative area. His family said, "oh, we forgot to tell you, he does that all the time."
- Choose a location that is convenient for you and the surgeon. For example, don't place an IV in the right hand if the patient is having a right-sided carpal tunnel release. Consider carefully before starting an IV in the foot of a patient with diabetes or significant soft tissue changes in the lower extremities. Some anesthesia providers will do it, but the podiatrists tend to advise against it.
- Use a tourniquet to engorge veins. A great technique before placing the tourniquet is to have the patient exercise the extremity against resistance

© 2006 Mayo Foundation for Medical Education and Research

for 20 seconds and then "hang" the extremity in a dependent position. This will provide a manyfold increase in blood flow to the extremity. To avoid cutting off arterial flow, do not make the tourniquet too tight. Put the tourniquet as close to the location of the vein that is being accessed as possible, so you don't forget to remove it. Consider the use of a forcing function as well—the person who puts the tourniquet on the patient is responsible for removing it—to make sure this happens, put a tourniquet on yourself or your pen or your stethoscope at the same time. Be especially careful if you have put a tourniquet on the lower leg, for some reason, these seem to be "forgotten" more often than tourniquets placed on the upper extremity.

- Flush your IV tubing before connecting it to the catheter to avoid letting air into the patient's circulation.
- Have gauze, tape, and dressings readily available and within your reach before you begin placing the IV. You don't want to lose a newly placed IV simply because you are fumbling with supplies. Have someone assist you whenever possible.
- If the patient shows signs of being a difficult stick, ask him if he can recommend a site.
- Only one person sticks the patient at a time!
- Advance your needle far enough that the catheter is within the vein. Remember that a flash of blood in the angiocath indicates that the *needle* has punctured the wall of a vein, but the catheter might still be outside. This is especially true in larger-bore IVs, in which there is 2 to 3 mm between the tip of the needle and the tip of the catheter.
- Give the patient reliable information. If you tell him that you will try only one more time before having someone else try, keep your word.
- Don't be greedy, the truism about the 18-gauge IV that runs versus the 16-gauge hematoma may be annoying when someone says it to you, but it **is** true.
- Recognize when it's "not your day" and don't be shy about having another anesthesia provider do the IV if you can't after about two (or so) tries.
- There are many individual styles of securing the IV once it is inserted, and this has actually been the subject of scientific inquiry. One study found that the "double-chevron" method, using two pieces of tape for the hub and the barrel of the needle, gave superior results (*Fig. 19.1*). Flat transparent dressings are generally superior to gauze dressings. Take care not to wrap the IV tubing circumferentially around the arm or hand, and don't make "purse handles" with extra long loops of unsecured tubing.

Although a single IV is adequate for some anesthetics, sometimes it is necessary to place additional ones. This is typically done after induction,

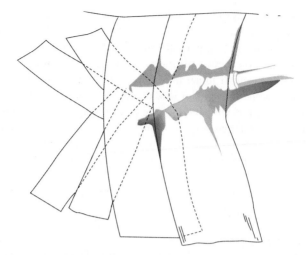

FIGURE 19.1. Preferred taping method. [Modified from Patel N, Smith CE, Pinchak AC, et al. Evaluation of different methods of securing intravenous catheters: measurement of forces during simulated accidental pullout. *Can J Anaesth.* 1995;42(6):504–510.]

because not only does it avoid patient discomfort, the vasodilating effects of general anesthesia will often make peripheral veins more obvious. Some indications for starting a second IV are

- The potential for large-volume blood loss. Although administration of medications can be done with small-caliber IVs, replacement of fluids and blood products is best done through large peripheral IVs, typically 18 gauge or larger. The larger the diameter of the catheter, the lower the resistance to flow, and the more rapidly you can push fluids. Always make sure to discuss the expected blood loss with the surgeons before the operation, and when in doubt, play it safe! Also, remember to obtain informed consent from your patient for all blood products.
- When patient positioning is such that obtaining additional IV access during surgery will be difficult. For example, if both arms will be tucked to the sides, it will be wise to start a second IV just in case one fails during the procedure.
- If you are planning to use a continuous infusion. Although it is not entirely necessary, it is sometimes preferred to use a dedicated IV at a constant rate for infusions, so that fluid and medication boluses do not disrupt the flow rate.

- Be confident and calm when starting an IV on an awake patient.
- Remember that peripheral IV skills can atrophy a bit even during a two-week vacation.
- Never argue with patients about their veins—if they insist they will be difficult, agree and tell them you will use the techniques used for children.
- Control the tourniquet!
- Exercise the extremity before placing the tourniquet.
- Make sure you are in the vein before trying to advance the catheter.
- Remember that the IV start is a chance to make a good impression, but unfortunately, it is also a chance to make an unfavorable impression.

SUGGESTED READINGS

Frey AM, Schears GJ. Why are we stuck on tape and suture? A review of catheter securement devices. *J Infus Nurs.* 2006;29(1):34–38.

Palmer D. Fewer patients dislodged peripheral intravenous catheters with transparent dressings than with gauze dressings. *Evid Based Nurs.* 1998;1:81.

Patel N, Smith CE, Pinchak AC, et al. The influence of tape type and of skin preparation on the force required to dislodge angiocatheters. *Can J Anaesth.* 1994;41(8):738–741.

Patel N, Smith CE, Pinchak AC, et al. Evaluation of different methods of securing intravenous catheters: measurement of forces during simulated accidental pullout. *Can J Anaesth.* 1995;42(6):504–510.

20

NEVER USE AN INTRAVENOUS LINE WITHOUT PALPATING AND INSPECTING IT VISUALLY

RYAN C. MCHUGH, MD AND JURAJ SPRUNG, MD, PHD

Intravenous (IV) infiltration is the unintentional extravascular leakage of IV fluid. Signs of infiltration include tissue edema, skin blanching or erythema, and skin temperature change. Patients may report pain and tightness around the IV site. Sites that are commonly infiltrated include the hand, forearm, and antecubital fossa, which are the most frequent sites of IV placement. Patient populations associated with higher rates of infiltration are critical care and oncology patients, owing primarily to the increased number of IV lines placed at a given time and the number of times that veins need to be accessed (e.g., repeated treatments with cytotoxic agents). Age groups at highest risk include the elderly and neonates. Neonates have small vessels and immature skin, whereas elderly persons have fragile vessels and skin. Placement of the IV outside the vessel in loose subcutaneous skin may mimic proper IV placement. Before use, every IV should be inspected visually for IV infiltration.

PERIOPERATIVE IV FLUID CONCERNS

Perioperative IV fluid therapies include crystalloids and colloids. Crystalloids are water-based solutions, usually with low-molecular-weight salts (vs. ions), whereas colloids contain high-molecular-weight proteins or glucose polymers. Another type of infusing material, called vesicants, has greater potential for substantial cellular injury. Vesicants include radiocontrast dyes, pressor agents, and chemotherapy solutions. In theory, colloid solutions may increase extravascular fluid content after infiltration by drawing fluid out of the cells, whereas any hypotonic solution may lead to cellular rupture after fluid absorption. Dyes act more like hypotonic solutions and include methylene blue and indocyanine green. Infiltration with these dyes may result in severe skin discoloration, but this effect is not permanent. The duration of discoloration is dependent on the rate of dye (fluid) reabsorption from the extracellular space, usually 12 to 24 hours. Hyaluronidase injected in multiple sites around the infiltration site has been used to treat mannitol infiltration.

INTRAOPERATIVE MONITORING

Before anesthetic induction, initial palpation of the IV site is recommended. If fluids (or medications) are administered by syringe extravascularly, they may elicit high pressure on injection, causing pain in awake patients. Relying on a free-flowing IV may lead to false positives, particularly in the elderly, for whom loose skin may allow easy infiltration. For catheters that are not located in an extremity, such as central lines, be mindful of which vein the catheter is expected to enter because infiltration will depend on its position in the body; extravasated fluid may leak into the arm, chest wall, or neck. Positive aspiration of blood must be achieved, providing the IV was placed in the major central vein. Transducing the catheter should be done to confirm venous placement of a central line.

If the extremity is exposed during surgery, continuous monitoring of the IV site for edema or blanching are necessary. Jewelry such as rings should be removed before surgery, especially for arms that are tucked in (placed along the body and covered with drapes) and arms in which the IV catheter has been placed. However, the frequent practice of tucking in arms requires careful IV monitoring. Should the IV stop flowing intraoperatively, full inspection of the IV site must be made. Facilitation of a sluggish IV by using "pressure bags" should not be done until the site is properly inspected for signs of possible extravascular infiltration.

CONSEQUENCES

Consequences of infiltration can be divided into pressure-related injuries and cellular irritant–related injuries. Pressure-related injuries may expose tissue to arterial ischemia, and irritant-related injuries may expose tissue to pH differences, osmotic differences, and direct toxicity. Severe consequences of either may include compartment syndrome, tissue necrosis, ulcers, and complex regional pain syndrome. Perioperatively, vigilance is required, particularly when administering antibiotics, vasopressors, cytotoxic drugs, osmotically active substances (total parenteral nutrition, hypertonic dextrose solutions), and cationic solutions (potassium, calcium, or bicarbonate salts).

TREATMENT OPTIONS

Simple maneuvers should be done initially. First, discontinue the IV infusion. Second, elevate the affected extremity, providing this elevation does not interfere with extremity perfusion (pulse oximetry can be placed on the extremity for perfusion assessment). Application of warm compresses, to decrease pain and swelling, may help for all fluids except vesicants. Warming a site extravasated with vesicant fluid may increase induration of the area and slow reabsorption. Ice compresses should be applied to a vesicant extravasation site for the first 24 hours, with subsequent moist heat thereafter until inflammation decreases.

Certain vesicants have specific antidotes. For example, norepinephrine extravasation can be treated with local infiltration of phentolamine.

Chemotherapeutic agents have specific antidotes depending on the agent infiltrated. Invasive techniques such as saline flushout and liposuction have been described. The worst cases may be treated by fasciotomy, débridement, and split skin grafting. However, a fairly recent study examining extravasation injuries in three hospitals recommended conservative treatment. A more recent study suggested prompt action and appropriate intervention should irritant injuries occur with vasopressors, hyperosmolar solutions, and concentrated electrolyte solutions in the perioperative period. If a substance is known to be an irritant, it should be used in a stable vein and in a vein without prior intravenous attempts.

CONCLUSIONS

After an injury occurs, management should fall into two categories, operative or nonoperative. Postinfiltration management should include frequent assessment and, most important, perfusion of the affected extremity. Ultimately, education of all perioperative staff on safe practices regarding intravenous access is the best approach to decrease the incidence of these complications.

TAKE HOME POINTS

- Be aware of which patients are at high risk for infiltration of the IV—the very young and elderly, ICU patients, and chemotherapy patients.
- Do *not* depend on the rate the IV is flowing to ensure that fluid will not extravasate—always inspect visually and palpate an IV before using it.
- Do *not* put a pressure bag on an IV that is suddenly running sluggishly—it is infiltrated until proven otherwise.
- Injuries are categorized as pressure-related or irritant-related. Some hospitals have policies involving peripheral infusion of soft tissue irritants such as potassium—know them.
- Treatment options range from conservative to invasive, depending partially on distal perfusion.
- Call the hospital pharmacy to see if there is a specific antidote.

SUGGESTED READINGS

Ford MD, Delaney KA, Ling LJ, et al, eds. *Clinical Toxicology.* Philadelphia: WB Saunders; 2001.

Gault DT. Extravasation injuries. *Br J Plast Surg.* 1993;46:91–96.

Kasper DL, Braunwald E, Fauci A, et al. *Harrison's Principles of Internal Medicine.* 16th ed. New York: McGraw-Hill; 2004.

Kumar MM, Sprung J. The use of hyaluronidase to treat mannitol extravasation. *Anesth Analg.* 2003;97:1199–1200.

Kumar RJ, Pegg SP, Kimble RM. Management of extravasation injuries. *ANZ J Surg.* 2001;71:285–289.

Miller RD, ed. *Miller's Anesthesia*. 6th ed. Philadelphia: Elsevier Churchill Livingstone; 2005.

O'Hara JF Jr., Connors DF, Sprung J, et al. Upper extremity discoloration caused by subcutaneous indigo carmine injection. *Anesth Analg*. 1996;83:1126–1128.

Roberts JR, Hedges JR, eds. *Clinical Procedures in Emergency Medicine*. 4th ed. Philadelphia: WB Saunders; 2004.

Schummer W, Schummer C, Bayer O, et al. Extravasation injury in the perioperative setting. *Anesth Analg*. 2005;100:722–727.

21

USE OF ULTRASOUND GUIDANCE FOR CANNULATION OF THE CENTRAL VEINS IMPROVES SUCCESS RATES, DECREASES NUMBER OF ATTEMPTS, AND LOWERS COMPLICATION RATES

MICHAEL AZIZ, MD

Ultrasound guidance for placement of central venous catheters is becoming the standard of care across medical disciplines. Doppler localization of vascular structures has been used for many years, and the literature has slowly come to prove the utility of ultrasound. Newer portable equipment has made ultrasound useful and practical at the bedside. The widespread use of ultrasound has been slower to occur than might be anticipated. The success rate for internal jugular cannulation by the landmark technique is impressive at 95% to 99%. Many clinicians with skilled hands do not feel that they need assistance in localizing a central vein because they have had such dramatic success with the landmark method. However, in reviewing the studies that document such widespread success for internal jugular cannulation, we find that they often require multiple attempts and have a significant complication rate. A review of the literature demonstrates that two-dimensional ultrasound guidance for central venous access improves the success rate, reduces the complication rate, and reduces the number of attempts when compared to landmark techniques.

Ultrasound guidance improves cannulation success rates. For the internal jugular vein there is a relative risk reduction of 86% for failed cannulation in adults, and risk reduction of 85% in infants. For the subclavian vein, data demonstrate a relative risk reduction of 86% for failed cannulation. For the femoral vein, there is a relative risk reduction of 73%. These data are compiled from meta-analysis of large randomized controlled trials and are statistically significant.

Ultrasound guidance also reduces the likelihood of complication during central venous cannulation. There is a relative risk reduction of 57%. With a complication rate of 5% in experienced hands and 11% in inexperienced hands, these findings stand to improve patient safety and outcome dramatically.

Ultrasound guidance reduces the number of attempts for venous cannulation. The relative risk reduction for successful cannulation on the first attempt is 41%. Ultrasound also decreases the time to successful cannulation.

ⓒ 2006 Mayo Foundation for Medical Education and Research

Some clinicians believe that ultrasound guidance adds time and burden to their procedures, but the evidence demonstrates fewer attempts and shorter times to successful venous cannulation.

The data presented above demonstrate a favored approach for ultrasound over landmark methods for central venous cannulation. Other meta-analyses have pooled data that include Doppler localization into the ultrasound group and could not demonstrate results as favorable. The Hind study demonstrates that Doppler localization (as opposed to two-dimensional ultrasound) is less successful and more time-consuming than even landmark methods. These data, therefore, support the use of two-dimensional ultrasound over Doppler localization and the landmark method.

There are several reasons why this author believes that the literature has come to prove that ultrasound guidance improves safety and success with venous cannulation. When the landmark method is used and a cannulation becomes difficult, subsequent ultrasound often demonstrates venous thrombosis or absence of a patent vein. This difficulty is completely avoided by using ultrasound first and guiding the choice of central vein based on visualized venous patency. I think direct visualization of a needle compressing a vein avoids carotid and pleural puncture. With the landmark method, at times the needle is passed directly through the vein and into the carotid artery without venous aspiration, because the vein becomes compressed from needle pressure. Ultrasound shows this compression occurring as the needle is passing and keeps one from passing the needle into deeper structures such as arteries, pleura, or nerves. Often, central lines are placed during states of hypovolemia, when veins are especially prone to collapse.

Widespread use of ultrasound guidance for central venous access remains limited for several reasons. Some institutions cannot justify the cost of high-resolution ultrasound equipment. I argue, however, that the health care system stands to save money from reduced complication costs. Other clinicians fear that the use of ultrasound will impair their ability to cannulate a vein in an emergency situation using the landmark method. Ultrasound does not affect our ability to use landmarks as well. As I teach these methods, I like to identify the landmarks and expected course of the vein before ultrasound identification. In this way, students gain skill in both methods. Also, in an emergency situation, an available ultrasound probe is likely to expedite venous cannulation, not slow it down. However, if a probe is not available in an emergency situation, the landmark methods become necessary.

Practice habits have varied to accommodate the above considerations. Some authors advocate the use of ultrasound only in situations that predict difficult central vein access, such as previous neck surgery, multiple previous cannulations, hypovolemia, existing catheters or pacemaker, and obesity. Other clinicians use ultrasound to confirm the landmark anatomy, then remove the probe from the field. Others use ultrasound only after failed attempts using the landmark method. In such scenarios, the landmark method skill is retained for emergency situations. Although these practices have merit, evidence favors a prepuncture ultrasound scan with ultrasound-directed needle placement and cannulation.

TAKE HOME POINTS

- Ultrasound guidance is becoming the standard of care in placement of central venous access.
- Even in studies in which success rate was extremely high using the landmark technique, ultrasound guidance decreased the number of attempts and complication rates.
- Ultrasound guidance for access can be used for infants as well as adults.
- Two-dimensional ultrasound guidance is a superior technique for central line placement over Doppler localization.
- Resistance to adopting ultrasound guidance as a standard technique is still prevalent—concerns that it slows line placement time are not supported by the literature.
- Maintain skill in the landmark technique by appreciating and outlining the pertinent anatomic landmarks before placing the ultrasound probe.

SUGGESTED READINGS

Goldfarb G, Lebrec D. Percutaneous cannulation of the internal jugular vein in patients with coagulopathies: an experienced based on 1,000 attempts. *Anesthesiology.* 1982;56:321–323.

Hind D, Calvert N, McWilliams R, et al. Ultrasonic locating devices for central venous cannulation: meta-analysis. *Br Med J.* 2003;327:361–364.

Schwartz AJ, Jobes DR, Greenhow DE, et al. Carotid artery puncture with internal jugular cannulation using the Seldinger technique: incidence, recognition, treatment, and prevention. *Anesthesiology.* 1979:51:S160.

Sznajder JI, Zveibil FR, Bitterman H, et al. Central vein catheterization: failure and complication rates by three percutaneous approaches. *Arch Intern Med.* 1986;146:259–261.

22

CENTRAL LINE PLACEMENT: NEVER NEGLECT THE BASICS

HASSAN M. AHMAD, MD

Intravenous (IV) access is a crucial part of anesthesia care, and placement and management of lines are important skills for both the anesthetist and anesthesiologist. Virtually all anesthetics require some degree of IV access, whether it is for induction of general anesthesia, administration of medications, fluid resuscitation, or blood sampling.

Before attempting to place a central line, be sure you are well versed on anatomic landmarks and appropriate techniques. This is never a benign procedure, so always make sure to weigh the risks and benefits and discuss them with the patient as part of your informed-consent process. Central line placement has been associated with several complications, including:

- Accidental arterial puncture with pseudoaneurysm or hematoma
- Pneumo- or hemothorax
- Venous air embolism
- Infection and sepsis
- Cardiac arrhythmias

The decision to place a central line is multifactorial. Always assess the overall clinical picture, and discuss with the surgeon and intensive care unit (ICU) staff if possible. Some of the indications for obtaining central venous access are

- Inability to obtain peripheral venous access.
- Cardiac arrest or "code" situation. In this case, a femoral approach is best, as it does not interfere with chest compressions or endotracheal intubation.
- Administration of certain medications. Generally, any medication that can cause direct damage to peripheral veins must be given centrally, for example, 3% saline. Also, highly concentrated vasopressors can cause vasospasm if given through a peripheral vein. Check with the pharmacy for other medications that need to be given centrally.
- Central venous pressure monitoring. Although not considered to be a highly accurate measure of volume status, it can be used in conjunction with other clinical signs to guide fluid management.
- Massive blood transfusion. As mentioned above, large-diameter catheters are preferred for rapid transfusion, but remember that the *length* of the catheter also contributes to resistance to flow. For example, a short

© 2006 Mayo Foundation for Medical Education and Research

16-gauge peripheral IV has much less resistance than a long 16-gauge central line. For rapid infusion of large volumes, a large-bore, short catheter, such as a Cordis or introducer sheath, is best.

- Potential need for a pulmonary artery catheter placement. A right-sided internal jugular or left-sided subclavian introducer is preferred.
- High risk of venous air embolism (VAE) during surgery. Be familiar with the clinical signs of VAE and potentially high-risk procedures. In addition to placement in the left-lateral decubitus position, flooding the surgical field with fluid, increasing FiO_2, and discontinuing nitrous oxide, aspirating through a central line may remove air from the right side of the heart. In this case, a multilumen catheter is preferred.

Some basic things *always* to remember when placing a central line:

- Be aware of coagulopathy, thrombocytopenia, or any other contraindication to a particular line (thrombosis, existing hardware, etc).
- Choose your site wisely. For example, in a patient with a right-sided pneumothorax, choose a right IJ or SC to avoid the risk of bilateral pneumothoraces.
- Place your patient in Trendelenburg position, or at least flat, when placing an internal jugular or subclavian line. This minimizes the risk of venous air embolism.
- Create a sterile field. Studies have shown that infection risk decreases significantly when proper sterile techniques, including a full body drape, are used.
- Be familiar with your supplies and have them ready and within your reach before you begin the procedure. Get an experienced nurse to help you whenever possible.
- Be aware of your patient's condition during the procedure. Draping can make an awake patient very anxious, and a head-down position can exacerbate orthopnea or gastric reflux. Use monitoring and inhaled oxygen whenever possible.
- Always have control of the guidewire!
- Confirm venous (versus arterial) placement. There are several ways to do this. The most accurate is ultrasound-guided placement. However, if you do not have access to that equipment and the clinical situation warrants central line placement, the options include a simple "drop-test," transducing a pressure tracing, or obtaining a radiograph. Do not use the line until you are convinced it is in the right place.
- Secure the line with sutures and a sterile dressing.

SUGGESTED READINGS

Black SM, Chambers WA. *Essential Anatomy for Anesthesia*. New York: Churchill Livingstone; 1997:37–70.

Pollard A, Johnson RV. Assessment of correct central venous line placement. *Anaesthesia.* 2002;57(12):1223.

Robinson JF, Robinson WA, Cohn A, et al. Perforation of the great vessels during central venous line placement. *Arch Intern Med.* 1995;155(11):1225–1228.

Stoelting RK, Miller RD. *Basics of Anesthesia.* 4th ed. New York: Churchill Livingstone; 2000:215–216.

23

APPROACH THE USE OF A PULMONARY ARTERY CATHETER WITH CAUTION

AMY V. ISENBERG, MD

The pulmonary artery (PA) catheter is an invasive hemodynamic monitor utilized to both diagnose and manage certain conditions. Optimally placed catheters give direct measurements of central venous, pulmonary artery, and pulmonary artery wedge pressures.

Features of the PA catheter (PAC) include a thermistor at the tip to estimate cardiac output (CO) and systemic and pulmonary vascular resistance, the ability to perform mixed venous oximetry, the option of pacing, and the measurement of right-heart cardiac output in order to infer left-heart output.

USES FOR THE PAC

The pulmonary artery catheter, although controversial, has demonstrated continued usefulness in differentiating shock states, defining the etiologies of respiratory and cardiac failure, and assessing intracardiac shunts and regurgitation of mitral and tricuspid valves. The PAC also has use in several specific surgical situations involving large fluid shifts or potential cardiac damage, such as liver transplantation, aortic cross-clamp cases, and large operating room (OR) cases involving renal-failure patients. Although PACs were traditionally used to guide therapy in patients with acute myocardial infarct, recent studies have shown that PAC tracings are marginally beneficial in sensing ischemia, except in the instance of intraoperative right ventricular ischemia.

Perioperative use of the pulmonary artery catheter is common in the intensive care unit (ICU) setting. Many patients in the ICU suffer multiple organ dysfunctions, and data from PACs are useful in detecting and defining various hemodynamic disturbances for therapy implementation. Infection becomes a greater risk with ICU use, particularly for more than 6 days.

RISKS OF THE PAC

Pulmonary artery catheterization may be complicated by adverse events that occur during access of the central venous system, positioning of the PA catheter, and catheter "residence". According to American Society of Anesthesiologists (ASA) 2003 data (*Table 23.1*), the most common complication in obtaining central venous access is postoperative neuropathy, followed by

ⓒ 2006 Mayo Foundation for Medical Education and Research

TABLE 23.1   ADVERSE EFFECTS ASSOCIATED WITH PULMONARY ARTERY MONITORING

COMPLICATION	REPORTED INCIDENCE (%)
Central venous access	
Arterial puncture	1.1–13
Postoperative neuropathy	5.3
Pneumothorax	0.3–1.1
Air embolism	0.3–4.5
Positioning of the PAC	
Minor dysrhythmias	4–68.9
Ventricular tachycardia or fibrillation	0.3–62.7
Right bundle branch block	0.1–4.3
Complete heart block (prior LBBB)	0–8.5
Complications associated with catheter residence	
Pulmonary artery rupture	0.1–1.5
Positive catheter tip cultures	1.4–34.8
Sepsis secondary to catheter residence	0.7–11.4
Thrombophlebitis	6.5
Venous thrombosis	0.5–66.7
Pulmonary infarction	0.1–5.6
Mural thrombus	28–61
Valvular or endocardial vegetations	2.2–100
Deaths attributed to PAC	0.02–1.5

Source: ASA Task Force on Pulmonary Artery Catherization. Practice guidelines for pulmonary artery catherization: an updated report by The American Society of Anesthesiologists Task Force on Pulmonary Catherization. *Anesthesiology.* 2003;99:998–1014.)

arterial puncture, air embolism, and pneumothorax. Placement of the PAC commonly causes minor dysrhythmias (4.7% to 68.9% reported incidence), followed by ventricular tachycardia or fibrillation, right bundle branch block, and complete heart block preceded by left bundle branch block; the catheter may also coil or knot. Once it is in place, the PAC can rupture the pulmonary artery (0.1% to 1.5% reported incidence), become infected and lead to sepsis, or cause thrombophlebitis, venous thrombosis, pulmonary infarction, mural thrombus, or valvular or endocardial vegetations. Deaths attributed to pulmonary artery catheters have a reported incidence of 0.02% to 1.5%.

SPECIAL ISSUES IN PAC INSERTION

Sterile technique, including use of mask, cap, sterile gloves and gown, and large sterile drape, must be applied to avoid complications with infection. Use of 2% chlorhexidine is recommended for skin preparation. Remember that insertion requires two people—one sterile person to "float" the catheter and a knowledgeable nonsterile person to assist with the transducers, flush, and balloon inflation. Also, a surprisingly common error is to forget to place the sterile sleeve on the catheter before insertion or to put in on backwards.

The right atrium is most easily accessed via the right internal jugular vein. The left internal jugular approach may be complicated by damage to the thoracic duct as well as by variable anatomy such as may exist in patients with congenital heart disease. Additionally, the left internal jugular vein may drain into a persistent left superior vena cava. Approach from the subclavian veins (higher risk of pneumothorax) or from various peripheral veins (higher risk of venospasm, which increases placement difficulty or thrombosis) may be sought as well.

The electrocardiograph (EKG) should be monitored continuously during placement of the PAC, and a defibrillator should be available. When the PAC has been inserted through the introducer, the balloon should be inflated at approximately 20 cm and should always been inflated as the catheter is advancing (and the balloon should always be deflated for withdrawal). Avoid coiling and knotting of the catheter (which can result in the need for surgical or radiologic intervention) by not inserting excessive lengths of catheter. The wave pattern should be monitored for its characteristic form as the catheter tip passes through the right atrium, right ventricle, pulmonary artery, and the wedge (*Fig. 23.1*). Persistent premature ventricular contractions may be suppressed with lidocaine. The right ventricular trace is commonly measured

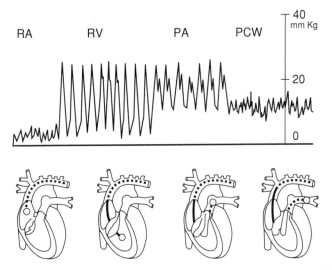

FIGURE 23.1. Picture of waveform change as catheter tip progresses. (From Dizon CT, Barash PG: The value of monitoring pulmonary artery pressure in clinical practice. *Conn Med.* 1977;41:622–625.)

at the 30- to 35-cm mark on the catheter, the PA trace at 40 to 50 cm, and the pulmonary capillary wedge pressure trace at 50+ cm. If the characteristic tracings are not readily observed, the balloon should be deflated and the catheter withdrawn to 20 cm.

The proximal port should reside in the right atrium in order to transduce right atrial pressure and to inject thermodilution fluid. The distal lumen, when properly seated, will transduce pulmonary artery pressure and pulmonary capillary wedge pressure.

The risk of pulmonary artery perforation can be minimized by not "overwedging" the balloon, by minimizing the number of balloon inflations, and by using proper balloon technique (inflate slowly and deflate passively). Do not leave the balloon inflated continuously. As balloon rupture can devastate patients with right-to-left intracardiac shunts, the anesthesiologist may use CO_2 in the balloon instead of air. Remember that PA rupture is more common in patients with pulmonary hypertension, partly because the PAC is more difficult to place.

In patients with known dysrhythmia, especially bundle branch blocks, external pacing/defibrillator pads placed before placing the catheter may help manage dysrhythmias induced by line insertion. Patients with left bundle branch block may be candidates for fluoroscopic placement of the PAC to expedite passage of the catheter through the right ventricle to reduce the chances of instigating a right heart block (which would leave the patient in complete heart block with the need for immediate transthoracic or transvenous cardiac pacing). Fluoroscopic guidance of insertion is also useful in patients with right atrial or ventricular dilatation, and in those with severe tricuspid regurgitation. Transesophageal echo may be useful in intubated patients in the OR or ICU setting to ascertain correct placement.

SPECIAL ISSUES IN PAC DATA INTERPRETATION

Unfortunately, intraobserver variation in data interpretation has been reported among critical care specialists and anesthesiologists. Proper utilization of the PAC necessitates knowing how best to position the catheter to optimize data generation as well as understanding what the data signify in different situations.

The transducer must be "zeroed" with atmospheric air. Correct equipment calibration requires that the transducer be level with the right atrium (approximately 5 cm below the sternal angle of Louis). Remember that wave damping may result from clot formation over the catheter tip, air bubbles, or tip against the pulmonary artery wall. Cardiac contractions causing catheter motion may lead to "fling" or "catheter whip." High-frequency components of the pressure-wave signals matching the resonating frequency of the fluid-filled monitoring system can result in harmonic resonance. The resonating frequency can be altered by changing the length of the tubing or using tubing made of a different material, preferably of a rigid, noncompliant type.

Spontaneous respiration may result in negative and positive pressure artifacts being transmitted to the PAC during inspiration and exhalation, respectively. Positive-pressure artifacts may be seen during mechanical ventilation. The degree of artifact is affected by lung and chest wall compliance, PAC position, and by the use of positive end-expiratory pressure (PEEP).

Although left atrial pressure is generally a good estimate of left ventricular end diastolic pressure (LVEDP), in mitral stenosis, left atrial pressure (LAP) is greater than LVEDP. LAP is also greater than LVEDP in mitral regurgitation, with systolic retrograde flow resulting in a large V wave on the PCWP tracing. Conversely, LVEDP is greater than LAP when there is retrograde flow from the aorta into the ventricle, as with aortic regurgitation and premature closure of the mitral valve.

Preload/left ventricular end-diastolic volume (LVEDV)/LVEDP measurements may be inaccurate with changes in compliance. Factors that decrease compliance include myocardial ischemia, restrictive cardiomyopathy/myocardial fibrosis, right-to-left interventricular septal shift, aortic stenosis, cardiac tamponade, effusion, inotropic drugs, and hypertension. Factors that increase compliance include vasodilators, congestive myopathies, left-to-right interventricular septal shift, and mitral and aortic regurgitation.

Problems with data interpretation occur when pulmonary vascular resistance is increased, reducing pulmonary blood flow and changing the relationship between PCWP and LAEDP. This relationship can also be modified in conditions such as acute/chronic lung disease, pulmonary emboli, hypoxia, acidosis, and hypoxemia. Drugs that increase pulmonary vascular resistance, and tachycardia (which shortens ventricular diastole), will increase pulmonary vascular resistance and affect the accuracy of the PAC data.

Finally, the PAC tip must be located in Zone 3 (PAP > PA < PVP), where there is an open fluid channel between the catheter tip and the left atrium. Supine patients will generally have the catheter at this level. However, PEEP and hypovolemia can alter the pressure relationships in this zone.

OUTCOMES ASSOCIATED WITH THE PAC

The effect of PAC monitoring remains controversial. The 1997 Pulmonary Artery Consensus Conference produced a statement concerning PAC use in cardiac and noncardiac surgery. PAC use demonstrated no benefit or uncertain benefit in patients undergoing cardiac surgery, low-risk aortic surgery, neurosurgery, or in surgical patients >65 years old. The experts supported use of PACs to reduce complications in patients undergoing peripheral vascular surgery and high-risk aortic valve surgery. It was recommended that in the absence of severe lung disease, pulmonary hypertension, or impaired right ventricular function, central venous pressure monitoring alone may be adequate to guide fluid management. The 2003 ASA guidelines offer suggestions for appropriate use of the PAC in the current OR and perioperative environment. New technology offering continuous cardiac output monitoring allows the ability to detect changes in ventricular performance as alterations occur; how this will change current clinical practice is still being discussed. Controversy continues over anesthesiologist preference for PAC versus transesophageal echocardiography (TEE) as well as the timing of PAC placement (before or after induction of anesthesia). As such, there is considerable variation in how the use of a PAC is "taught" to anesthesia students.

TAKE HOME POINTS

- The risk/benefit ratio for use of a PAC favors certain specific indications, e.g., sepsis, persistent hypotension of unknown etiology, fluid management in the anuric patient, and "special" cases (acute anterior myocardial infarction, high aortic cross-clamp, liver transplantation).
- Insertion requires sterile technique and two people.
- Do not overwedge the catheter, and *always inflate the balloon carefully!*
- Remember that as experience increases, anesthesia providers tend to have increasing respect for the possible morbidity and mortality incurred with the use of these catheters.
- Expect that anesthesiologists will use the measured and calculated values differently in managing care—do not be shy about asking why some practitioners may feel the cardiac output is the single most important value and others may more carefully follow left ventricular stroke work index.

SUGGESTED READINGS

ASA Task Force on Pulmonary Artery Catherization. Practice guidelines for pulmonary artery catherization: an updated report by The American Society of Anesthesiologists Task Force on Pulmonary Catherization. *Anesthesiology*. 2003;99:998–1014.

DiNardo JA, Monitoring. Anesthesia for Cardiac Surgery, Appleton and Lange, Stamford, CT, 1990.

Hollenberg M, Mangano DT, Browner WS, et al. Predictors of postoperative myocardial ischemia in patients undergoing noncardiac surgery. The Study of Perioperative Ischemia Research Group. *JAMA*. 1992;268:205.

Lee TL. Pitfalls of pulmonary artery pressure monitoring. In: Faust ed. *Anesthesiology Review*. Churchill Livingston; 2002.

Murphy G, Vender J. Monitoring the anesthetized patient. In: Barash P, ed. *Clinical Anesthesia*. 5th ed. Philadelphia: Lippincott Williams & Wilkins; 2006.

Pulmonary Artery Catheter Consensus Conference: consensus statement. *Crit Care Med*. 1997;25(6):901.

24

AVOID TECHNIQUE-RELATED CENTRAL VENOUS CATHETER COMPLICATIONS BY USING MODERN TOOLS

J. SAXON GILBERT, MD AND KAREN HAND, MD

Placement of central venous catheters is a routine procedure in modern anesthesia care. The somewhat routine nature of this procedure should not lull the anesthesia provider into complacency regarding the importance of meticulous attention to technique. Of the many thousands of central venous catheters placed each year, the U.S. Food and Drug Administration (FDA) estimates that approximately 10% will be associated with a complication, 52% of which are related to practitioner technique. The cost of these complications to the U.S. health care system exceeds $1 billion annually.

In anesthesia practice, right internal jugular vein cannulation is most commonly selected. This is because of the relatively straight path to the superior vena cava, increased distance from the cupola of the lung (vs. left side), and absence of the thoracic duct on the right side. The potential for nerve, vessel, or lung injury exists for any approach to central venous catheterization, including the right internal jugular approach. The subclavian approach increases the risk of pneumothorax because of the proximity of the pleura to the subclavian vein. In addition, if the subclavian artery is punctured, it is not possible to control hemorrhage with direct pressure. Femoral vein cannulation is associated with increased risk of infection, but can be a good alternative if the line is intended for rapid volume infusion. Peripherally inserted central catheters can also be used. Catheter length hinders this option for the purpose of rapid volume infusion.

Although infections are responsible for approximately 75% of catheter complications, American Society of Anesthesiologists (ASA) closed claims data indicate that technical complications during placement are the most deadly. Pneumothorax, wire or catheter embolization, air embolism, extravasation of fluid or blood into the neck, and a variety of cardiac and vascular injuries may occur. Of these, direct arterial injury and vascular injury resulting in cardiac tamponade or hemo/hydrothorax have the worst mortality (*Table 24.1*). In addition to site of catheter placement, the risk of pneumothorax can be diminished by using ultrasonic guidance and properly angling the needle away from the pleura on initial approach to the vessel. Wire embolization is avoided by using a technique of catheter insertion that permits one hand to continuously control the wire until it is removed. Catheter embolization is

ⓒ 2006 Mayo Foundation for Medical Education and Research

TABLE 24.1   OVERALL COMPLICATIONS AND FATALITIES
              FOR THE PERIODS 1978–1989 AND 1990 AND
              LATER

COMPLICATIONS	1978–1989	1978–1989 FATALITIES	1990 & LATER	1990 & LATER FATALITIES
Cardiac tamponade	10	8	2	2
Wire or catheter embolism	10	0	0	0
Vascular injuries	16	9	16	7
Hemothorax	6	6	5	3
Hydrothorax	3	1	1	1
Carotid artery injury	5	1	9	3
Subclavian artery injury	2	1	1	0
Pulmonary artery rupture	4	4	1	1
Pneumothorax	7	1	3	0
Air embolism	2	1	1	1
Fluid extravasation in neck	0	0	3	1
Total	49	23	26	12

prevented by taking care to avoid withdrawing the catheter at any time over a needle with a cutting bevel, which can shear the tip. Air embolization is of particular concern when the patient is breathing spontaneously or when the insertion site is above the level of the heart. Avoid this complication by using the Trendelenburg position (which improves identification of neck vessels as well), occluding the catheter/introducer with a gloved finger, and taking care to eliminate air from the catheter itself with aspiration and flushing either before or after insertion. The risk of fluid or blood extravasation is avoided by ensuring that the skin nick for the introducer does not lacerate the vein being cannulated, and by suturing the catheter securely to avoid the tip slipping. Cardiac tamponade usually results from a catheter with the tip inside the right atrium or angled against the wall of the superior vena cava, which can erode through the thin-walled atrium or vessel. This usually occurs after hours or days. The most serious direct vascular injury is caused by the inadvertent insertion of the catheter or introducer sheath directly into an artery that was mistaken for a vein.

Eliminating life-threatening vascular complications entails correct positioning of the introducer and catheter within the appropriate central vein. Fortunately, modern tools are available to assist the anesthesia provider in correct placement and definitive confirmation that the catheter will be inserted into a vein and not an artery. Subjective methods of ascertaining correct placement such as evaluation of the pulsatile quality or color of the blood are unreliable. This is because they can depend on variable factors such as oxygen saturation of the blood or arterial/venous pressure. Use of two-dimensional ultrasound as a guide to initial venous puncture is the best means of avoiding insertion complications. A 2001 review of the literature by the Agency for Healthcare Research and Quality revealed that use of ultrasound for placement of central venous catheters improved catheter insertion success rate, diminished the number of venipuncture attempts, and reduced the number of overall line complications. The best means of confirming correct line placement is a two-step process: step one is to tranduce the pressure in the vessel before placing the introducer (ensure that it is not an arterial waveform), and step two is to confirm proper placement via a chest radiograph either intraoperatively or at the end of the procedure. A retrospective study of 1,021 central lines by Jobes et al. revealed that among 43 cases of arterial puncture, five resulted in inadvertent placement of 8.5-French catheters in the carotid artery and one patient subsequently died. Conversely, in a prospective study of 1,284 central line placements in which the line was transduced after insertion, unrecognized arterial puncture was detected in 10 patients and there were no inadvertent arterial cannulations.

TAKE HOME POINTS

- Beside infections, the majority of central venous catheter complications are secondary to technical problems.
- Minimizing serious complications related to central venous catheter insertion can be accomplished by using the techniques discussed above.
- Strict aseptic technique and avoiding confusion between artery and vein are paramount.
- Using modern tools such as two-dimensional ultrasound and pressure transducers has been shown to reduce the number of life-threatening complications.
- Keep in mind the primary dictum of medical practice when inserting central lines: First, do no harm!

SUGGESTED READINGS

Bowdle, TA. Central line complications from the ASA Closed Claims Project. *ASA Newsletter.* 1996;60(6):22–25.

Bowdle, TA. Central line complications from the ASA Closed Claims Project: an update. *ASA Newsletter.* 2002;66(6):11–12, 25.

Jobes DR, Schwartz AJ, Greenhow DE, et al. Safer jugular vein cannulation: recognition of arterial puncture and preferential use of the external jugular route. *Anesthesiology.* 1983;59:353–355.

Rothschild JM. Ultrasound guidance of central vein catheterization. Evidence report/technology assessment, no. 43. Making health care safer. A critical analysis of patient safety practices. Agency for Healthcare Research and Quality Publication 10-E058. 2001:245–253.

www.venousaccess.com

25

DON'T OVERFLUSH LINES

JULIE MARSHALL, MD AND PETER ROCK, MD, MBA

Anesthesiologists become experts at the placement of lines for access and monitoring, but the routine care and maintenance of these lines may be less familiar. It is important to remember that unintentional overflushing of arterial and central lines happens commonly (especially during the busier intervals in a procedure) and can lead to significant complications. Also, patients not infrequently come to the operating room (OR) or intensive care unit (ICU) with indwelling devices already in place. These may under certain circumstances be accessed for use in the OR, provided that the anesthesia providers have a plan and proceed carefully.

Overzealous flushing of arterial lines may lead to retrograde emboliza-tion of air or clot into the central arterial circulation. It has been shown that the saline volume needed to reach the subclavian-vertebral artery junction from a radial artery averages just 6.6 mL, with a range from 3 to 12 mL. Arterial catheter continuous-flush devices deliver 3 mL/hour of saline, often with heparin, at a pressure of 300 mm Hg. Flushing the line through the flush valve or with a syringe can increase the volume and rate of delivery. Continuous-flush devices have been reported to deliver 0.8 to 4.7 mL/second when flushing an arterial line by opening the flush valve (commonly referred to as the "pigtail"). An increased rate of delivery, smaller patient size (in-fants), and increased flush volume all increase the potential for embolization of air bubbles into the central arterial circulation. To decrease the risk of em-bolization, all air should be removed from the arterial line. The drip chamber in the flush bag should be completely filled with fluid to decrease the chance of entraining air. Volume and rate of flush should be limited by opening the flush valve for only 2 to 3 seconds at a time. When flushing an arterial line with a syringe, the volumes should be small, 1 to 3 mL, and the flush should be done slowly. Both the injection port and the syringe should be free of air. Emboli may also occur from a clot in the arterial line or from arterial thrombi at the end of the catheter. If the line is not cleared following blood draws, small clots may be found in arterial lines or stopcocks. These small clots can be embolized with a forceful flush. Thrombi may form on the tip of the arterial catheter, which may also embolize with forceful flushing. These emboli have the possibility of entering the central circulation or embolizing peripherally to cause tissue ischemia. Care should be taken to monitor for clots in the line and avoid forceful flushing.

© 2006 Mayo Foundation for Medical Education and Research

Central lines and vascular access devices are common in the OR and ICU population. Lumens not connected to continuous infusions require intermittent flushing to remain patent or before being put into use. Every line that remains patent is one less line you will have to replace. As with arterial lines, there is risk of air and clot embolization with excessive flushing of lines and/or lack of vigilance in eliminating air and clot from circuits and injections. Infection from indwelling catheters is a serious and frequent occurrence. Maintaining aseptic technique by using alcohol to clean the access port before flushing or accessing lines is required to decrease this risk. *Before flushing, the line should be aspirated and the old blood that has been sitting in the line should be discarded.* There are two reasons to do this—first, there is no reason to flush into the circulation blood that may have formed clots or be colonized with bacteria that found a nice culture medium of old blood. Second, large-bore indwelling catheters such as the double-lumen Groshong or Shiley catheters that are used for dialysis access will have between 2,500 and 5,000 units of heparin in each lumen. The frequency and volume of flush varies among institutions and depends on the type of catheter. Typically, central lines list the volume on the packaging or on the lumen of the catheter. Groshong catheters need to be flushed weekly; other central lines often need to be flushed more than once per day to remain patent. Saline or heparinized flush may be used, depending on institution preference. When in doubt, consult the ICU or dialysis services at your practicing institution; they will be able to advise you.

Patients may come to the operating room with vascular access devices, such as Port-A-Cath, Q-Port, or Infuse-A-Port, that may be used for infusions. These can be useful devices for anesthesiologists in patients with poor venous access. However, there are also several caveats to accessing these ports. First, why was the device placed? How has it been maintained, and when was it last accessed? Is it currently in use for ongoing chemotherapy treatments? Second, you must know how to access the device. Again, maintaining aseptic technique is necessary, using sterile gloves and cleaning the port site with alcohol. Palpate the skin to find the port septum, which may be on the top or the side of the device. To avoid damage to the septum, a noncoring needle (usually a right-angle Huber needle) is used to access the port. The needle is pushed through the septum until it hits the bottom of the reservoir. Aspirate for blood and discard the old blood, flush with saline, and apply a sterile dressing. The needle can be connected to an infusion or an extension set and flushed as your institution directs. Before deaccessing, the port is flushed with a heparinized solution to maintain patency. It is important to use the right amount of heparin, as an excessive amount may lead to unintentional systemic anticoagulation. If you are unsure about whether the port can or should be used and how to deaccess it, contact the oncology service. Usually, the oncology or chemotherapy nurses will be able to advise you. Remember that these needles and ports are designed for slow drips, not for boluses, because chemotherapy is generally given over several hours. They will not look or infuse the way a normal "induction IV" does, and caution must be taken when using them to induce a patient.

Indwelling lines for access and monitoring are necessary and useful devices in anesthesiology. However, these lines have the potential for complications. Knowing the proper methods of care and access will decrease these risks and improve perioperative patient care.

TAKE HOME POINTS

- The volume of the arterial tree from radial artery to vertebral artery is only about 6 cm!
- Never "power flush" the arterial line either by hand or via a prolonged flush through the valve. This can fill the fill the 6-cm volume in 1 to 2 seconds.
- Don't flush a line if there are visible air bubbles or clots in either the central or arterial line.
- Remember that there is a *significant* amount of heparin in the lumens of the common in-dwelling catheters—always withdraw from them before you flush.
- Vascular access ports must be accessed with a noncoring needle to avoid damaging the diaphragm.

SUGGESTED READINGS

Bedford RF. Complication of intensive cardiovascular monitoring. In: Gravenstein N, Kirby RR, eds. *Complications in Anesthesiology*. 2nd ed. Philadephlia: Lippincott-Raven; 1996.

Cohen N, Brett CM. Arterial catherization. In: Benumof J, ed. *Clinical Procedures in Anesthesia and Intensive Care*. Philadelphia: JB Lippincott; 1992:375–389.

Lowenstein E, Little JW, Lo HH. Prevention of cerebral embolization from flushing radial-artery cannulas. *N Engl J Med*. 1971;285:1414–1415.

Morray J, Sandra T. A hazard of continuous flush systems for vascular pressure monitoring in infants. *Anesthesiology*. 1983;58:187–189.

Perucca R. Infusion monitoring and catheter care. In: Hankins J, Lonsway RAW, Hedrick C, Perdue MB, eds. *Infusion Therapy in Clinical Practice*. Philadelphia: WB Sanders; 2001:389–397.

Seneff MG. Arterial line placement and care. In: Irwin RS, Cerra FB, Rippe JM, eds. *Intensive Care Medicine*. 4th ed. Vol. 1. Philadelphia: Lippincott-Raven; 1999:36–46.

26

DO NOT USE THE SUBCLAVIAN VEIN FOR CENTRAL ACCESS OF ANY TYPE IN A PATIENT PLANNED FOR DIALYSIS

MICHAEL J. MORITZ, MD AND CATHERINE MARCUCCI, MD

There are about 300,000 hemodialysis patients in the United States today, and the number is increasing by about 4% to 5% annually. The increasing incidences of diabetes mellitus and hypertension, and the relative scarcity of renal transplants (still only about 10,000 annually in the United States) mean that hemodialysis will continue to be required. For many patients who will never receive a transplant, hemodialysis must be considered a life-long treatment. Because the critical nature of vascular access for hemodialysis is amplified by length of time on treatment, provision and maintenance of vascular access will remain one of the greatest problems in dialysis medicine.

In the most optimal situation, permanent dialysis access is placed in advance of dialysis. However, more commonly, patients present with an acute need for dialysis that requires temporary dialysis access via a percutaneous catheter. Anesthesiologists will usually be confronted with this situation as part of the intensive care management of a patient. If there is any thought that the patient may go on to require chronic dialysis, it is imperative that the temporary access not compromise the vasculature. The preferred sites for temporary access catheter placement are the internal jugular veins or the femoral veins—*not* the subclavian veins.

Temporary percutaneous dialysis catheters are associated with significant damage to the cannulated vein, and there is a very real risk of acute or delayed thrombosis or stenosis of the vein. Dialysis catheters in subclavian veins have been associated with a rate of thrombosis/stenosis of 50% to 70%, versus 0 to 10% for catheters placed in the internal jugular veins. Patients with subclavian vein occlusion may have spontaneous recanalization after 3 to 6 months and can also be treated with angioplasty and stent placement, but the vein will never be completely normal. Remember that permanent hemodialysis access involves an arterial-to-venous connection, either as a fistula (direct artery-to-vein connection) or with a prosthetic graft between the artery and vein. The longest-lasting and most successful access is placed in the upper extremity because of lower infection rates and better patient comfort. Permanent hemodialysis access will create high flow through the vessels of the upper extremity, and the success and function of the site is highly dependent on adequate venous outflow from the access site to the

© 2006 Mayo Foundation for Medical Education and Research

right atrium. Decreased venous outflow can also create profound edema that can be limb-threatening.

Although the risk of injury to the subclavian vein is less with smaller catheters such as sheaths for pulmonary artery catheters and triple- or single-lumen central lines, subclavian vein cannulation with these lines should be avoided for the same reasons. Remember that subclavian thrombosis or stenosis (even if clinically silent) results in loss of all potential access sites in the ipsilateral extremity.

TAKE HOME POINTS

- Many renal failure patients will never receive a kidney transplant and will require lifelong dialysis.
- Temporary access secured in the perioperative period for dialysis and other reasons must not compromise the vasculature of the upper extremity.
- For this reason, catheters (especially dialysis cathers) should be preferentially placed in the internal jugular veins.

SUGGESTED READINGS

Bander SJ, Schwab SJ. Central venous angioaccess for hemodialysis and its complications. *Semin Dial.* 1992;5:121–128.
Cimochowski GE, Worley E, Rutherford WE, et al. Superiority of the internal jugular over the subclavian access for temporary hemodialysis. *Nephron.* 1990;54:154–161.

27

REMEMBER THAT INADVERTENT INTRA-ARTERIAL INJECTION IS NOT RARE

MICHAEL S. N. HOGAN, MB, BCH, SURJYA SEN, MD
AND JURAJ SPRUNG, MD, PHD

The estimated incidence of iatrogenic complication from accidental intra-arterial (IA) injection of drugs is between 1 in 3,440 and 1 in 56,000 anesthetics administered. The potential complications range from none to severe tissue ischemia and necrosis necessitating amputation. All anesthesia providers should be aware of risk factors, signs and symptoms, available therapeutic modalities, and preventive measures for IA drug injection during anesthesia. Commonly used anesthetic drugs and inadvertent IA injection effects are shown in *Table 27.1*.

RISK FACTORS FOR IA INJECTION

- Patients who are unable to report pain on injection. Patients during general anesthesia, comatose patients, or patients with altered mental status, and very young pediatric patients.
- Pre-existing vascular anomalies of the forearm. The most common arterial anomaly of the upper limb is a high-rising radial artery resulting in a superficial branch (prevalence, 1% to 14%). This anomaly results in the radial artery ending in a thin superficial palmar branch that can be mistakenly cannulated (*Fig. 27.1, Left*). Another common anomaly (1% prevalence) is the antebrachialis superficialis dorsalis artery (*Fig. 27.1, Right*). The radial artery bifurcates in the forearm, resulting in an anomalous superficial branch between the index finger and thumb. Often, this branch will cross underneath a terminal branch of the cephalic vein, just superficial to the radial styloid process—a common site for insertion of intravenous (IV) catheters (called the "intern vein").
- High-risk anatomic locations, where arteries and veins lie in close proximity.
  - Antecubital fossa: brachial artery may be cannulated rather than the median basilic vein.
  - Groin: femoral artery cannulation rather than femoral vein.
- Multiple infusions through several IV lines with numerous ports (patients in the intensive care unit).
- Miscellaneous factors. Morbid obesity, darkly pigmented skin, multiple attempts at line placement, placement of lines under nonideal situations (central line during operations and/or without ultrasonographic

TABLE 27.1	EFFECTS OF IA INJECTION OF COMMONLY USED ANESTHETIC AGENTS
DRUG	**EFFECT OF IA INJECTION**
Midazolam	Initial discoloration but no long-term effect
Promethazine, chlorpromazine	Gangrene
Thiopental	Chemical endarteritis, immediate vasoconstriction, thrombosis, tissue necrosis, endothelial cell destruction
Etomidate	No reports of necrosis
Ketamine	Proximal skin necrosis
Propofol	Pain, cutaneous hyperemia
Lidocaine	Used therapeutically, no adverse effects
Penicillin	Gangrene
Cefazolin, ceftazidime	Arteriospasm and distal necrosis
Meperidine	Gangrene
Sodium bicarbonate	Edema, erythema, pain; tissue necrosis
Metoclopramide	Discoloration but no long-term effect
Phenytoin	Cyanosis, digital artery occlusion, gangrene
Atracurium	Marked ischemia but full recovery
Dextrose solution	Gangrene
Calcium chloride	No adverse effects reported Used therapeutically to localize insulinoma
Ephedrine, phenylephrine, epinephrine, succinylcholine, vecuronium, rocuronium, fentanyl, oxymorphone, hydromorphone, ketorolac, ondansetron, atropine, glycopyrrolate, neostigmine	No reports available

IA, intra-arterial.

guidance), those with a pre-existing arterial or venous catheter who present for urgent resuscitation (trauma).

SIGNS AND SYMPTOMS OF ARTERIAL CANNULATION

- Bright red backflow and/or pulsatile blood into an IV catheter
- Backflow of blood into the IV tubing, even with the fluid bag at a higher level than the catheter insertion site
- Increase in blood pressure on an indwelling arterial catheter with ipsilateral "IV" bolus
- Distal (e.g., nail bed) signs of ischemia (pallor) and skin mottling with "IV" fluid bolus
- Greater-than-expected pain with injection

PATHOPHYSIOLOGY

Although the underlying pathophysiologic mechanisms to explain the sequelae of an IA drug injection remain unclear, a few concrete conclusions can be drawn.

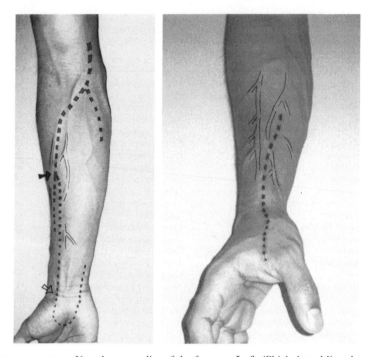

FIGURE 27.1. Vascular anomalies of the forearm. **Left:** Thick dotted line shows abnormal artery. *Open arrow,* normal branching point of radial artery; *closed arrow,* anomalous high-rising radial artery. **Right:** Thick dotted line shows anomalous antebrachialis superficialis dorsalis radial artery. Thin black lines show typical venous pattern. The abnormal artery course is in close proximity to commonly cannulated veins. (From Sen S, Chini EN, Brown MJ. Complications after unintentional intraarterial injection of drugs: risks, outcomes, and management strategies. *Mayo Clin Proc.* 2005;80:783–795. Used with permission of Mayo Foundation for Medical Education and Research.)

- Not all medications cause ischemia by the same mechanism. Some may cause crystallization and mechanical blockage of blood flow, whereas others may be directly toxic to the endothelium.
- Regardless of the mechanisms involved, thrombosis seems to be the common end point.

TREATMENT OPTIONS

Most treatment modalities are based on maintaining distal perfusion to the involved extremity. Management should be based on the following principles:

- Immediately stopping administration of the offending agent
- Cessation or reversal of arterial spasm

- Maintaining or re-establishing blood flow to distal extremities
- Treating any sequelae of vascular injury or ischemia (edema, compartment syndrome, infection, necrosis, gangrene)
- Symptomatic relief

Step 1: Maintain the IA Catheter **in Situ.** When an inadvertent IA injection occurs, the first instinct may be to remove the catheter, but maintaining the arterial catheter has several advantages. First, the catheter should be cleared of any remaining drug, either by opening the catheter to atmosphere to allow backflow of blood or by simply aspirating with a syringe. This should be followed by slow infusion of heparinized saline to help maintain catheter patency. If there is any doubt regarding the catheter site (i.e., arterial vs. venous), confirm placement by drawing a sample for arterial blood gas analysis or by transducing the line. Maintaining the IA catheter will also allow immediate delivery of specific medications to the site of injury, including contrast dye for angiography. If the larger-bore IA catheter was placed inadvertently, removing the catheter may also require surgical intervention to suture the large hole in the artery.

Step 2: Identify Potential for Injury. Certain clinical indicators can be roughly correlated with progressive tissue injury. Treiman et al. developed a "tissue ischemia score" based on signs and symptoms at presentation of 48 patients with IA injections. Patients were assigned a 0 for the absence or a 1 for the presence of four symptoms: cyanosis, cool extremity, delayed capillary refill, and sensory deficit. Of patients who had a tissue ischemia score of 2 or lower, 92% had a normal outcome. Of patients who had a score higher than 2, only 41% had a normal outcome in the involved extremity; the others had tissue necrosis or permanent neurologic dysfunction.

Step 3: Initiate Anticoagulation. Administration of heparin seems to be broadly accepted as the initial treatment of IA injections. There is no consensus on the initial bolus amounts to use, appropriate target ranges for the activated partial thromboplastin time (aPTT), or duration of therapy, but an initial loading dose of 60 U/kg with subsequent aPTT goals of 1.5 to 2.3 times higher than normal seem prudent. Of course, this must be balanced against the risk of hemorrhage in a postoperative patient. The duration of therapy can then be guided by resolution of symptoms, angiographic evidence of clot resolution, or the need for surgical intervention.

Step 4: Symptomatic Relief. Increased sympathetic vascular tone, edema distal to the site of injury, muscle injury or forced flexion contractures, temperature hypersensitivity, and paresthesias may all contribute to ongoing pain. Multiple case reports suggest that oral analgesics, elevation, massage, and passive motion devices can be critical to treatment and recovery.

Step 5: Specific Interventions. After implementing the first four steps, it is important to determine whether any other specific intervention is needed. The following interventions have been used with varying degrees of success:

- Local anesthetic injection: IA lidocaine (without epinephrine) to prevent or treat reflex vasospasm
- Extremity sympatholysis: stellate ganglion/axillary plexus blocks
- Arterial vasodilators: calcium-channel blockers (nicardipine)
- Thromboxane synthase inhibitors: topical aloe vera, methimazole, aspirin, methylprednisolone
- Iloprost: a prostacyclin analog used for various ischemic conditions
- IA papaverine: induces vascular smooth muscle relaxation by increasing intracellular cyclic adenosine monophosphate levels
- IA thrombolytics
- Hyperbaric oxygen therapy
- Corticosteroids: mainstay of treatment for any condition involving inflammation.

PREVENTION OF IA INJECTION

- Be aware of the risk and maintain a high index of suspicion when placing any intravascular catheter, particularly in antecubital and cephalic veins.
- Look for signs of arterial cannulation as outlined above.
- Use caution and maintain an index of suspicion with all pre-existing lines.
- Palpate target veins before IV placement.
- Do not tie a tourniquet tight enough to occlude arterial flow.
- Use clear labeling of arterial line at all injection ports.
- Color-code lines and injection ports.
- Remove unnecessary injection ports or stopcocks. If an injection port is necessary, keep it as close to the patient as possible.
- Trace each extension line back to the site of the cannula before injecting any medications.

Despite recognition of accidental IA injections for many decades, these cases still commonly occur. As always, the best solutions are prevention and continuous vigilance. Clinicians should be aware of risk factors for IA injection, the associated signs and symptoms, the underlying pathophysiology, and available treatment options. Such awareness will help decrease the incidence, delays in diagnosis, and resulting complications of this medical error.

TAKE HOME POINTS

- Remember that inadvertent IA injection is not rare.
- IA happens because you mistake an artery for a vein line on insertion of the cannula or because you mistakenly inject into the wrong stopcock.

- Develop techniques for making sure you do not get venous and arterial lines and/or stopcocks mixed up—red and blue tape at injection ports, etc. Minimize the number of ports.
- Do not take out the catheter if there is an inadvertent injection.
- Inform the necessary people (surgeons, etc.) and start treatment as soon as possible.

SUGGESTED READINGS

Book LS, Herbst JJ. Intra-arterial infusions and intestinal necrosis in the rabbit: potential hazards of umbilical artery injections of ampicillin, glucose, and sodium bicarbonate. *Pediatrics.* 1980;65:1145–1149.

Cohen SM. Accidental intra-arterial injection of drugs. *Lancet.* 1948;2:361–371, 409–416.

Doppman JL, Chang R, Fraker DL, et al. Localization of insulinomas to regions of the pancreas by intra-arterial stimulation with calcium. *Ann Intern Med.* 1995;123:269–273. Erratum in: *Ann Intern Med.* 1995;123:734.

Murphy EJ. Intra-arterial injection of metoclopramide, midazolam, propofol and pethidine. *Anaesth Intensive Care.* 2002;30:367–369.

Ohana E, Sheiner E, Gurman GM. Accidental intra-arterial injection of propofol. *Eur J Anaesthesiol.* 1999;16:569–570.

Sen S, Chini EN, Brown MJ. Complications after unintentional intra-arterial injection of drugs: risks, outcomes, and management strategies. *Mayo Clin Proc.* 2005;80:783–795.

Sivalingam P. Inadvertent cannulation of an aberrant radial artery and intra-arterial injection of midazolam. *Anaesth Intensive Care.* 1999;27:424–425.

Treiman GS, Yellin AE, Weaver FA, et al. An effective treatment protocol for intraarterial drug injection. *J Vasc Surg.* 1990;12:456–465.

Wood SJ, Abrahams PH, Sanudo JR, Ferreira BJ. Bilateral superficial radial artery at the wrist associated with a radial origin of unilateral median artery. *J Anat.* 1996;189:691–693.

Zveibil FR, Monies-Chass I. Accidental intra-arterial injection of ketamine. *Anaesthesia.* 1976;31:1084–1085.

28

AVOID ERRORS IN INVASIVE BLOOD PRESSURE MEASUREMENT

MICHAEL S. N. HOGAN, MB, BCH AND
JURAJ SPRUNG, MD, PHD

Monitoring of a patient's blood pressure (BP) is crucial to the safe conduct of any surgical procedure. This chapter focuses on invasive arterial-line BP monitoring and some of the common errors associated with inaccurate readings.

For an arterial monitoring system to provide an accurate reading of the measured waveform, it must have an appropriate natural frequency and damping (*Fig. 28.1A*). Briefly, each measuring system has a natural frequency about which it oscillates. This frequency is proportional to the stiffness of the tubing and the transducer diaphragm and to the cross-sectional area of the catheter. It is inversely proportional to the catheter length and fluid density. If the frequency of the pressure wave being measured approaches the natural frequency of the system, the system distorts the measurements by excessive amplification (ringing or resonance) of the incoming waveform. This may overestimate the systolic BP by as much as 25% and underestimate the diastolic BP by 10% (the mean pressure is not affected). Damping counteracts this phenomenon.

Several problems can occur in this interaction between the natural frequency and damping parameters. Overdamping decreases the frequency response too much, underestimating the systolic BP and overestimating the diastolic BP (*Fig. 28.1B*). Blood clots, air bubbles in the tubing, and kinked catheters are common causes of an overdamped system. Underdamping, or hyperresonance, occurs when long connecting lines (>1.4 m) or small-diameter tubing (<1.5 mm internal diameter) are used or when the catheter is too large for the vessel (e.g., 18-gauge catheter in a small radial artery). This overestimates the systolic BP and underestimates the diastolic BP. Underdamping may also cause the appearance of additional, small, nonphysiologic pressure waves on the tracing (*Fig. 28.1C*). Slow degradation in the dynamic response also may occur over time (decrease in the natural frequency with increase in the damping coefficients), causing underdamping. Fortunately, this problem can be easily rectified with periodic manual flushing of the system.

Problems within the system that lead to inaccurate measurements are usually due to problems with the mechanical connection components (i.e., the catheter, fluid-filled tubing, or the stopcock). To prevent these mechanical problems, several steps should be followed.

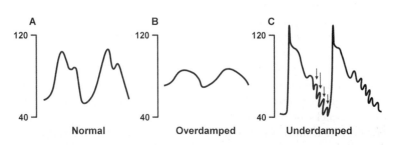

FIGURE 28.1. Arterial blood pressure (BP) waveform tracings. A: Normal. B: Overdamped tracing, causing underestimated systolic BP and overestimated diastolic BP. C: Underdamped tracing, causing overestimated systolic BP and underestimated diastolic BP. Extra nonphysiologic waveforms on the underdamped tracing reflect hyperresonance of the measuring system (*arrows*).

- Choose the proper size arterial cannula (20 gauge for radial or brachial, 18 gauge for femoral).
- Optimize the frequency response of the measuring system by using tubing that is short (maximum length, 120 cm), wide (1.5 to 3.0 mm internal diameter), and rigid.
- Use only one stopcock per line. Keep the tubing, stopcocks, and domes free of bubbles and clots. Avoid kinks in the tubing.
- If arterial BP is overdamped:
  - Try flushing the line.
  - Keep the entire mechanical coupling system flushed with heparinized saline to prevent development of clots (1 U of heparin per milliliter of normal saline) at 1 to 3 mL/hour.
  - Be sure that the flushing system of the arterial line is adequately pressurized.
- If arterial BP is underdamped:
  - Use a resonance overshoot eliminator (commercial product).
  - Temporarily put a small air bubble in the system (do not forget to withdraw it immediately after measurement is accomplished). This can help to estimate the "real" BP, but this is a controversial technique that not all authors recommend.
- Use a transducer with the highest possible frequency response.
- Zero the arterial line to atmospheric pressure to provide a reference point. By convention, the transducer is placed level with the right atrium or midaxillary line. For a sitting patient, the transducer is placed at the level of the brain (ear). Check frequently for improper zeroing and drift. Every time the measured BP is "out of expected range," quickly check that the transducer is zeroed (open the transducer to air and see if the baseline goes

to zero; waiting for the digital reading to confirm the proper "zeroing" numerically is not necessary. Readjust the transducer after every change in patient positioning.

Anesthesiologists often have no control over the inherent natural frequency and damping coefficients present in monitoring systems. Furthermore, clinical circumstances sometimes require longer extension tubing or extra stopcocks for blood sampling and flushing. In these circumstances, the fast-flush test, described in *Fig. 28.2*, is a convenient bedside method for determining system performance parameters. The damping coefficient may be determined as described in the legend of *Fig. 28.2*.

In the clinical situation, if there are two different arterial BP readings (e.g., noninvasive vs. invasive, left arm vs. right arm) and/or two different waveforms (e.g., femoral vs. radial), it may not be clear which pressure to "trust." The phenomenon of distal pulse amplification can affect the morphology and detail of the arterial waveform and can often give important diagnostic information. In short, pressure waveforms recorded simultaneously from different arterial sites will have different morphologies. This difference is due to the physical characteristics of the vascular tree—specifically, impedance and harmonic resonance. As the arterial pressure wave travels toward the periphery, the arterial upstroke steepens, the systolic peak increases, the dicrotic notch appears later, the diastolic wave becomes more prominent, and the end-diastolic pressure decreases. This results in higher systolic pressure, lower diastolic pressure, and wider pulse pressure. In addition, a substantial difference between peripherally measured BP (radial artery) and more centrally measured BP may temporarily exist in specific conditions such as after cardiopulmonary bypass surgery. However, despite these differences, the mean arterial pressure between central and peripheral readings should be roughly the same. Ultimately, the pressure that can more adversely affect outcome (e.g., low systolic BP in a patient with critical aortic stenosis) is the one that should be "believed."

During the course of a surgery, if significant hypotension occurs, the following steps should be performed:

- Look for other obvious signs of hypotension:
  - Sudden decrease in end-tidal CO_2 (indicates low cardiac output and poor perfusion of pulmonary vasculature)
  - Poorly palpable radial pulse (can indicate systolic BP <55 to 65 mm Hg)
- Check the result against a cuff pressure. If a substantial discrepancy exists:
  - Check the transducer position. Having the patient higher than the transducer produces falsely high readings and vice versa. The magnitude of the error is exactly equal to the difference in hydrostatic pressure between the patient and the transducer (1 mm Hg = 1.3 cm H_2O).

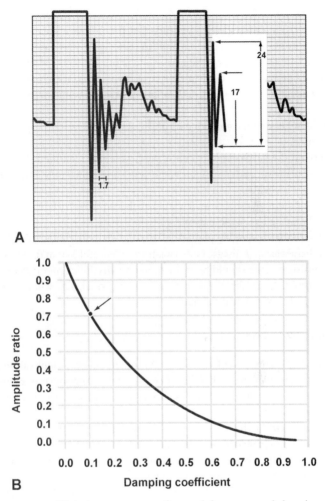

FIGURE 28.2. Clinical measurement of natural frequency and damping coefficient with the fast-flush test. **A:** Two square-wave fast-flush artifacts interrupt an arterial pressure waveform recorded on standard 1-mm grid paper at a speed of 25 mm/second. Natural frequency is determined by measuring the period of one cycle of adjacent oscillation peaks (1.7 mm). The damping coefficient is determined by measuring the heights of adjacent oscillation peaks (17 and 24 mm). From these measurements, a natural frequency of 14.7 Hz (1 cycle/1.7 mm × 25 mm/s = 14.7 cycle/second) and an amplitude ratio of 0.71 may be calculated. **B:** The amplitude ratio corresponds to a damping coefficient of 0.11, suggesting overdamping (an optimally damped system has a damping coefficient of 0.6 to 0.7). (From Mark JB. *Atlas of Cardiovascular Monitoring.* New York: Churchill Livingstone; 1998:112–113. Used with permission.)

- Zero the reference value on the monitor. Open the stopcock to air and inspect the monitor screen to ensure that the pressure trace overlies the zero pressure line on the screen and that the digital pressure value equals zero. (Note that checking the zero value is not the same as "zeroing the arterial line," which is done at the start of the procedure.) If the pressure is not equal to zero, baseline drift of the electrical circuit's transducer has occurred.
- Double-check all the components of the system (electrical plug-ins, loose attachments, etc.).
- Interrupt the surgical course until the problem is identified. In extreme cases, ask the surgeon to palpate some of the abdominal or thoracic vessels if any are accessible.
- Do not assume an overdamped waveform, because the "overdamped wave-form" may be true hypotension.
- Be aware that severe "hypotension" on one extremity may reflect severe peripheral vascular disease (subclavian stenosis), and that in these patients BP measurements should be made on both extremities (noninvasively, or by palpating the radial pulse) before deciding which side will be used for placing the invasive arterial line.

TAKE HOME POINTS

- Measuring systems oscillate around a natural frequency, which can amplify a measured waveform, if the frequencies are close. Damping can counteract this, but be aware that a variety of factors can cause either underdamping or overdamping.
- Problems within the system that lead to inaccurate measurements are usually due to problems with the mechanical connection components.
- Pressure waveforms recorded simultaneously from different arterial sites will have different morphologies. This difference is due to the physical characteristics of the vascular tree—specifically, impedance and harmonic resonance.
- The mean arterial pressure between central and peripheral readings should be roughly the same.
- If the blood pressure measurement decreases suddenly, do not assume an overdamped waveform, because the "overdamped waveform" may be true hypotension.

SUGGESTED READINGS

Faust RJ, ed. *Anesthesiology Review*. New York: Churchill Livingstone; 2002.
Mark JB, Slaughter TF. Cardiovascular monitoring. In: Miller RD, ed. *Miller's Anesthesia*. 6th ed. Philadelphia: Churchill Livingstone; 2005:1265–1362.

29

REMEMBER THAT LOSS OF A PATENT HEMODIALYSIS FISTULA IN THE PERIOPERATIVE PERIOD IS A SERIOUS EVENT FOR THE PATIENT AND REQUIRES IMMEDIATE COMMUNICATION WITH THE SURGEONS

ANAGH VORA, MD AND STEVEN J. BUSUTTIL, MD, FACS

Chronic renal insufficiency/failure (CRI/F) is a leading cause of morbidity and mortality in a growing percentage of the U.S. population. Most causes of end-stage renal disease stem from two major comorbid conditions—diabetes mellitus and hypertension. The ultimate end result of CRF is reliance on hemodialysis for maintenance of renal function. The use of hemodialysis fistulas has both improved the quality and prolonged the lives of CRF patients, although there are associated complications (*Table 29.1*).

HEMODIALYSIS FISTULAS

Hemodialysis fistulas or ports for dialysis are surgically created communications between the native artery and vein in an extremity. Direct communications between artery and vein are called native arteriovenous fistulas (AVFs). Polytetrafluoroethylene (PTFE) and other materials (Dacron, polyurethane) are used or have been used as a communication medium between the artery and the vein and are termed prosthetic hemodialysis access arteriovenous grafts (AVGs). The patency rates for AVFs are about four times greater than for AVGs. The access that is created is routinely used for hemodialysis two to five times per week. Preservation of a patent well-functioning dialysis fistula is one of the most challenging issues for the dialysis patient. As many as 25% of hospital admissions in the dialysis population have been attributed to vascular access problems, including fistula malfunction and thrombosis.

In fact, only 15% of dialysis fistulas remain patent and can function without problems during the entire period of a patient's dependence on hemodialysis. The majority of patients who have native fistulas placed will be problem free with their fistulas for a mean of 3 years after creation, whereas prosthetic PTFE grafts usually last only about a year before indications of failure or thrombosis are noted.

Long-term secondary patency rates are reportedly 7 years in the forearm, 3 to 5 years in the upper arm for native fistulas, and about 1 year for prosthetic grafts after multiple interventions to treat the underlying stenosis and thrombosis.

ⓒ 2006 Mayo Foundation for Medical Education and Research

TABLE 29.1 **COMPLICATIONS OF HEMODIALYSIS FISTULAS**

- Hemodynamic complications—congestive heart failure
- Arterial steal syndrome
- Carpal tunnel syndrome
- Infection
- Noninfectious fluid collections—seroma, lymphocele, hematoma
- Aneurysm, pseudo-aneurysm

ARTERIOVENOUS FISTULA FAILURE

The underlying cause of AVF failure in the nonacute setting or outpatient setting is invariably thrombosis due to venous anastomosis in prosthetic grafts or anastomosis of the outflow vein in native fistulas (*Table 29.2*). The pathophysiology behind this failure is the eventual intimal hyperplasia at the anastomosis site. Future therapy is directed at halting the intimal growth of anastomotic vessels, using technology similar to that employed with drug-eluting cardiac stents.

The main cause of AVF thrombosis in the acute care setting, particularly the perioperative period, is almost always low flow, usually caused by hypotension and/or poor cardiac output. A sudden decrease in blood pressure can lead to platelet aggregation, sledging, and eventual thrombosis. An important secondary cause for the loss of a patent fistula is excessive external pressure on the AVF, usually as a result of monitoring or positioning. Remember also that surgical patients are in a hypercoagulable state—this may also predispose to thrombotic events.

It is imperative that anesthesia providers recognize the clinical signs of impending AVF thrombosis. It is wise to evaluate the fistula as thoroughly as possible *before* starting the anesthetic. Remember that dialysis patients are often the best source for information on their personal fistula histories.

Clinical signs of impending AVF thrombosis include the following:

- Loss of thrill
- Increase pulsatility (water-hammer pulse)
- Direct palpation of stenosis

TABLE 29.2 **CAUSES OF AVF THROMBOSIS**

- Poor cardiac outflow (hypotension)—sudden decrease in blood pressure can lead to platelet aggregation, sledging, and eventual thrombosis.
- Excessive pressure on AVF (blood pressure measurement)
- Hypercoagulable state
- Progressive inflow stenosis
- Venous outflow stenosis

- Insufficient inflow, such as stenosis in the supplying native artery or proximally in the subclavian or brachiocephalic artery
- Identification of high venous pressures or low flow according to the protocol provided by the specific type of hemodialysis machine—try to ascertain whether there were problems with the duration of treatment or volume of fluid removed in the last dialysis run before surgery.
- Ipsilateral arm edema and/or collateral venous pathways suggestive of a central venous stenosis

Similarly, the care of AVFs during anesthesia requires the very close attention of the practitioner:

- Maintain normotension—hypotension may lead to clot formation and thrombosis.
- Maintain heart rate—symptomatic bradycardia may decrease coronary output and lead to thrombosis.
- Do *not* place the noninvasive blood pressure cuff on the AVF arm—compression can limit inflow/outflow and promote thrombosis.
- Do *not* perform venipuncture on the AVF arm—local clotting factors may favor thrombosis. If you get stuck for sites for line placements, consult with the surgeons and/or vascular surgeons before the start of the operation. Emergency situations may involve broaching the integrity of the vasculature of the extremity that has the fistula—if so, expect that the fistula may be lost and make proactive plans.
- Actively feel and *document* presence of a thrill at regular intervals during the procedure—presence confirms a functioning AVF.
- Consider regional anesthesia when appropriate to minimize fluctuations in blood pressuer and heart rate.
- Document the thrill when signing the patient out in the PACU or ICU.
- Communicate immediately with the surgeon if there is a change in AVF status (this usually means the loss of the thrill)

TREATMENT OF AVF THROMBOSIS

Unfortunately, thrombosis of dialysis access is not an uncommon event during the perioperative period. Historically, treatment of AVF thrombosis involved surgical thrombectomy with ongoing hospital admission. Typically, surgical treatment resulted in sacrificing a portion of the outflow vein.

Multiple treatment options are now available and depend on the patient's co-morbid conditions, the availability of the appropriate surgical personnel, the availability of radiologic support, and previous fistula treatment (*Table 29.3*). Often, a radiologic intervention is considered most favorable if possible. Patients may thus sometimes go directly from the PACU to interventional radiology. Alternatively, other dialysis access, such as a double-lumen Shiley, may be placed in the immediate postoperative period. Occasionally,

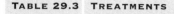

TABLE 29.3   TREATMENTS

- Thrombolysis
  - With angioplasty
  - Without angioplasty
- Percutaneous thrombectomy
  - With angioplasty
  - Without angioplasty
- Surgical thrombectomy
  - With revision
  - Without revision

treatment is deferred until the patient is clinically and hemodynamically stable.

TAKE HOME POINTS

- Native AVFs are less prone to thrombosis than grafts.
- Loss of the graft is a serious perioperative event for the patient.
- Low flow states caused by hypotension, low cardiac output, and external compression are the most significant causes of fistula thrombosis. If there is a new or existing hemodialysis fistula, think carefully before lowering the blood pressure aggressively with propofol, labetalol, or hydralazine.
- Maintain high vigilance for hemodynamics and positioning.
- Don't be afraid to consult the surgeons about the preferred sites for both venous and arterial line placement.
- Check for the thrill at regular intervals and let the surgeons know immediately if the thrill is lost.
- One final point—what you feel when lightly palpating the fistula is *not* a bruit—*by definition*, a bruit is an abnormal sound heard when placing a stethoscope over an artery.

SUGGESTED READINGS

Maya ID, Oser R, Saddekni S, et al. Vascular access stenosis: comparison of arteriovenous grafts and fistulas. *Am J Kidney Dis.* 2004;44(5):859–865.

Swedberg SH, Brown BG, Sigley R, et al. Intimal fibromuscular hyperplasia at the venous anastomosis of PTFE grafts in hemodialysis patients. Clinical, immunocytochemical, light and electron microscopic assessment. *Circulation.* 1989;80(6):1726–1736.

Zibari GB, Rohr MS, Landreneau MD, et al. Complications from permanent hemodialysis vascular access. *Surgery.* 1988;104(4):681–686.

FLUIDS, RESUSCITATION, AND TRANSFUSION

30

HYPERTONIC SALINE: THE "SOLUTION" TO THE SOLUTION PROBLEM?

LAVINIA M. KOLARCZYK, MD AND PATRICK J. FORTE, MD

Analogous to the variety of beverages in your supermarket's soda aisle, there exist numerous choices for fluids for patients. What is best for your patient's needs? What fluid is appropriate for specific situations? How much fluid should be administered? Although these questions may seem trivial, the knee-jerk reflex for most residents is to use a fluid that they feel most comfortable administering. Let us wade out of the "normal saline" pool and explore the clinical uses of hypertonic saline.

Fluids became the focus of prehospital resuscitation research more than 75 years ago. The same clinical problems encountered with fluid resuscitation efforts then remain the focus of today's research. The search continues for an "ideal" fluid, i.e., one that is inexpensive, generates sustained hemodynamic effects with minimal peripheral or pulmonary edema, and is effective even in small volumes.

Traditionally, isotonic crystalloids such as lactated Ringer's solution and normal saline have been considered first-line treatment for trauma patients. Although these fluids are inexpensive, readily available, nonallergenic, noninfectious, and efficacious in restoring total body fluid, they lack oxygen-carrying capacity and coagulation capability, and they have limited intravascular half-life. A proposed solution to the "solution problem" is to augment the osmotic properties of traditional resuscitation fluids. In theory, this would extend the intravascular half-life and reduce the amount of third spacing. The "ideal" fluid search then focused on osmotic properties, and hypertonic saline (with and without colloid) became a prime subject of research.

Hypertonic saline already had a role in the trauma setting, as it was used for patients with increased intracranial pressure secondary to traumatic head injury. Of note, mannitol (an osmotic diuretic and cerebral arteriolar vasoconstrictor) was traditionally used as first-line therapy in this patient population, but it was associated with rebound intracranial hypertension. It was believed that this effect was due to intravascular dehydration and an inability to maintain cerebral perfusion pressure when diuresis was not matched by appropriate fluid administration. Hypertonic saline became the agent of choice, as it served a dual purpose as a diuretic and a resuscitative agent.

© 2006 Mayo Foundation for Medical Education and Research

TABLE 30.1	HYPERTONIC SALINE: BEYOND PLASMA VOLUME EXPANSION
Vasoregulatory effects	Counteracts vasospasm occurring after traumatic brain injury through its vasodilatory effects. Improves microvascular perfusion by attenuating leukocyte–endothelial interactions.
Immunologic effects	Changes in extracellular sodium that occur after injury may be attenuated by hypertonic saline, which is thought to depress leukocyte adherence and neutrophil margination.
Neurochemical effects	Changes in excitatory neurotransmitters that occur after injury may be attenuated by hypertonic saline, which stimulates adrenocorticotropin and cortisol release.

Further research in the use of hypertonic saline in the trauma setting revealed that it had vasoregulator, immunologic, and neurochemical effects (*Table 30.1*). Hypertonic saline increases blood pressure and cardiac output secondary to plasma volume expansion, and it is also thought to stimulate adrenocorticotropin and cortisol release. Hypertonic saline is also believed to counteract vasospasm occurring after traumatic brain injury through its vasodilatory effects. On a molecular level, hypertonic saline has been shown to improve microvascular perfusion by attenuating leukocyte–endothelial interactions. It has also been suggested that hypertonic saline can provide protection from bacterial illness by attenuating changes in extracellular sodium and excitatory neurotransmitters that occur after injury. These changes are thought to depress leukocyte adherence and neutrophil margination.

Although the most common concentration of hypertonic saline used clinically is 3%, the concentrations studied in clinical trials ranges from 1.7% to 29.2%. In spite of concern for hypertonicity, acute increases in serum sodium levels to 155 to160 mEq have not been shown to be harmful to most patients.

Another clinical problem with hypertonic saline is the transient nature of the resulting hemodynamic improvement (30 to 60 minutes) when it is used as a resuscitative fluid, much like traditional resuscitative fluids. Proposed strategies to lengthen the hemodynamic effects of hypertonic saline include longer infusion times, subsequent or concomitant infusion of blood or conventional fluids, and adding 6% dextran to the hypertonic saline. Despite the claims surrounding the addition of colloid, there remains no clear answer as to the best strategy to lengthen hemodynamic effects of hypertonic saline.

The reality is that the clinical efficacy of hypertonic saline resuscitation versus conventional fluids remains unclear because many prehospital studies compared only single boluses of experimental and control fluids. Furthermore, misleading conclusions exist about the clinical responses to different types of fluid resuscitation (including hypertonic saline with and without colloid additives). This is likely the result of studies comparing two or more regimens that alter more than one variable.

In addition to the use of hypertonic saline in the prehospital and trauma setting, it has several well-established roles. These include the care of patients with severe, symptomatic hyponatremia (<115 to 120 mEq) and in the fluid management of critical burn injuries. Nontraditional uses of hypertonic saline include stimulation of expectoration, which has been implemented in the care of patients with cystic fibrosis. Hypertonic saline has also been used in the treatment of tricyclic antidepressant (TCA) toxicity. Rapid, cataclysmic clinical deterioration may occur shortly after TCA overdose. Traditionally, sodium bicarbonate is used to reverse TCA cardiotoxicity (dysrhythmias), but hypertonic saline has also been shown to do this. Furthermore, in the setting of hemodynamic instability generated by TCA toxicity, hypertonic saline may be especially useful for a hypotensive patient.

Support for hypertonic saline is growing in the prehospital and trauma setting based on recent research into its beneficial effects at the cellular and molecular levels. Hypertonic saline may come to be viewed as a "drug" instead of a simple fluid, which will bring about more research into the adequate "dose" and "timing of administration." This may ultimately clarify its clinical role and clear up the misleading conclusions that currently exist about its clinical efficacy in the trauma setting.

TAKE HOME POINTS

- Hypertonic saline has documented vasoregulatory, immunologic, and neurochemical effects—it may come to be viewed more as a drug than a simple fluid.
- The use of hypertonic saline has been driven by the resuscitation issues encountered with burn, trauma, and critically ill patients. Seek out senior providers in these areas to gain clinical expertise.
- From her personal use of 3% hypertonic saline, the editor recommends establishing a baseline serum sodium before initiating therapy. An infusion (typically 1 to 2 mL/hour) is then started via central access, with an initial serum sodium value checked at 30 minutes and then at regular intervals (usually 60 minutes). Consider discontinuation if the serum sodium increases 10 to 15 mEq above baseline or at 155 mEq, whichever is reached first.

SUGGESTED READINGS

Barash PG, Cullen BF, Stoelting RK. *Clinical Anesthesia*. 4th ed. Philadelphia: Lippincott Williams & Wilkins; 2001:177–179.

Gosling P. Salt of the earth or a drop in the ocean? A pathophysiological approach to fluid resuscitation. *Emerg Med J*. 2003;20:306–315.

Miller RD. *Miller's Anesthesia*. 6th ed. Churchill Livingstone; 2005:1785–1786, 1826.

Morgan GE, Mikhail S, Murray MJ. *Lange Clinical Anesthesiology*. 4th ed. New York: McGraw-Hill; 2006.

31

REMEMBER THAT THE SYNTHETIC COLLOID SOLUTIONS HAVE DISTINCT PROPERTIES AND RISK/BENEFIT RATIOS

IVAN V. COLAIZZI, MD AND RAYMOND M. PLANINSIC, MD

Before an anesthesia provider can consider the colloid solutions in general and the hetastarch products in particular, he or she must first have an understanding of the basics of perioperative fluid therapy. Perioperative fluid therapy includes the replacement of pre-existing fluid deficits, maintenance requirements, and surgical losses.

Normal maintenance requirements (*Table 31.1*) are what the body needs to keep up with urine production, losses from the respiratory tract or skin, and gastrointestinal (GI) secretions. Because these losses are hypotonic meaning that the fluids lost have a lower osmolality than the cells in the body.

Fluid deficits may come from a variety of sources. First, the great majority of patients who come to the operating room have fasted for at least 6 hours. For the average 70-kg man this calculates to a deficit of (110 mL/hour × 6) or 660 mL. For many GI procedures, patients may also get a preoperative bowel cleansing preparation. This may increase fluid losses by 1 to 2 L. Increased insensible losses also occur as a result of increased sweating, respiratory losses from fevers, as well as in any patient who has been breathing nonhumidified gases. Finally, patients who have diarrhea, vomiting, diuresis, or bleeding will have fluid depletion as well as electrolyte disturbances.

For surgical losses, the anesthesia provider has to be very vigilant. Underestimating surgical blood loss can have devastating consequences. The first obvious place to look is in the suction canister or at the sponges. Remember that a 4 × 4 sponge may hold 10 mL of blood and a full-sized, soaked laparotomy pad may represent 100 mL of blood loss. In addition, one must take into account the irrigation solution used. Good communication with the scrub nurse for estimating this fluid solution use is essential. With the increased use of cell salvage techniques, a second suction canister may be present. However quick visual estimation of blood losses may account for only one third of the "real blood loss." There may be a significant amount not accounted for in the tubing, on the drapes/floor, or on the surgeon/scrub nurse. Once an estimate of surgical blood loss has been made, a good rule for replacement volume for surgical blood loss (when not using blood products) is 1:3 for crystalloid solutions and 1:1 for colloid solutions. This means that

© 2006 Mayo Foundation for Medical Education and Research

TABLE 31.1 FLUID MAINTENANCE ESTIMATES

WEIGHT (KG)	RATE (ML/KG/H)
0–10	4
Next 10–20	2
Each kg >20	1

Fluid Estimates Calculation
Example 1. 100-kg person.
$(10 \times 4) + (10 \times 2) + (80 \times 1) = 140$ mL/h
Example 2. 23-kg child
$(10 \times 4) + (10 \times 2) + 3 = 63$ mL/h

if there is a 300-mL blood loss, one could correct this loss by giving 900 mL of crystalloid or 300 mL of colloid.

What are colloid solutions? Basically, they are solutions of high-molecular-weight substances administered to maintain intravascular volume. They last intravascularly from 3 to 6 hours. Some indications for use are for fluid resuscitation before blood products are available or in patients with severe hypoalbuminemia.

There are many different types of colloid solutions. One of the most familiar to anesthesia providers is albumin, which is available in 5% and 25% solutions. The albumin protein is relatively stable and is heated to 60°C for 10 hours. It is heated to potentially remove HIV, hepatitis, etc. Albumin is one of the most expensive solutions because it is derived from blood donations. Recently, Pentastarch and Hespan (Hetastarch) have been increasingly popular because of the lower cost. Both are composed of chains of glucose molecules to which hydroxylated ethyl ether groups have been added to resist degradation. The average molecular weight of Hespan is 450,000. Hetastarch comes in a 6% solution of either NaCl (Hespan) or LR (Hextend) (*Table 31.2*). Pentastarch, which has a slightly smaller molecular

TABLE 31.2 HESPAN VERSUS HEXTEND

	HES/BS (HEXTEND)	HES/NS (HESPAN)
HES (g/dL)	60	60
Na (mEq/L)	143	154
Cl (mEq/L)	124	154
Lactate (mEq/L)	28	—
Ca (mEq/L)	5	—
K (mEq/L)	4	—
Mg (mEq/L)	0.9	—
Dextrose (mg/L)	99	—

TABLE 31.3 HETASTARCH VERSUS PENTASTARCH		
	HETASTARCH	PENTASTARCH
pH	5.5	5
Avg. MW	450,000	264,000
Intravascular half-life	25.5 h	2.5 h
Elimination	Renal	Renal
Coagulation effects	Increases PT, PTT, bleeding time	Increases PT, PTT, bleeding time
Liver effects	Temporarily increases amylase, increases indirect bilirubin	Temporarily increases amylase
Maximum dose	15–20 mL/kg, max. 1 L	15–20 mL/kg, max. 1 L

Avg. MW, average molecular weight; PT, prothrombin time; PTT, partial thromboplastin time.

size, was developed secondary to the fact that the large Hespan molecules are sequestered in the reticuloendothelial system (RES), the kidney, and the liver. Although this has not been shown clinically, it may impair the RES. For a comparison of Hetastarch to Pentastarch (both in NaCl solution) see *Table 31.3.*

The polyhydroxylated starches have relative contraindications in patients with coagulopathies, fluid overload, or renal impairments, and both produce rare hypersensitivity reactions. Hespan has been shown to have a decreased inflammatory response compared to albumin preparations. However, there was evidence that showed possible impaired coagulation with Hespan as compared to albumin, particularly in cardiac surgery. The question was raised: If one put the Hetastarch in a balanced salt (BS) solution (i.e., Hextend), can the coagulation issues be avoided? One must also be aware that Hespan/normal saline (HES/NS) solution can cause a hyperchloremic metabolic acidosis because it is not a balanced salt solution (similar to giving too much normal saline). In June 2002 the U.S. Food and Drug Administration (FDA) Blood Products Advisory Committee recommended that Hespan/balanced salt solution (HES/BS) (a) should not have a warning label for bleeding, (b) is pharmacologically different from HES/NS, (c) is equivalent to 5% albumin, and (d) is superior to HES/NS.

Gan and colleagues studied 120 patients undergoing major elective surgery who received HES/NS or HES/BS intraoperatively. *Table 31.4* compares these solutions in patients who needed blood transfusions. No statistical differences between groups were found for volume of HES, crystalloid, packed red blood cells (PRBC), fresh frozen plasma (FFP), platelets, or cryoprecipitate infused, or estimated blood loss. However, in the subgroup of patients who received intraoperative blood transfusions, there were significant differences in the mean heart rate and estimated blood loss. In

TABLE 31.4   HESPAN VERSUS HEXTEND IN PATIENTS NEEDING BLOOD TRANSFUSIONS

	HES/NS (N = 25)	HES/BS (N = 31)	P VALUE
Heart rate, beats/min	85	78	0.049
EBL, mL	$2,516 \pm 1,856$	$1,560 \pm 99$	0.02
PRBC, mL	$1,516 \pm 1,397$	$1,040 \pm 639$	
FFP, mL	288 ± 697	73 ± 202	
Platelets, mL	83 ± 205	7 ± 38	
Cryoprecipitate, mL	4 ± 20	0	

HES/NS, Hespan/normal saline; HES/BS, Hespan/balanced salt solution; EBL, estimated blood loss; PRBC, packed red blood cells; FFP, fresh frozen plasma.

addition, the thromboelastogram (TEG) r-time was measured. Patients who received ≥ 20 mL/kg of HES/NS had a statistically significant change in r-time from baseline to the end of surgery ($p = 0.01$). Patients who received HES/BS or <20 mL/kg of HES/NS did not have a significant change in r-time.

Bennett-Guerro and colleagues included 200 perioperative (intraoperative plus 24 hours postoperative) coronary artery bypass graft and/or valvular heart surgery patients in a study comparing 5% albumin, HES/NS, and HES/BS administration. No differences between the albumin and HES/BS groups were identified. There was a statistically significant difference between the HES/BS and HES/NS groups for the number of units of PRBC and FFP transfused (*Table 31.5*). Serum creatinine measured 1 week postoperatively was also significantly different between the two groups (*Table 31.5*). Finally, *Table 31.6* includes several additional studies that support the

TABLE 31.5   CORONARY ARTERY BYPASS GRAFT AND/OR VALVULAR HEART SURGERY PATIENTS

	5% ALBUMIN	HES/NS	HES/BS
PRBC transfused, U	2 (0–2)	4 (2–6)[a]	2 (0–2)
FFP transfused, U	0 (0–4)	3 (0–6)[a]	0 (0–4.5)
Platelets transfused, U	0 (0–6)	6 (0–9)	0 (0–6)
Preoperative Scr, mg/dL		1.0 ± 0.3	1.0 ± 0.2
Postoperative Scr, mg/dL		1.5 ± 0.7[a]	0.9 ± 0.2

HES/NS, Hespan/normal saline; HES/BS, Hespan/balanced salt solution; PRBC, packed red blood cells; FFP, fresh frozen plasma; Scr, serum creatinine.
[a] $p < 0.05$ between HES/NS and HES/BS groups.

TABLE 31.6 COMPARISON OF 5% ALBUMIN, HES/NS, AND HES/BS

	PRODUCTS COMPARED	PATIENT POPULATION	RESULTS
Petroni et al.	HES/BS, 5% albumin/LR	Perioperative cardiac surgery patients ($n = 28$)	No difference in chest tube output, pre/postoperative Hct, or blood transfusions
Gan et al.	HES/BS, 5% albumin/NS	Perioperative GU surgery patients ($n = 25$)	No significant difference in PT, aPTT, Factor VIII, vWF, or platelet function
Roche AM	HES/BS, HES/NS, LR	In vitro TEG r-time	75% dilution of human blood: HES/BS-diluted blood samples had similar r-time as fresh blood; HES/NS-diluted samples failed to clot.

HES/NS, Hespan/normal saline; HES/BS, Hespan/balanced salt solution; Hct, hematocrit; GU, genitourinary; PT, prothrombin time; PRBC, packed red blood cells; FFP, fresh frozen plasma; aPTT, activated partial thromboplastin time; TEG, thromboeslastogram.

FDA Blood Product Advisory Committee's recommendations on the use of HES/BS.

There are several possible adverse reactions one should be aware of when giving Hetastarch products: volume overload, pulmonary edema, congestive heart failure, anaphylactic or anaphylactoid reactions (particularly with a corn allergy), hemodilution, nausea/vomiting, peripheral edema, submaxillary and parotid glandular enlargement, mild influenzalike symptoms, headaches, muscle pain, and pruritus. When giving Hetastarch in a NaCl solution, there is direct inhibition of Factor VIII, prolongation of activated partial thromboplastin time (aPTT), prothrombin time (PT), clotting and bleeding times, as well as increased risk of hyperchloremic metabolic acidosis.

Hetastarch products are available in 500-mL bags. The dosage and rate of administration depend on the clinical situation as well as the dynamics of the patient. A maximum of 1,000 mL of the HES/NS product should be used in a 24-hour period. There is no recommended maximum amount of Hextend®.

TAKE HOME POINTS

- Hespan is a colloid that can last intravascularly from 3 to 6 hours.
- Hespan has relative contraindications in patients with coagulopathies, fluid overload, or renal impairments and may produce hypersensitivity reactions.

- Hetastarch comes in a 6% solution of either NaCl (Hespan or HES/NS) or LR (Hextend or HES/BS).

- In June 2002 the FDA Blood Products Advisory Committee recommended that HES/BS (a) should not have a warning label for bleeding, (b) is pharmacologically different from HES/NS, (c) is equivalent to 5% albumin, and (d) is superior to HES/NS.

SUGGESTED READINGS

Barash PG, Cullen BF, Stoelting RK. *Clinical Anesthesia*. 5th ed. Philadelphia: Lippincott Williams & Wilkins; 2005.

Bennett-Guerrero E, Frumento RJ, Mets B, et al. Impact of normal saline based versus balanced-salt intravenous fluid replacement on clinical outcomes: a randomized blinded clinical trial. *Anesthesiology*. 2001;95:A147.

Bennett-Guerrero E, Manspeizer HE, Frumento RJ, et al. Impact of normal saline-based versus balanced salt fluid replacement on postoperative renal function: randomized trial preliminary results. *Anesth Analg*. 2001;92:SCA129.

Boldt J, Schölhorn T, Mayer J, et al. The value of an albumin-based intravascular volume replacement strategy in elderly patients undergoing major abdominal surgery. *Anesth Analg*. 2006;103(1):191–199.

Faust RJ, Cucchiara RF, eds. *Anesthesiology Review*. 3rd ed. Churchill Livingstone; 2001.

Gan TJ, Bennett-Guerrero E, Phillips-Bute B, et al. Hextend, a physiologically balance plasma expander for large volume use in major surgery: a randomized Phase III clinical trial. *Anesth Analg*. 1999;88:992–998.

Gan TJ, Wright D, Robertson C, et al. Randomized comparison of the coagulation profile when Hextend or 5% albumin is used for intraoperative fluid resuscitation. *Anesthesiology*. 2001;95:A193.

Morgan GE, Makhail MS, Murray MJ. *Clinical Anesthesiology*. 3rd ed. New York: McGraw-Hill/Appleton & Lange; 2001.

Niemi TT, Suojaranta-Ylinen RT, Kukkonen SI, et al. Gelatin and hydroxyethyl starch, but not albumin, impair hemostasis after cardiac surgery. *Anesth Analg*. 2006;102(4):998–1006.

Petroni KC, Green R, Birmingham S. Hextend is a safe alternative to 5% human albumin for patients undergoing elective cardiac surgery. *Anesthesiology*. 2001;95:A198.

Roche AM, Mythen MG, James MFM. Comparison of the coagulation effects of balanced electrolyte versus saline-based fluid haemodilution using TEG® *in vitro*. *Anesthesiology*. 2001;95:A199.

U.S. Food and Drug Administration. FDA Blood Products Advisory Committee. 13–14 June 2002. BioTime. www.fda.gov/ohrms/dockets/ac/02/briefing/BPAC. 50802.doc. Accessed December 10, 2003.

32

PROTECT THE KIDNEYS, NOT THE "UOP"

MICHAEL P. HUTCHENS, MD, MA

It is axiomatic in anesthesiology that abundant, or at least physiologically normal, intraoperative urine output (UOP) is essential to good postoperative renal outcome. Although it is true that the best monitor of intraoperative renal function is UOP, this is unfortunately true only in the sense that there is no other monitor of even passable use. One should not confuse poor data from a bad monitor with excellent data (such as from end-tidal capnography) from a monitor that demands action. Unfortunately, the differential diagnosis of intraoperative oliguria is not hypovolemia alone.

Clearly, slavish devotion to producing a UOP of 3 mL/kg/hour in an anuric renal failure patient during a lengthy bowel procedure will predictably produce pulmonary edema and ultimately congestive heart failure. A more probable situation is that in which large volumes of fluid are administered to a physiologically normal patient in an attempt to correct presumed hypovolemia in an oliguric patient who in fact has a kinked Foley catheter or an unsuspected urinary tract injury in the surgical field. In the first case, delayed diagnosis of the kinked catheter and volume resuscitation will result in an overdistended bladder and ultimately obstructive renal failure. In the second, renal function may be unaffected.

It has been frequently observed that patients undergoing laparoscopic surgery have lower-than-expected intraoperative UOP. Aggressive volume resuscitation in these patients may or may not increase their UOP. Euvolemia or slight relative hypervolemia may be necessary to ensure adequate blood pressure in this setting (because of increased intrathoracic pressure reducing return to the right heart). But does the reduced UOP reflect a danger to the kidney? Early laparoscopists thought this was the case—that pneumoperitoneum caused renal vein and parenchymal compression, which resulted in oliguria and eventually renal injury. There is now good evidence to show otherwise. In multiple studies in animal models, pneumoperitoneum of 15 mm Hg or less (the upper limit for most laparoscopic procedures is 15 mm Hg) predictably reduces UOP but does not result in significant changes in ultrasound, pathologic, or chemical indicators of renal function. This question has also been evaluated in humans. As laparoscopic gastric bypass was being developed, Nguyen et al. reported on renal physiology in more than 100 patients assigned randomly to either laparoscopic or open gastric bypass. Despite longer operative time and 64% lower intraoperative UOP in

© 2006 Mayo Foundation for Medical Education and Research

the laparoscopic group, there was no significant difference in postoperative blood urea nitrogen (BUN), creatinine, antidiuretic hormone (ADH), aldosterone, or renin levels, strongly suggesting that the reduced UOP reflects a reversible noninjurious physiologic consequence of pneumoperitoneum.

Similarly, the development of the laparoscopic donor nephrectomy offered an opportunity to study the effect of pneumoperitoneum directly in both the retained and the transplanted (hence stressed) kidney. Hawasli et al. studied the effect on donated and retained kidneys of two different levels of pneumoperitoneum (10 and 15 mm Hg). They found no difference in UOP or other indices of renal function between the groups. Importantly, the transplanted kidneys functioned equally well whether harvested at high or low pressure. Intraoperative UOP is generally controlled aggressively with fluids, hypervolemia, and diuretics during donor nephrectomy, so it is impossible to assess relative oliguria in this population, but studies have shown that the laparoscopic donor operation produces allograft function that is equivalent to that of the open operation.

Laparoscopic surgery is not the only setting in which relative oliguria may not be harmful. Patients undergoing radical head and neck surgery have also been observed to have relative oliguria intraoperatively. Priano et al. studied "dry" versus "wet" resuscitation strategies in head/neck surgery patients with normal preoperative renal function, finding that resuscitation of more than 1 L/hour produced a UOP of 1.3 mL/kg/hour; half dose resuscitation was associated with significantly less UOP (.4 mL/kg/hour). Both groups had normal intraoperative and postoperative hemodynamics, and normal postoperative renal function.

The anesthetic doctrine of "plentiful pee," then, has important exceptions. This is the case because a "normal" UOP is a second-line surrogate marker for instantaneous renal function, analogous to depending on the surgeons' assessment of blood color to measure adequacy of oxygenation. New technologies such as continuous renal ultrasound and near-infrared regional oximetry offer some hope of improving the monitoring of intraoperative renal function. In the meantime, we must use the monitor we have with intelligence, sophistication, and a high level of skepticism.

TAKE HOME POINTS

- Urine output is a poor monitor of renal function, but it's the only one we have in the operating room.
- Laparoscopic surgery patients can have low intraop UOP without detriment to postoperative renal function.
- Radical head and neck surgery patients can have low intraoperative UOP without detriment to postoperative renal function.

SUGGESTED READINGS

Hawasli A, Oh H, Schervish E, et al. The effect of pneumoperitoneum on kidney function in laparoscopic donor nephrectomy. *Am Surg*. 2003;69(4):300–303.

Nguyen NT, Perez RV, Fleming N, et al. Effect of prolonged pneumoperitoneum on intraoperative urine output during laparoscopic gastric bypass. *J Am Coll Surg*. 2002;195(4):476–483.

Priano LL, Smith JD, Cohen JI, et al. Intravenous fluid administration and urine output during radical neck surgery. *Head Neck*. 1993;15(3):208–215.

33

DO NOT TREAT LACTIC ACIDOSIS WITH BICARBONATE

PRASERT SAWASDIWIPACHAI, MD

Lactic acidosis is one type of anion-gap metabolic acidosis (AGMA). It occurs when the tissue metabolism has to undergo anaerobic metabolism, which produces significant amounts of lactic acid.

Lactic acidosis occurs at the cellular level (mitochondria) when the oxygen delivery to the tissue is inadequate or the cells cannot utilize the oxygen. Many causes of lactic acidosis are recognized, the most common being a result of low oxygen delivery because of shock (septic, hypovolemic, cardiogenic, or neurogenic), severe anemia, or severe hypoxemia. It also can occur from exposure to drugs (e.g., metformin, antiretroviral therapy, acetaminophen, salicylates, cocaine, valproic acid, sulfasalazine, isoniazid [INH], 5-fluorouracil [5-FU]), toxins, and sugar alcohols (sorbitol, xylitol, fructose).

Many systemic diseases can also be complicated by lactic acidosis, including diabetes mellitus, alcoholism, pancreatitis, cancer, infections, vitamin B_1 deficiency, short-gut syndrome, malabsorption syndrome, etc. Certain rare inborn errors in metabolism (e.g., Von Gierke disease, methylmalonic aciduria, pyruvate dehydrogenase deficiency) can also be responsible for lactic acidosis.

The best treatment of lactic acidosis is to treat the underlying causes. This often includes volume expansion, correcting anemia, increasing cardiac performance, and correcting hypoxemia. If the cause is detected and treated promptly, the lactic acidosis should gradually subside. The severity of acidemia (arterial pH) can be used to follow the effectiveness of the intervention.

Alkali therapy (especially sodium bicarbonate) should not be given in lactic acidosis. Although it may initially correct the deranged laboratory value, it actually worsens the clinical condition. The exogenous bicarbonate will result in a significant amount of CO_2, which can move freely between the compartments (including across the blood–brain barrier), whereas the bicarbonate does not. This creates disequilibrium of strong ions. Many studies in both animal and human cells have confirmed the increase in intracellular acidosis after bicarbonate therapy. Bicarbonate administration is widely accepted in acidosis associated with chronic loss of bicarbonate (e.g., renal

© 2006 Mayo Foundation for Medical Education and Research

tubular acidosis, pancreatic transplantation, diarrhea) but not in lactic acidosis.

One final thought is that mild to moderate systemic acidosis is not as deleterious as was once thought. The growing use of permissive hypercapnia in acute respiratory distress syndrome (ARDS) patients has shown that many adult patient have no change in cardiac contractility even when systemic pH is as low as 7.15.

TAKE HOME POINTS

- Lactic acidosis is the final common pathway resulting from a number of conditions and diseases, such as shock, severe anemia, severe hypoxemia, drug exposure, diabetes mellitus, and inborn errors of metabolism
- Treat the underlying cause, not the numbers!
- Sodium bicarbonate will "fix the number" on a short-term basis, but it actually worsens the clinical situation by increasing intracellular acidosis.
- Mild to moderate systemic acidosis may not be as deleterious as was once thought.

SUGGESTED READING

Forsythe SM, Schmidt GA. Sodium bicarbonate for the treatment of lactic acidosis. *Chest.* 2000;117:260–267.

34

CONSIDER THE USE OF TRIS-HYDROXYMETHYL AMINOMETHANE (THAM) TO TREAT REFRACTORY OR LIFE-THREATENING METABOLIC ACIDOSIS

LEANDER L. MONCUR, MD AND ELLIOTT R. HAUT, MD, FACS

You just assumed care of a 35-year-old man with severe septic shock and acute respiratory distress syndrome (ARDS) resulting from necrotizing pancreatitis and aspiration pneumonia. He has a combined metabolic and respiratory acidosis secondary to his underlying pancreatitis and permissive hypercapnia from the appropriate ventilatory strategy necessary for treatment of ARDS. His arterial pH remains <7.15 and mean arterial pressure (MAP) is 50 mm Hg despite being on a sodium bicarbonate ($NaHCO_3$) drip and multiple vasoactive agents. His serum sodium is 165 mEq/L and his serum creatinine is 1.0 mg/L. Your critical care attending physician suggests stopping the bicarbonate infusion and switching to tris-hydroxymethyl aminomethane (THAM) instead.

Acidemia, in critically ill patients, can have devastating consequences if it is not corrected in a timely fashion. These major adverse consequences often include impairment of cardiac contractility, cardiac arrhythmias, elevated pulmonary artery pressures, decreased responsiveness to catecholamines, hyperventilation, insulin resistance, hyperkalemia, increased metabolic demands, and changes in mental status. The role of buffers in treating severe acidosis (i.e., arterial pH <7.20) remains controversial. Sodium bicarbonate is the most commonly used buffer used to treat severe acidosis in North America, but the use of sodium bicarbonate is not without consequences. Its use can be associated with hypernatremia, hyperosmolality, volume overload, and exacerbation of acidosis through an increase in CO_2 production.

THAM is a biologically inert weak base that has a greater buffering capacity than sodium bicarbonate (pK_a 7.8 vs. pK_a 6.8, respectively). THAM is effective in buffering severe metabolic acidosis, permissive hypercapnia associated with Acute Lung Injury/Acute Respiratory Distress Syndrome (ALI/ARDS), and mixed acidoses. THAM can buffer both metabolic acids ($THAM + H^+ = THAM^+$) and respiratory acids ($THAM + H_2CO_3 = THAM^+ + HCO_3^-$). Unlike sodium bicarbonate, THAM does not generate CO_2 but uses CO_2 to generate bicarbonate and also buffers other sources of protons in body fluids, such as lactic acid.

© 2006 Mayo Foundation for Medical Education and Research

Currently, there are few clinical trials regarding the efficacy of THAM in treating severe acidosis in critically ill patients. The literature supports consideration for the use of THAM in patients with the following acid–base disturbances: severe metabolic acidosis and hypernatremia, extreme levels of permissive hypercapnia in patients with ALI/ARDS at maximum ventilatory support, treatment of dilutional acidosis intraoperatively, and failure of sodium bicarbonate to correct metabolic acidosis. The usefulness of THAM has been limited because of its serious side effects, including hyperkalemia, hypoglycemia, ventilatory depression, local injury with intravenous extravasation, and hepatic necrosis in neonates.

ADMINISTRATION OF THAM

THAM is available in several preparations. THAM base solution has a pH $= 10.4$ and should be administered only through a central venous catheter. THAM acetate solution (0.3 mol/L concentration is titrated to pH $= 8.4$ with acetic acid) can be administrated peripherally because it does not cause venous irritation. THAM also comes as a citrate syrup. It is indicated for use in patients with life-threatening acidemia (defined as pH 7.1 to 7.2, paCO$_2$ <35 mm Hg, and lactic acid >10 mEq/L) to temporarily or permanently normalize the acid–base status. THAM should be administered as a loading dose of 2 to 4 mmol/kg over 20 minutes, followed by a constant infusion of 0.5 to 1 mmol/kg/hour for 4 to 10 hours. The estimated dose of THAM is calculated as follows:

$$\text{Volume of 0.3 mol/L THAM (mL)} = \text{lean body weight (kg)} \times \text{base deficit (mEq/L)}$$

THAM is excreted by the kidneys, as THAM$^+$ (the protonated form), through glomerular filtration as a nonreabsorbable cation paired with an anion by the kidneys. It has an osmotic diuretic effect, increasing the excretion of urinary sodium and chloride. THAM can accumulate in patients with renal failure and produce an "osmolar gap" with pseudohyponatremia. Renal clearance of THAM is 2% greater than that of creatinine. At steady state, if no drug accumulates, the rate of THAM elimination must equal the rate of THAM infusion. It is recommended that the THAM plasma concentration be maintained ≤ 6 mmol/L. To calculate maximum infusion rate,

$$\text{Infusion rate of THAM (mmol/hr)} = 0.06 \times \text{creatinine clearance (ml/min)} \times \text{THAM plasma level (desired)}$$

THAM should generally be avoided in evolving renal failure, but if it is used, it must be monitored closely and stopped if hyperkalemia and an osmolar gap begin to develop.

- The primary goal in the treatment of metabolic acidosis is reversing the underlying cause.
- THAM may represent a viable alternative to sodium bicarbonate in treating severe metabolic acidosis.
- THAM should be used with extreme caution in patients with renal insufficiency.
- Hyperkalemia, hypoglycemia, and ventilatory depression should be actively watched for in patients receiving THAM.

SUGGESTED READINGS

Adrogue HJ, Madias NE. Management of life-threatening acid-base disorders (first of two parts). *N Engl J Med.* 1998;338:26–34.

Hoste EA, Colpaert K, Vanholder RC, et al. Sodium bicarbonate versus THAM in ICU patients with mild metabolic acidosis. *J Nephrol.* 2005;18:303–307.

Kallet RH, Jasmer RM, Luce JM, et al. The treatment of acidosis in acute lung injury with tris-hydroxymethyl aminomethane (THAM). *Am J Respir Crit Care Med.* 2000;161:1149–1153.

Nahas GG, Sutin KM, Fermon C, et al. Guidelines for the treatment of acidemia with THAM. *Drugs.* 1998;55(2):191–224.

35

USE THE PRINCIPLES OF "DAMAGE CONTROL ANESTHESIA" IN THE CARE OF THE MASSIVELY BLEEDING PATIENT AND ASK THE SURGEONS TO IMPLEMENT "DAMAGE CONTROL SURGERY" IF NECESSARY

T. MIKO ENOMOTO, MD AND MICHAEL P. HUTCHENS, MD, MA

Intraoperative life-threatening hemorrhage must be controlled with teamwork between the surgeons and anesthesiologist. With the realization that ongoing hemorrhage after injury leads to derangements in the body's ability to maintain hemostasis and homeostasis, trauma surgeons have evolved the concept of "damage control surgery," which proposes that definitive repair or fixation can in many cases be delayed until the patient has been resuscitated to the goals of appropriate blood composition, normalization of acid–base status, and normothermia. Among the anesthesia provider's roles in the care of the massively bleeding patient is to implement the accompanying concept of "damage control anesthesia" and help the nontrauma surgical team recognize that the magnitude of hemorrhage may require altering the surgical goals and plan.

At its most basic, damage control anesthesia seeks to mitigate the effects of the lethal triad of acidosis, hypothermia, and coagulopathy. Hypothermia results from infusion of intravenous (IV) fluids, and convective and conductive heat losses. Coagulopathy, resulting from depletion of clotting factors by ongoing hemorrhage, is exacerbated by hypothermia and acidosis, leading to further bleeding and hypotension. Resulting poor perfusion furthers acidosis, and the classic "downward spiral" ensues.

Dutton identifies the essentials of damage control anesthesia as: (a) control of the airway and ventilation, (b) control of bleeding, (c) preservation of homeostasis, and (d) analgesia and sedation. Indeed, these are similar to routine anesthetic care, but there are a few key differences.

Fluid resuscitation needs to focus not only on replacing circulating volume, but also on maintaining the appropriate blood composition in terms of oxygen-carrying capacity, clotting potential, and chemistry. This requires large-bore IV access, usually considered to be a minimum of two 18-gauge or larger IVs, and frequent laboratory analysis of blood. The desired end points or goals of volume resuscitation are currently being re-examined in light of recent evidence suggesting that hypotensive resuscitation may be beneficial. Strategies for hypotensive resuscitation include delayed resuscitation, in

© 2006 Mayo Foundation for Medical Education and Research

which fluid resuscitation is delayed until after control of the site of bleeding, and permissive hypotension, in which resuscitation is continuous but with a goal of a subnormal blood pressure. In a landmark study, Bickell et al. demonstrated a survival advantage to limited volume replacement until the time of operative intervention in the setting of penetrating torso trauma. A proposed mechanism for the advantage of hypotensive resuscitation is that, by limiting fluid volume, regional vasoconstriction and lower blood pressure allow the adhesion of the fragile platelet–fibrin clot. In addition, the composition of the blood, including coagulation factors, is minimally diluted. Limited infusion of fluids reduces the development of hypothermia.

Of course, the potential benefit of hypotensive resuscitation in the multiply injured trauma patient must be weighed against the risk of worsening hypoperfusion, resulting in increased acidosis and ischemic organ damage. Hypotension resulting from hemorrhagic shock is thought to be a significant mechanism for the "second hit hypothesis," which adds ischemic injury to the initial insult in the setting of traumatic brain injury. In practice, blood pressure is typically used as one of the main parameters guiding resuscitation, but there is abundant animal and clinical data that blood pressure is not an accurate gauge of tissue oxygenation.

Diligent attention must be paid to maintaining normothermia: Keep the ambient temperature warm despite medical team discomfort, warm all IV fluids using a rapid infuser with inline air detection and heat exchanger, place a convective warmer where possible, and minimize the length of exposure of internal organs and raw surfaces.

Blood products should be replaced in the appropriate proportions, guided by cell counts and coagulation studies. Active repletion of calcium and other electrolytes must be pursued, guided by frequent chemistries. In the setting of active bleeding, the platelet count should generally be maintained >100K, and the international normalized ratio (INR) kept <1.4. These goals should be adjusted based on the clinical situation.

In addition to direct control of a bleeding vessel, there are many methods of achieving hemostasis. Packing of venous bleeding or diffuse oozing, or clamping of arterial bleeding, can be used as a temporizing measure while the patient is warmed, resuscitated, and stabilized. In the setting of some types of bleeding, such as that resulting from pelvic trauma, angiographic embolization may be the safest and fastest way to control the bleeding without causing further damage. For diffuse bleeding from raw surfaces, novel topical hemostatic agents, such as fibrin glue, chitosan (HemCon), modified rapid deployment hemostat (MRDH), or QuikClot, continue to become available. In the setting of diffuse coagulopathic bleeding not controlled by replacement with blood products, administration of recombinant factor VIIa (rFVIIa) should be considered. rFVIIa is postulated to jump-start the initiation phase of coagulation in a site-specific manor, and has been shown to be of benefit in trauma patients who fail standard methods of correcting coagulopathy. Significant drawbacks include great expense and a small risk of thrombotic complications.

Perhaps the most important thing that the anesthesiologist can do to prevent lethal hemorrhage is to communicate with the surgical team. If the patient is unstable, the surgeons must be made aware of this.

TAKE HOME POINTS

- Damage control surgery was developed for the case of massively bleeding patients whose medical status is compromised by the hemorrhage. It is based on delay of the definitive repair.
- Damage control anesthesia involves correction of coagulopathy, acidosis, and establishment of normothermia.
- Become familiar with the concept of "limited resuscitation" and "limited infusion" techniques as applied to trauma patients.
- Remember that blood pressure is not necessarily an accurate indicator of tissue oxygenation.

SUGGESTED READINGS

Bickel WH, Wall MJ, Pep PE, et al. Immediate versus delayed fluid resuscitation for hypotensive patients with penetrating torso injuries. *N Engl J Med.* 1994;331:1105–1109.

Boffard KD, Riou B, Warrant B, et al. Recombinant factor VIIa as adjunctive therapy for bleeding control in severely injured trauma patients: two parallel randomized, placebo-controlled, double-blind clinical trials. *J Trauma.* 2005;59:8–18.

Dutton RP. Damage control anesthesia. *Int Trauma Care (ITACCS).* 2005;197–201.

Schreiber MA. Coagulopathy in the trauma patient. *Curr Opin Crit Care.* 2005;11:590–597.

36

Learn from the care of the combat victim: Ask the surgeons to consider damage control surgery for the bleeding patient

Surjya Sen, MD

Damage control surgery is defined as operative management that employs a staged approach to the severely injured patient. It seeks to avoid "physiologic burnout" seen with the lethal triad of hypothermia, acidosis, and coagulopathy. Definitive therapy for the patient's problem or injury is deferred to give preference to the stopping of hemorrhage and the control of contamination by using the simplest and most rapid means possible. Temporary wound closure methods are employed initially, with a plan to return the patient to the operating room after physiologic abnormalities have been corrected (or at least stabilized) in an intensive care setting.

Historical Perspective
Traditionally, it was believed that the operative management of a patient should provide definitive care even if the physiologic condition of a patient was deteriorating (especially if the physiologic deterioration was due to a problem that was the focus of the operation). In the early 1900s, this dogma was challenged in management of battlefield victims with exsanguinating injuries. J. H. Pringle introduced the techniques for the temporization of hepatic hemorrhage for trauma by using liver packs and vascular compression. However, because of poor outcomes, these techniques fell out of favor until the 1970s and 1980s, when they were reintroduced with "abbreviated laparotomies." These procedures were used to temporize the source of bleeding in trauma victims so that they could return later to the operating room, after their coagulopathies had been corrected. By the 1990s, damage control surgery (coined by Rotondo in 1993) had gained popularity not only for application toward soldiers in combat settings, but also for trauma victims in civilian settings.

Applicability to Noncombat Situations
Although damage control surgery offers evident advantages in a combat situation (faster evacuation times, better use of limited resources, and more efficient management of a large number of casualty victims who may present simultaneously), it also has applicability in civilian traumas. Abbreviated

---

© 2006 Mayo Foundation for Medical Education and Research

surgeries allow the surgical, anesthesia, and intensive care teams to steer clear of irreversible physiologic end points such as uncontrolled hemorrhage from disseminated intravascular coagulopathy. Avoiding life-threatening abnormalities such as hypothermia, coagulopathy, and acidosis are the primary end points for the care providers. Once these have been met, the patient is returned to the operating room for definitive management.

BASICS OF THE PROCEDURE (THREE STAGES)

The following outlines the damage control procedure.

Initial Management

■ Initiation of advanced trauma life support (ATLS) protocols
■ Proper patient selection
  • Patients with injuries that are technically difficult
  • Patients who will require extensive, multistep surgical procedures
  • Patients with exsanguinating blood loss
  • Patient in whom delaying definitive repair will not result in death

Stage 1 (the damage control operation)

■ Abdominal injury
  • The abdomen is usually packed with a goal to tamponade bleeding while maintaining organ perfusion.
  • Vascular injuries may be treated with ligation, temporary intraluminal shunts, or intravascular balloon catheters.
  • Hollow viscus injuries are often resected (reanastomosis is postponed).
  • Biliopancreatic injuries can be temporized with closed suction drainage.
  • Renal damage is often best treated with radical nephrectomy.
  • Closure: Temporary closure is employed.
■ Thoracic injury
  • Usually involves the placement of chest tubes.
  • Management of cardiac tamponade.
  • Lobectomies or pneumonectomies are often performed.

Stage 2 (resuscitation)

■ Patients are returned to the intensive care unit (ICU) for correction and management of
  • Acidosis
  • Hypothermia
  • Coagulopathy

Stage 3 (definitive operation)

■ Exact timing of the reoperation has not been standardized.
■ Patients who return in less than 72 hours tend to have lower morbidity and mortality.
■ A thorough exploration is performed to ensure that no injuries have been missed.

COMPLICATIONS

Complications following damage control surgery tend to not be specific to this type of procedure, but rather to the population of surgical and critically ill patients. Local complications include abscesses, fistulas, necrosis, and pseudocysts; systemic complications include acute respiratory distress syndrome (ARDS), abdominal compartment syndrome, and multiple organ failure.

OUTCOMES

The reported incidence of ARDS and multiple organ failure in this patient population ranges from 14% to 53%. The best predictors of mortality tend to be the *initial pH* upon return to the ICU (for stage 2) and the *worst partial thromboplastin time PTT* from hospital admission to ICU admission. Overall mortality following damage control surgery varies, but the trend has shown a progressive decrease, from as high as 67% (in 1983) to as low as 10% (in 2001).

TAKE HOME POINTS

■ Damage control surgery has applicability in both the combat and noncombat situation. It can be employed in the treatment of trauma victims and even in elective operations when unforeseen complications lead to the destabilization of normal physiologic homeostasis.

■ The central focus of damage control surgery attempts to delay definitive therapy while prioritizing the management of coagulopathies, maintaining normothermia, and correcting acid–base abnormalities.

■ Patients who undergo definitive therapy within 72 hours tend to have better outcomes.

SUGGESTED READINGS

Abikhaled JA, Granchi TS, Wall MJ, et al. Prolonged abdominal packing is associated with increased morbidity and mortality. *Am Surg.* 1997;63(12):1109–1113.

Aoki N, Wall MJ, Granchi T, et al. Predictive model for survival at the conclusion of a damage control laparotomy. *Am J Surg.* 2000;180:540–545.

Pringle J. Notes on the arrest of hepatic hemorrhage due to trauma. *Ann Surg.* 1908;48:541–549.

Rotondo MF, Schwab W, McGonigal MD, et al. Damage control: an approach for improved survival in exsanguinating penetrating abdominal injury. *J Trauma.* 1993;35(3):375–383.

Schreiber MA. Damage control surgery. *Crit Care Clin.* 2004;20:101–118.

Sebesta MAJ. Special lessons learned from Iraq. *Surg Clin N Am.* 2006;86:711–726.

37

KNOW WHAT SCREENING TESTS ARE PERFORMED ON VOLUNTEER DONOR BLOOD

ANDREW M. GROSS, MD

Donated blood is subjected to a rigorous series of tests before it is deemed safe for transfusion. The list of tests performed by the Red Cross seems ever expanding, and this has resulted in an overall safer blood supply and fewer transfusion-associated risks. Blood testing consists of screening for infectious disease as well as ABO screening, Rh screening, and testing for various red-cell antibodies.

Infectious disease screening is accomplished two ways. An initial level of screening is by self-report of previous diseases and living or travel situations. Since March 2005, all blood donors in the United States must complete a 54-question survey called the Universal Donor Survey. For example, donors are asked if they have had oral surgery in the last 3 days (to eliminate the possibility of transient bacteremia of mouth pathogens) or have ever had certain blood-borne infections such as malaria or babesiosis (both intracellular erythrocyte parasites). They are also queried about residence in Europe during the interval that may increase the epidemiologic risk for bovine spongiform encephalopathy. Affirmative answers on the test can disqualify the donor temporarily or permanently.

Serum tests for infectious disease entities include HIV-1 and -2, hepatitis C (HCV), hepatitis B (HBV), human T-lymphocyte virus (HTLV)-I and -II, West Nile virus, and *Treponema palladium* (syphilis). Alanine aminotransferase is also tested as a laboratory marker of infectious disease. All viruses are initially tested for by enzyme-linked immunoassay (ELISA). An initial positive result is then rechecked in two separate ELISA tests, and if one of those two subsequent tests is also positive, the blood is discarded. Only if both are negative is the blood taken out of special quarantine and subjected to further testing.

A new method of testing blood was started in 1999. Nucleic acid testing or NAT is used to screen blood for the presence of HIV, HCV, and, as of 2003, West Nile virus. Nucleic acid testing is done by polymerase chain reaction (PCR) or transcription-mediated amplification (TMA). As both of these are fairly expensive tests, most commonly nucleic acid testing is done on a minipool sampling. This involves pooling multiple donations, and if an infection is present, then all of the individual donations in the pool are tested. This supersensitive assay is responsible for detecting HIV an average

ⓒ 2006 Mayo Foundation for Medical Education and Research

of 11 days earlier than other forms of testing, and in concert with ELISA and Western blot tests for anti-HIV antibodies, has decreased the risk of transfusion-related infection to 1 in 2 million in the United States, 1 in 5 million in Germany, and 1 in 10 million in Canada. HCV infection has been dramatically reduced using nucleic acid testing, from 1 in 100,000 in 1996 to 1 in 2 million in the United States in 2005. Nucleic acid testing results in a decrease from an average of a 70-day window for undetectable infection using ELISA screening for HCV antibodies to an 8- to 10-day window of undetectable infection.

Blood infected with HBV is screened for by hepatitis B surface antigen and core antigen testing. The latency period of about 60 days results in a higher amount of undetected virus in the donor pool and thus HBV infection risk remains the highest among the diseases tested for—estimates vary from 1 in 60,000 to 1 in 270,000. HTLV-I and -II are screened for by ELISA and confirmed by Western blot or PCR. The resulting infection rate is estimated at 1 in 2 million for HTLV. Syphilis is also screened for by a number of serologic assays varying from lab to lab using highly sensitive specific anti-gens for *T. palladium*. Finally, cytomegalovirus (CMV) is screened for only in a select number of cases, because of the need for CMV-negative blood for transplant recipients and the immunosuppressed population, especially HIV-infected individuals.

In addition to infectious agents, blood type testing is still of critical importance, and all blood donations are screened for ABO type using anti-A and anti-B antibodies. Each unit is also tested for the presence of a D antigen. Those who have the D antigen are said to be Rh-positive, and those without, Rh-negative. Blood types and Rh type are rechecked in individual hospital blood banks before dispensing units for transfusion, as the result of a mislabeled or improperly tested unit could be catastrophic or even fatal. Some but not all donated blood is subsequently screened for red-cell antigens. These antigens include the remainder of the Rh system in addition to the D antigen and the more minor groups (e.g., Duffy, Kell, Big E, Kidd). Special units that are negative for all of these antigens are stored for donation to people who have preformed antibodies to these groups. Cross-matching is done in the blood bank at individual hospitals to determine which antigens are present in donated blood versus which antigens and antibodies are present in the recipient. Donated blood is itself screened for antibodies to the minor blood groups by exposing it to control red cells that have sed antigens present on their surface. The components that have preformed antibodies cannot be given to a recipient with the corresponding antigen, as major complications can arise.

Blood transfusions are a crucial part of practicing anesthesiology. Many critically ill patients' lives will depend on receiving transfusions that are safe and properly administered. In order for an informed decision to be made by both physician and patient, it is important to understand the risks of blood administration. Transfusions are still a source of anxiety for patients, and knowing how to alleviate that fear is of the utmost importance. Most anxiety surrounding blood transfusion stems from patients' fears of contracting an infectious disease, and although the risk is low, it is not zero. Of understandable concern to patients is the risk of acquiring a disease from an "emerging" condition such as Lyme, ehrlichiosis, or Chagas disease; all conditions that are well established in the United States. These and other conditions with known or probable blood transmission can be debilitating or fatal if acquired and are not tested for in the blood supply in the United States. When discussing the risks of acquiring these diseases (or yet-unknown diseases; thousands of patients died from AIDS acquired through blood transfusions), it is incumbent to tell patients that self-report measures have never been proven to be fail-safe screening procedures for preventing transmission of blood-borne pathogens.

TAKE HOME POINTS

- Screening of volunteer donor blood starts with the Universal Donor Survey—this is strictly a "self-report" instrument that attempts to indirectly screen for such blood-borne diseases as malaria and babesiosis. For a true positive diagnosis, both these disease require a thin-smear erythrocyte analysis, which is not performed on donated blood. In Lyme-endemic areas, such as Connecticut, it has been determined that a certain percentage of volunteers presenting for blood donation are actually asymptomatic carriers of the babesia parasite. Transfusion-related transmission of the disease has been reported.
- The first level of serologic testing is by ELISA—this is intended to screen against viral and spirochetal organisms.
- Nucleic acid testing is usually done on pooled samples and has increased the sensitivity of the serologic testing process.
- The blood supply has increased in safety in recent years, but of course is not completely safe, and the risks should not be minimized or "glossed over" in discussions with the patient. A good approach is to discuss the relative risks of transfusion vs. significant perioperative events linked to anemia, such as retinal ischemia and visual loss.

SUGGESTED READINGS

American Association of Blood Banks. *Standards for Blood Banks and Transfusion Services.* 18th ed. Bethesda, MD: American Association of Blood Banks.

Chiavetta JA, Escobar M, Newman AM, et al. Incidence and estimated rates of residual risk for HIV, hepatitis C, hepatitis B and human T-cell lymphotropic viruses in blood donors in Canada, 1990–2000. *Can Med Assoc J.* 2003;169:767.

Dodd RY, Notar EP, Stramer SL. Current prevalence and incidence of infectious disease markers and estimated window period risk in the American Red Cross blood donor population. *Transfusion.* 2002;42:975.

Pealer LN, Marfin AA, Petersen LR, et al. Transmission of West Nile virus through blood transfusion in the United States in 2002. *N Engl J Med.* 2003;349:1236.

Stramer SL, Glynn SA, Kleinman SH, et al. Detection of HIV-1 and HCV infections among antibody-negative blood donors by nucleic acid-amplification testing. *N Engl J Med.* 2004; 351:760.

38

TRANSFUSION OF PACKED RED BLOOD CELLS REQUIRES A CAREFUL RISK–BENEFIT ANALYSIS

HEATHER A. ABERNETHY, MD AND
MICHAEL P. HUTCHENS, MD, MA

Transfusing allogenic red blood cells is an intervention that has both life-saving and life-threatening potential. Anesthesia providers are familiar with the deleterious effects of acute hemorrhagic anemia: Reduced cardiac output associated with severe blood loss can result in tissue hypoxia and eventually organ dysfunction and failure. Consequences of anemia depend on the patient's ability to compensate for these physiologic changes. Because hemoglobin values are readily determinable in most intraoperative settings, it is tempting to transfuse packed red blood cells based on a number. However, the down sides to transfusion are more complex than just acute transfusion reaction alone. In order to fully assess the risks and benefits of transfusion, anesthesiologists must have a thorough understanding of their patient's current medical condition and co-morbidities as well as the current literature on transfusion.

Laboratory experiments indicate that extreme hemodilution is well tolerated in healthy animals. Animals subjected to acute hemodilution tolerate decreasing hemoglobin concentrations down to around 5 g/dL, with ischemic electrocardiographic changes and depressed ventricular function noted at these levels. However, acute hemodilution is tolerated less well in animal models of coronary stenosis—ischemic electrocardiographic changes and depressed cardiac function are seen at hemoglobin concentrations between 7 and 10 g/dL. Human data regarding the limits of anemia tolerance are inadequate and often conflicting.

Guidelines regarding red cell transfusion have been presented by the American Society of Anesthesiologists Task Force on Blood Component Therapy. The authors strongly recommend reading the document in its entirety. The Task Force consensus states that transfusion is rarely indicated when hemoglobin concentration is greater than 10 g/dL and is almost always indicated when it is less than 6 g/dL, especially when the anemia is acute. Determining the need to transfuse for levels in between these numbers should take into account the individual's risks of potential damage from possible inadequate oxygen delivery.

© 2006 Mayo Foundation for Medical Education and Research

A patient's likelihood of complications from anemia must be weighed against the risks of red cell transfusion. Some of the known risks of transfusion include threat of infection such as HIV, hepatitis B or C, or cytomegalovirus (CMV). Other, unquantified infectious risks almost certainly exist. There is also a danger of hemolytic or nonhemolytic reactions, allergic reactions, transfusion-related acute lung injury, and anaphylactic shock with any blood product transfusion. Despite numerous safeguards, transfusion mishaps due to human (often clerical) error remain the most common cause of serious transfusion reaction.

Numerous studies suggest that patients who are transfused more liberally have worse outcomes, in both the short and long term. Specific perioperative hazards associated with liberal transfusion include increased delirium and worsened pulmonary function. Some studies have shown increased postoperative infection, mortality, and length of stay. The seminal TRICC trial of 1998 concluded that intensive care unit (ICU) patients who received transfusions to maintain their hemoglobin greater than 9 g/dL (rather than greater than 7 g/dL) had increased mortality. These effects are thought to be secondary to immunomodulation from leukocytes in stored blood. There is speculation that routine transfusion of leukodepleted blood may reduce some of these adverse outcomes. Another important sequela of red blood cell transfusion is decreased long-term survival of some cancer patients, again possibly mediated by an alteration of immunologic status, although this is not borne out in large-scale studies.

Note: An interesting aspect to this discussion is whether anesthesiologists can and/or should use ICU studies as guideline for intraoperative transfusion practices. The question is do ICU patients comprise a similar cohort for the average same-day-admit patient (ASA 1-3) that we routinely care for? It is the senior author's opinion that although the data on transfusions are complicated, confusing, and occasionally contradictory, the power of the aggregate data is quite large. The author feels that a combination of this power and what can reasonably be taken as "expert consensus" justifies a more restrictive approach to transfusion.

It is still true that the best therapy for the perioperative anemic patient who is exsanguinating is blood transfusion. This is a clinical situation that is usually readily recognized by anesthesia providers. However, it is the patient with a relatively stable hemoglobin in the range between 6 and 10 g/dL that presents a clinical conundrum. Patients with risk factors for organ dysfunction, such as severe coronary artery disease, known carotid artery stenosis, a history of transient ischemic attack (TIA), or renal insufficiency will least tolerate anemia and are therefore thought to be most likely to benefit from a more liberal transfusion strategy, although slim evidence supports this conclusion. As the risk of anemia to the patient is that of oxygen supply–demand imbalance, a rational transfusion strategy should include the full armamentarium of strategies to optimize oxygen balance. If clinically appropriate, pharmacologic reducers of oxygen demand, such as optimal anesthesia, opioids, and beta-blockers, should be used. It is reasonable to deliver high concentrations of inspired oxygen for short periods of increased oxygen demand. Nontransfusion strategies to increase red cell mass, such as intraoperative autotransfusion, acute normovolemic hemodilution, or preoperative autologous donation and retransfusion, should be considered. Antifibrinolytics such as aminocaproic acid, aprotinin, or tranexamic acid may be considered in cases in which exuberant fibrinolysis is a known consequence, such as liver transplant or cases involving cardiopulmonary bypass.

Remember also that patients with coronary or cerebrovascular disease are not the only ones who may not tolerate sudden decreases in hematocrit. Patients undergoing spinal surgery with prolonged intraoperative hypotension, perioperative anemia, and facial swelling are at risk of developing posterior ischemic optic neuropathy (PION). PION follows infarction of the posterior portion of the optic nerve and can result in the devastating complication of postoperative visual loss. This list of risk factors is based on retrospective analyses and a very small number of actual cases; it is not clear that transfusion alone can prevent PION, and experts are in disagreement on this topic. Nonetheless, the best available data suggest that it is prudent to closely monitor these patients and consider a different threshold for red cell blood transfusion.

Generally, experienced anesthesia providers do not transfuse packed red blood cells without discussing the ongoing clinical situation (as possible) with the surgeons and notifying them that transfusion is planned. Because the intraoperative period can be busy, one way to handle the situation is to talk with the surgeons in the preoperative period and outline the parameters that would trigger a transfusion. This is a situation in which it is necessary to consider closely the surgeons' opinions; however, it is unusual for a surgeon to disagree with a thought-out and well-articulated plan.

TAKE HOME POINTS

- It is no longer axiomatic that blood is the best intravenous fluid.
- Although it is not possible to state with certainty that transfusion is hurtful, the preponderance of evidence suggests that the outcomes of transfusion are complex and deleterious and may outweigh the advantages of simple resolution of perioperative anemia.
- Don't forget about the important consideration of postoperative visual loss and the role that anemia may plan in its etiology.
- Talk to the surgeons!

SUGGESTED READINGS

Chen A, Carson J. Perioperative management of anaemia. *Br J Anaesthesia*. 1998;81(suppl 1): 20–24.

Dunker S, Hsu H, Sebag J, Sadun A. Perioperative risk factors for posterior ischemic optic neuropathy. *J Am Coll Surg*. 2002;194:705–710.

Hebert P, McDonald B, Tinmouth A. Clinical consequences of anemia and red cell transfusion in the critically ill. *Crit Care Clin*. 2004;20:225–235.

Hebert P, McDonald B, Tinmouth A. Overview of transfusion practices in perioperative and critical care. *Vox Sang*. 2004;87(suppl 2):209–217.

Hebert P, Wells G, Blajchman M, et al. A multicenter, randomized controlled clinical trial of transfusion requirements in critical care. *N Engl J Med*. 1999;340:409–417.

Practice guidelines for blood component therapy: a report by the American Society of Anesthesiologists Task Force on Blood Component Therapy. *Anesthesiology*. 1996;84:732–747.

Schreiber G, Burch M, Kleinman S, Korelitz J. The risk of transfusion-transmitted viral infections. *N Engl J Med*. 1996;334:1685–1690.

Shander A, Knight K, Thurer R, et al. Prevalence and outcomes of anemia in surgery: a systematic review of the literature. *Am J Med*. 2004;116(suppl 7A):58–69.

Strumper-Groves D. Perioperative blood transfusion and outcome. *Curr Opin Anaesthesiol*. 2006; 19(2):198-206.

39

Jehovah's Witnesses and transfusion: Ethical issues

ROSE CHRISTOPHERSON, MD, PhD

The issues surrounding transfusion of Jehovah's Witnesses should be examined in the broader context of medical ethics. Two aspects of medical ethics are important in this discussion: informed consent, and Do Not Resuscitate (DNR) orders. Patients are normally informed about their treatment plans. They have the right to refuse any care, as long as they are both competent and have capacity to make health care decisions. Many Jehovah's Witnesses refuse transfusion of blood or some blood products because of their interpretation of certain passages in the Bible. Because other patients have the same right to refuse blood transfusion, it is not appropriate to argue with patients about their reasons for refusal. If they are competent, they have the right to refuse.

It is important to determine whether the patient is competent and has the capacity to make medical decisions, and to determine exactly what the patient refuses. Some patients are willing to accept reinfusion of their own blood, or transfusion of some blood components such as fresh frozen plasma. Jehovah's Witnesses are as diverse a group as any other religious group. It is wrong to assume from the fact that a patient is a Jehovah's Witness that she or he refuses blood transfusion. It is also important that there is no coercion of the patient, intended or unintended, because of the presence of family members or clergy. This is best done by speaking with the patient alone. It is important, in obtaining informed consent, to make it very clear that patients do not necessarily die as a result of withholding of transfusion. They may have strokes, myocardial infarction, or other organ damage. Thus the patient needs to understand that, if transfusion is withheld, she or he may emerge from the anesthetic with permanent impairment.

All participating caregivers must understand the patient's wishes and agree to the same plan. Surgeons have been known to refuse to perform surgery on patients who refuse transfusion. The type of surgery to be performed, urgency of the surgery, and likelihood of blood loss are all important. Participating nurses must agree with the plan. Even though the anesthesiologist will give or withhold blood products, if the patient dies or has some other adverse outcome related to anemia, all on the care team will share the pain of this bad, and in a sense avoidable, outcome.

© 2006 Mayo Foundation for Medical Education and Research

Often, Do Not Resuscitate (DNR) orders are suspended in the perioperative period. Transfusion of blood or blood products is often part of resuscitation. DNR orders are on most patients' charts because of some terminal disease the patient has. When these patients need surgery for palliation or for some unrelated problem, they are generally willing to have their DNR orders cancelled for the perioperative period. They may need airway management or administration of resuscitation medicines to maintain appropriate vital signs during surgery. Their DNR status will resume after surgery.

Jehovah's Witnesses, on the other hand, are often quite healthy, and they may want every form of resuscitation other than blood transfusion. The situation can be even more troubling if the Jehovah's Witness wants transfusion withheld from a child or an elderly parent. Thus the refusal of a Jehovah's Witness, or of any other patient, of perioperative transfusion is somewhat contrary to accepted hospital procedures related to perioperative resuscitation.

It is not surprising if anesthesiologists feel uncomfortable about caring for Jehovah's Witnesses. We are asked to agree to things that we do not otherwise agree to. We are asked, potentially, to allow a patient to bleed to death while withholding the red cells, platelets, or fresh frozen plasma that would deliver oxygen to their tissues or even help stop the bleeding. Physicians or other caregivers may feel that they are asked to compromise their own religious or other deeply held moral beliefs. In fact, this is true. The patient's wishes have some priority over the physician's wishes, simply because treating patients against their will is battery and is not permitted.

However, it is not clear that a caregiver who refuses to anesthetize a patient because of the patient's unwillingness to receive blood is necessarily doing wrong. In some cases it is obvious that the patient is very unlikely to survive a procedure without transfusion. If at all possible, the caregiver should find another anesthetist, who is willing to agree to the patient's wishes. Lists of colleagues who are willing to withhold transfusion are helpful. It is never possible to avoid this conflict completely. Sometimes anesthesiologists will have to decide whether their duty to give the anesthetic and do their best to keep patients in good condition without transfusion outweighs their personal religious or moral beliefs.

Finally, we turn to patients who cannot make health care decisions. This includes unconscious patients; incompetent patients; and children. Some of these patients may have a document stating what interventions may be made on their behalf, e.g., a living will. Some Jehovah's Witnesses may carry a wallet card, which may state that they refuse blood. However, if such documentation cannot be found, given the diversity of beliefs among Jehovah's Witnesses, it should be assumed that transfusion is permissible. In the case of children, there is legal controversy (www.virtualmentor.org). If surgery is elective, it is probably best to obtain consultation from both an ethics committee and a hospital attorney.

TAKE HOME POINTS

- The issues involved in the care of Jehovah's Witness patients are rooted in the medical ethics problems of informed consent and DNR orders.
- Do not argue with a Jehovah's Witness patient about his or her reasons for refusal of blood or blood products.
- Jehovah's Witnesses are as diverse a group as any other religious group. It is wrong to assume from the fact that a patient is a Jehovah's Witness that she or he refuses blood transfusion.
- Always speak to the Jehovah's Witness in a confidential location.
- Accept that there may be varying levels of discomfort among the anesthesia and operating room teams. It is never possible to avoid this conflict.
- Unconscious, incompetent, and pediatric Jehovah's Witness patients are a special situation—consult the ethics and legal staffs.

MANAGEMENT STRATEGIES FOR JEHOVAH'S WITNESS PATIENTS—THE BASIC 3 PART APPROACH

1) Minimize Losses
   - Consider staging complex procedures so that time between operations can allow some recovery for patients
   - Apply damage control surgery principles to minimize bleeding as a first objective, then return later for definitive treatment
   - Minimize blood draws
   - Avoid anticoagulants and antiplatelet agents as much as possible
   - Consider Recombinant Factor VIIa to decrease the need for further transfusions and improve hemostasis
   - Employ the use of hemostatic surgical devices like electrocautery, ultrasonic scalpels and tourniquets
   - Utilize pharmacologic agents such as fibrin glues as blood vessel sealants and antifibrinolytics
   - Consider using strategies such as normovolemic hemodilution, controlled hypotension and continuous recovery cell salvage devices
2) Increase Production
   - For planned elective cases, use recombinant human erythropoetin to improve reticulocytosis and increase normboblast production
   - Supplement with IV iron, folate and vitamin B12

3) Stabilization and substitutions
- When bleeding is suspected, take decisive interventional steps early to quickly control blood loss
- Supplement oxygen and resuscitate fluid losses aggressively to improve oxygen delivery
- Manage coagulopathies early
- In select cases, consider blood substitutes such as Polyheme and Hemospan (still in clinical trials)

SUGGESTED READINGS

Hung T, Tong M, van Hasselt CA. Jehovah's Witnesses and surgery. *Hong Kong Med J.* 2005;11(4):311–312.

McInroy A. Blood transfusion and Jehovah's Witnesses: the legal and ethical issues. *Br J Nurs.* 2005;14(5):270–274.

Remmers PA, Speer AJ. Clinical strategies in the medical care of Jehovah's Witnesses. *The American Journal of Medicine.* 2006;119:1013–1018.

Rogers DM, Crookston KP. The approach to the patient who refuses blood transfusion. *Transfusion.* 2006;46(9):1471–1477.

Medications

40

BEWARE OF THE MECHANICAL BOWEL PREP

JAMES C. OPTON, MD

Mechanical bowel preparation (MBP) is commonly used for colonoscopy and elective colorectal surgery. Its goal is to rid the colon of solid fecal material. It is believed that the "clean" bowel has a lower bacterial load and has a lower risk of contaminating the wound and peritoneal cavity during surgery. The prepped bowel is much easier to manipulate during surgery and enables the surgeon to perform intraoperative colonoscopy. Disruption of the anastomosis and the sequela of an anastomotic leak may be attenuated by the MBP as well. Other surgeries in which the MBP is commonly used include abdominal and pelvic operations involving the aorta, kidneys, bladder, and reproductive structures. Absolute contraindications to the mechanical bowel prep include complete bowel obstruction and free perforation.

For colonoscopy and elective colorectal surgery, MBP is the standard of care worldwide. Historically, agents such as castor oil, senna, bisacodyl, and magnesium citrate have all been used in conjunction with a low-residue diet. Whole-gut lavage with large volumes of isotonic solutions via a nasogastric tube has also been used. However, this technique has been associated with side effects including electrolyte abnormalities, abdominal distention, nausea, and vomiting. Whole-gut lavage with mannitol has also been used, but this practice has been shown to be associated with catastrophic intraoperative explosions when gases produced from fermentation of mannitol by *Escherichia coli* were ignited by electrocautery. Currently, the two most widely used agents for MBP are polyethylene glycol and sodium phosphate.

Polyethylene glycol (PEG) was developed in the 1980s as an oral agent for MBP. It is an iso-osmotic, nonabsorbable sodium sulfate–based solution that cleans the bowel by washout of ingested material without significant fluid and electrolyte shifts. Patients are required to drink at least 2 to 4 L of solution along with additional fluids. Abdominal cramping, nausea, and vomiting are common side effects, and patients are typically prescribed prophylactic antiemetics.

Sodium phosphate (NaP) was developed in response to patient dissatisfaction with PEG and has generally been found to be more tolerable and associated with a higher rate of compliance. NaP is a hyperosmotic electrolyte solution that provides high-quality bowel cleansing while avoiding

© 2006 Mayo Foundation for Medical Education and Research

the need to ingest large volumes of solution. It can be taken in two 45-mL doses or in a series of 40 tablets. Abdominal cramping, nausea, and vomiting are common side effects.

Because NaP is a hyperosmolar solution, a watery diarrhea is induced with its administration. A negative fluid balance can ensue, which can lead to hypovolemia that may become especially evident at the induction of anesthesia if adequate fluid replacement has not taken place. PEG, on the other hand, leaves the fluid balance virtually unaffected. Water and electrolytes are neither absorbed nor excreted from the bowel. Therefore, patients do not usually exhibit hemodynamic instability during the induction of anesthesia. For these reasons NaP may have a narrower therapeutic index than PEG, especially in patients who may be vulnerable to shifts in intravascular volume. NaP has been linked more frequently than PEG to serious electrolyte and metabolic derangements. Most commonly reported are transient decreases in pH, magnesium, calcium, and potassium. Hypernatremia and hyperphosphatemia can also occur, because these solutions contain 48 g of monobasic sodium phosphate and 18 g of dibasic sodium phosphate per 100 mL of solution. Although most patients are not clinically affected by these electrolyte abnormalities, NaP should be avoided in patients with renal disease, congestive heart failure, ascites, and in those who cannot adequately hydrate themselves. Furthermore, severe hyperphosphatemia and associated electrolyte and metabolic derangements following administration of NaP have been reported, as well as at least one case report of fatal hypocalcemic, hyperphosphatemic, metabolic acidosis following sequential NaP enema administration.

Cleansing the bowel before colorectal surgery with some form of MBP is a major surgical dogma with a long-standing history. However, this view has recently come into question. Several prospective, randomized trials comparing preprocedural MBP (with NaP and/or PEG) to no bowel prep have shown no difference in rates of postoperative wound infection, abscess formation, or anastomotic leakage. In fact, some of the studies have shown an increased rate of anastomotic complications in the MBP group. It has also been repeatedly demonstrated that the frequency of anastomotic leakage is no higher in patients with penetrating trauma to the bowel who do not undergo MBP due to the urgency of surgery than it is for scheduled patients who do undergo preoperative MBP. The same comment holds true for patients with obstructive lesions in the colon, in whom preoperative MBP is contraindicated. As more such data become available, the use of the MBP may evolve into an "as indicated" procedure. However, when a "clean view" of the colon is necessary, such as for colonoscopy (whether intraoperative or in the gastrointestinal [GI] laboratory), MBP will likely remain a standard practice.

TAKE HOME POINTS

- Remember that bowel preps are not used just for abdominal surgeries; ask all patients having surgery on internal viscera if they have done a prep.
- The polyethylene glycol bowel preps have trade names such as Golytely and Nulytely.
- The sodium phosphate bowel preps have trade names such as Fleets Phospha-Soda.
- Polyethylene preps can cause significant upper GI distress and vomiting; look for upper GI loss of potassium and disruptions in acid/base status and consider preinduction antiemetics and cricoid pressure.
- Sodium phosphate preps can cause significant electrolyte depletion from lower GI losses; consider checking preinduction potassium levels, especially if the patient is also on a diuretic or digoxin.
- Patients who have had a NaP prep may also need extra intravenous fluid replacement at the time of induction.

SUGGESTED READINGS

American Society of Colon & Rectal Surgeons Homepage. American Society of Colon & Rectal Surgeons. www.fascrs.org. 1 Apr 2006.

American Society for Gastrointestinal Endoscopy Homepage. American Society of Gastrointestinal Endoscopy. www.askasge.org. 1 Apr 2006.

Baum E, Sherman Y, Well R, et al. Is mechanical bowel preparation mandatory for elective colon surgery? *Arch Surg.* 2005;140:285–288.

Kirby R. *Clinical Anesthesia Practice.* 2nd ed. Philadelphia: WB Saunders; 2002:1188–1189.

Pekka R, Miettinen J, Laitinen ST, et al. Bowel preparation with oral polyethylene glycol electrolyte solution vs. no preparation in elective open colorectal surgery. *Dis Colon Rectum.* 2000;43:669–675.

Pitcher DE, Ford SR, Nelson TM, et al. Fatal hypocalcemic, hyperphosphatemic, metabolic acidosis following sequential sodium phosphate-based enema administration. *Gastrointest Endosc.* 1997;46:266–268.

Slim K, Vicaut E, Panis Y, et al. Meta-analysis of randomized clinical trials of colorectal surgery with or without mechanical bowel preparation. *Br J Surg.* 2004;91:1125–1130.

Tan HL, Leiw QY, Loo S, et al. Severe hyperphosphatemia and associated electrolyte and metabolic derangement following the administration of sodium phosphate for bowel preparation. *Anaesthesia.* 2002;57:478–483.

Townsend C. *Sabiston Textbook of Surgery.* 17th ed. Philadelphia: WB Saunders; 2004:1416–1417.

Zmora O, Mahajna A, Bar-Zakai B, et al. Colon and rectal surgery without mechanical bowel preparation: A randomized prospective trial. *Ann Surg.* 2003;237:363–367.

Zmora O, Pikarsky AJ, Wexner SD. Bowel preparation for colorectal surgery. *Dis Colon Rectum.* 2001;44:1537–1546.

41

BEWARE THE ANTIBIOTIC BOWEL PREP

JAMES C. OPTON, MD, CATHERINE MARCUCCI, MD,
AND NEIL B. SANDSON, MD

Bowel preparation for elective colorectal surgery typically consists of mechanical bowel prep, oral antibiotics, and intravenous antibiotics. Mechanical bowel prep is discussed elsewhere; this chapter focuses on perioperative antibiotics for colorectal surgery. Other surgeries for which antibiotic bowel preparation is commonly used include abdominal and pelvic operations involving the aorta, kidneys, bladder, and reproductive structures.

Infectious complications are the leading cause of morbidity and mortality in colorectal surgery. The most common infectious complications include wound infection, intra-abdominal or pelvic abscess, and anastamotic leaks. Offending micro-organisms are typically endogenous colonic flora and include *Bacteroides fragilis*, *Clostridia*, *Escherichia coli*, *Klebsiella*, *Proteus*, and *Pseudomonas*. The logical goals of perioperative antibiotics include decreasing fecal load and bacterial count in the colonic lumen and achieving therapeutic tissue levels of antibiotics in the event that contamination occurs.

Oral antibiotics act on colonic flora intralumenally to decrease bacterial load when the lumen is opened, promoting less contamination and fewer infectious complications. Although there are many conflicting studies on the utility of oral antibiotics in this setting, >70% of surgeons use them as part of their bowel preparation. A combination of neomycin plus erythromycin or metronidazole are the most commonly used agents. The oral antibiotics used are typically given the day before surgery. At the senior author's hospital, the regimen includes three doses of erythromycin of 1 g each on the day before surgery. Although some oral antibiotics are not well absorbed from the gut, there is significant systemic absorption of erythromycin following oral administration.

One underappreciated problem that may arise with this protocol is the occurrence of unanticipated drug–drug interactions. Through two distinct mechanisms, erythromycin is likely to raise the blood levels of a large number of other drugs. First, erythromycin is a potent inhibitor of both intestinal and hepatic forms of the most important of the cytochrome P450 enzymes, CYP3A4. As such, it inhibits the metabolism of the broad array of CYP3A4 substrates, leading to increases in the blood levels of such drugs. Significant examples of CYP3A4 substrates include alprazolam, carbamazepine,

© 2006 Mayo Foundation for Medical Education and Research

cyclosporine, methadone, and quinidine, to name just a few. Second, erythromycin also inhibits the functioning of the extruding P-glycoprotein transporter. Thus, inhibition of this transporter also leads to increased levels of P-glycoprotein substrates, such as carbamazepine, cyclosporine, digoxin, morphine, phenytoin, tacrolimus, and tricyclic antidepressants. Drug toxicities are a clear concern when a patient is taking any of these drugs and they also receive a bowel preparation that includes erythromycin. Additionally, inferential reasoning also implicates metronidazole as a P-glycoprotein inhibitor, so the same toxicity concerns would be present when P-glycoprotein substrates are co-administered with metronidazole.

The goal of intravenous antibiotics is to provide therapeutic tissue levels at the time of exposure if contamination occurs. Agents traditionally used have covered colonic microflora. In the past, the triad of an aminoglycoside, a penicillin, and clindamycin or metronidazole has been used to cover Gram-negative bacteria, enterococci, and anaerobes, respectively. However, with the development of cephalosporins, aminoglycosides are no longer commonly used, avoiding the potential toxicity of this class of antibiotics. The majority of surgeons administer a second-generation cephalosporin that is active against both aerobic and anaerobic colonic bacteria within 1 hour of skin incision and continue it for up to two doses for the first 24 hours postoperatively. Continuing prophylaxis beyond the first 24 hours postoperatively has not been shown to be of any additional benefit and increases the risk of side effects, bacterial resistance, and *Clostridium difficile* colitis.

TAKE HOME POINTS

- There are many conflicting studies on the utility of oral antibiotics in this setting, however, >70% of surgeons use them as part of their bowel preparation.
- Erythromycin is a potent inhibitor of both intestinal and hepatic forms of the most important of the cytochrome P450 enzymes, CYP3A4.
- It will inhibit the metabolism of CYP3A4 substrates, such as alprazolam, carbamazepine, cyclosporine, methadone, and quinidine, leading to increases in the blood levels of such drugs.
- Erythromycin also inhibits the functioning of the extruding P-glycoprotein transporter. Thus, inhibition of this transporter also leads to increased levels of P-glycoprotein substrates, such as carbamazepine, cyclosporine, digoxin, morphine, phenytoin, tacrolimus, and tricyclic antidepressants.
- Cephalosporins do not inhibit or induce the metabolism of other drugs.

SUGGESTED READINGS

Abbott Laboratories. Erythromycin (package insert). North Chicago, IL: Abbot Laboratories; 2000.

Cozza KL, Armstrong SC, Oesterheld JR. *Drug Interaction Principles for Medical Practice: Cytochrome P450s, UGTs, P-Glycoproteins.* Washington, DC: American Psychiatric Publishing; 2003:45–55.

Sandson NB. *Drug Interactions Casebook: The Cytochrome P450 System and Beyond.* Washington, DC: American Psychiatric Publishing; 2003:243–245.

Zmora O, Pikarsky AJ, Wexner SD. Bowel preparation for colorectal surgery. *Dis Colon Rectum.* 2001;44:1537–1549.

Zmora O, Wexner S, Hajjar L, et al. Trends in preparation for colorectal surgery: Survey of the members of the American Society of Colon and Rectal Surgeons. *Am Surg.* 2003;69: 150–154.

42

BE AWARE OF THE DRUGS THAT REQUIRE SLOW INTRAVENOUS ADMINISTRATION

MAGGIE JEFFRIES, MD AND LAUREL E. MOORE, MD

The speed at which intravenous (IV) medications can be administered is often overlooked and can have devastating consequences. The drug package inserts contain information on administration, but these are frequently unavailable to anesthesiologists and the information included is not always appropriate for anesthetized patients. We often rely on pharmacists to relay important information regarding the IV administration of particular medications. As anesthesia providers, however, we frequently prepare medications for administration without pharmacy intervention. The purpose of this chapter is to review common medications that need to be administered slowly or that have other special considerations. The chapter is not intended to be used for dosing of medications. This is by no means an all-inclusive list; our intention is to cover commonly used medications that are at high risk for being administered inappropriately.

The following medications *must* be given slowly when they are administered intravenously: Phenytoin, protamine, vancomycin, potassium chloride, clindamycin, thymoglobulin, furosemide, gentamicin, and oxytocin.

PHENYTOIN (DILANTIN)

Phenytoin is a neurologic and cardiac depressant and is one of the most dangerous medications we administer intraoperatively. For status epilepticus, the maximum rate of IV administration is 50 mg/min (for children, 1 to 3 mg/kg/min up to a max of 50 mg/min). Because we generally give the medication prophylactically in the operating room, it is recommended to administer phenytoin much more slowly in anesthetized patients (e.g., max. 10 to 20 mg/min). Elderly patients and patients with cardiovascular disease should also receive the medication more slowly. If phenytoin is given rapidly IV, asystole and cardiovascular collapse is possible, but more commonly hypotension, bradycardia, and cardiac dysrhythmias are seen. These effects may be related to the diluent (propylene glycol) and may be minimized by using fosphenytoin. The dose must also be adjusted in those with hypoalbuminemia and liver disease. It is advised that the medication be diluted in *normal saline* to a final concentration of 1 to 10 mg/mL and be administered with an infusion pump. Extravasation of this medication can cause severe soft tissue injury, and it is therefore recommended to inject phenytoin into

© 2006 Mayo Foundation for Medical Education and Research

a large vein through a large-gauge IV catheter. Be sure to flush the line before and after administration with normal saline. This medication may be piggybacked, but there is a high potential for precipitation in the presence of other medications, so a 0.22-μm filter should be used.

PROTAMINE

Protamine is administered frequently in cardiac and vascular anesthesia to reverse the anticoagulant effects of heparin. Administer protamine slowly, no faster than 50 mg over 10 minutes. Severe hypotension, bradycardia, pulmonary hypertension, and an anaphylactic reaction can result if protamine is given by IV push. Patients at increased risk of severe reactions include diabetics taking insulin, patients with fish sensitivities, men who have undergone vasectomy, and patients who have been previously exposed to protamine. Dilution of the medication is not necessary.

VANCOMYCIN

Administration of vancomycin should be no faster than 10 mg/min and should be administered with the use of an infusion pump. "Red man" syndrome (erythematous rash on face and body) may occur, and if so, the infusion rate should be reduced. Rapid IV infusion has been reported to cause hypotension and, rarely, cardiac arrest. Vancomycin may cause soft tissue injury if it extravasates. When possible, a large-gauge IV catheter or central line should be used for administration.

POTASSIUM

Potassium may precipitate cardiac arrhythmias if serum concentrations increase too rapidly. In general, the maximum speed of administration is 40 mEq/h. The patient should have electrocardiogram (EKG) monitoring in place before administration. This medication causes venous irritation, so infusion via large IV catheters is preferred. If it is not prepackaged, potassium must be diluted.

CLINDAMYCIN

Clindamycin should be diluted before administration to a concentration of no more than 18 mg/mL. Do not "push" clindamycin intravenously, because it can cause profound hypotension. Infuse over 10 to 60 minutes at a rate no greater than 30 mg/min. This medication can cause thrombophlebitis at the injection site.

THYMOGLOBULIN

Thymoglobulin (lymphocyte immune globulin or antithymocyte globulin rabbit) is often used in renal transplant patients at increased risk for rejection. Administration is through a 0.22-μm filter and is infused over at least 6 hours for the first infusion to decrease the development of fever and/or chills. Hypertension is a known side effect, but hypotension may be noted intraoperatively. Administration through a central line or other high-flow vein is preferred to decrease the risk of thrombosis or thrombophlebitis. Patients may be premedicated with corticosteroids, Tylenol, and/or antihistamines to reduce side effects.

FUROSEMIDE (LASIX)

Lasix should also be administered slowly over 1 to 2 minutes. Administer no faster than 4 mg/min if large doses are to be given. There have been reports of acute hypotension and sudden cardiac arrest after IV administration. Ototoxicity has been associated with rapid IV infusion. Renal impairment, concurrent administration of other ototoxic medications, and excessive doses increase the risk of ototoxicity.

GENTAMICIN

Gentamicin has a small therapeutic window, which can make dosing challenging. Dosing adjustments in situations of renal impairment are particularly important. Aminoglycosides in general are associated with both nephrotoxicity and ototoxicity. It is thought that toxicity is related to the dose given and the duration of therapy. There have been reports of hypotension after administration of an aminoglycoside, and it is therefore recommended that gentamicin be diluted and administered slowly. Gentamicin can potentiate neuromuscular blockade.

OXYTOCIN (PITOCIN)

There are multiple uses of Pitocin for obstetric patients. Infusions of Pitocin for induction of labor are managed by the obstetric staff, but anesthesia staff are often asked to administer this medication during caesarian sections and in hemorrhagic emergencies. Dilute Pitocin in either a 0.9% normal saline or lactated Ringer's solution and administer slowly. Rapid administration may cause arrhythmias and/or hypertension in the mother. Uterine hyperactivity as severe as uterine hypertonicity, tetanic contraction, and uterine rupture is also possible. Be aware that Pitocin has an antidiuretic effect that may result in water intoxication, with convulsions, coma, or death.

OTHER PEARLS TO AVOID COMMON ERRORS INVOLVING IV ADMINISTRATION IN THE OPERATING ROOM

- The following IV-administered products must be given through a filter: *All* blood products—packed red blood cells, platelets, fresh frozen plasma, cryoprecipitate, etc.
- Pressors that require dilution for administration include the following (with recommended final concentration): Phenylephrine (100 mcg/mL),

ephedrine (5 mg/mL), and epinephrine (non–cardiac arrest situation, 10 and 100 mcg/mL).

■ Label all medications carefully!

TAKE HOME POINTS

■ One of the most important tasks for the anesthesia provider is to give dangerous drugs in a precision—this includes not only giving the correct dose of a drug, but giving it at an appropriate rate

■ Rapid administration of certain drugs can have fatal consequences

■ Do not accept information from the neurosurgeons as to the appropriate rate of phenytoin infusion—know the limiting rate yourself and personally insure it is not being exceeded. If the surgeons insist they cannot continue on with the case until the infusion is complete, then advise them they may have to adjust their expectations about how rapidly the case will proceed, but do not speed up the rate of the infusion. The editors are personally aware of several cases with fatal outcomes due to excessively rapid administration of phenytoin. In one case, it effectively ended the career of the anesthesia provider.

■ Protamine is used in the heart rooms, where it is commonly given via central access and invasive monitoring allows for close inspection of the hemodynamic effects. Somewhat more dangerous is a request by the surgeons for "50 of protamine" in a peripheral vascular case at the end of surgery, when the high-vigilance times of the case (placement and removal of the crossclamp are over). The request is typically made because the patient "is oozy" and so that the surgeons can close. Often the anesthesia provider is requested to give it via a peripheral IV.

■ The key to controlling the rate of potassium chloride infusion is to have a policy to always use an infusion pump (NOT just an infusion set with a piece of tape over the Cair clamp).

SUGGESTED READINGS

Byerly WG, Horton MW. IV administration of phenytoin. *J Gen Intern Med.* 1989;4(5):432–444.
Seifert HA, Jobes DR, Ten Have T, et al. Adverse effects after protamine administration following cardiopulmonary bypass in infants and children. *Anesth Analg.* 2003;97(2):383–389.

43

REMEMBER THAT SMOKING CESSATION AND RE-INITIATION ARE IMPORTANT VARIABLES IN THE PERIOPERATIVE PERIOD

NEIL B. SANDSON, MD AND CATHERINE MARCUCCI, MD

It has been estimated that at least one third (and probably closer to one half) of all patients presenting for surgery are smokers, which predisposes them to significant postoperative respiratory complications. As such, patients are usually counseled to stop smoking before surgery and may even be prescribed a nicotine patch as therapy.

Certainly, a few patients achieve the recommended goal of smoking cessation 4 to 6 weeks before surgery, but by far the greater number do not manage to stop smoking until the day before or even the morning of surgery ("No, I don't smoke, I quit two hours ago"). Acute smoking cessation has the paradoxic action of transiently increasing airway secretions due to improved mucociliary transport, but the balance of effects on the pulmonary and cardiovascular systems is beneficial. These include a decrease in blood carbon monoxide levels as well as a rightward shift in the oxygen–hemoglobin dissociation curve and an increase in tissue oxygenation. However, anesthesia providers must be aware of the unintended consequences of smoking cessation—balanced against the obvious benefits is the fact that the polycyclic aromatic hydrocarbons in smoked tobacco act as strong inducers of the P450 1A2 enzyme, moderate inducers of P450 2E1, and inducers of some not yet well characterized phase II enzymes. Abrupt cessation of smoking may cause alterations in the blood levels and/or end organ effects of various medications, possibly in ways that could produce inconvenience or even harm to patients.

Only smoked tobacco acts as an enzymatic inducer. Rather, it is the polycyclic aromatic hydrocarbons that must be smoked in order to induce metabolic enzymes. The P450 1A2 enzyme catalyzes the metabolism of a number of substrates that are of clinical relevance in the perioperative period. These include cyclobenzaprine, flecainide, propranolol, theophylline, and R-warfarin (*Table 43.1*). In the days following smoking cessation, the decreased availability of P450 1A2 decreases the metabolic clearance of these 1A2 substrates, leading to significantly increased blood levels. These increases in substrate levels can produce frank toxicity (such as with theophylline) and otherwise complicate perioperative management. There have been cases of increased bleeding attributable to smoking cessation in patients who

© 2006 Mayo Foundation for Medical Education and Research

TABLE 43.1	DRUGS THAT INTERACT WITH CYTOCHROME P450 1A2	
1A2 SUBSTRATES	1A2 INHIBITORS	1A2 INDUCERS
Caffeine		
Clozapine	Caffeine	Carbamazepine
Cyclobenzaprine	Cimetidine	Modafinil
Flecainide	Ciprofloxacin	Rifampin
Fluvoxamine	Ethinylestradiol	Tobacco (smoked)
Haloperidol	Fluvoxamine	
Mexiletine	Grapefruit juice	
Olanzapine	Mexiletine	
Propranolol	Norfloxacin	
Tacrine	Ofloxacin	
Theophylline	Ticlopidine	
(R-)Warfarin		

take warfarin. The effects of smoking cessation may be mimicked by the abrupt introduction of inhibitors of P450 1A2, such as caffeine, cimetidine, ethinylestradiol, and many of the fluoroquinolones (*Table 43.1*). Other inducers of 1A2 (besides tobacco smoking) include carbamazepine, rifampin, and modafinil (*Table 43.1*).

Although smoked tobacco produces a less potent induction effect at P450 2E1 than at 1A2, smoking cessation can still lead to decreased metabolism and increased blood levels of notable 2E1 substrates, including acetaminophen, ethanol, and the "flurane" inhalational anesthetics.

Awareness of the pharmacokinetic issues arising from abrupt smoking cessation can help the careful clinician avoid drug toxicity that might otherwise develop in the perioperative period.

TAKE HOME POINTS

- For the majority of smokers who present for surgery, the perioperative period is characterized by abrupt smoking cessation.
- The polycyclic aromatic hydrocarbons in smoked tobacco act as strong inducers of the P450 1A2 enzyme, moderate inducers of P450 2E1, and inducers of some not yet well characterized phase II enzymes.
- Abrupt cessation of smoking may cause alterations in the blood levels and/or end organ effects of various medications, especially substrates of P450 1A2, such as cyclobenzaprine, flecainide, propranolol, theophylline, and R-warfarin.
- Re-initiation of smoking after discharge from the hospital will re-induce P450 1A2, leading to increased clearance of 1A2 substrates and a corresponding decrease in blood levels. In the days following re-initiation of

smoking, dosages of 1A2 substrates that were decreased following smoking cessation will need to be increased to their original levels.

SUGGESTED READINGS

Desai HD, Seabolt J, Jann MW. Smoking in patients receiving psychotropic medications: A pharmacokinetic perspective. *CNS Drugs.* 2001;15(6):469–494.

Evans M, Lewis GM. Increase in international normalized ratio after smoking cessation in a patient receiving warfarin. *Pharmacotherapy.* 2005;25(11):1656–1659.

Kroon L. Drug interactions and smoking: Raising awareness for acute and critical care providers. *Crit Care Nurs Clin North Am.* 2006;18(1):53–62.

Lee BL, Benowitz NL, Jacob P 3rd. Cigarette abstinence, nicotine gum, and theophylline disposition. *Ann Intern Med.* 1987;106(4):553–555.

Zevin S, Benowitz NL. Drug interactions with tobacco smoking: An update. *Clin Pharmacokinet.* 1999;36(6):425–438.

44

CONSIDER INSULIN THERAPY TO CORRECT PERIOPERATIVE HYPERGLYCEMIA IN BOTH DIABETIC *AND* NONDIABETIC PATIENTS

HEATHER A. ABERNETHY, MD AND
SERGE JABBOUR, MD, FACP, FACE

Outcome studies have shown evidence of an association between hyperglycemia in the perioperative period and adverse events. These include a longer length of hospital stay as well as higher incidences of surgical site infection, pneumonia, infections of intravascular devices, sepsis, acute renal failure, blood product transfusion, neurocognitive dysfunction after cardiac surgery, and mortality. The effects of hyperglycemia are known to be mediated through a number of mechanisms: impaired neutrophil and monocyte function, endothelial cell dysfunction, production of interleukin-6 (IL-6) and tumor necrosis factor-alpha (TNF-α) by mononuclear cells, induction of platelet activity, and elevated levels of fibrinogen and von Willebrand factor. The tasks for the anesthesia provider are (a) to treat vigorously both preoperative and perioperative hyperglycemia in patients who are known to be diabetic—it has been suggested that diabetic patients having elective surgery should have glycemic control optimized to yield a HgbAIC of less than 7%—and (b) to be vigilant in watching for possible instances of hyperglycemia in patients without a previous diagnosis of diabetes (diagnosed or undiagnosed metabolic syndrome, perioperative steroid use, etc.)

To do this, the anesthesiologist must be aware that the definition of hyperglycemia is changing. It varies depending on the study, but in general the window of normoglycemia is narrowing—several outcome studies have defined hyperglycemic patients as those having a blood glucose of 150 mg/dL or higher. Also, in 2004, the American Association of Clinical Endocrinologists issued a position statement recommending intravenous insulin therapy in critically ill and non–critically ill patients during the perioperative period and for labor and delivery patients. Members of the consensus panel agreed on 110 mg/dL as the acceptable upper limit of blood glucose during the perioperative period, mainly for critically ill patients, and 100 mg/dL for labor and delivery patients.

The DIGAMI trial was one of the first trials devised to examine whether managing hyperglycemia would improve patient outcomes. Diabetic patients with an acute myocardial infarction were enrolled and randomized to routine care of hyperglycemia versus intravenous insulin for at least 24 hours

© 2006 Mayo Foundation for Medical Education and Research

followed by four daily subcutaneous injections continuing for 3 months after discharge. Patients were followed for a mean of 3.4 years. Mortality at that time was 11% lower in the intensive insulin therapy group (33% vs. 44%). The greatest benefit was seen in those without prior insulin use and without a prior cardiac history. The results of this study led to the investigation of intensive insulin therapy in other populations. One important study (by Van den Berghe) of mechanically ventilated patients admitted to a surgical intensive care unit (ICU) was stopped early because of the significant reduction in mortality in patients managed with intensive insulin therapy in the immediate postoperative period.

It has been suggested that insulin therapy per se may have a positive effect on reducing adverse outcomes, apart from its effect on the glycemic state. Insulin increases nitric oxide levels, inhibits free fatty acids, and reduces levels of inflammatory cytokines. In both the DIGAMI and Van den Berghe trials, the differences in blood glucose levels between the outcome groups were only approximately 50 mg/dL. Other studies have shown an improvement in outcomes in patients who had no change in blood glucose levels but who received insulin therapy.

It seems likely that hospitals will continue the current trend of writing and implementing formal protocols to treat hyperglycemia in the ICUs and on the floors. Management of diabetes in the immediate preoperative period and intraoperatively will remain the task of the anesthesia provider, however. An infusion is usually recommended over subcutaneous injections, because infusion is more effective over a wide range of insulin requirements. Typical infusion dosing is 1 U of regular insulin/mL crystalloid (mix 100 U of regular insulin in 100 mL of 0.9% saline), given with a piggyback solution. The lines should be flushed with 20 mL of insulin infusion to saturate the insulin-binding sites in the tubing. *First check a baseline blood glucose*, then infuse at a fairly slow rate if the initial value is not between 80 and 150 mg/dL. A simple calculation for starting insulin in the operating room (OR) is to divide the blood glucose by 100 and then round to the nearest 0.5 U for both the bolus dose and the infusion rate. The blood glucose level should be checked at least hourly until it is stable, to assure it is within the desired range. Aiming for tight glucose control may increase the risk of hypoglycemia; therefore, strict monitoring is mandatory, as hypoglycemia under anesthesia is difficult to diagnose.

TAKE HOME POINTS

- The association between hyperglycemia in the perioperative period and adverse events has been demonstrated by outcome studies.

- Diabetic patients should have both preoperative and perioperative optimization of the diabetic state. The target HgbA1C goal is 7 or lower.
- The anesthesia provider must also be vigilant and guard against hyperglycemia in patients who have *not* been diagnosed previously as having diabetes.
- Be aware that the definition of a hyperglycemic state is changing. Endocrinologists now consider 110 mg/dL to be the upper limit of acceptable blood glucose.
- Management of diabetes in the immediate preoperative period and intraoperatively is the task of the anesthesia provider.
- For now, the mainstay of glucose control involves the use of low-dose insulin infusions.

SUGGESTED READINGS

American College of Endocrinology Position Statement on inpatient diabetes and metabolic control. *Endocrine Pract.* 2004;10(1):77–82.

Brown D. Glycemic control during the perioperative period: how sweet is too sweet? *ASA Newsl.* 2004;68(8).

Krinsley JS. Effect of an intensive glucose management protocol on the mortality of critically ill adult patients. *Mayo Clinc Proc.* 2004;79(8):992–1000.

Malmbreg K, Norhammar A, Wedel H, et al. Glycometabolic state at admission: important risk marker of mortality in conventionally treated patients with diabetes mellitus and acute myocardial infarction: long-term results from the Diabetes and Insulin-Glucose Infusion in Acute Myocardial Infarction (DIGAMI) study. *Circulation.* 1999;99(20):2626–2632.

Pembrook L. Surgical-site infections reduced by tight peri-op glucose control. *Anesthesiol News.* 2005;31(11):1–6.

Umpierrez GE, Isaacs SD, Bazargan N, et al. Hypergycemia: an independent marker of in-hospital mortality in patients with undiagnosed diabetes. *J Clin Endocrinol Metab.* 2002;87(3):978–982.

Van Den Berghe G, Wouters P, Weekers F, et al. Intensive insulin therapy in critically ill patients. *N Eng J Med.* 2001;345:1359–1367.

45

STOP METFORMIN BEFORE ELECTIVE SURGERY OR INTRAVASCULAR CONTRAST DYE STUDY TO DECREASE THE RISK OF LACTIC ACIDOSIS

SERGE JABBOUR, MD, FACP, FACE AND
MICHAEL J. MORITZ, MD

Metformin is an insulin-sensitizing agent that has been in use for more than 50 years. Chemically, metformin is a biguanide. Its main action is to increase peripheral glucose utilization and decrease hepatic glucose release. In overweight patients with Type 2 diabetes, metformin has been shown to lower cardiovascular and diabetes-related deaths and has been considered the oral hypoglycemic agent of choice. It is also indicated to treat the insulin resistance of polycystic ovary syndrome. Metformin is excreted renally and has a half-life of 1.5 to 5 hours. Metformin is available as the branded drugs Glucophage, Glucophage XR tablets, Fortamet tablets, and Riomet liquid. It is also a component of three combination drugs: Glucovance, Metaglip, and Avandamet.

Lactic acidosis is a high-anion-gap acidosis. Lactate is produced by anaerobic glycolysis, and the development of lactic acidosis requires over-production, slowed breakdown, or both. At high blood levels, metformin produces severe refractory lactic acidosis by the uncoupling of oxidative glycolysis, thus driving cellular mechanisms toward anaerobic metabolism.

Lactic acidosis associated with metformin is rare but has a mortality of 50%. The risk with chronic use in the outpatient setting ranges from 1/1,000 to 1/30,000 patient-years. Patients in the acute care setting, however, incur an additional risk because they are exposed to situations, such as transient or ongoing renal insufficiency, that may lead to drug accumulation and increases in drug levels. As such, surgery or exposure to iodinated radiologic contrast dye (seen with angiography and intravenous contrast for computed tomography scan) must prompt discontinuation of metformin. Other clinical situations that may precipitate lactic acidosis in patients taking metformin include advanced age, dehydration, liver disease, congestive heart failure, chronic alcohol abuse or binge drinking of alcohol, shock with tissue hypoperfusion (septic, cardiogenic, etc.), and hypoxia.

At present, there are no outcome studies pertaining to the administration of metformin in the perioperative period. Generally, endocrinology consultants recommend that metformin be withheld on the day of surgery

© 2006 Mayo Foundation for Medical Education and Research

or contrast dye study only or at most for 24 hours. This represents a change in current opinion from as recently as 5 years ago and is based on both pharmacodynamic studies and the very important competing issue of improved perioperative outcomes due to tighter perioperative glucose control. For both surgical and radiology patients, the drug should be held for at least 48 hours and restarted only after renal function is known to be normal. Additionally, surgical patients should have resumption of adequate oral caloric intake.

SUGGESTED READINGS

Bailey CJ, Turner RC. Metformin. *N Engl J Med*. 1996;334:574–579.

Brown JB, Pedula MS, Barzilay J, et al. Lactic acidosis rates in type 2 diabetes. *Diabetes Care*. 1998;21:1659–1663.

Nisbet JC, Sturtevant JM, Prins JB. Metformin and serious adverse events. *AMJ*. 2004;180:53.

Thomsen HS, Morcos SK. Contrast media and metformin: guidelines to diminish the risk of lactic acidosis in non-insulin-dependent diabetics after administration of contrast media. ESUR Contrast Media Safety Committee. *Eur Radiol*. 1999;9:738–740.

46

REMEMBER THAT ADMINISTRATION OF ANGIOTENSIN SYSTEM INHIBITORS WITHIN 10 HOURS BEFORE SURGERY IS A SIGNIFICANT INDEPENDENT RISK FACTOR FOR HYPOTENSION IN THE POSTINDUCTION PERIOD[*]

THOMAS B. O. COMFERE, MD AND
JURAJ SPRUNG, MD, PHD

In general, the decision to withdraw medications with cardiovascular effects before surgery depends on the risk balance between the deleterious interaction of the drug with anesthetics and possible morbidity resulting from hemodynamic effects that may occur in the absence of these medications.

Drugs that affect the renin–angiotensin system, such as angiotensin-converting enzyme inhibitors (ACEIs) and angiotensin II receptor subtype 1 antagonists (ARAs), are often used in the management of hypertension, congestive heart failure, and chronic renal failure. These drugs may interfere with the regulation of arterial blood pressure by several different mechanisms, including sympathetic blockade, decrease in responsiveness to α_1-adrenergic agonists, impaired degradation of bradykinin (which promotes vasodilation), and inhibition of the receptor binding of angiotensin II.

Current practice guidelines recommend the perioperative continuation of therapies that have potential for myocardial protection, such as β-adrenoceptor-blocking drugs and calcium-channel blockers. Other drugs that are generally recommended to be continued are those with a potential for rebound hypertension with withdrawal, such as α_2-adrenoceptor agonists.

In the case of perioperative ACEI/ARA therapy, clear guidelines are not available. Severe intraoperative hypotension has been observed in patients treated with preoperative ACEIs and ARAs, and adequate perioperative management of antihypertensive therapy in patients receiving angiotensin-system blockers has been debated.

Preoperative withdrawal of ACEI/ARA therapy has been proposed on the basis of several reports of intraoperative hypotension, which has been reported to be refractory to common measures such as fluid boluses or intravenous ephedrine and phenylephrine. Several small, controlled, randomized

---

[*]Portions of this chapter were previously published in Comfere T, Sprung J, Kumar MM, et al. Angiostensin system inhibitors in a general surgical population. *Anesth Analg* 2005;100:636–644. Used with permission.

studies showed an increased frequency of hypotension after the induction of anesthesia when ACEI/ARA therapy was continued through the morning of surgery compared with discontinuation of therapy the night before surgery.

Angiotensin-system inhibition has also been shown to increase vasopressor requirements after cardiopulmonary bypass. Vasopressin or vasopressin analogs such as terlipressin have been advocated in patients on ACEI/ARA therapy to treat hypotension that is refractory to other measures.

Despite reports of intraoperative hypotension, some authors have recommended continued perioperative ACEI/ARA therapy for its potentially beneficial effects. Possible benefits are a decrease in ischemia-related myocardial cell damage in cardiac surgery and improved renal function in patients undergoing cardiopulmonary bypass, as measured by an improvement in urinary excretion of sodium.

In a recent large clinical trial by Comfere et al., the timing of the last ACEI or ARA dose was a major determinant of the frequency of postinduction hypotension. During the first 30 minutes after anesthetic induction, moderate hypotension (systolic blood pressure <85 mm Hg) was more frequent in patients whose most recent ACEI/ARA dose was taken within 10 hours (60%) compared with those whose last dose was taken more than 10 hours before induction (46%).

These findings can be explained by the elimination half-lives of ACEI/ARA drugs (*Table 46.1*). Specifically, a 10-hour interval between

TABLE 46.1	ELIMINATION HALF-LIVES OF ANGIOTENSIN-CONVERTING ENZYME INHIBITORS (ACEIs) AND ANGIOTENSIN-RECEPTOR ANTAGONISTS (ARAs)	
DRUG	ACTIVE METABOLITE	HALF-LIFE, H
ACEI		
Benazepril	Benzaprilat	≈ 11
Enalapril	Enalaprilat	≈ 11
Lisinopril		≈ 12
Quinapril	Quinaprilat	≈ 2
Fosinopril	Fosinoprilat	≈ 12
Ramipril	Ramiprilat	Range, 9–18
ARA		
Candesartan		Range, 5.1–10.5
Losartan	E-3174	Range, 6–9
Valsartan		Range, 6–9

Source: Modified from Comfere T, Sprung J, Kumar MM, et al. Angiotensin system inhibitors in a general surgical population. *Anesth Analg.* 2005;100:636–644. Used with permission.

the last dose and anesthetic induction corresponds to the average half-life of an ACEI or ARA and appears to be sufficient to decrease the incidence of hypotensive episodes after anesthetic induction. In humans, most ACEIs are eliminated renally via glomerular filtration or tubular secretion. Renal insufficiency may have a substantial effect on the half-life of certain ACEIs, and the altered pharmacokinetics of ACEIs in chronic renal failure may be a potential hazard; thus, abstinence for longer than 10 hours before surgery may be considered in patients with renal insufficiency.

In the study by Comfere et al., there was no clinically significant effect of timing of the last ACEI/ARA dose on preanesthetic arterial blood pressures, and both study groups had moderate preoperative hypertension regardless of when the last ACEI/ARA dose was taken.

TAKE HOME POINTS

- In patients receiving chronic ACEI/ARA therapy who receive general anesthesia, the administration of these drugs within 10 hours before anesthesia is a significant independent risk factor for the development of moderate hypotension within 30 minutes after induction in a common clinical setting.
- Anecdotally, hypotension in a setting of ACEI/ARA premedication was described in several case reports as being refractory to the usual therapeutic interventions. However, in a large clinical trial, all episodes of hypotension responded to conventional therapy, such as fluid boluses and intravenous ephedrine or phenylephrine, and thus seemed to be of little clinical consequence.
- Preoperative withholding of ACEI/ARA therapy should be considered for patients who may be especially prone to hypotension-induced complications (e.g., patients with severe aortic stenosis or cerebrovascular disease).
- No trial to date has demonstrated any deleterious effects of a short interruption of ACEI/ARA therapy in the immediate perioperative period.

SUGGESTED READINGS

Behnia R, Molteni A, Igic R. Angiotensin-converting enzyme inhibitors: mechanisms of action and implications in anesthesia practice. *Curr Pharm Des.* 2003;9:763–776.

Boccara G, Ouattara A, Godet G, et al. Terlipressin versus norepinephrine to correct refractory arterial hypotension after general anesthesia in patients chronically treated with renin-angiotensin system inhibitors. *Anesthesiology.* 2003;98:1338–1344.

Boldt J, Rothe G, Schindler E, et al. Can clonidine, enoximone, and enalaprilat help to protect the myocardium against ischaemia in cardiac surgery? *Heart.* 1996;76:207–213.

Brabant SM, Bertrand M, Eyraud D, et al. The hemodynamic effects of anesthetic induction in vascular surgical patients chronically treated with angiotensin II receptor antagonists. *Anesth Analg.* 1999;89:1388–1392.

Comfere T, Sprung J, Kumar MM, et al. Angiotensin system inhibitors in a general surgical population. *Anesth Analg.* 2005;100:636–644.

Licker M, Schweizer A, Hohn L, et al. Cardiovascular responses to anesthetic induction in patients chronically treated with angiotensin-converting enzyme inhibitors. *Can J Anaesth.* 2000;47:433–440.

Pigott DW, Nagle C, Allman K, et al. Effect of omitting regular ACE inhibitor medication before cardiac surgery on haemodynamic variables and vasoactive drug requirements. *Br J Anaesth.* 1999;83:715–720.

Tuman KJ, McCarthy RJ, O'Connor CJ, et al. Angiotensin-converting enzyme inhibitors increase vasoconstrictor requirements after cardiopulmonary bypass. *Anesth Analg.* 1995;80:473–479.

47

BE AWARE THAT MANY DRUGS COMMONLY GIVEN IN THE PERIOPERATIVE PERIOD HAVE SIGNIFICANT P-GLYCOPROTEIN TRANSPORT PUMP ACTIVITY

NEIL B. SANDSON, MD

In today's medical climate, the anesthesiologist must be prepared to function as a specialist in perioperative medicine. This includes (among many other tasks) a thorough knowledge of the drugs commonly given not just in the operating room (OR), but in the perioperative period, including routes of administration, dosing, and the specifics of drug elimination. Although discussions of pharmacokinetic drug handling most often focus on issues of metabolism and excretion, the emerging importance of the P-glycoprotein transporter highlights the relevance of absorption and distribution as well. The P-glycoprotein transporter is an ATP-dependent pump that extrudes various compounds (substrates) from protected intracellular domains. For instance, P-glycoprotein lines the lumen of the small intestine. When a P-glycoprotein substrate is absorbed across its concentration gradient into the cytosol of an enterocyte, this transporter acts to then extrude that drug out of the enterocyte and back into the gut lumen. Insofar as this process moves the drug against its concentration gradient, it requires ATP. P-glycoprotein also lines the blood–brain barrier, acting as one of the constituents that minimizes access of xenobiotic substances to the central nervous system. In a manner analogous to the small intestine, P-glycoprotein substrates diffuse from the vasculature into the cytosol of blood–brain barrier capillary endothelial cells, but the pump then acts to extrude them back into the vasculature. Significant P-glycoprotein substrates include carbamazepine, corticosteroids, cyclosporine, dexamethasone, digoxin, morphine, ondansetron, phenytoin, risperidone, tacrolimus, and tricyclic antidepressants. Dose-finding studies to determine effective doses of these and other P-glycoprotein substrates have already incorporated these effects.

Many compounds act to inhibit the action of the P-glycoprotein. Thus, P-glycoprotein inhibitors decrease the efflux of P-glycoprotein substrates from enterocytes into the gut lumen. The net effect of this process is that in the presence of a P-glycoprotein inhibitor, there will be greater systemic absorption of substrates at given doses. Similarly, at given intravascular

© 2006 Mayo Foundation for Medical Education and Research

concentrations of P-glycoprotein substrates, there will be more influx past the blood–brain barrier and into the central nervous system. In these instances, drug toxicity may be a concern. Significant P-glycoprotein inhibitors include atorvastatin, erythromycin, fluoxetine, lidocaine, lovastatin, midazolam, omeprazole, propranolol, simvastatin, tricyclic antidepressants, and verapamil. For instance, there are reports that co-administration of digoxin with a number of P-glycoprotein inhibitors, including atorvastatin, fluoxetine, and verapamil, among others, will reliably raise serum digoxin levels.

A smaller number of compounds act as inducers of the production of the P-glycoprotein transporter. When an inducer causes increased presence of the transporter, this leads to enhancement of the pump's action on substrates. Thus, in the presence of P-glycoprotein inducers there will be a decrease in substrate blood levels and less influx from the systemic vasculature into the central nervous system. In these instances, loss of drug efficacy may be a concern. Significant P-glycoprotein inducers include aspirin, rifampin, St. John's wort, and trazodone. It has been established that co-administration of rifampin and/or St. John's wort with digoxin will decrease serum digoxin levels through this mechanism.

These lists include a fraction of the known P-glycoprotein substrates, inhibitors, and inducers, and each month a growing number of drugs are found to have a functional relationship with this transporter system. When a patient is taking a P-glycoprotein substrate with a narrow therapeutic index, such as digoxin or tacrolimus, it is prudent to attend to the presence, addition, or deletion of P-glycoprotein inhibitors or inducers from the patient's regimen. A list of known P-glycoprotein substrates, inhibitors, and inducers may be found at www.mhc.com/Cytochromes.

TAKE HOME POINTS

- Today's anesthesia provider must expand her knowledge base beyond that of the basic anesthetic drugs.
- The P-glycoprotein transporter is an ATP-dependent pump that is relevant in the absorption and distribution of a number of important drugs in the perioperative period.
- There are both inducers and inhibitors of the P-glycoprotein transport pump.
- Be aware of the co-administration of both inhibitors and inducers of the P-glycoprotein pump when the patient is on a drug with a narrow therapeutic window, such as digoxin.

SUGGESTED READINGS

Cozza KL, Armstrong SC, Oesterheld JR. *Drug Interaction Principles for Medical Practice: Cytochrome P450s, UGTs, P-Glycoproteins.* Washington, DC: American Psychiatric Publishing; 2003:45–55.

Jaffrezou JP, Chen G, Duran GE, et al. Inhibition of lysosomal acid sphingomyelinase by agents which reverse multidrug resistance. *Biochim Biophys Acta.* 1995;1266(1):1–8.

Weiss J, Dormann SM, Martin-Facklam M, et al. Inhibition of P-glycoprotein by newer antidepressants. *J Pharmacol Exp Ther.* 2003;305(1):197–204.

48

ACKNOWLEDGE THE COMPLEX MEDICAL AND LEGAL ISSUES SURROUNDING OFF-LABEL DRUG USE

ANGELA M. PENNELL, MD

Imagine this scene: Your healthy, 5-year-old patient has just emerged from anesthesia after a routine, 30-minute case for PE tube placement. She is ventilating spontaneously and her vital signs are stable. As you leave the operating room (OR), she becomes agitated, screaming and thrashing on the stretcher and inconsolable. Pondering your options for treating her emergence delirium, you acknowledge that she does not have an intravenous (IV) line. Quickly, you administer 2 mcg/kg of intranasal clonidine. She becomes calm and quiet and you are thankful she is no longer a risk to herself. Her parents are reassured, the postanesthesia care unit (PACU) nurses are able to care for their new patient efficiently, and you move on to your next case without interruption. This was a successful and safe intervention, wasn't it? Perhaps so, but intranasal clonidine use is not described in the U.S. Food and Drug Administration (FDA) package insert.

The practice of anesthesiology reflects a mastery of pharmacology. Not only is the proper indication for and administration of a particular drug important to the anesthesia provider, but also the ability to co-administer agents or even to use them in novel ways. The most responsible and safest approach to this practice is to acknowledge drug labels created by the FDA and then strive to apply those guidelines to clinical practice. If a drug is used beyond those conditions described on its label, it is considered off-label.

The FDA regulates many aspects of drug development, research, safety, marketing, and labeling. The drug label is a summary of data collected by clinical trials. Therefore, in order to achieve approval for specific uses of a drug there must be evidence-based data to support it. Obviously, we cannot anticipate every detail of our patient population. So, based on medical literature, drugs are frequently used beyond the specific guidelines listed in the drug label for dose, route, indication, regimen, or patient population. How common is this practice? Sources site up to 23% of prescriptions being written for off-label use. This trend is not necessarily harmful, but, rather, reflects a lack of well-controlled study data held by the FDA (the study has not been done or there is no financial incentive to develop new indications,

© 2006 Mayo Foundation for Medical Education and Research

e.g., isobaric spinal bupivacaine). Further, if there is a known adverse effect of an off-label drug use, it will be listed in the Contraindications, Warnings, or Precautions section of the label.

According to the FDA, "once a product has been approved for marketing, a physician may prescribe it for uses in treatment regimens or patient populations that are not included in approved labeling. Valid new uses for drugs already on the market are often first discovered through serendipitous observations and therapeutic interventions." It is important to realize that the FDA does not seek to restrict a physician's decision to use a drug off-label and the *Physicians' Desk Reference* (PDR) also acknowledges this use. Interestingly, the publisher of the PDR, Medical Economics, also publishes an "off-label treatment guide." So, there is acknowledgement that this use has an important place in patient care. Currently in the United States, the physician has no ethical or legal obligation to educate the patient on FDA regulatory status when a drug is used. However, it is the physician's responsibility to be aware of details in the drug label, including pharmacology, toxicology, and chemistry (buffers, preservatives, antioxidants, and incompatibility with other drugs).

Anesthesiologists must also consider the unfortunate litigious climate of medicine. Drug manufacturers, the FDA, and the PDR all recognize the clinically observed safe and effective uses of a variety of medicines although they may not be supported by well-controlled, evidence-based data. However, courts and judges may have the ultimate authority over a physician's ability to practice off-label pharmacology and the liability for doing so (e.g., gabapentin and suicide risk). To be found liable for off-label drug use, the patient must prove that the anesthesiologist committed a breach of duty of care, that the breach resulted from a failure to reach the standard of care required by the law, and that the breach of duty resulted in injury. Based on the importance and well-recognized practice of off-label drug use per a physician's discretion, for a drug manufacturer to assert that it warned against unapproved uses is disingenuous. However, harm incurred to a patient related to an off-label use of a medication may ultimately be the prescriber's responsibility.

In general, there is a growing feeling that off-label drug use is the newly discovered gold mine of malpractice attorneys. The "learned intermediary" doctrine used by pharmaceutical manufacturers to protect them from liability asserts that they have provided the physician with warnings about a drug via the drug label. Hence, the physician now has the duty to warn the patient about that drug's hazards. Of course, this issue is really very complex. Ultimately, the FDA package insert must list the side effect of which the patient complains and there must be a way to prove that the patient was not adequately warned or was misled by the physician about those side effects. And,

TABLE 48.1 EIGHT DRUGS AND THEIR APPROVED AND OFF-LABEL USES

	PROPOFOL	FENTANYL	BUPIVACAINE	CLONIDINE	KETAMINE	LORAZEPAM	SUFENTANIL	NEURONTIN
Description	Propofol is a hindered phenol compound with IV general anesthetic properties. The drug is unrelated to any of the currently used barbiturate, opioid, benzodiazepine, arylcyclohexylamine, or imidazole IV anesthetic agents.	Binds stereospecific receptors at multiple CNS sites; increases pain threshold; alters pain perception; inhibits ascending pain pathways.	Blocks both the initiation and conduction of nerve impulses by decreasing the neuronal membrane's permeability to sodium ions, which results in inhibition of depolarization with resultant blockade of conduction.	Stimulates α_2-adrenoreceptors in brainstem to activate inhibitory neuron–decreased sympathetic outflow from CNS; decreased PVR, renal vascular resistance, HR, BP. Relief of epidural pain at spinal presynaptic, postjunctional α_2-adrenoreceptors by preventing transmission of pain signals.	Blockade of neuronal postsynaptic NMDA receptor. Direct action on cortex and limbic system. Stimulates release of endogenous catecholamines that maintain BP and HR. Reduces polysynaptic spinal reflexes.	Benzodiazepine—Binds to GABA receptors, increasing permeability to Cl$^-$ ions and enhancing inhibitory effects on neuronal excitation.	Binds opioid receptors in CNS to open K$^+$ channels and inhibiting Ca^{2+} channels; increases pain threshold; alters pain perception; inhibits ascending pain pathways; short-acting narcotic.	Mechanism of action unknown; similar properties to other anticonvulsants; structurally similar to GABA.

(continued)

TABLE 48.1 (CONTINUED)

	PROPOFOL	FENTANYL	BUPIVACAINE	CLONIDINE	KETAMINE	LORAZEPAM	SUFENTANIL	NEURONTIN
Approved uses	Induction of anesthesia for inpatient or outpatient surgery in patients aged ≥3 y; maintenance of anesthesia for inpatient or outpatient surgery in patients aged >2 mo; in adults, for the induction and maintenance of monitored anesthesia care sedation during diagnostic procedures; treatment of agitation in intubated, mechanically ventilated ICU patients.	Injection: Sedation, relief of pain, preoperative medication, adjunct to general or regional anesthesia. Transdermal: Management of moderate-to-severe chronic pain. Transmucosal (Actiq): Management of breakthrough cancer pain. Sedation for minor procedures/analgesia: For children aged 1–12 y; for children aged >12 y, refer to adult dosing. Continuous sedation/analgesia: For children aged 1–12 y. Chronic pain management: For children aged ≥2 y (opioid-tolerant patients). Transdermal: Refer to adult dosing.	Local anesthesia: Infiltration: 0.25% infiltrated locally; maximum: 175 mg. Caudal block (preservative-free): 15–30 mL of 0.25% or 0.5%. Epidural block (other than caudal block; preservative-free): Peripheral nerve block: 5 mL of 0.25% or 0.5%; max.: 400 mg/d Sympathetic nerve block. Retrobulbar anesthesia. Spinal anesthesia: Preservative-free solution of 0.75% bupivacaine in 8.25% dextrose.	Acute hypertension, hypertension. Pain management: Epidural infusion: Starting dose: 30 mcg/h; titrate as required for relief of pain or presence of side effects; minimal experience with doses >40 mcg/h; should be considered an adjunct to intraspinal opiate therapy. Warning against using as epidural for perioperative, obstetric, or postpartum pain because of possible bradycardia or hypotension. ADHD in children	Induction and maintenance of general anesthesia; sedation; analgesia.	Nausea/vomiting w/chemotherapy; status epilepticus; anxiety; preanesthesia for amnesic effect.	10–50 mcg/kg for induction w/10–50 mcg PRN. Pediatrics: ages 2–12 y, 10–25 mcg/kg induction; 1–2 mcg/kg maintenance (total dose).	Adjunct for partial seizures with and without secondary generalized seizures in patients aged >12 y. Adjunct therapy for partial seizures in pediatric patients aged 3–12 y. Management of postherpetic neuralgia in adults.

Off-Label Uses	Postoperative antiemetic; refractory delirium tremens (case reports); conscious sedation. Infusions faster than 40 mg q 10 s or 20 mg q 10 s for elderly, debilitated, ASA III or IV patients.	Epidural or intrathecal. Children aged <2 y.	Isobaric intrathecal. Pediatric patients aged <12 y.	Pediatric emergence delirium. Heroin or nicotine withdrawal; severe pain; dysmenorrhea; vasomotor symptoms associated with menopause; ethanol dependence; prophylaxis of migraines; glaucoma; diabetes-associated diarrhea; impulse-control disorder; ADHD; clozapine-induced sialorrhea.	Obstetric patients. Pediatric patients aged <16 y.	Agitation-IV. Insomia: short-term therapy. Ethanol detoxification. Psychogenic catatonia. Partial complex seizures.	Intrathecal.	Chronic pain. Bipolar disorder. Social phobia. Postoperative pain.

IV, intravenous; CNS, central nervous system; PVR, pulmonary vascular resistance; HR, heart rate; BP, blood pressure; ICU, intensive care unit; ADHD, attention-deficit/hyperactivity disorder.

in countries such as England, cases are being decided in favor of patients who claim that they were given inadequate information about a drug and, therefore, did not give informed consent. In situations in which there are alternative, FDA-approved medications to a drug being used off-label and purportedly resulting in harm, it might be difficult to convince a jury that the decision of the physician was sound. Thus, in England, physicians must now obtain informed consent for prescribed medicines, especially those used off-label. This includes risks and benefits, information about "approved" alternatives, education about the meaning of off-label drug use, and the lack of testing existing for that use. In England, to use a drug off-label is then justified only if there is no approved alternative and not because the use is more convenient or less costly.

Of note, it is illegal for drug manufacturers to market off-label uses of their products. An interesting example of this involves Neurontin (gabapentin), originally manufactured by Parke-Davis (now controlled by Pfizer). This drug underwent scrutiny beginning in 2005 when concerns were raised about increased suicide rates among patients taking the drug not for seizures, but for other medical conditions including chronic pain. The FDA has asked Pfizer to analyze its study data for evidence of suicide risk. Attorneys are requesting that the FDA attach a black-box warning addressing suicide risk. To date, there is no clear evidence of increased suicide risk in those using Neurontin outside its FDA-approved treatment of seizure disorder. The final decision is expected in 2007. It should be recognized that it is also illegal for drug representatives to discuss off-label use, and this information should be obtained from the medical literature. The ultimate decision to use a drug off-label is appropriately made by an individual physician for an individual patient.

In general, off-label drug use by a licensed physician is a common and widely recognized practice. The decision to do so should be based on current medical literature and with the acknowledgment that there is not a better, FDA-approved drug available. In addition, consideration should be given to current legal action surrounding the drug. For anesthesiologists who primarily administer drugs in the hospital setting, it may also be wise to educate and inform the patient via literature included with the consent for care received upon admission. *Table 48.1* describes eight drugs and their approved and off-label uses.

SUGGESTED READINGS

Babhair SA, Tariq M, Abdullah, ME. Comparison of intravenous and nasal bioavailability of clonidine in rodents. *Res Commun Chem Pathol Pharmacol.* 1990;67(2):241–248.

Barnett M. The new pill pushers: Big Pharma warily watches lawsuit over "off-label" prescription drug marketing. *USNews.com.* 26 April 2004.

Chang NS, Simone AF, Schultheis LW. From the FDA: What's in a label? A guide for the anesthesia practitioner. *Anesthesiology.* 2005;103(1):179–185.

Donnelly AJ, Baughman VL, Gonzales JP, et al. *Anesthesiology and Critical Care Drug Handbook.* 6th ed. Hudson, Ohio: Lexi-Comp; 2004.

Pringle E. Off-label prescribing of prescription drugs: Pfizer embroiled in massive lawsuit over off-label use of Neurontin. *Health.* 1 June 2006. www.onlinejournal.com/artman/publish/article_860.shtml.

Saj S. Medico-legal controversies in the management of preterm labour: "Off-label" medicines. Ferring Pharmaceuticals; 2005. http://oblink.com/display.asp?page= PresentationTranscript_shah_COGI2005.

Tesoro S, Mezzetti D, Marchesini L, et al. Clonidine treatment for agitation in children after sevoflurane anesthesia. *Anesth Analg.* 2005;101(6):1619–1622.

Thornton RG. Defending claims related to prescribing drugs or using medical devices. *Proc (Bayl Univ Med Cent).* 2002;15(1):102–104. www.pubmedcentral.nih.gov/articlerender. fcgi?artid=1276346.

Washington Post examines how many off-label uses for Rx drugs are not based on solid evidence. www.medicalnewstoday.com/medicalnews.php?newsid=43904. Accessed May 2006.

Editors' Note: We recommend strict on-label use for drugs administered in the intrathecal space, and advise against the use of certain lidocaine preparations and isobaric bupivacaine for spinals. Remember, it is easy to establish that isobaric bupivacaine is not only off-label but "against-label", as the vials are plainly marked as "Not for Spinal Anesthesia"—do you want to be forced to read that in a deposition or court of law? Another good example of the off-label controversy concerns the use of certain lidocaine spinals. There has been quite a bit of fallout at very respected institutions regarding off-label use of lidocaine, even with IRB approval. One of the many articles that appeared about this can be found at Anesth Analg. 2002 Sep;95(3):757–9.

49

REMEMBER THAT THE UNTHINKABLE *IS* POSSIBLE—FOLLOW THESE PRINCIPLES IN THE EVALUATION AND TREATMENT OF PATIENTS SUFFERING FROM NERVE AGENT POISONING

DANIEL J. BOCHICCHIO, MD, FCCP

It's rush hour on a warm June afternoon. While walking past a television in the operating room (OR) lounge, a news flash breaks into today's soap opera. A reporter at the baseball stadium approximately 7 miles away from your hospital is describing a plane crash. A small crop-dusting aircraft flew low over the grandstands and crashed into the press box. Apparently, some form of toxic chemical was being released by the aircraft at the time of the crash. The scene on television is chaotic. The news camera pans toward the stadium exits, where there are numerous dead bodies. Several individuals are staggering about. Several collapse onto the sidewalk. One victim vomits, collapses, and begins seizing. The chemical is tentatively identified as a "nerve agent." Absolute chaos is an appropriate description for the scene at the trauma center closest to the disaster. The press is estimating as many as 1,000 causalities, with >100 dead at the scene. You hear over the public address system that the hospital is implementing its mass casualty disaster plan. You have just been informed that your hospital can expect >100 casualties. Among the casualties are numerous police, fire, and emergency medical personnel. In an effort to evacuate the site rapidly, some victims may not have received adequate decontamination.

Thirty minutes later you receive your first victim from the scene. A 28-year-old woman, while attempting to flee, fell and was trampled by the crowd. She now presents with multiple contusions and abrasions for a laparotomy and possible splenectomy. She is awake and alert but appears very anxious, tremulous and tearful. Her blood pressure is 119/74 mm Hg, pulse 118 beats/min, respirations 32/min with mild dyspnea. While the staff in the emergency department is performing a brief focused physical exam, she vomits and voids on the stretcher.

The patient's respiratory condition begins to deteriorate. She is promptly brought to the OR. You are informed that the agent has been identified as Sarin. You consider that the luckiest moment in your life is when the anesthesiologist who is covering the intensive care unit (ICU) this week comes over to help you start your case. He is a colonel in the Army Reserves with a specialty in chemical warfare.

© 2006 Mayo Foundation for Medical Education and Research

He induces general endotracheal anesthesia. You notice that the airway pressure at 7-mL/kg tidal volume is 52 cm H_2O. There are copious secretions noted in the no. 8 endotracheal tube. The surgeons are asking to begin. The patient's blood pressure is 134/67, pulse is 110 beats/min, SaO_2 is 92% by pulse oximetry on 100% inspired oxygen. Approximately 30 minutes after induction, your anesthesia technician begins to complain of blurry vision and rhinorrhea.

The surgical procedure, an exploratory laparotomy and splenectomy, requires 1 hour to complete. It is without significant surgical complication. The patient is brought to the postanesthesia care unit (PACU). In the PACU there are again copious secretions noted in the endotracheal tube. Your ICU colleague says he will give more antidote (in the chaos, you were not completely clear that "antidote" had been given in the first place) and asks you to resuction the airway. After a few more minutes the spontaneous respirations appear much less labored and the secretions are improving. Your senior colleague decides not to extubate at this time and leaves you to care for the patient while he goes downstairs to help there. The nurse in pre-op holding calls you to come quickly; your next patient is apneic and seizing. She also confirms that there are hundreds of patients downstairs who need care.

How do you approach this mass casualty situation? What is meant by decontamination? What is meant by "the antidote?" How will you do the anesthesia for the next patient? Can you keep yourself safe?

DISCUSSION

Chemical warfare agents are chemicals that have direct toxic effects on mammalian tissue. The modern era of chemical warfare began on the French battlefields of World War I. On April 22, 1915, the German Army attacked the Allied positions with chlorine gas. The bombardment caused 15,000 Allied casualties, with 5,000 dead. In 1936, Dr. Gerhard Schrader discovered the highly toxic effects of the pesticide Tabun on mammalian tissue. This was quickly followed by the discovery of several more nerve agents. Although these highly toxic compounds have been in existence for 70 years, the vast majority of civilian health professionals have received little if any education or training on the medical management of victims of nerve agent poisoning.

Accordingly, most physicians and other health care providers caring for chemical casualties in recent conflicts lacked any formal training in this area. There are case reports of casualties contaminated with mustard agent in the Iraq–Iran war having been evacuated as far as hospitals in France without adequate decontamination. Lack of adequate knowledge to deal with the problem under the stress of a mass casualty situation will have a serious negative effect on survivability. There is nothing unique about the pathophysiology of chemical injury that is beyond the understanding of properly trained clinicians. The principles of rapid, thorough decontamination, self-protection, and an understanding of the actions of antidotes are the keys to effective chemical casualty care.

Nerve agents are the most toxic chemical weapons known. They exert their biologic effect by inhibiting the enzyme acetylcholinesterase (AChE), thereby precipitating a cholinergic crisis. There are two major classes, the carbamates and the organophosphates (OPs). Among the former are neostigmine, physostigmine, pyridostigmine, and several commercially available insecticides. The OPs include the "military" nerve agents and several insecticides. Five OP AChE inhibitors are recognized as military nerve agents (NAs). They are commonly known as Tabun (North Atlantic Treaty Organization [NATO] designation: GA), Sarin (NATO: GB), Soman (GD), GF, and VX. The agents GF and VX do not have common names. The "G" agents were developed in Nazi Germany by Gerhard Schrader and his associates while researching insecticides for the conglomerate IG Farben between 1936 and 1944. VX was developed by the British in 1954 while searching for a replacement for the insecticide DDT. A nerve agent, given adequate time, will irreversibly bind all three forms of AChE.

The binding of NAs to AChE prevents the degradation of acetylcholine (ACh). The toxic effects of NAs are a result of massive excess of ACh. The symptoms are related to both the dose and the route of exposure. Inhalation of vapor causes immediate symptoms. If the vapor concentration (mg/m^3) and exposure time are significantly high, then the onset will be immediate and death may occur in minutes. Nerve agents are readily absorbed through intact skin and will penetrate clothing. The onset of symptoms after skin exposure to liquid agent can be delayed. Onset of systems depends on the amount of exposure, the promptness of decontamination, and temperature, moisture, and location on the body. Time of onset can range from several minutes up to 12 to 18 hours (Sidel et al., 1997).

All NAs are liquid at standard atmospheric conditions. The G–series agents are more volatile than VX and constitute a significant vapor hazard, whereas VX presents predominately a liquid hazard. Sarin (GB) is the most volatile of the G–agents and has a vapor pressure (2.1 mm Hg. at 20°C) that is close to that of water. Nerve agents are essentially colorless, odorless, and tasteless liquids. The G-agents are less persistent than VX, with $t_{1/2}$ of several hours to a few days. The $t_{1/2}$ of VX can be a week or longer. Nerve agents may be dispersed via several types of delivery systems. Identification of NAs can be accomplished using several detection systems. These detectors may not be immediately available to the initial civilian responders. Initial identification will likely be made by recognition of the clinical symptoms of toxicity until the arrival of civilian or military hazardous materials (HAZMAT) teams.

The toxic effects of cholinergic poisoning occur in the central, autonomic, and peripheral nervous systems. The most immediately life-threatening are the respiratory compromise resulting from increased airway resistance, central nervous system (CNS)-mediated respiration depression, and paralysis. At higher exposures, apnea, seizures, and coma occur. Of particular concern to health care providers are the ophthalmic symptoms of miosis, blurred vision, diminished visual acuity, and loss of accommodation. These symptoms can occur after minimal exposure to vapor and can severely affect patient care. In the 1995 Sarin attack on the Tokyo subway, miosis was the most common symptom among victims and health care providers. Miosis was reported by >90% of victims.

If the toxic agent is not immediately identified, secondary contamination may pose a significant risk to emergency response personnel. Decontamination should occur as close to the site of exposure as possible to limit the spread of contamination and reduce the time to initial treatment. A hospital receiving potentially contaminated casualties should establish a "hot zone," where casualties can receive adequate decontamination before being permitted entry into the facility. This area is best located in a well-ventilated open area outside the hospital. A "dirty dump" site must be established downwind from the treatment facility.

Decontamination begins with removal of the victim's clothing. The goal is the physical removal and chemical degradation of the chemical agent. Casualties should be decontaminated with copious amounts of tepid soap and water. The victim's hair may become a source of contamination and may require cutting to facilitate decontamination. Avoid hot water, harsh chemicals, strong soaps, and stiff brushes. Care should be taken to avoid causing vasodilatation or mechanical damage to the skin, as this may enhance absorption of nerve agents. Mild alkaline solutions and chlorine releasing agents such as diluted (0.5% hypochlorite) household bleach will neutralize NAs more quickly that plain soap and water. This solution is contraindicated in open injuries of the eye, abdomen, or brain.

In spite of decontamination stations, contaminated patients may find their way into the emergency department, operating room, intensive care unit, or any other hospital location if not controlled. Contaminated medical electronic equipment may not be recoverable. Secondary injury to health care providers will seriously degrade medical capabilities and add to the casualty numbers. *Institutional and individual self-protection is of critical importance. Latex gloves, surgical masks, and gowns are not protective.* Butyl rubber gloves and gowns or chemical-protective overgarments must be worn by all personnel caring for all casualties whose contamination status is unknown. "Off-gassing" of volatile nerve agent from clothing and, to a much lesser extent, skin poses a vapor threat, and appropriate respiratory protection must be worn.

For chemically injured patients, the fundamental principles of resuscitation do not change. Establish an airway and provide adequate gas exchange and circulatory support. However, to this must be added: Terminate the exposure and decontaminate the victim. The exact sequence in which these occur can be greatly influenced by the situation. The cornerstones of pharmacologic management consist of three classes of drugs: Atropine, an anticholinergic; pralidoxime (2-PAM), a pyridinium oxime; and the benzodiazepines. The actions of atropine and the oximes may be synergistic. Atropine is extremely effective at blocking the effects of excess ACh at peripheral muscarinic sites. Atropine will improve the bronchoconstriction, bronchorrhea, nausea, vomiting, diarrhea, and bradycardia. Atropine will not alleviate many of the ocular disturbances or prevent skeletal muscle paralysis. The oxime 2-PAM reactivates AChE by breaking the AChE–NA bond. The NA bound to 2-PAM is unable to attack and bind AChE. The 2-PAM reactivation of AChE is most apparent in improved skeletal muscle strength. It should be noted that reactivation of AChE by oximes will occur only if this treatment is given before the chemical process of aging of the AChE–NA bond. Once the AChE–NA bond has aged, the oxime cannot reactivate the enzyme. Thereafter, recovery of function depends on synthesis of new AChE. The aging half-time varies from a few minutes for Soman to 48 hours for VX. The aging half-time for Sarin is 5 hours. Benzodiazepines are used to decrease convulsant activity associated with severe exposure.

Simplicity should be the goal for any mass-casualty treatment protocol. The U.S. Army Chemical Casualty Care Division of the Medical Research Institute of Chemical Defense offers a practical approach to medical management initially developed for battlefield use. Remember that exposure to NAs generally occurs via one of three routes—inhalation of vapor, liquid on skin, or ingestion. Because of the large absorptive capacity of the respiratory system, exposure to vapor rapidly produces symptoms. Exposed patients present with acute-onset miosis, copious rhinorrhea, dyspnea, apnea, and ultimately, convulsions and death. Depending on the severity of the exposure, the time course of events may vary from a few seconds to a few minutes. Victims exposed to high concentrations of vapor are unlikely to survive, so you probably won't be seeing these patients in the surgical suite. The time to onset of symptoms following dermal exposure may be highly variable.

Exposures are characterized by the severity of the intoxication as well as the route. Intoxication can be mild to moderate or severe. A mild vapor exposure might present with miosis, dim vision, rhinorrhea, salivation, anxiety, and/or mild dyspnea. The presence of severe respiratory distress, loss of bowel or bladder control, generalized muscle fasciculation, convulsions, or apnea implies severe poisoning. Mild to moderate dermal exposure may present with localized muscle twitching and sweating at the exposure site, anxiety, nausea, vomiting, and a feeling of weakness. Severe liquid exposure would include all of the aforementioned symptoms, plus severe dyspnea, generalized muscle twitching, seizures, loss of consciousness, apnea, and loss of bowel and bladder control. For mild to moderate intoxication in an adult, 2 to 4 mg of atropine by intravenous (IV) bolus plus 600 to 1200 mg of pralidoxime IV over 30 minutes would be the initial therapy. For severe intoxication, 6 mg of atropine with 1,800 mg pralidoxime plus 10 mg Diazepam IV is the recommended initial therapy. Atropine is titrated to an improvement in symptoms as generally indicated by a reduction in secretions and the ability to oxygenate and ventilate the victim. Nebulized [beta]-agonists should be administered to help treat NA-induced bronchoconstriction. It should be noted that nerve agent–induced miosis is resistant to parenterally administered atropine and therefore is not a good indicator of full atropinization. If intravenous access is unavailable, then both antidotes may be given intramuscularly. Civilian physicians may see military-style, U.S. Food and Drug Administration–approved, Atro-Pen MARK I kits used in a NA attack. Many municipalities are acquiring them for emergency responders and other providers. The kits contain two autoinjectors: One containing 2 mg of atropine and another containing 600 mg of pralidoxime chloride. Autoinjectors are a superior delivery method for intramuscular antidotes and can quickly achieve high serum concentrations. Using this dosing method, casualties would receive one, two, or three MARK I kits intramuscularly (IM), with or without diazepam, based on the severity of the exposure. Additional atropine would then be titrated to clinical response at 10- to 15-minute intervals. Children are more susceptible to the effects of NAs. Resuscitation of pediatric victims of NA exposure poses a greater challenge. Dosing is weight-based, and intravascular access may be difficult. The current recommendations are atropine 0.05 to 0.1 mg/kg, pralidoxime 25 to 50 mg/kg, and Diazepam 0.05 to 0.3 mg/kg IV/IM.

Victims with combined injuries are at higher risk of mortality. Nerve agent intoxication reduces the cardiopulmonary response to physical trauma. Penetrating trauma provides a direct portal of entry for NAs. Examination and evaluation of a toxic, traumatized patient may be a particular challenge. The anesthetic management of the NA-intoxicated, traumatized patient is based on a very small number of cases and is therefore largely unknown. General endotracheal anesthesia may be the safest anesthetic technique. Inhaled volatile anesthetics are potent bronchodilators and relax skeletal muscle. This should facilitate ventilation and provide acceptable surgical conditions. The high risk of nausea and vomiting will require airway protection during the induction of anesthesia. Selection of induction agents can be a challenge. Sodium thiopental or propofol may worsen the hemodynamic instability of the NA-intoxicated patient. Ketamine may offer some advantages. Ketamine is commonly used to induce anesthesia in the hemodynamically compromised patient and is a potent analgesic. The bronchodilation and mild increase in heart rate may be beneficial. Atropine should be given before the ketamine to avoid central apnea. The skeletal muscle relaxation choices may also be restricted. NA-induced inhibition of plasma cholinesterase and the unique structure of succinylcholine may cause its duration of action to become unpredictable. The positive chronotropic effect of pancuronium may make it a better choice. Using neostigmine to reverse the effects of the neuromuscular blockade may prove problematic. Careful monitoring of the neuromuscular blockade is recommended. Perioperative pain management may require opioids. The histamine-releasing potential of morphine may make it a poor selection. Histamine release can exacerbate the bronchoconstriction and hypotension associated with NAs. Fentanyl has potential vagotonic effects and may worsen the bradycardia. The use of meperidine as an analgesic has been suggested because of its lack of histamine release and its tendency to cause an increase in heart rate.

TAKE HOME POINTS

- The medical management of mass-casualty events poses some of the greatest challenges to the health care delivery system.
- Mass-casualty situations involving chemical, biologic, or radiologic weapons present an even greater threat.
- One fact is certainly not debatable: Lack of preparedness on the part of the health care community will not improve the outcome of such an event. With proper training and preparation, the human costs of a chemical attack can be mitigated.
- Nerve agents are odorless, tasteless, colorless liquids—the term "nerve gas agent" is a common misnomer.
- Individual self-protection is critically important—standard OR garb *does not* provide an adequate barrier to contamination.
- Ask what the nerve agent mass-casualty plans are for your location—do not assume it can't happen!

SUGGESTED READINGS

Ben-Abraham RB, Rudick V, Weinbrom AA. Practical guidelines for acute care of victims of bioterrorism: Conventional injuries and contaminant nerve agent intoxication. *Anesthesiology*. 2002;97:989–1004.

Holstage CP, Kirk M, Sidell FR. Chemical warfare, nerve agent poisoning. *Crit Care Clin*. 1997;13(4):923–939.

Marrs TC, Maynard RL, Sidell FR. *Chemical Warfare Agents: Toxicology and Treatment*. New York: Wiley; 1996.

Medical Management of Chemical Casualties Handbook. 3rd ed. Chemical Casualty Care Division, United States Army Medical Research Institute for Chemical Defense (USAMRICD). June 2000. Available at: http://ccc.apgea.army.mil/reference_materials/handbooks/RedHandbook/001TitlePage.htm.

Rotenburg JS, Newmark J. Nerve agent attacks on children: Diagnosis and management. *Pediatrics.* 2003;112:648–658.

Sidell FR, Takafuji ET, Franz DR. *Textbook of Military Medicine, Part I, Medical Aspects of Chemical and Biological Warfare,* Washington, DC: Office of the Surgeon General, Borden Institute; 1997. Available at: http://ccc.apgea.army.mil/reference_materials/textbook/HTML_Restricted/index.htm.

50

USE BICARBONATE AS A BUFFER TO LOCAL ANESTHETICS, ESPECIALLY FOR SKIN INFILTRATION

HOOMAN RASTEGAR FASSAEI, MD AND STEVEN L. OREBAUGH, MD

Local anesthetics reversibly block impulse conduction along nerve axons and other excitable membranes that utilize sodium channels as the primary means of action potential generation. The local anesthetics used clinically consist of a lipid-soluble, substituted benzene ring linked to an amine group via an alkyl chain containing either an amide or an ester linkage.

Local anesthetics are weak bases (pK$_a$ 7.6 to 9). These agents are poorly soluble in water and therefore are usually marketed in acidic hydrochloride salt solutions (pH 3 to 6). In this form, the local anesthetic rapidly becomes reduced to a cationic form. This process is readily reversible, and the relative proportions of neutral base and ionized form will equilibrate as described by the Henderson-Hasselbach equation:

$$\text{Log}(\text{cationic form}/\text{uncharged form}) = pK_a - pH$$

The proportions of the drug that exist in each form depend on the pH of the solution and the pK$_a$, or dissociation constant, of the particular drug. This dissociation constant (pK$_a$) denotes the pH at which the ionized and neutral forms of the molecule are present in equal amounts. Since the pK$_a$ of most local anesthetics is in the range of 7.6 to 9.0, the larger fraction in the body fluids at physiologic pH will be the charged, cationic form.

Local anesthetics reversibly block conduction of action potentials by interacting with the intracellular portion of the voltage-gated sodium channels. It is the charged form of the local anesthetic molecule that appears to interact with this portion of the channel. The local anesthetic must first penetrate the lipid-rich neural cell membrane as the uncharged, lipid-soluble form.

BUFFERING LOCAL ANESTHETICS TO DECREASE ONSET TIME

Local anesthetics are administered in an acidic solution, so most of the agent is in the ionized form, which is lipophobic. Therefore, the drug must first be converted to the nonionized form in sufficient quantity to enter the nerve cell. This depends on the pK$_a$ of the local anesthetic and the pH of the tissue. Once inside the nerve cell, the lower pH converts the drug back into the ionized form, which is then able to block the sodium channels.

© 2006 Mayo Foundation for Medical Education and Research

Increasing the pH of the carrier solution of local anesthetics with sodium bicarbonate will favor the formation of a more neutral base form of the drug. This uncharged molecule is more capable of diffusing through the cell membrane and will theoretically result in more rapid nerve blockade.

The addition of sodium bicarbonate to local anesthetic solutions has been reported to decrease the time of onset of conduction blockade. Alkalinization of solutions of bupivacaine or lidocaine accelerates the onset of brachial plexus and epidural blockade in some studies but not others. In addition, a recent animal study suggests that alkalinization of lidocaine decreases the duration of peripheral nerve blocks if the solution does not also contain epinephrine.

BUFFERING LOCAL ANESTHETICS TO DECREASE PAIN ON INJECTION

The acidity of the commercial preparations of local anesthetics makes them painful to inject into the skin or subcutaneous tissues. There are several studies that show adding bicarbonate to lidocaine attenuates pain on skin infiltration.

The mechanism of pain reduction is unknown but probably relates to an increase in pH. If H^+ ions themselves cause pain, sodium bicarbonate would decrease pain merely by decreasing H^+ concentration. Consistent with this idea, commercial lidocaine with epinephrine (pH 4.15) has a low pH and is more painful than is lidocaine with added epinephrine (pH 6.4). However, the cause of pain on skin infiltration is probably more complex and depends on factors other than pH alone. For example, procaine (pH 4.3) is more acidic but less painful than lidocaine (pH 6.3). Alternatively, the pain–reducing effect of sodium bicarbonate may represent a shift of the equilibrium between the ionized and nonionized forms of lidocaine, favoring formation of the nonionized form. The more rapid diffusion of the nonionized form may result in rapid inhibition of pain transmission, thereby preventing nociceptive impulses from being fully appreciated.

How to Prepare Buffered Lidocaine for Skin Infiltration

- Add 1 mL of sodium bicarbonate at a concentration of 1 mEq/mL to 9 mL plain lidocaine 1%.
- Add 1 mL of sodium bicarbonate at a concentration of 1 mEq/mL to 4 mL plain lidocaine 2% (will increase the pH from approximately 6.2 to 7.26).

Buffering local anesthetic solutions decreases their shelf life. Most amides and amines are chemically unstable in the buffered, uncharged form and are subject to photodegradation and aldehyde formation. Buffered lidocaine remains active for only 1 week when stored at room temperature, and for a few weeks when refrigerated.

- Local anesthetics are weak bases that are poorly soluble in water. They are marketed in acidic salt solutions to improve stability and shelf life.
- Buffering with bicarbonate solution increases the neutral (nonionized) fraction, which can cross the lipid-rich neural cell membrane and then be converted to the ionized form to act on the sodium channel.
- Some (but not all) studies have shown that buffering local anesthetic decreases the onset time for brachial plexus and epidural blocks.
- Buffering local anesthetics *will* decrease "pain of injection." Palmon et al. found that the addition of bicarbonate had a greater overall effect than needle size in decreasing the pain associated with the intradermal injection of lidocaine. It is hoped that increased use of buffered lidocaine for intravenous starts and needle placement for nerve blocks will decrease the necessity of the warning, "A little stick and a burn here, Mr. Johnson."

SUGGESTED READINGS

Barash PG. *Clinical Anesthesia.* 5th ed. Philadelphia: Lippincott Williams & Wilkins; 2006: 459–460.

Brogan GX Jr, Giarrusso E, Hollander JE, et al. Comparison of plain, warmed, and buffered lidocaine for anesthesia of traumatic wounds. *Ann Emerg Med.* 1995;26(2):121–125.

Colaric KB, Overton DK, Moore T. Pain reduction in lidocaine administration through buffering and warming. *Am J Emerg Med.* 1998;16(4):353–356.

Jackson T, McLure H. Pharmacology of local anesthetics. *Ophthalmol Clin N Am.* 2006;19: 155–161.

Katzung BG. *Basic & Clinical Pharmacology.* 8th ed. New York: McGraw-Hill; 2001:436–446.

McKay W, Morris R, Mushlin P. Sodium bicarbonate attenuates pain on skin infiltration with lidocaine, with or without epinephrine. *Anesth Analg.* 1987;66(6):572–574.

Miller RD, ed. *Miller's Anesthesia.* 6th ed. Elsevier Churchill Livingstone; 2005:585.

Palmon SC, Lloyd AT, Kirsch JR. The effect of needle gauge and lidocaine pH on pain during intradermal injection. *Anesth Analg.* 1998;86:379–381.

Sinnott CJ, Garfield JM, Thalhammer JG, et al. Addition of sodium bicarbonate to lidocaine decreases the duration of peripheral nerve block in the rat. *Anesthesiology.* 2000;93(4): 1045–1052.

51

Consider Perioperative Clonidine Administration—It Has Anxiolytic, Antiemetic, and Analgesic Properties

Bryan J. Fritz, MD and Shashank Saxena, MD

Clonidine, originally introduced clinically as a nasal decongestant and subsequently used as a centrally acting antihypertensive, has become increasingly utilized for its anesthetic properties. The sedative effects of α_2-agonists have been known since their introduction. In fact, a volunteer once slept for an entire day following a dose of intranasal clonidine. Human and animal studies performed in the late 1960s demonstrated a profound reduction in minimum alveolar concentration (MAC) when inhalation agents were administered concurrently with α_2-receptor agonists such as clonidine. α-Receptor agonists have been utilized in veterinary medicine for many years as a regional anesthetic, but only relatively recently have they been employed in human patients. Tamsen and Gordh injected a parenteral preparation of clonidine epidurally into two patients in 1984, after they first established its safety in animals. Since that time a large body of research has explored both the safety and the clinical benefits of clonidine as an analgesic; however, it is only approved by the U.S. Food and Drug Administration (FDA) to treat hypertension and in the treatment of cancer pain. Though it is more popular in Europe, clonidine is used off-label in the United States for many other benefits.

Chemical Properties/Pharmacology

Clonidine, an imidazoline, is a partial α_2-aerometric receptor agonist that acts primarily presynaptically and inhibits norepinephrine release in the nucleus tractus solitarii of the medulla oblongata. It is not highly selective at α-receptors, as it has a selectivity ratio of approximately 200:1 for α_2- to α_1-receptors, respectively. Furthermore, clonidine is able to interact with nonadrenergic imidazoline receptors found in the brain, kidney, and pancreas. α_2-Adrenergic receptors function through G-protein mechanisms. Four subtypes exist, and all activate well-defined intracellular cascades. Clonidine was first thought to exhibit its effects primarily through presynaptic receptors in the medulla, though it is now known to act both directly in spinal preganglionic sympathetic neurons as well as in the dorsal horn by pre- and postsynaptic mechanisms.

© 2006 Mayo Foundation for Medical Education and Research

PHYSIOLOGIC EFFECTS

The primary affect of clonidine is sympatholytic, but—possibly because it binds with many different receptors—the drug has various actions beyond antihypertensive properties, such as sedation, anxiolysis, analgesia, and as an adjunct with other anesthetics. Clonidine causes a decrease in central sympathetic outflow, thereby lowering arterial pressure. At low doses, clonidine has an anxiolytic effect on the central nervous system (CNS), though at higher doses it can be anxiogenic and cause hypertension, most likely as a result of α_1-activity. Little effect is exerted on the respiratory system, save a small reduction in minute ventilation. α_2-Receptors of β-cells in the pancreas are stimulated and cause a temporary inhibition of insulin release. This has not been proven to be problematic in a clinical setting. Clonidine has the added benefit for anesthesia of an antisialagogue effect.

DOSING/DURATION OF ACTION

The high lipid solubility of clonidine allows rapid and complete absorption after oral administration. Less than 50% is metabolized hepatically to inactive metabolites, with the remaining drug excreted unchanged by the kidneys. Orally, the peak plasma level is reached in 1 to 1.5 hours. It readily crosses the blood–brain barrier with an elimination half-life of 30 minutes after epidural injection of 150 mcg. In general, hemodynamic effects peak at around 1 to 2 hours and last approximately 6 to 8 hours. Sedation occurs in a dose-dependent fashion within 20 minutes regardless of the route of administration. These effects can last 4 to 6 hours. Dosing information on clonidine is shown in *Table 51.1*.

ANTIHYPERTENSIVE EFFECTS

Hypertensive patients usually respond to clonidine with a more profound drop in blood pressure than do normotensive patients. Though clonidine reduces heart rate, it seems to have little effect on the baroreceptor reflex, thus accompanying orthostatic hypotension and profound bradycardia are produced less frequently than with other antihypertensive drugs. Researchers have shown an attenuation of the stress response to direct laryngoscopy when a minimum dose of 4 mcg/kg clonidine is administered intravenously (IV) preoperatively. Further studies have shown a possible benefit in reducing perioperative cardiac ischemia, though conflicting reports exist. Rapid discontinuation of clonidine can precipitate a hypertensive crisis, so clonidine should be continued throughout the perioperative period.

SEDATION/REDUCTION IN ANESTHETIC REQUIREMENTS

Although clonidine is not used as a sole anesthetic agent, it has been used as a premedication in numerous studies. It is especially useful in pediatrics. In

TABLE 51.1	DOSING INFORMATION FOR CLONIDINE
Hypertension	Oral (adults): Initially, 0.1 mg PO twice daily; increase by 0.1–0.2 mg/d PO until desired effect is achieved (usual dosage range 0.2–0.6 mg/d PO). Children: Initially, 5–10 mcg/kg/d PO in divided doses every 8–12 h. Increase gradually (every 5–7 d) to 5–25 mcg/kg/day PO in divided doses every 6 h. Maximum dosage is 0.9 mg/d. Transdermal (adults only): Initially, apply one patch (delivers 0.1 mg/24 h) patch to an intact area of hairless skin on the upper arm or torso, once every 7 d. Adjust dosage every 1–2 wk.
Neuraxial pain control	Adults: Initially, 30 mcg/h by continuous epidural infusion in combination with opioid analgesics. Dosage titration is based on pain relief and adverse events; max. rate is 40 mcg/h. In clinical trials, bolus doses of epidural clonidine range from 100 to 900 mcg/dose. Intrathecal: Clonidine in doses of 25–40 mcg/h (600–960 mcg/d) has been used to manage chronic-pain patients.
Pediatric anesthesia	Given orally preoperatively (4 mcg/kg), decreases intraoperative anesthetic requirements and postoperative opioid consumption. The epidural or caudal dose is 1–2 mcg/kg, which may be followed by an infusion of 0.05–0.33 mcg/kg/h. It may cause sedation and hypotension when given via the epidural route.
Regional anesthesia	Dose of 0.5 mcg/kg or more enhances and prolongs the effect of local anesthetics used for brachial plexus block, peribulbar and retrobulbar blocks, and IV regional anesthesia. An intra-articular dose of 150 mcg enhanced postoperative analgesia in patients undergoing knee arthroscopy. Hemodynamic effects, namely, bradycardia and hypotension, increase with doses of 1.5 mcg/kg or more.

comparison to benzodiazepines, clonidine produces a state of sedation similar to sleepiness rather than amnesia. Subjects are more easily roused when asked to perform tasks. Clonidine has also been shown to be an effective anxiolytic. A reduction in halothane MAC by as much as 50% has been demonstrated experimentally with clonidine. This effect has largely borne out clinically with other inhaled anesthetics. Other studies have demonstrated reductions in opioid, benzodiazepine, barbiturate, and propofol requirements.

ANALGESIA

Oral, epidural, intrathecal, and parenteral administration of clonidine all produce analgesia and potentiate the action of other agents, thus enhancing motor and sensory blockade. This corresponds to a reduced side-effect profile in most instances. Epidural administration is most common, as a number of studies have demonstrated epidural clonidine to be an efficacious adjunct to opioid and local anesthetic injection in the management of acute postoperative pain. Studies have also demonstrated epidural clonidine to be superior to IV use for pain control after orthopedic surgery. Intrathecal clonidine seems to provide no additional benefit to epidural clonidine, as it provides no additional analgesia but does cause a greater incidence of hypotension. Also popular for use as an adjunct in regional anesthesia, clonidine prolongs duration of peripheral nerve blocks at small doses but does run the risk of prolonging motor blockade. Chronic pain treatment with clonidine has several benefits, including the avoidance of opioids in patients who may become dependent or addicted with long-term use. Clonidine is approved in the United States for the treatment of intractable cancer pain.

OTHER USES

Additional off-label uses are particularly interesting to the anesthesiologist. Clonidine has been shown to decrease postoperative nausea and vomiting. It is an effective antisialagog. Some studies have shown clonidine to be an efficacious alternative to meperidine for postoperative shivering. A decrease in intraocular pressure has been reported with the use of clonidine during ophthalmic surgery. Hyperactive children with manic symptoms have been treated with the drug. Clonidine has also been used in the treatment of opioid, benzodiazepine, and alcohol withdrawal, as well in smoking cessation.

SIDE EFFECTS/CONTRAINDICATIONS

Clonidine's side-effect profile makes it a useful adjunct in anesthesiology. Common side effects that are often desirable perioperatively include dry mouth and sedation. Abrupt discontinuation of clonidine can produce a withdrawal syndrome possibly resulting in nausea, insomnia, headaches, and restlessness. Severe sudden cessation can result in profound hypertension and tachycardia. As stated above, clonidine is a very mild respiratory depressant at indicated doses and does not appear to potentiate opioid-induced respiratory depression. In the event of an overdose, clonidine has been reported to act as a more significant respiratory depressant. Furthermore, in high doses, α_1-activation can cause anxiety and this limits its use as a sedative. Although it is well established that intrathecal or epidural administration of clonidine is not neurotoxic, these routes are not recommended in pregnancy because they can cause hypotension. Clonidine is classified as a pregnancy category C drug. The contraindication includes hypersensitivity to clonidine hydrochloride or any component of the formulation. It should be avoided in patients with perioperative hypovolemia, spontaneous bradycardia, atrioventricular block, or prolonged P-R interval. Transdermal patch may contain conducting metal (e.g., aluminum); therefore it should be removed prior to

MRI. Due to the potential for altered electrical conductivity, the transdermal patch should be removed before cardioversion or defibrillation.

TAKE HOME POINTS

- Clonidine serves as a useful drug to the anesthesiologist beyond its use as an antihypertensive.
- It is useful as a sedative, especially in pediatric anesthesia.
- Although it is not used as a sole anesthetic, clonidine reduces the dose requirements in epidural, intrathecal, and peripheral nerve blocks.
- Clonidine is approved for cancer pain and serves as an off-label adjunct in the treatment of other chronic pain syndromes. It is also used in the treatment of opioid and nicotine withdrawal.
- Clonidine has additional benefits as an antisialagogue, antiemetic, and in reducing postoperative shivering.
- When the recommended dose is used, clonidine has very few side effects or contraindications.
- Newer, more selective α_2-agonists such as dexmedetomidine are likely to find more widespread use by the anesthesiologist.

SUGGESTED READINGS

Bergendahl H, Lonnqvist PA, Eksborg S. Clonidine in paediatric anaesthesia: Review of the literature and comparison with benzodiazepines for premedication. *Acta Anaesthesiol Scand.* 2006;50:135–143.

Brislin RP, Rose JB. Pediatric acute pain management. *Anesthesiol Clin North Am.* 2005;23(4): 789–814.

Eisenach JC, De Rock M, Klimscha W. Alpha sub 2-adrenergic agonists for regional anesthesia: A clinical review of clonidine (1984–1995). *Anesthesiology.* 1996;85(3):655–674.

Habib AS, Gan TJ. Role of anesthetic adjuncts in post operative pain management. *Anesthesiol Clin North Am.* 2005;23(1):85–107.

Khan ZP, Ferguson CN, Jones RM. Alpha-2 and imidazoline receptor agonists. *Anaesthesia.* 1999;54:146–165.

Miller RD, ed. *Miller's Anesthesia.* 6th ed. New York: Churchill Livingstone; 2005:650–651.

Catapres-TTS prescribing information, Boehringer Ingelheim Pharmaceuticals Inc., Ridgefield, CT 06877 USA, Revised: February 14, 2006.

52

Consider Chloroprocaine for Regional Blockade When Appropriate—It Is a Rapid-Onset Local Anesthetic with Low Systemic Toxicity

Joshua M. Zimmerman, MD and
Randal O. Dull, MD, PhD

2-Chloroprocaine is an ester local anesthetic introduced into clinical practice in 1951; the initial paper described >200 successful spinal anesthetics. Despite its initial use in spinal anesthetics, 2-chloroprocaine found its greatest use in labor epidurals because of its rapid metabolism and low toxicity to both mother and fetus. The widespread use and availability of intrathecal lidocaine, however, apparently prevented most anesthesiologists from adopting 2-chloroprocaine as their spinal drug of choice. After decades of use, a report of 8 patients who suffered neurologic deficits after "epidural" anesthesia with 2-chloroprocaine was published. It appears that at least half of these patients had inadvertently received intrathecal administration, and this raised the question of neurotoxicity. It was not clear at the time whether the etiology was the local anesthetic or the sodium bisulfite preservative. A flurry of publications have attempted to address this issue of toxicity, establish a dose–response curve, and evaluate various adjuncts to 2-chloroprocaine as an effective spinal anesthetic and as a replacement for intrathecal lidocaine.

Chemical Properties
2-Chloroprocaine contains a lipophilic aromatic ring bound to a hydrophilic tertiary amine by an ester linkage.

Clinical Pharmacology
Like all local anesthetics, chloroprocaine inhibits the generation and propagation of nerve impulses by increasing the threshold for electrical excitation, slowing conduction, and reducing the rate of rise of the action potential. Being an ester, 2-chloroprocaine is metabolized by plasma cholinesterase (and red cell esterase, to a lesser extent) into an alcohol and a *para*-aminobenzoic acid. Chloroprocaine is metabolized much more quickly than procaine or tetracaine, contributing to its low systemic toxicity. Its plasma half-life is approximately 21 seconds in adults and 43 seconds in neonates. Any condition, however, that inhibits the activity or quantity of pseudo-cholinesterase will prolong action and increase toxicity (e.g., liver disease,

© 2006 Mayo Foundation for Medical Education and Research

atypical cholinesterase). The kidney is the primary route of excretion for chloroprocaine metabolites.

CLINICAL USE

Intrathecal Use. Though chloroprocaine was initially described as a spinal anesthetic, it has fallen into disfavor in the past two decades because of concerns about neurotoxicity. This notion has recently been challenged by a series of studies. The future of 2-chloroprocaine as a medication for intrathecal use is currently in flux, and further studies are underway to further define its use. It was initially shown that 2-chloroprocaine was an appropriate substitute for intrathecal lidocaine, providing similar quality, height, and duration of block when compared to equal doses of lidocaine. A later study showed that 30, 45, and 60 mg of 2-chloroprocaine yielded mean maximal block heights of T7, T5, and T2 and block duration of 98, 116, and 132 minutes, respectively. When 20 mcg of fentanyl was added, the duration of sensory but not motor blockade was lengthened (by 25 minutes). When epinephrine was added to 2-chloroprocaine, a transient flulike syndrome was reported, leading to the recommendation to avoid this combination. When compared to other local anesthetics for ambulatory surgery, 2-chloroprocaine provides adequate duration and quality of blockade, with significantly faster resolution than bupivacaine and less risk of transient neurological syndrome (TNS) than lidocaine. Considerable controversy still surrounds the issue of potential neurotoxicity of spinal 2-chloroprocaine. The prevailing conclusion of a series of animal studies was that the preservative sodium bisulfite, possibly in combination with low pH, was responsible for several early episodes of irreversible blockade. However, at least one study suggests that 2-chloroprocaine may itself be neurotoxic, and that sodium bisulfite may actually be neuroprotective.

Epidural Use. Because of its low toxicity and rapid onset, chloroprocaine has been used effectively for years as an epidural anesthetic. When a 3% solution is used, an epidural dose of 15 mL will provide analgesia to T10, and 20 mL will yield a level to T4 with a rapidity that approaches that of subarachnoid anesthesia. The duration of action is short, however, with chloroprocaine lasting only 30 to 50 minutes even when epinephrine is added. These properties can be used to good effect in the delivery suite—chloroprocaine can be used to "repaint" an epidural block after delivery when the labor block has worn off and episiotomy repair will be extensive or when a small surgical procedure, such as tubal ligation, is planned after delivery.

Formulations of 2-chloroprocaine containing ethylenediamminetetraacetic acid (EDTA) were associated with severe low back pain on injection. It was hypothesized that the EDTA chelated calcium in the paraspinous muscle, inducing local muscle spasm. Formulations are now available that do not contain EDTA.

Topical Use. Although it is not an "on-label" use, 2-chloroprocaine provides rapid topical anesthesia for skin incisions. Because of its rapid plasma clearance, direct administration of 2-chloroprocaine into incisions appears to be safe and effective. This is the "splash block" that anesthesiologists with many years of experience may refer to.

TAKE HOME POINTS

- Chloroprocaine is an ester local anesthetic with a plasma half-life of 21 seconds in adults and 43 seconds in neonates.
- Whether chloroprocaine should be used as a local anesthetic for intrathecal purposes is still debatable (it may actually be neurotoxic).
- Using chloroprocaine with epinephrine as an additive is not recommended—especially with spinal anesthesia.
- For epidural use, chloroprocaine provides an excellent safety index. Further, it has a rapid onset that comes close to that seen with intrathecal use of local anesthetics.
- Typical anesthetic levels with a 3% epidural solution are T10 with 15 mL and T4 with 20 mL.
- Chloroprocaine can be useful to supplement an epidural when short-acting anesthesia is necessary for an episiotomy repair.
- Because of its rapid plasma clearance, it can even be administered directly into an incision (as a "splash block").

SUGGESTED READINGS

Coda B, Bausch S, Haas M, Chavkin C. The hypothesis that antagonism of fentanyl analgesia by 2-chloroprocaine is mediated by direct action on opioid receptors. *Regional Anesth.* 1997;22:43–52.

Corke BC, Carlson CG, Dettbarn W-D. The influence of 2-chloroprocaine on the subsequent analgesic potency of bupivacaine. *Anesthesiology.* 1984;60:25–27.

Foldes FF, McNall PG. 2-Chloroprocaine: A new local anesthetic agent. *Anesthesiology.* 1952;13:287–296.

Gissen AJ, Datta S, Lambert DL. The chloroprocaine controversy: Is chloroprocaine neurotoxic? *Regional Anesth.* 1984;9:135–145.

Grice SC, Eisenach JC, Dewan DM. Labor analgesia with epidural bupivacaine plus fentanyl: Enhancement with epinephrine and inhibition with 2-chloroprocaine. *Anesthesiology.* 1990;72:623–628.

Kouri ME, Kopacz DJ. Spinal 2-chloroprocaine: A comparison with lidocaine in volunteers. *Anesth Analg.* 2004;98:75–80.

Kuhnert BR, Kuhnert PM, Prochaska AL, Gross TL. Plasma levels of 2-chloroprocaine in obstetric patients and their neonates after epidural anesthesia. *Anesthesiology.* 1980;53:21–25.

Ravindran RS, Bond VK, Tasch MD, et al. Prolonged neural blockade following regional analgesia with 2-chloroprocaine. *Anesth Analg.* 1980;59:447–451.

Reisner LS, Hochman BN, Plumer MH. Persistent neurologic deficit and adhesive arachnoiditis following intrathecal 2-chloroprocaine injection. *Anesth Analg.* 1980;59:452–454.

Smith KN, Kopacz DJ, McDonald SB. Spinal 2-chloroprocaine: A dose-ranging study and the effect of added epinephrine. *Anesth Analg.* 2004;98:81–88.

Taniguchi M, Bollen AW, Drasner, K. Sodium bisulfite: Scapegoat for chloroprocaine neuro-toxicity? *Anesthesiology.* 2004;100(1):85–91.

Vath JS, Kopacz DJ. Spinal 2-chloroprocaine: The effect of added fentanyl. *Anesth Analg.* 2004;98:89–94.

Wang BC, Hillman DE, Spielholz NI, Turndorf H. Chronic neurological deficits and Nesacaine-CE—an effect of the anesthetic, 2-chloroprocaine, or the antioxidant, sodium bisulfite? *Anesth Analg.* 1984;63:445–447.

Yoos JR, Kopacz DJ. Spinal 2-chloroprocaine: A comparison with small-dose bupivacaine in volunteers. *Anesth Analg.* 2005;100:566–572.

53

CONSIDER USING KETAMINE WHEN APPROPRIATE—IF MANAGED CAREFULLY, THE BENEFITS WILL USUALLY OUTWEIGH THE POTENTIAL SIDE EFFECTS

ELIZABETH E. COSTELLO, MD

In 1970, 8 years after it was first synthesized, ketamine was released for clinical use in the United States. Initially ketamine was believed to be the "ideal" anesthetic, providing amnesia, analgesia, immobility, and loss of consciousness. Shortly after its use became widespread, however, there were many reports of patients emerging from anesthesia with hallucinations and recalling vivid dreams. The discovery of "emergence reactions" led many practitioners to avoid using ketamine for routine cases. However, ketamine remains an important tool in the anesthesiologist's armamentarium, as it is a versatile drug that can be given by almost any route and can provide analgesia, sedation, or general anesthesia depending on the dose administered. Originally, ketamine was indicated as an anesthetic as well as an analgesic for cardiac surgery, trauma, obstetric analgesia, as well as for dressing changes in burns patients.

Ketamine is different from other anesthetics in that it induces a state of dissociate anesthesia, whereby higher centers in the brain are unable to perceive auditory, visual, or painful stimuli. There is a dose-related loss of consciousness and profound analgesia. Patients' eyes remain open and they often maintain reflexes, although corneal, cough, and swallow reflexes cannot be assumed to be protective. In addition, patients have anterograde amnesia and have no recall of surgical procedures. There is a rapid onset of action, as the drug crosses the blood–brain barrier quickly secondary to low molecular weight, high lipid solubility, and a pK_a near physiologic pH. Following intravenous (IV) administration, onset is seen in 30 seconds, with peak action in 60 seconds. The anesthetic effects of ketamine following a usual induction dose (1 to 2 mg/kg) remain for 10 to 15 minutes only. Drug plasma levels required for anesthesia and amnesia are 0.7 to 2.2 mcg/mL, with awakening occurring at levels of 0.5 mcg/mL. Although the anesthetic duration of action of ketamine is short, the analgesic effects last much longer, as a plasma level of only 0.1 mcg/mL is required for analgesic effects to be seen.

Ketamine interacts with N-methyl-D-aspartate (NMDA), opioid, nicotinic, muscarinic and calcium-channel receptors. It is the antagonistic action

© 2006 Mayo Foundation for Medical Education and Research

222

at NMDA receptors that produces the majority of ketamine's effects, including analgesia, amnesia, and the psychomimetic side effects. It also has effects on both central and spinal opioid receptors, with μ-receptors contributing to analgesia and κ-receptors to the psychomimetic effects. On a larger scale, ketamine leads to inhibition of thalamocortical pathways and stimulation of the limbic system.

Ketamine acts differently from other anesthetic drugs in relation to both the respiratory and cardiac systems. Ketamine does not depress respiration unless it is given in a large rapid bolus, and CO_2 responsiveness is maintained at or close to normal levels. The major respiratory advantage of ketamine is that it causes profound bronchodilation, to the same degree as inhalation agents. This makes ketamine an excellent choice of induction agent in asthmatic patients. It has even been used to treat refractory cases of status asthmaticus.

Unlike other anesthetic agents, ketamine does not depress the cardiac system. On induction with ketamine, increases in heart rate, blood pressure, and cardiac output are seen. The mechanism of the cardiovascular effects is sympathetic stimulation and inhibition of both intraneuronal and extraneuronal uptake of catecholamines. Because it is indirect stimulation that leads to these effects, in the catecholamine-depleted patient, ketamine can have the opposite effect, as the drug also has a direct myocardial depressant effect that is normally masked by its sympathetic activity. Ketamine's effects on the heart lead to an increase in cardiac oxygen consumption, thus making it a poor choice for patients with ischemic cardiac disease. Patients with pulmonary hypertension are also poor candidates for ketamine, as the drug causes a greater increase in pulmonary vascular resistance than systemic vascular resistance.

A variety of patients can benefit from the use of ketamine as an induction agent, especially ASA class 4 patients with respiratory and cardiac dysfunction, excluding cardiac ischemia. The bronchodilating effects of ketamine make it particularly helpful for patients with severe bronchospastic disease. The other niche where ketamine has been found to be interesting is with patients with hemodynamic compromise secondary to hypovolemia or cardiomyopathy. This includes such diagnoses as sepsis, trauma, cardiac tamponade, and restrictive pericarditis. The only caveat is that if these patients are catecholamine-depleted, the direct myocardial depressant effects may be seen. In tamponade, the benefit of ketamine is that it maintains the heart rate and right atrial filling pressures through its sympathetic stimulation. Patients who require frequent, brief procedures, such as burn patients undergoing dressing changes, can benefit from the use of ketamine as a sedative, because subanesthetic doses can be used with good analgesia and rapid return to normal function. It can be used as an adjunct to regional anesthesia, as a sedative prior to painful blocks, or to position patients already in pain. The main advantage is the profound analgesia without respiratory depression or hypotension. Because of these properties, ketamine is useful in emergency medicine, war zones, entrapment situations, and high-altitude anesthesia.

Pediatric anesthesia includes another subset of patients who benefit from the use of ketamine. Intramuscular ketamine (7 to 9 mg/kg) remains in use for induction of anesthesia in uncooperative pediatric patients. Children with neuromuscular disorders also benefit from the use of ketamine as a maintenance agent, as volatile agents should be avoided in these children, who are at increased risk of malignant hyperthermia. Children with congenital heart defects leading to right-to-left shunt do well with ketamine as an induction agent for cardiac surgery, as it increases systemic vascular resistance and does not reverse the shunt. Finally, ketamine is useful for pediatric sedation, as it produces analgesia and sedation with a low incidence of complications. Emergence reactions are much less common in the pediatric population than in adults.

A more controversial area for ketamine is its use in neurosurgical patients. It had previously been thought that ketamine increased intracranial pressure and cerebral blood flow and was therefore contraindicated in patients at risk for elevated intracranial pressure. However, recent studies have shown that if benzodiazepines are given with ketamine and normocapnea is maintained, there is no elevation in intracranial pressure and so ketamine may have a role in neurosurgery. Additionally, blockade of NMDA receptors may be neuroprotective, as it can decrease cell destruction and necrosis following cerebral ischemia. The role of ketamine in neurosurgery has not yet been decided, and further research will determine its utility.

Recently, ketamine has received much attention for its use as an analgesic. It has been used as an adjunct in both acute postoperative pain management as well as in chronic pain, including both neuropathic and refractory cancer pain. The analgesic effects of ketamine are due to several mechanisms. The primary mechanism is NMDA-receptor antagonism leading to suppression of pain transmission to higher centers in the brain. Ketamine also prevents the development of tolerance to acute opioid administration and development of increased pain sensitivity secondary to opioid-induced hyperalgesia by its NMDA antagonism. By this mechanism it also prevents the "windup" phenomenon, which is an increase in dorsal horn activity due to repetitive and constant C-fiber stimulation. There is some evidence that ketamine also acts directly on opioid receptors in the brain and spinal cord, contributing to its analgesic effect.

For postoperative pain control, ketamine can be given preincision, postincision, or as a part of the postoperative pain regimen. Subanesthetic doses of ketamine (0.1 to 0.3 mg/kg) produce analgesia, and the analgesic effects of an induction dose of ketamine are seen for several hours following an initial bolus dose. The goal of pre-emptive analgesia is to decrease post-operative pain by interrupting nociceptive pathways. NMDA receptors are responsible for pain memory and "windup," so ketamine, an NMDA antagonist, can prevent the massive nociceptive afferent impulses from reaching the brain. However, at the present time there is some controversy regarding the efficacy of pre-emptive ketamine and whether it is able to reduce total opioid requirements postoperatively. If it is given intraoperatively, it has been shown that ketamine is a much more effective analgesic when given as an infusion rather than as a single bolus dose at the time of induction. Anesthesia providers who have a lot of sedation cases report that a ketamine infusion coupled with a low- to moderate-dose propofol infusion (known sometimes in the vernacular as "P-K anesthesia") has good efficacy in a wide range of surgical cases. Postoperatively, ketamine has been added to Patient Controlled Analgesic (PCAs) (1 to 2 mcg/kg/h) and has been shown to decrease the total amount of morphine required as well as to decrease side effects.

Ketamine has been used as an additive with local anesthetics for epidural or caudal use, and patients receiving ketamine in this form require less postoperative opioid than those receiving only local anesthetics. However, racemic ketamine is not preservative-free, and the preservative benzethonium chloride may be neurotoxic. S(+)-ketamine is an isolated stereoisomer that is preservative-free and shows potential for future neuraxial use. However, in the United States, ketamine is available only in racemic form. In Europe, S(+)-ketamine has gained in popularity and is a more potent anesthetic associated with more rapid emergence and a lower incidence of emergence reactions.

Although it has many advantageous properties, no drug is without its adverse reactions. Ketamine has a fairly notorious side-effect profile, which may lead to hesitance in using this drug. The emergence reactions seen with ketamine include visual, auditory, and proprioceptive illusions that can illicit fear or excitement in patients. An illustrative clinical anecdote was related by one of the Certified Registered Nurse Anesthetist (CRNA) advisers to this book: The anesthetist was using ketamine as a partial induction agent, and just as the patient lost consciousness, one of the operating room (OR) staff mentioned that he had killed a large black snake in his yard that morning. On emergence, the patient related that he had had vivid and severely unpleasant "dreams" under anesthesia about black snakes. The anesthetist now uses the power of suggestion in a positive way before the administration of ketamine—she tells her patients they may have vivid dreams and asks them to imagine their favorite or a very pleasant "brightly colored place"—e.g., a sunny tropical beach or brilliant fall foliage. She also requests that there be no excessive chatter or loud noises at induction. It is also well recognized that the concomitant use of benzodiazepines reduces the risk of emergence reactions, and virtually all practitioners who use ketamine preadminister a benzodiazepine.

Ketamine also causes profuse salivation in some patients, which can be a problem in the unprotected airway with the possibilities of laryngospasm and aspirations. It is recommended to pretreat these patients with an anti-sialagogue such as glycopyrrolate. Atropine is to be avoided, as it can cause an increased risk of delirium on emergence. However, with appropriate use and proper patient selection, ketamine has proven to be beneficial for a variety of procedures and patient populations.

TAKE HOME POINTS

- Although ketamine went through a period of "unpopularity," it is actually a valuable drug that every anesthesia provider should be familiar with and comfortable using.
- It can be given by a number of routes and acts at a number of receptors. It can be used for sedation, amnesia, anesthesia, and pain relief.
- Consider it especially in cases when sedation/anesthesia is needed for short periods of intense surgical or procedural stimulus, such as dressing changes, burn treatments, or removal of K-wires.
- It is valuable as an adjunctive agent in both general anesthetic and sedation cases.
- Actively manage the potential side effects, particularly the possibilities of hallucinations—reassure and discuss beforehand with the patient, always give a benzodiazepine, and ensure a quiet, calm anesthetizing location.
- Contraindications to ketamine include:
  - Elevated ICP
  - Open eye injury – ketamine increases IOP
  - As sole anesthetic in ischemic cardiac disease
  - Vascular aneurysm – don't want sudden change in arterial pressure
  - Psychiatric disorders like schizophrenia
  - History of adverse reaction to ketamine or pcp
  - If post op delirium could be from other cause–delirium tremens, head trauma
- Factors that increase risk of delirium include:
  - Age >16 years
  - Dose >2 mg/kg
  - Pre-existing personality problems

SUGGESTED READINGS

Kohrs R, Durieux ME. Ketamine: Teaching an old dog new tricks. *Anesth Analg*. 1998;87:
1186–1193.

Lin C, Durieux ME. Ketamine and kids: An update. *Pediatr Anesth*. 2005;15:91–97.

Miller RD, ed. *Miller's Anesthesia*. 6th ed. Philadelphia, PA: Churchill Livingstone; 2005.

White PF. The changing role of non-opioid analgesic techniques in the management of postoperative pain. *Anesth Analg*. 2005;101(5S):S5–S22.

54

DEXMEDETOMIDINE CAN BE A USEFUL DRUG, BUT WILL IT BE UNIVERSALLY APPLICABLE?

EVAN T. LUKOW, DO, MIRIAM ANIXTER, MD AND TETSURO SAKAI, MD, PHD

Sedative-hypnotic and analgesic agents (benzodiazepines, propofol, and opioids) form an integral part of anesthesia to provide patients' comfort and safety in the operating room (OR) and the intensive care unit (ICU). a_2-Adrenergic receptor agonists have been used increasingly as a new armamentarium to provide sedative/hypnotic, analgesic, anxiolytic, and sympatholytic effects in the perioperative and critical care settings.

WHAT IS DEXMEDETOMIDINE?

Dexmedetomidine (Precedex; Abbott Labs, Abbott Park, IL, USA) is a relatively selective a_2-adrenergic receptor agonist (eight times more specific for the a_2-adrenoreceptor compared to clonidine). Compared to other a_2-adrenergic agonists such as clonidine, dexmedetomidine has a shorter half-life (2 hours for intravenous dexmedetomidine versus 8 to 12 hours for peroral clonidine).

HOW DOES DEXMEDETOMIDINE WORK?

Dexmedetomidine stimulates a_2-adrenoreceptors in the locus ceruleus of the brainstem to provide sedation. It also provides analgesia by stimulating a_2-adrenoreceptor in the central and peripheral nervous systems. Dexmedetomidine causes sympatholysis via central and peripheral mechanisms. Following intravenous (IV) administration, dexmedetomidine undergoes rapid redistribution, with a distribution half-life of 6 minutes and an elimination half-life of 2 hours. Dexmedetomidine exhibits linear kinetics in the dosing range of 0.2 to 0.7 mcg/kg/h when administered through IV infusion for 24 hours. Dexmedetomidine is 94% protein-bound and undergoes nearly complete biotransformation in the liver to inactive metabolites that are excreted in the urine.

POTENTIAL BENEFITS OF DEXMEDETOMIDINE

During a continuous infusion within its therapeutic level, dexmedetomidine provides unique sedation (patients appear to be asleep but are readily aroused), analgesic-sparing effect, and minimal depression of respiratory function. Dexmedetomidine has no pharmacokinetic or cytochrome P450 enzyme drug–drug interactions.

© 2006 Mayo Foundation for Medical Education and Research

COMPLICATIONS/CONTRAINDICATIONS

Hypotension, hypertension, nausea, bradycardia, fever, and vomiting are most frequently observed adverse events associated with dexmedetomidine. The net effect of α_2-adrenergic agonists, exerted via central and spinal receptors, is sympatholytic (or "provagal"). Therefore, caution should be exercised in patients with pre-existing severe bradycardia disorders or severe ventricular dysfunction, in whom sympathetic tone is critical for maintaining hemodynamic balance. Clinical events of bradycardia and sinus arrest have been associated with dexmedetomidine administration in young, healthy volunteers with high vagal tone or with different routes of administration including rapid IV/bolus administration (www.fda.gov/cder/foi/label/1999/21038lbl.pdf). Transient hypertension has also been observed, primarily during the loading infusion, associated with initial peripheral vasoconstriction effects of dexmedetomidine prior to its central nervous system (CNS)–mediated vasodilatory effect.

Recent clinical studies, however, demonstrated more reliable control of heart rate and blood pressure in patients undergoing surgery with appropriate doses of dexmedetomidine. Dose reduction should be considered in patients with impaired liver and renal function. Dexmedetomidine is contraindicated in patients with a known hypersensitivity to the drug, which has not been reported so far.

FDA-APPROVED USES

In 1999, dexmedetomidine was approved by the U.S. Food and Drug Administration (FDA) for sedation of adult patients who are intubated and mechanically ventilated in the intensive care setting. Dexmedetomidine should be administered by continuous infusion not to exceed 24 hours.

How to Administer Dexmedetomidine

Dexmedetomidine is supplied in 2-mL vials each containing 100 mcg of drug/mL (200 mcg total) and should be diluted with 48 mL of sterile water or 0.9% sodium chloride to a final concentration of 4 mcg/mL. Dexmedetomidine is recommended to be administered as a loading dose of 1 mcg/kg over 10 to 20 minutes, followed by a maintenance infusion of 0.2 to 0.7 mcg/kg/h, titrated to the desired sedation scale.

CLINICAL APPLICATIONS OF DEXMEDETOMIDINE

Intensive Care Unit. Because of its nonopioid mechanism of analgesia and lack of respiratory depression, dexmedetomidine has been used in the critical care setting for sedation. It is not necessary to discontinue dexmedetomidine infusion before extubation. The use of dexmedetomidine is not limited to the ICU, and a growing body of literature has described the effectiveness of the drug in perioperative settings.

Operating Room. Compared to placebo or propofol infusion, dexmedetomidine infusion was reported to provide more stable hemodynamics for patients who underwent cardiac and vascular surgeries. Dexmedetomidine seems to attenuate the stress-induced sympathoadrenal response seen with laryngoscopy, intubation, and surgery. It potentiates the anesthetic effects of varieties of intraoperative anesthetic drugs. This anesthetic-sparing effect of dexmedetomidine can be translated into a more rapid recovery from anesthesia. Dexmedetomidine may also be useful as an anesthetic adjunct in patients who are susceptible to narcotic-induced respiratory depression, such as morbidly obese patients, in whom the opioid-sparing effects of dexmedetomidine have proven extremely useful. Also, in the difficult-airway realm, dexmedetomidine has been used as a single-agent sedative along with topical anesthesia for awake fiber-optic intubation. It has been used as an adjunct in monitored anesthesia care. Some studies have demonstrated the effective use of dexmedetomidine in awake craniotomy, or even as a sole anesthetic for minor procedures.

Pediatrics. Dexmedetomidine has gained significant attention for the treatment of emergence delirium, which is a frequent phenomenon in children recovering from general anesthesia. Dexmedetomidine has been shown to reduce the incidence of emergence delirium when administered as a single dose of 1 mcg/kg intraoperatively approximately 30 minutes before the end of the procedure. Treatment of existing emergence delirium is also effective, with 0.125 mcg/kg bolus and repeated doses as needed, which avoids unnecessary oversedation. Continuous infusions have also been studied, and both treatment options have not shown any increase in prolonging time to extubation or time to discharge from the postanesthesia recovery unit. Dexmedetomidine may prove to be very useful in children with underlying neurologic disorders, who often develop agitation or adverse hemodynamic or respiratory reactions with opioids or benzodiazepines. Dexmedetomidine has also become a viable option for pediatric ICU sedation, much as in the adult population. This has allowed for avoiding the prolonged use of propofol for sedation, minimizing the possibilities of "propofol infusion syndrome." Though dexmedetomidine is not currently approved by the FDA for use in the pediatric population, it may offer an additional choice for the sedation of children both postoperatively and in the ICU. The efficacy of non-IV administration (intramuscular, per-oral, and buccal) of the drug has also been suggested.

CLINICAL CONTROVERSY

Many investigators have demonstrated a variety of off-label clinical applications of dexmedetomidine as described above. A few studies also suggest caution in the usage of dexmedetomidine. The provagal effect of dexmedetomidine was demonstrated by Ebert and associates, with augmentation of baroreceptor response to phenylephrine and preservation of baroreceptor response to nitroprusside. This "provagal" effect of dexmedetomidine was considered to be a contributory factor in cardiac arrest of an adult patient, reported by Ingersoll-Weng and others, who underwent sternotomy with a thoracic epidural anesthesia and preoperative pyridostigmine. We had a pediatric patient who developed hypotension without bradycardia with low-dose dexmedetomidine in the presence of baclofen (unpublished observation). The delayed recovery can be a problem with dexmedetomidine. Jalowiecki and colleagues counseled against the use of dexmedetomidine as a sole agent for procedural sedation, in light of hemodynamic instability and the need for prolonged recovery. Koroglu and associates compared the sedative, hemodynamic, and respiratory effects of dexmedetomidine and propofol in children undergoing magnetic resonance imaging. In the study, they found the onset of sedation, recovery, and discharge time were significantly longer in the dexmedetomidine group, although the decrease of mean blood pressure, heart rate, and respiratory rate from the baseline were smaller in the dexmedetomidine group compared to the propofol group.

There is significant synergism of opioids with dexmedetomidine. Therefore, one should be cautious against overdosing with dexmedetomidine in the presence of opioids, which can result in delayed emergence. In practice terms, the use of dexmedetomidine may be cumbersome because of the need for a loading dose, controlled continuous infusion, and titration of the dosage to prevent overdosing.

Dexmedetomidine is, at the present time, approved by the FDA only for sedation in mechanically ventilated adult patients who are being monitored in the ICU. Large prospective clinical studies are needed to further elucidate and confirm the effectiveness of the off-label uses of dexmedetomidine.

TAKE HOME POINTS

- Dexmedetomidine, a newer selective a_2-adrenergic receptor agonist, decreases sympathetic tone with attenuation of the neuroendocrine and hemodynamic responses to anesthesia and surgery, reduces anesthetic and opioid requirements, and provides sedation and analgesia without respiratory depression.
- Dexmedetomidine is recommended to be given as a loading dose of 1 mcg/kg over 10 to 20 minutes, followed by a maintenance infusion of 0.2 to 0.7 mcg/kg/h for a total duration of not more than 24 hours.
- Dexmedetomidine is currently approved for intubated and mechanically ventilated adult patients in the ICU. However, it has demonstrated its effectiveness in other surgical settings.

SUGGESTED READINGS

Aantaa R, Jalonen J. Perioperative use of α_2-adrenoceptor agonists and the cardiac patient. *Eur J Anaesthesiol.* 2006;23:361–372.

Anttila M, Penttila J, Helminen A, et al. Bioavailability of dexmedetomidine after extravascular doses in healthy subjects. *Br J Clin Pharmacol.* 2003;56:691–693.

Coursin DB, Coursin DB, Maccioli GA. Dexmedetomidine. *Curr Opin Crit Care.* 2001;7: 221–226.

Ebert TJ, Hall JE, Barney JA, et al. The effect of increasing plasma concentrations of dexmedetomidine in humans. *Anesthesiology.* 2000;93:382–394.

Grant SA, Breslin DS, MacLeod DB, et al. Dexmedetomidine infusion for sedation during fiberoptic intubation: A report of three cases. *J Clin Anesth.* 2004;16:124–126.

Hall JE, Uhrich TD, Barney JA, et al. Sedative, amnestic, and analgesic properties of small-dose dexmedetomidine infusions. *Anesth Analg.* 2000;90:699–705.

Hofer RE, Sprung J, Sarr MG, et al. Anesthesia for a patient with morbid obesity using dexmedetomidine without narcotics. *Can J Anesth.* 2005;52:176–180.

Ingersoll-Weng E, Manecke G, Thistlewaite PA. Dexmedetomidine and cardiac arrest. *Anesthesiology.* 2004;100:738–739.

Jalowiecki P, Rudner R, Gonciarz M, et al. Sole use of dexmedetomidine has limited utility for conscious sedation during outpatient colonoscopy. *Anesthesiology.* 2005;103:269–273.

Jorden VS, Pousman RM, Sanford MM, et al. Dexmedetomidine overdose in the perioperative setting. *Ann Pharmacother.* 2004;38:803–807.

Koroglu A, Teksan H, Sagir O, et al. A comparison of the sedative, hemodynamic, and respiratory effects of dexmedetomidine and propofol in children undergoing magnetic resonance imaging. *Anesth Analg.* 2006;103:63–67.

Ramsay MAE, Luterman DL. Dexmedetomidine as a total intravenous anesthetic agent. *Anesthesiology.* 2004;101:787–790.

Shukry M, Clyde MC, Kalarickal PL, et al. Does dexmedetomidine prevent emergence delirium in children after sevoflurane-based general anesthesia? *Pediatr Anesth.* 2005;15:1098–1104.

Tobias JD, Berkenbosch JW. Sedation during mechanical ventilation in infants and children: Dexmedetomidine versus midazolam. *South Med J.* 2004;97:451–455.

www.fda.gov/cder/foi/label/1999/21038lbl.pdf

www.medsafe.govt.nz/profs/datasheet/p/Precedexinf.htm

55

CHECK FOR HISTORY OF MIGRAINE BEFORE GIVING ONDANSETRON, ESPECIALLY IN CHILDREN

MICHAEL J. MORITZ, MD

Serotonin, or 5-hydroxytryptamine (5-HT) is a neurotransmitter derived from the amino acid tryptophan. Systemic 5-HT affects the cardiovascular, respiratory, and gastrointestinal systems, with vasoconstriction being the typical vascular response. Thus, 5-HT antagonists will cause vasodilation. In the gastrointestinal system, most serotonin receptors are of the 5-HT3 type. Thus, 5-HT antagonists will cause vasodilation. In the gastrointestinal system, most serotonin receptors are of the 5-HT3 type. The strongest stimulus for emesis from both chemotherapy and postoperatively is serotonin release from the gut enterochromaffin cells. This release stimulates afferent vagal fibers via their 5-HT3 receptors that activate the vomiting center in the brainstem (chemoreceptor trigger zone). Thus, serotonin antagonists decrease nausea and cause vasodilation.

The three 5-HT3 antagonist drugs available in the United States are ondansetron (Zofran), granisetron (Kytril), and dolasetron (Anzemet). These 5-HT3 receptor antagonists are the most effective antiemetic drugs available. All three drugs are similar in effectiveness, cost, and side-effect profiles.

The 5-HT3 antagonists have relatively few side effects. The most common side effect is headache, occurring in 10% to 20% of patients receiving doses to prevent chemotherapy-induced emesis and in 10% of patients receiving the lower doses used for postoperative nausea and vomiting. In children in particular, a personal or family history of migraine headache leads to a much higher risk of ondansetron-related migraine at the antiemetic dosing for chemotherapy.

The interplay of the 5-HT3 receptor, vasodilation, and vasoconstriction can be seen in the management of migraine. The treatment of migraine blocks the vasodilation that causes the headache, typically with serotonin agonists. For example, sumatriptan succinate (Imitrex) is a 5-HT1 agonist that causes vasoconstriction. Because the 5-HT3 antagonists cause vasodilation, their use should be considered carefully in patients susceptible to migraines.

ⓒ 2006 Mayo Foundation for Medical Education and Research

- The strongest stimulus for emesis from both chemotherapy and postoperatively is serotonin release from the gut enterochromaffin cells.
- In the gastrointestinal system, most serotonin receptors are of the 5-HT3 subtype.
- Serotonin has multiple systemic effects; the most typical vascular response is vasoconstriction.
- The 5-HT3 antagonists generally have relatively few side effects; however, anesthesia providers should be aware of the interplay of the 5-HT3 receptor and vasodilation, as it plays a role in the pathogenesis of migraine-type headaches, especially in children.

SUGGESTED READINGS

American Society of Health System Pharmacists. Therapeutic guidelines on the pharmacologic management of nausea and vomiting in adult and pediatric patients receiving chemotherapy or radiation therapy or undergoing surgery. *Am J Health Syst Pharm.* 1999;56:729–764.

Khan, RB. Migraine-type headaches in children receiving chemotherapy and ondansetron. *J Child Neurol.* 2002;17:857–858.

Ondansetron hydrochloride. In: Nissen D, ed. *Mosby's Drug Consult.* 13th ed. St. Louis: Mosby; 2003.

56

REMEMBER THAT NOT ALL BLUE-COLORED COMPOUNDS ARE THE SAME

CHAUNCEY T. JONES, MD

There are many blue dye compounds, and each is used for a variety of purposes. Their uses include food coloring, dye for materials, antiseptics, tissue stains, chemical reaction indicators, and to treat diseased aquarium life. Blue dyes are also used in humans for both diagnostic and therapeutic purposes. These dyes include methylene blue, patent blue, isosulfan blue, and indigo carmine. While these substances are all blue in color, they are distinct compounds and have widely varying properties, uses, and adverse effects (*Table 56.1*).

METHYLENE BLUE

Synonyms: Methylthionium chloride, tetramethylthionine chloride, urolene blue, swiss blue, solvent blue

Molecular formula: $C_{16}H_{18}ClN_3S$

Molecular weight: 319.85

Structure:

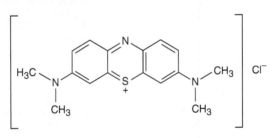

Methylene blue has been used in many clinical situations in humans. It is used primarily as an antidote for both chronic methemoglobinemia (e.g., occurring with dapsone therapy) and acute methemoglobinemia. At low concentrations it promotes the reduction of methemoglobin (the ferric form of hemoglobin) to hemoglobin by acting as a cofactor for the enzyme NADPH-methemoglobin reductase. The recommended dose is 1 to 2 mg/kg administered intravenously (IV). The dose may be repeated after 1 hour if symptoms persist.

Methylene blue has been used as a sentinel lymph node tracer for breast cancer and may be as efficacious and have fewer side effects than other

ⓒ 2006 Mayo Foundation for Medical Education and Research

TABLE 56.1	**BLUE DYE COMPOUNDS**	
BLUE COMPOUND	**COMMON USES**	**ADVERSE EFFECTS**
Methylene blue	■ Antidote for metHgb ■ Sentinel lymph node tracing ■ Genitourinary antiseptic ■ Septic shock ■ Cyanide toxicity	■ Hypertension ■ Chest pain ■ Anemia ■ Bladder irritation ■ Transient, false SpO_2 decrease ■ Headaches, diaphoresis, abdominal pain

Patent blue	■ Sentinel lymph node tracing
	  • Breast cancer
	  • Melanoma
	  • Endometrial cancer
	  • Colon cancer
		■ Severe anaphylaxis
		■ Prolonged, false SpO_2 decrease

Isosulphan blue	■ Tumor marking ■ Lymphangiography	■ Urticarial reactions ■ Anaphylaxis ■ Transient, false SpO_2 decrease

Indigo carmine	■ Urology
	  • Locate ureteral orifices during cystoscopy
	  • Test anastomoses
	  • Identify transected ureters intraoperatively
		■ Mild elevation of blood pressure
		■ Relatively low side-effect profile
		■ Transient, false SpO_2 decrease

Indocyanine green	■ Ophthalmology
	  • Macular surgery
	  • Cataract surgery
	■ Blood volume, cardiac output determinations
	■ Infrared therapy for colon cancer
		■ Can be toxic to eye unless thoroughly washed out
		■ Transient, false SpO_2 decrease

Blue #1	FDA black box warning against use in enteral feeds for detecting aspiration	■ Refractory hypotension ■ Metabolic acidosis (acts as a mitochondrial toxin) ■ Worse in patient with increased gastrointestinal permeability ■ Death

blue dyes more traditionally used for this purpose. It has also been used as a genitourinary antiseptic and for topical virus therapy. The antimicrobial effect is presumed to be secondary to its oxidative/reduction properties.

Although it is not the treatment of first choice, at high concentrations methylene blue can be used to treat cyanide toxicity by converting ferrous hemoglobin to ferric methemoglobin. Methemoglobin combines with cyanide to form cyanmethemoglobin. This serves as an alternative pathway for cyanide and prevents it from combining with cytochrome oxidase, which results in cyanide toxicity.

Possible side effects of methylene blue include hypertension; chest pain; headache; confusion; dizziness; diaphoresis; anemia; discoloration of skin, urine, and feces; nausea; vomiting; abdominal pain; and bladder irritation. The increase in blood pressure caused by methylene blue is so pronounced that it was historically used as a treatment for septic shock, before the era of modern-day vasopressors.

Methylene blue can also transiently decrease pulse oximetry readings by causing the oximeter to interpret methylene blue as deoxygenated blood. It is sometimes used by anesthesia personnel as an indicator dye or "marker" to denote a special situation in the operating room, such as an IV bag that has had succinylcholine added to it or to provide a visual cue to diagnose an endotracheal cuff leak. Be aware, however, that the high side-effect profile of methylene blue mandates careful consideration of this type of use.

PATENT BLUE
Synonyms: Sulphan blue, blue v, disulphine blue, food blue 3, acid blue 1
Molecular formula: $C_{27}H_{31}N_2NaO_6S_2$
Molecular weight: 566.67
Structure:

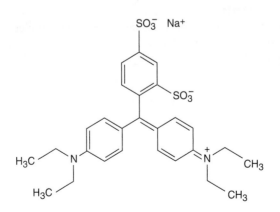

In humans, patent blue is used primarily for lymphangiography and sentinal node biopsy. When a tumor is identified, dye is injected into the tumor and peritumoral tissue. The dye is then taken up by the lymphatics that drain that region. The first lymph node that absorbs dye is the sentinal lymph node. This node is then biopsied and checked for malignancy. This information is used for staging, to decide whether more extensive lymph node dissection is needed, and to determine the need for other ajuvant therapies. This modality is most commonly used in breast cancer but is also used for other cancers, such as melanoma, endometrial cancer, and colon cancer. Before the development of sentinal node biopsies, radical lymph node dissections were routinely performed for breast cancer. Patent blue can also be used in conjunction with radiolabeled materials as an alternative method of identifying sentinal nodes.

The side-effect profile of patent blue is of considerable concern to users. It has been cited as causing severe anaphylaxis in humans and its use is limited in certain countries, including the United States. In addition, pulse oximetry readings can be artificially reduced for prolonged periods with higher doses of patent blue. This is likely because the dye is being injected subcutaneously versus intravascularly as with methylene blue.

ISOSULPHAN BLUE

Isosulfan blue (also called lymphazurin) is the 2,5-disulfophenyl isomer of patent (or sulphan) blue and is also used for tumor marking and lymphangiography for sentinal node biopsies.

Though it is generally thought to be safer than sulfan blue, it has been cited as causing an array of allergic reactions ranging from mild urticaria to severe anaphylaxis. Preoperative prophylaxis appears to reduce the severity but not the incidence of these reactions. Isosulfan blue has similar affects as patent blue on transiently decreasing pulse oximetry readings.

INDIGO CARMINE

Synonyms: Sodium indigotin disulfonate, soluble indigo blue, indigotine, Acid Blue 74, FD&C Blue No. 2
Molecular formula: $C_{16}H_8N_2Na_2O_8S_2$
Molecular weight: 466.35
Structure:

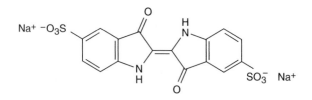

Indigo carmine is excreted unaltered by the kidneys. This excretion is relatively fast, and blue urine can be seen as quickly as 5 to 10 minutes after administration. It was once used as a kidney test to rule out obstruction before more sophisticated modalities became available. It currently is used to locate ureteral orifices during cystoscopy, to test cystourethral anastomosis, and to identify transected ureters intraoperatively. Typically, a 5-mL one-time dose of indigo carmine is administered intravenously.

This compound has a relatively low side-effect profile. Mild elevations in blood pressure have been reported. Indigo carmine can cause a transient decrease in pulse oximetry readings.

INDOCYANINE GREEN
Synonyms: Fox Green, Cario–Green
Molecular formula: $C_{43}H_{47}N_2NaO_6S_2$
Molecular weight: 774.98
Structure:

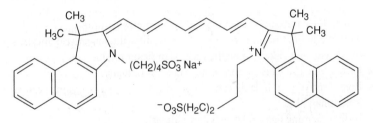

Despite its name, indocyanine green is often grouped with the blue dyes. In humans, indocyanine green is most commonly used for eye surgery, specifically for macular hole and cataract surgery. It can be toxic to the eye if not thoroughly removed at the end of surgery. Its tissue-toxic effects have been used for therapeutic purposes in the photo–oxidative destruction of colon cancer cells with infrared light. It can also be used as a diagnostic aid in blood volume determination and cardiac output via its absorption properties. Indocyanine green may cause a transient decrease in pulse oximetry if it is injected intravascularly.

FDA BLACK BOX WARNING!
In September 2003, the U.S. Food and Drug Administration (FDA) issued a Public Health Advisory ("Black Box Warning") against the use of blue dye to color enteral feeds as a means to detect pulmonary aspiration. Though this practice had been in effect for about 30 years, it had been previously uninvestigated by the FDA. The report specifically targets FD&C Blue No. 1, which is used in much lower concentrations in foods, cosmetics, and drugs. This compound is also known as Blue #1 and Steri-Blue. Blue #1

was temporally associated with several effects. These included discoloration of skin, urine, feces, serum, refractory hypotension, metabolic acidosis, and death. The most susceptible patient population was the critically ill and those with increased gut permeability (i.e., patients with sepsis, trauma, burns, inflammatory bowel disease). The exact reason for severe side effects is not known, but Blue No. 1 is known to be a mitochondrial toxin, which could lead to severe metabolic acidosis. Finally, the FDA states that other blue dyes such as methylene blue and FD&C Blue No. 2 (indigo carmine) may have similar or even worse toxicity than Blue No. 1 and are not appropriate replacements. Some experienced hospital pharmacists are now recommending that the above-described blue dyes not be used when contact with the gastrointestinal tract is possible.

TAKE HOME POINTS

- These compounds are all blue in color, but they have a wide variety of properties.
- Most blue compounds can affect pulse oximetry readings.
- Methylene blue has a high side-effect profile (under general anesthesia, hypertension is likely to be the most significant one).
- Patent blue can cause severe anaphylaxis in humans.
- Preoperative prophylaxis can reduce the severity of reactions seen with isosulphan blue.
- Indigo carmine has a relatively low side-effect profile.
- Indocyanine green must be thoroughly washed out after eye surgery.
- Blue compounds should not be used as markers in enteral feeds.

SUGGESTED READINGS

Acheson D, ed. FDA Public Health Advisory: Reports of blue discoloration and death in patients receiving enteral feedings tinted with the dye, FD&C Blue No. 1. September 29, 2003.

Braunwald E, ed. *Harrison's Principles of Internal Medicine.* 15th ed. New York: McGraw-Hill; 2001:2612.

Cheng S, Yang T, Ho J, et al. Ocular toxicity of intravitreal indocyanine green. *J Ocul Pharmacol Ther.* 2005;21:85–93.

Crisci A, Young M, Murphy B, et al. Ureteral reimplantation for inadvertent ureteral injury during radical perineal prostatectomy. *Urology.* 2003;62:941.

Eldrageely K, Vargas M, Khalkhali I, et al. Sentinel lymph node mapping of breast cancer: A case-control study of methylene blue tracer compared to isosulfan blue. *Am Surg.* 2004;70:872–875.

Miller R, ed. *Miller's Anesthesia.* 6th ed. Philadelphia: Elsevier Churchill Livingstone; 2004:1450–1452.

Montgomery L, Thorne A, Van Zee K, et al. Isosulfan blue dye reactions during sentinel lymph node mapping for breast cancer. *Anesth Analg.* 2002;95:385–388.

Morgan G, ed. *Clinical Anesthesiology.* 3rd ed. New York: McGraw-Hill; 2002:110, 227–228, 238.

O'Neil M, ed. *The Merck Index.* 13th ed. Whitehouse Station, New Jersey: Merck; 2001:6085, 4973, 4988, 9080.

Raut C, Hunt K, Akins J, et al. Incidence of anaphylactoid reactions to isosulfan blue dye during breast carcinoma lymphatic mapping in patients treated with preoperative prophylaxis: Results of a surgical prospective clinical practice protocol. *Cancer*. 2005;104:692–699.

Rodier J, Routiot T, Mignotte H, et al. Lymphatic mapping and sentinel node biopsy of operable breast cancer. *World J Surg*. 2000;10:1220–1225.

Schneider F, Lutun P, Hasselmann M, et al. Methylene blue increases systemic vascular resistance in human septic shock. *Intensive Care Med*. 1992;18:309–311.

Vokach-Brodsky L, Jeffrey S, Lemmens H, et al. Isosulfan blue affects pulse oximetry. *Anesthesiology*. 2000;93:1002–1003.

Waters G, Geisinger K, Garske D, et al. Sentinel lymph node mapping for carcinoma of the colon: A pilot study. *Am Surg*. 2000;66:943–945.

57

DO NOT FORGET THAT LINEZOLID IS A MONOAMINE OXIDASE INHIBITOR (MAOI) AS WELL AS AN ANTIBIOTIC

NEIL B. SANDSON, MD

Linezolid is one of the more recently developed antibiotics, and it is gaining increasing use in the treatment of infections caused by multiply resistant gram-positive organisms. An important, often underappreciated, feature of linezolid is its action as a weak, reversible inhibitor of monoamine oxidase. Lack of recognition of the possibility of significant MAOI-based interactions has led to unfortunate results in hospitalized patients.

To review briefly, the enzyme monoamine oxidase is critically important in the metabolism of the monoamines, which include all of the catecholamines deriving from tyrosine (epinephrine, norepinephrine, and dopamine) as well as serotonin. Inhibition of monoamine oxidase via pharmacologic agents can result in greatly increased catecholamine levels. Co-administration of an MAOI with a sympathomimetic agent, or with any medication that increases the activity or availability of catecholamines, creates the danger of a hypertensive crisis. Similarly, combining MAOIs with serotonergically active compounds may lead to a central serotonin syndrome, characterized by flushing, diarrhea, myoclonus, fever, delirium, seizures, and possibly autonomic collapse and death. Patients who take MAOIs must also adhere to a tyramine-free diet (no aged cheeses, aged or fermented meats, broad bean pods, chianti wine, sauerkraut, or most soybean products) in order to avoid a potential hypertensive crisis.

The most commonly prescribed monoamine oxidase inhibitors (MAOIs) are the antidepressant medications phenelzine (Nardil) and tranylcypromine (Parnate), both potent and irreversible inhibitors of monoamine oxidase. These drugs have been in clinical use for decades and are generally readily recognized by anesthesia providers. Clinical practice concerning the administration of phenelzine and tranylcypromine in the perioperative period has undergone some evolution over the years—generally, most practitioners do not withhold these drugs in the perioperative period, but in order to minimize the danger of a hypertensive crisis instead advocate careful and titrated administration of sympathomimetics.

© 2006 Mayo Foundation for Medical Education and Research

Because linezolid is a reversible and less potent inhibitor of monoamine oxidase than phenelzine or tranylcypromine, it was hoped that the same pharmacodynamic interactions would not be seen. Unfortunately, such has not been the case. Since its introduction, there have been numerous reports of central serotonin syndrome when linezolid has been combined with selective serotonin reuptake inhibitors. There has also been one report of intractable intraoperative hypertension occurring in a patient on a combination of linezolid and bupropion (an antidepressant that inhibits the reuptake of both norepinephrine and dopamine).

Therefore, the same caveats that we apply to the administration of adrenergic and serotonergic drugs to patients receiving the traditional MAOIs should also apply to patients on linezolid. For patients who are receiving linezolid in the perioperative period, it is likely that pressor agents would produce exaggerated and possibly dangerous responses. These agents include ephedrine, isoproterenol, and phenylephrine. It is important to note that rapid increases in desflurane concentration have been described as causing a paradoxical increase in sympathetic activity, including increases in plasma norepinephrine as well as the clinical effects of hypertension and tachycardia. Therefore, the author recommends that desflurane be avoided as well. Serotonergic drugs that are contraindicated for patients on linezolid include meperidine and dextromethorphan.

If the patient is on linezolid or has been in the previous 2 weeks, it is important to either craft an anesthetic plan that minimizes the use of agents that would interact with an MAOI, or to communicate with the treatment team as to possible alternative antibiotic agents that might be used. It is important to review the patient's medication regimen before surgery, as an interaction between monoaminergically active medications and linezolid may become apparent only during the sympathetic activity that may accompany painful surgical maneuvers. Although there have been no case reports of linezolid–tyramine interactions, avoidance of high-tyramine foods while taking linezolid is prudent.

Remember also that there are actually several drugs with a degree of MAOI activity. One such drug is a new antidepressant in the form of transdermal selegiline (trade name Emsam), approved by the U.S. Food and Drug Administration (FDA) in March 2006. This antidepressant is likely to find widespread clinical use, so anesthesia providers will probably be encountering this drug in patients' preoperative medication panels. Traditionally, selegiline is an oral drug that is used to treat Parkinson disease. At low doses, neither of these forms of selegiline requires a tyramine-free diet. However, use of these drugs at any dose dictates the same perioperative concerns as with linezolid, phenelzine, or tranylcypromine.

- Linezolid is frequently used in the perioperative setting for the treatment of resistant gram-positive organisms.
- Anesthesia providers must be aware that linezolid is an inhibitor of monoamine oxidase.
- Although linezolid is a weak, reversible inhibitor of MAO, it has the same potential for deleterious interactions as phenelzine (Nardil) and tranyl-cypromine (Parnate).
- Other drugs with a degree of MAOI activity have recently been approved, such as transdermal selegiline (trade name Emsam), an antidepressant that is likely to find widespread use.

SUGGESTED READINGS

Bristol-Myers Squibb Company. *Emsam.* New York: Bristol-Myers Squibb; 2006.
Evers AS, Maze M. *Anesthetic Pharmacology: Physiological Principles and Clinical Practice.* Philadelphia: Churchill Livingstone; 2004.
Marcucci C, Sandson NB, Dunlap JA. Linezolid-bupropion interaction as possible etiology of severe intermittent intraoperative hypertension? *Anesthesiology.* 2004;101(6):1487–1488.
Pfizer, Inc. *Nardil.* New York: Pfizer; 2003.
GlaxoSmithKline. *Parnate.* Research Triangle Park, NC: GlaxoSmithKline; 2001.

58

BE ALERT FOR THE SIGNS AND SYMPTOMS OF PERIOPERATIVE DIGOXIN TOXICITY, ESPECIALLY IF THE PATIENT IS AT RISK FOR ELECTROLYTE DEPLETION

GRACE L. CHIEN, MD

Digoxin is a semisynthetic steroid glycoside derived from the plant *Digitalis lanata* (common name: Grecian foxglove). It is used for the treatment of systolic dysfunction and some arrhythmias. By reversibly inhibiting the Na–K ATPase pump, digoxin increases the availability of intracellular calcium and subsequently increases cardiac contractility. This increase shifts the Frank–Starling curve to the left in both healthy and failing myocardium. Digoxin also reduces circulating levels of norepinephrine and thus increases parasympathetic tone. This in turn reduces sinoatrial nodal automaticity and atrioventricular nodal conduction. With its neurohumoral-modulating effects, digoxin has been used to treat some re-entrant paroxysmal supraventricular tachycardias.

Digoxin toxicity develops when there is an overload of intracellular calcium in both systolic and diastolic states, and this may cause significant arrhythmias. According to Mahdyoon et al., digoxin toxicity occurred in 0.8% and possible toxicity occurred in another 4% of the population. Factors that increase the risk of digitalis intoxication are renal insufficiency, electrolyte abnormalities (hypokalemia, hypomagnesemia, and hypercalcemia), acute myocardial ischemia, advanced age, hypothyroidism, and pulmonary disease. Pharmacokinetic interactions with other drugs can also affect digoxin levels. Remember that digoxin is a substrate of the P-glycoprotein transporter, so inhibitors and inducers of this transporter will raise and lower serum digoxin levels respectively (see Chapter 47).

Signs of digoxin toxicity may appear at a level of 2 ng/mL, and the incidence of toxicity increases with plasma concentration. Plasma concentration reaches steady state between 6 and 12 hours after the last dose, and thus digoxin levels are best measured within this time. Signs of digoxin toxicity may be very nonspecific. Patients may present with confusion, dizziness, ventricular ectopy, tachycardia, visual disturbances, depression, anxiety, apathy, gynecomastia, or simply a rash.

Dangerous signs of digoxin toxicity include atrioventricular (AV) nodal block, bradycardia, ventricular arrhythmia, thrombocytopenia, delirium,

ⓒ 2006 Mayo Foundation for Medical Education and Research

and hallucinations. For patients under general anesthesia, the main warning signs of toxicity are electrocardiogram (EKG) changes. Digoxin toxicity can cause many types of dysrhythmias but does not usually cause atrial flutter, atrial fibrillation, or Mobitz type II second-degree AV block. However, digoxin toxicity can superimpose on the underlying cardiac pathology. For example, digoxin may create an unusually slow ventricular response to atrial fibrillation. Digoxin can also increase both atrial and ventricular ectopic activity and induce junctional tachycardia. Premature ventricular contraction is often the first sign of digoxin toxicity, progressing to ventricular bigeminy, fascicular tachycardia, ventricular tachycardia, and fatal ventricular fibrillation.

One arrhythmia that is almost pathognomonic for digoxin toxicity is bidirectional ventricular tachycardia (*Fig. 58.1*). The pattern resembles bigeminy except that the R–R interval is regular because all of the beats arise from a single ventricular focus. Patients with the rare disorder of familial catecholaminergic polymorphic ventricular tachycardia may also show this EKG pattern. Digoxin toxicity may cause AV junctional rhythms with escape rates of 30 to 50 beats/min. When the patient's heart rate is 50 to 60 beats/min, an escape rhythm may be in play. With an accelerated junctional rhythm of 60 to 120 beats/min, nonparoxysmal junctional tachycardia is seen. The enhanced vagal tone created by digoxin may generate first-degree, second-degree type I, and third-degree heart blocks.

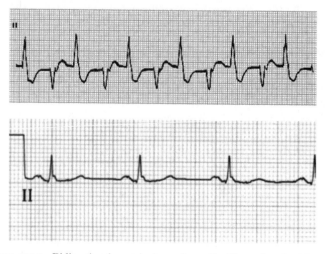

FIGURE 58.1. Bidirectional ventricular tachycardia. (Reproduced with permission, © UpToDate at www.uptodate.com.)

Of course, the first-line treatment for digoxin toxicity is to avoid it. Anesthesia providers should pay special attention to both digoxin levels and serum electrolytes in a patient who has had a bowel prep. Remember that a patient who has even low-normal serum potassium may be at increased risk of digoxin toxicity, even at "therapeutic" digoxin levels. Most clinicians aim for a serum potassium of around 4.0 mEq/L at the time of induction; this is supported by a classic scattergraph in Opie's *Drugs for the Heart*. Also, be aware that a common time to see digoxin-induced arrhythmias is at induction or just after induction. Keep close surveillance of the EKG during this time and do not disrupt the patient's acid–base status with untoward adjustments in ventilation.

Other treatment of digoxin toxicity depends on the symptoms of the patient. Impending cardiac arrest necessitates the ABCs (airway, breathing, and circulation). Bradycardia can be treated with atropine. Transvenous cardiac pacing and β-receptor agonists should be avoided because they may precipitate other cardiac arrhythmias. Administering activated charcoal within 6 to 8 hours postingestion may ameliorate digoxin toxicity. If hyperkalemia coexists with digoxin toxicity, calcium should not be given in the usual fashion for hyperkalemia, because it may potentiate digoxin toxicity. Hypomagnesemia should be treated promptly, because it also potentiates cardiac glycoside toxicity.

The most specific and effective treatment for digoxin toxicity is digoxin-specific Fab fragments (Digibind). Digibind is indicated in patients with life-threatening arrhythmias associated with digoxin, patients with hemodynamic instability, patients with severe bradycardia, patients whose plasma potassium levels are >5 mEq/L, patients with plasma concentration >10 ng/mL, ingestion of >10 mg of digoxin in adults or >4 mg in children, or digoxin-toxic rhythm in the setting of an elevated digoxin level. Digibind binds to intravascular and interstitial digoxin, causing diffusion of digoxin from the intracellular to the extracellular space. Bound digoxin cannot reassociate with the inhibitory site on the α-subunit of Na–K-ATPase, rendering it ineffective. Dosing of Digibind is as follows:

$$\text{Vials of digoxin-specific Fab fragments} = \text{digoxin level (ng/mL)}$$
$$\times \text{ mass (kg)}/100.$$

The digoxin and digoxin-specific Fab fragment complex is rapidly excreted in urine with an elimination half-life of 15 to 20 hours. In patients with renal failure, dialysis can effectively eliminate Fab fragment-digoxin complexes. In contrast, digoxin has not been shown to be effectively eliminated by dialysis.

- Digoxin is a steroid glycoside with multiple cardiac and neurohumoral actions.
- Digoxin toxicity is not rare—known risk factors include advanced age, acute myocardial infarction, renal insufficiency, and electrolyte abnormalities, all of which are factors commonly seen in surgical patients.
- Digoxin serum levels are mediated by the P-glycoprotein transporter.
- There are multiple signs of digoxin toxicity in the unanesthetized patient; in patients under anesthesia, the first sign is usually an EKG abnormality, often PVCs.
- If the patient is on digoxin and has had a bowel prep, ensure electrolyte repletion before the start of the anesthetic.
- Do not give calcium to treat hyperkalemia in a digoxin-toxic patient.
- The most specific and effective treatment for digoxin toxicity is Digibind.

SUGGESTED READINGS

Bigger JT Jr. Digitalis toxicity. *J Clin Pharmacol*. 1985;25(7):514–521.

Dec GW. Digoxin remains useful in the management of chronic heart failure. *Med Clin North Am*. 2003;87(2):317–337.

Doherty JE. Digitalis glycosides. Pharmacokinetics and their clinical implications. *Ann Intern Med*. 1973;79(2):229–238.

El-Salawy SM, Lowenthal DT, Ippagunta S, et al. Clinical Pharmacology and Physiology Conference: Digoxin toxicity in the elderly. *Int Urol Nephrol*. 2005;37(3):665–668.

Gheorghiade M, van Veldhuisen DJ, Colucci WS. Contemporary use of digoxin in the management of cardiovascular disorders. *Circulation*. 2006;113(21):2556–2564.

Kelly RA, Smith TW. Recognition and management of digitalis toxicity. *Am J Cardiol*. 1992;69(18):108G–1G; disc 18G–19G.

Mahdyoon H, Battilana G, Rosman H, et al. The evolving pattern of digoxin intoxication: Observations at a large urban hospital from 1980 to 1988. *Am Heart J*. 1990;120(5):1189–1194.

Opie LH, Gersh BJ. *Drugs for the Heart*. 4th ed. Philadelphia: WB Saunders; 2001; 153.

Priori SG, Napolitano C, Memmi M, et al. Clinical and molecular characterization of patients with catecholaminergic polymorphic ventricular tachycardia. *Circulation*. 2002;106(1):69–74.

Rabetoy GM, Price CA, Findlay JW, et al. Treatment of digoxin intoxication in a renal failure patient with digoxin-specific antibody fragments and plasmapheresis. *Am J Nephrol*. 1990;10(6):518–521.

Reisdorff EJ, Clark MR, Walters BL. Acute digitalis poisoning: The role of intravenous magnesium sulfate. *J Emerg Med*. 1986;4(6):463–469.

Smith TW. Digitalis. Mechanisms of action and clinical use. *N Engl J Med*. 1988;318(6):358–365.

Smith TW, Antman EM, Friedman PL, et al. Digitalis glycosides: Mechanisms and manifestations of toxicity. Part III. *Prog Cardiovasc Dis*. 1984;27(1):21–56.

Taboulet P, Baud FJ, Bismuth C, et al. Acute digitalis intoxication—is pacing still appropriate? *J Toxicol Clin Toxicol*. 1993;31(2):261–273.

59

EXERCISE CARE IN THE USE OF AMIODARONE AND ALTERNATIVE ANTIARRHYTHMICS FOR THE TREATMENT OF ATRIAL FIBRILLATION

MUHAMMAD DURRANI, MD, ALAN CHENG, MD, AND EDWIN G. AVERY, IV, MD

Atrial fibrillation is a common arrhythmia in both the intensive care unit (ICU) and perioperative cardiothoracic surgery settings. The mainstay of therapy is rate control, with beta-blockers being the first-line agents. In more acute clinical situations that involve significant hemodynamic deterioration, synchronized, direct-current cardioversion is immediately indicated. Frequently, however, the decision is made to use rhythm-converting agents, such as amiodarone. Amiodarone is a complex antiarrhythmic agent (predominantly class III) that shares at least some of the properties of each of the other three Vaughn-Williams classes of antiarrhythmics. Amiodarone is commonly used for the treatment and prevention of persistent atrial and ventricular tachyarrhythmias, although it is approved by the U.S. Food and Drug Administration (FDA) only for management of ventricular arrhythmias. It is one of the few agents that can be used safely in individuals with congestive heart failure. Contraindications to amiodarone include severe sinus node dysfunction with marked sinus bradycardia or syncope, second- or third-degree heart block, known hypersensitivity to its contents, cardiogenic shock, and probably severe chronic lung disease.

Amiodarone is highly lipid-soluble, extensively distributed in the body, and highly concentrated in many tissues, especially in the liver and lungs. After variable (30% to 50%) and slow gastrointestinal (GI) absorption, amiodarone is very slowly eliminated with a half-life of about 25 to 110 days. The onset of action after oral administration is delayed, and a steady-state drug effect may not be established for several months unless large loading doses are used. Amiodarone undergoes extensive hepatic metabolism to the pharmacologically active metabolite, desethylamiodarone (DEA). Amiodarone is excreted not by the kidneys but rather by the lacrimal glands, the skin, and the biliary tract. Neither amiodarone nor DEA is dialyzable.

Amiodarone is both an antiarrhythmic and a potent vasodilator. Amiodarone lengthens the effective refractory period by prolonging the action-potential duration in all cardiac muscles, including bypass tracts (class III activity). It also has a powerful class I antiarrhythmic effect that works by inhibiting inactivated sodium channels at high stimulation frequencies.

© 2006 Mayo Foundation for Medical Education and Research

Amiodarone slows phase 4 depolarization of the sinus node as well as conduction through the atrioventricular node. It also decreases Ca^{2+} current (class IV effect) and transient outward delayed rectifier and inward rectifier K^+ currents. Amiodarone noncompetitively blocks α- and β-adrenergic receptors (class II effect); this effect is additive to competitive receptor inhibition by beta-blockers.

There is a risk of hypotension with intravenous amiodarone administration, more common with rapid administration. Other notable acute effects include bradycardia, hypokalemia, interactions with medications such as Coumadin and digoxin, and, rarely, torsades de pointe. There is a risk of pulmonary toxicity with high doses, starting with pneumonitis and leading to pulmonary fibrosis. Other organ systems affected by amiodarone therapy include the thyroid (hypothyroidism or hyperthyroidism), the central nervous system (proximal muscle weakness, peripheral neuropathy and neural symptoms), and the gastrointestinal tract (nausea 25%, elevated liver functions), and it may cause testicular dysfunction, corneal microdeposition, and photosensitive slate-gray or bluish skin discoloration.

Agents that can be considered as alternatives to amiodarone for the treatment of atrial fibrillation depend on the patient's cardiac history, as individuals with reduced left ventricular systolic function are especially prone to the proarrhythmic effects of certain antiarrhythmic agents. Some commonly used alternatives include ibutilide, dofetilide, and sotalol. Strong consideration should be given to obtaining consultation with a cardiac electrophysiologist before initiating these agents.

Ibutilide prolongs repolarization by inhibition of the delayed rectifier potassium current (Ikr) and by selective enhancement of the slow inward sodium current. This drug is efficacious in the termination of atrial fibrillation and flutter with both single and repeated intravenous infusions. It is as effective as amiodarone in cardioversion of atrial fibrillation. The proarrhythmic effect resulting in torsades de pointe is higher in individuals with heart failure, those with bradycardia, nonwhite subjects, women, and in those given the drug for atrial flutter rather than atrial fibrillation. The risk of this is greatest during or shortly after the infusion of the drug (within 1 hour) and wanes rapidly after administration because the half-life (2 to 12 hours) of this agent is short. The patient should be monitored for at least 4 hours after the start of the infusion.

Dofetilide prolongs the action potential and QTC in a concentration-related manner. Dofetilide exerts its effects solely by inhibition of the rapid component of the delayed rectifier potassium current Ikr. Dofetilide has stronger evidence in its favor for acute cardioversion of atrial fibrillation than for maintenance thereafter, according to a meta-analysis. It can be given to patients with depressed function but needs to be initiated while being continuously monitored on telemetry for the first 3 days of therapy because this too, like ibutilide, carries a risk of proarrhythmia. The risk of torsades de pointes can be reduced by establishing or maintaining normal serum potassium and magnesium levels, predose adjustment of renal function, and post-dose reduction based on QT_C (ideally, baseline $QT_C < 429$ milliseconds). Administration of dofetilide requires that the hospital and the prescriber be trained as confirmed administrators. Further information can be found at www.tikosyn.com.

Sotalol has combined class II and class III properties, is active against a variety of arrhythmias, and has the ability to produce profound bradycardia or prolongation of the QT interval. Of the many indications, sotalol is most commonly used for maintenance of sinus rhythm after cardioversion for atrial fibrillation and for reducing ventricular tachyarrhythmias. Despite its ability to prevent tachyarrhythmias, sotalol (like any other antiarrhythmic) can also be proarrhythmic because of its ability to profoundly prolong the QT interval. As a result, initiation of this drug should occur while the patient is closely monitored. Sotalol is contraindicated in patients with reduced creatinine clearance (<40 mL/min) and asthma. It should be avoided in patients with serious conduction defects, in patients with bronchospastic disease, and when there are evident risks of proarrhythmia.

The use of these antiarrhythmic medications must be undertaken in a clinical environment with the appropriate resources to deal with the complications that may accompany their use. Specifically, these drugs should be used only in care settings with immediately available emergency resuscitation equipment (e.g., a code cart with emergency drugs, airway mechanisms, and pacing devices) as well as personnel appropriately trained (e.g., anesthesiologists, intensivists, or cardiologists) to use this equipment.

SUGGESTED READINGS

Miller MR, McNamara RL, Segal JB, et al. Efficacy of agents for pharmacologic conversion of atrial fibrillation and subsequent maintenance of sinus rhythm: A meta-analysis of clinical trials. *J Fam Pract.* 2000;49(11):1033–1046.

Opie LH, Gersh BJ. *Drugs for the Heart.* 6th ed. Philadelphia: Elsevier;2005:218–274.

60

USE EXTREME CAUTION WHEN ADMINISTERING MILRINONE IN RENAL FAILURE

YING WEI LUM, MD AND EDWIN G. AVERY, IV, MD

MECHANISM OF ACTION

Milrinone is a selective inhibitor of peak cAMP phosphodiesterase III isozyme in cardiac and vascular smooth muscle. Its inhibitory action on phosphodiesterase results in increased cAMP levels, which in turn increases contractility in cardiac muscle and stimulates vasodilation in blood vessels. This causes an increase in cardiac output and a decrease in pulmonary wedge pressure. These hemodynamic changes are obtained without excessive changes in heart rate or increase in myocardial oxygen consumption.

INDICATIONS

Milrinone's use has been best studied in patients with congestive heart failure. It appears to be very efficacious in nonhypotensive patients with acute nonischemic cardiomyopathy despite treatment with diuretics. These patients benefit from an enhancement in contractility and afterload reduction. Additionally, milrinone is known to provide enhanced diastolic function. Duration of therapy should last for 48 to 72 hours. There are no studies to date that support its use for a longer period. Long-term oral therapy with milrinone has been associated with increased mortality.

DOSE

The recommended dose in patients with normal renal function is a 50-mcg/kg bolus followed by a continuous infusion at 0.375 to 0.75 mcg/kg/min. Because milrinone is excreted mainly through the kidneys, its dose in patients with renal impairment should be adjusted accordingly (by surface area) (CrCl denotes creatinine clearance):

CrCl 50 mL/min/1.73 m^2: Administer 0.43 mcg/kg/min.
CrCl 40 mL/min/1.73 m^2: Administer 0.38 mcg/kg/min.
CrCl 30 mL/min/1.73 m^2: Administer 0.33 mcg/kg/min.
CrCl 20 mL/min/1.73 m^2: Administer 0.28 mcg/kg/min.
CrCl 10 mL/min/1.73 m^2: Administer 0.23 mcg/kg/min.
CrCl 5 mL/min/1.73 m^2: Administer 0.2 mcg/kg/min.

An immediate improvement in hemodynamics is seen within 5 to 15 minutes after initiation of therapy. The mean half-life of milrinone is

© 2006 Mayo Foundation for Medical Education and Research

approximately 2.4 hours, and patients reach a steady-state plasma milrinone concentration (200 ng/mL) within 6 to 12 hours of a continuous maintenance infusion of 0.50 mcg/kg/min. The impact of the half-life of milrinone is clinically important, as the effects of the drug cannot be "turned off" rapidly as can those of many of the other commonly used inotropic agents, such as epinephrine.

CAUTION

Milrinone decreases atrioventricular nodal conduction time, allowing a potential for increased ventricular response rates (up to 3.8%) for patients with supraventricular arrhythmias. Ventricular arrhythmias (ventricular ectopy, sustained and nonsustained ventricular tachycardia) have also been reported in up to 12% of patients. Life-threatening ventricular arrhythmias appear to be related to the presence of other underlying factors such as a preexisting arrhythmia and/or metabolic abnormalities. Extreme caution must be used in patients with renal compromise. Fatal ventricular arrhythmias developed in six of nine patients in a recent study of the pharmacokinetics of milrinone in patients on continuous venovenous hemofiltration (CVVHD). These patients were oliguric (<400 mL/24 h) and had a serum creatinine of >2.0 mg/dL. All patients received 0.25 mcg/kg/min of milrinone and developed a mean steady-state concentration of 845 ng/mL; four times higher than that of patients with normal renal function. The high protein-binding affinity of milrinone and decreased urinary excretion could have contributed to this high concentration, thereby leading to the increased incidence of ventricular arrhythmias.

TAKE HOME POINTS

- Milrinone is a phosphodiesterase inhibitor that acts primarily on cardiac and vascular smooth muscle. Its effects are to enhance diastolic function, increase cardiac output, and decrease pulmonary wedge pressure.
- Milrinone is given intravenously for a period of 48 to 72 hours. It has a mean half-life of 2.4 hours—it cannot be turned off as most inotropes can.
- Extreme caution must be used in patients with renal failure because of the potential development of life-threatening arrhythmias.
- For patients with renal compromise, the milrinone dose must be adjusted on a sliding scale.

SUGGESTED READINGS

Taniguchi T, Shibata K, Saito S, et al. Pharmacokinetics of milrinone in patients with congestive heart failure during continuous venovenous hemofiltration. *Intensive Care Med.* 2000;26(8):1089–1093.
http://milrinone.com.

61

USE MEPERIDINE WITH CAUTION

NEIL B. SANDSON, MD

Meperidine (Demerol) was the first phenylpiperidine analgesic to come onto the market in the United States. Through the years it has been used extensively as a narcotic analgesic as well as a favored drug for sickle-cell crises, shaking chills, and various surgical uses. However, in more recent years, a growing number of clinicians are recognizing that the benefits of meperidine probably do not justify the risks.

Meperidine has disadvantages compared to other narcotics, even when given as monotherapy. It will provide adequate analgesia for the surgical patient on initial dosing, but the risk–benefit ratio then shifts somewhat. Meperidine has a half-life of only 3 to 5 hours. The primary metabolite, normeperidine, has a half-life of 15 to 20 hours, but it is only half as effective an analgesic as meperidine. A significant problem is that normeperidine has neuroexcitatory properties. So, when meperidine is given in repeated doses, which is often required given the relatively short-lived nature of its analgesic effect (for postoperative pain), there is a tendency for patients to experience irritability, tremors, muscle twitching, and new-onset seizures. Normeperidine toxicity can even prove fatal, especially in individuals with hepatic and/or renal impairment, because of their greater susceptibility to normeperidine accumulation.

Other problematic issues with the use of meperidine involve the likelihood of troublesome drug–drug interactions (DDIs). The first set of DDI concerns that must be considered by the anesthesia provider are pharmacodynamic in nature. As a serotonergically active agent, meperidine can act synergistically with other serotonergic drugs (such as fluoxetine, paroxetine, sertraline, and other selective serotonin reuptake inhibitors) or with monoamine oxidase inhibitors (phenelzine, tranylcypromine, selegiline, and linezolid) to produce a potentially lethal central serotonin syndrome (*Table 61.1*). This was the primary cause of the death of Libby Zion in the 1984 case that generated national attention for a number of years. She visited a New York emergency department and received meperidine for her shaking chills, even though she was known to be taking phenelzine. She developed a fever of 107.6°F in the course of her serotonin syndrome and eventually expired. Her death then became a rallying point around the issue of house staff work hours, as it was suspected that the resident who ordered the meperidine would have known better had he been better rested.

© 2006 Mayo Foundation for Medical Education and Research

TABLE 61.1   MEPERIDINE DRUG–DRUG INTERACTIONS (DDIs)

MECHANISM OF DDI	INTERACTING DRUGS	CLINICAL CONSEQUENCES
Pharmacodynamically synergistic serotonergic effects	Selective serotonin reuptake inhibitors (citalopram, escitalopram, fluoxetine, fluvoxamine, paroxetine, sertraline) Monoamine oxidase inhibitors (linezolid, phenelzine, selegiline, tranylcypromine) Theoretically, other serotonergically active drugs (dextromethorphan, tricyclic antidepressants, venlafaxine, etc.)	Central serotonin syndrome (nausea, diarrhea, fever, flushing, autonomic instability, diaphoresis, myoclonus, seizures, coma, death)
Inhibition of P450 2B6 and/or 3A4	Azole antifungal agents (fluconazole, ketoconazole, etc.) Cimetidine Ciprofloxacin Diltiazem Erythromycin Fluoxetine Fluvoxamine Paroxetine Protease inhibitors (acute ritonavir, saquinavir, etc.) Sertraline Verapamil	Excessive narcotic effects (sedation, respiratory depression, delirium)
Induction of P450 2B6 and/or 3A4	Barbiturates Carbamazepine Phenytoin Prednisone Rifampin Ritonavir (chronic) St. John's wort	(a) Decreased analgesia; (b) increased production of neurotoxic normeperidine metabolite

Pharmacokinetic DDIs are also quite problematic when using meperidine. Meperidine is metabolized (demethylated) into normeperidine primarily by the cytochrome P450 enzymes 2B6 and 3A4. This gives rise to two main concerns. First, any of the numerous *inhibitors* of these enzymes are likely to yield excessive narcotic effects, such as oversedation, respiratory depression, and delirium. Inhibitors of these enzymes include such drugs as azole antifungals, ciprofloxacin, diltiazem, erythromycin, fluoxetine, paroxetine, protease inhibitors, sertraline, and verapamil, to name a few (*Table 61.1*).

The second of these pharmacokinetic concerns involves interactions with enzymatic *inducers* of these P450 enzymes. These inducers generate both decreases in meperidine levels, with associated loss of analgesic efficacy, as well as increased production of the normeperidine metabolite with its associated neurotoxicity. Inducers of these P450 enzymes include barbiturates, carbamazepine, phenytoin, prednisone, rifampin, ritonavir (chronically administered), and St. John's wort.

There are anesthesia providers who "like" meperidine, have used it often, and feel they have never had a patient with a significant interaction. There is also the occasional patient who claims that only meperidine helps him or her with an acute or chronic pain syndrome. Finally, it is still not infrequent that an anesthesia provider will get a call from the postanesthesia care unit (PACU) asking for a verbal meperidine order for a patient who is shivering. *In any of these situations, it is incumbent that the provider ascertain that there is no possibility of a significant pharmacodynamic or pharmacokinetic DDI.* Failing to do so will both endanger the patient and leave the practitioner open to medical and legal censure, should an interaction arise.

One final note: In late 2006, this author's hospital removed meperidine from its formulary, as have many other hospitals. With the availability of safe, effective warming devices to combat patient shivering and newer-generation analgesic drugs, it was the consensus opinion of the staff physicians that meperidine was no longer a necessary agent in the pharmacologic armamentarium.

TAKE HOME POINTS

- Meperidine has a short half-life (3 to 5 hours). Its primary metabolite, normeperidine, has much less therapeutic value and a half-life of 15 to 20 hours.
- Even with monotherapy, neurotoxicity is a concern with repeated doses.
- Patients on multidrug therapy including meperidine are at risk for both pharmacodynamic and pharmacokinetic DDIs.
- *Never* give meperidine to a patient who is taking a serotonergic drug or a monoamine oxidase inhibitor.
- Meperidine is metabolized by the P450 3A4 and 2B6 enzyme subsystems.
- Pharmacokinetic DDIs involve the interaction of both inhibitors and inducers of these enzymes.
- Do not give a verbal order for meperidine unless you have verified that the patient is not being co-administered any of the drugs in *Table 61.1.*

SUGGESTED READINGS

Beckwith MC, Fox ER, Chandramouli J. Removing meperidine from the health-system formulary—frequently asked questions. *J Pain Palliat Care Pharmacother.* 2002;16(3): 45–59.

Latta KS, Ginsberg B, Barkin RL. Meperidine: A critical review. *Am J Ther.* 2002;9(1):53–68.

Piscitelli SC, Kress DR, Bertz RJ, et al. The effect of ritonavir on the pharmacokinetics of meperidine and normeperidine. *Pharmacotherapy.* 2000;20(5):549–553.

Ramirez J, Innocenti F, Schuetz EG, et al. CYP2B6, CYP3A4, and CYP2C19 are responsible for the in vitro N-demethylation of meperidine in human liver microsomes. *Drug Metab Dispos.* 2004;32(9):930–936.

Intraoperative and Perioperative

62

WASH YOUR HANDS!

JAMES W. IBINSON, MD, PhD AND DAVID G. METRO, MD

You've heard it since you were too young to remember: *"Wash your hands!"* Despite that, many anesthesia providers practice poor habits in this area. Although most anesthesiologists on direct questioning will "know" the benefits of good hand hygiene, their habits may leave something to be desired. We must remember that hand hygiene (handwashing *and* glove use) benefits not only you but also your patients.

Although the absolute indications for ideal handwashing practice is not known (because of the lack of controlled studies), the Centers for Disease Control and Prevention (CDC) state that health care workers (HCWs) should "decontaminate hands before having direct contact with patients," after "contact with body fluids or excretions, mucous membranes, non-intact skin, and wound dressings," and even after "contact with a patient's intact skin" (*Table 62.1*). These recommendations are based on their findings that "Handwashing is the single most important procedure for preventing nosocomial infections" (Boyce and Pittet, 2002).

The American Society of Anesthesiologists (ASA) has also published guidelines for hand hygiene using the above findings as justification. Stating that "strict adherence to handwashing and aseptic technique remains the cornerstone of prevention of catheter-related infections," the ASA recommends that hands be washed before and after any patient contact, as indicated in *Table 62.2*. Their statement details the use of both hand cleansing and glove use. For this discussion, both will be included in the term "hand hygiene."

As obvious as the above standards may seem, anesthesiologists have repeatedly been shown to be among the worst of physicians for adherence to hand hygiene standards. Pittet et al. (2004) demonstrated that anesthesiologists showed proper hand hygiene only 23% of the time. In a survey of anesthesiologists in the United Kingdom, El Mikatti et al. stated that only 36.4% washed their hands between cases. Studies show that anesthesiologist hand hygiene rates increase, however, when they perceive an infectious threat. Tait and Tuttle (1995) showed that when treating patients thought to be carrying HIV or HBV, 95% of HCWs washed their hands, versus only 58% of HCWs for the exact same patients when knowledge of HIV or HBV status was not known. This suggests the HCWs understand the importance of hand hygiene in preventing the transmission of disease but fail to appreciate its importance in routine contact. Although it is noted that

© 2006 Mayo Foundation for Medical Education and Research

TABLE 62.1 CDC RECOMMENDATIONS FOR ACTIVITIES THAT REQUIRE HANDWASHING

1) Decontaminate hands before having direct contact with patients.
2) Decontaminate hands before donning sterile gloves when inserting a central intravascular catheter.
3) Decontaminate hands before inserting indwelling urinary catheters, peripheral vascular catheters, or other invasive devices that do not require a surgical procedure.
4) Decontaminate hands after contact with a patient's intact skin (e.g., when taking a pulse or blood pressure, or lifting a patient).
5) Decontaminate hands after contact with body fluids or excretions, mucous membranes, nonintact skin, and wound dressings even if hands are not visibly soiled.
6) Decontaminate hands if moving from a contaminated-body site to a clean-body site during patient care.
7) Decontaminate hands after contact with inanimate objects (including medical equipment) in the immediate vicinity of the patient.
8) Decontaminate hands after removing gloves.
9) Before eating and after using a restroom, wash hands with a nonantimicrobial soap and water or with an antimicrobial soap and water.

---

these studies may be somewhat dated, clear evidence that hand hygiene has improved within anesthesiology is not available.

The reasons for this poor compliance have been studied extensively and include logistical barriers (sink/antiseptic hand-rub location) and a heavy workload resulting from overcrowding and understaffing of patient care areas. These issues need to be addressed on an administrative as well as an individual level. The open layout of most postanesthesia care units (PACUs)

TABLE 62.2 SUMMARY OF RECOMMENDATIONS OF THE ASA FOR HAND HYGIENE

1) Wash hands before performing invasive procedures.
2) Wash hands after touching blood, body fluids, secretions, excretions, and contaminated items, whether or not gloves are worn.
3) Wash hands immediately after gloves are removed, between patient contacts, and when otherwise indicated to avoid transfer of micro-organisms to other patients or environments.
4) It may be necessary to wash hands between tasks and procedures on the same patient to prevent cross-contamination of different body sites.
5) Waterless handwashing solutions may be considered when the anesthesiologist cannot leave the room.
6) Appropriate barrier precautions such as gloves, fluid-resistant masks, face shields, and gowns must be used routinely with all patients.
7) Remove gloves and gowns promptly after use, before touching noncontaminated items and environmental surfaces, and wash hands before seeing another patient.

and many intensive care units (ICUs) also seems to lower hand hygiene compliance. Pittet et al. (2003) found that only 19.6% of HCWs cleaned their hands properly when admitting a new patient to the PACU.

Anesthesiologists who do not follow recommended hand hygiene practice in terms of glove use most commonly cite a loss of touch as the reason. Several studies have investigated this claim. Tiefenthaler et al. (2006) showed that touch sensitivity as tested by filament force on the fingertip required for sensation is indeed reduced with either standard single-use protective gloves or sterile surgical gloves. Two-point discrimination, on the other hand was not significantly different. No difference was found between the two glove types. Kopka et al. (2005) examined single-use protective gloves, standard sterile surgical gloves, and extrathin surgical gloves in terms of skin-pressure sensation. They found no significant difference between standard protective and surgical gloves but did note an improvement when using extrathin surgical gloves. Although these studies may support the case against glove use in terms of sensation, arguments for routine use are strengthened by the finding that approximately 10% of all patients undergoing surgery can be infected with infectious viruses or methicillin-resistant *Staphylococcus aureus*, and that *glove use can prevent up to 98% of blood-borne pathogens.* CDC and ASA recommendations on this are clear, and the Occupational Safety and Health Administration (OSHA) requires gloves as part of its standard precautions.

TAKE HOME POINTS

- Both the CDC and the ASA recommend that hands be cleaned before and after all contact with patients and potentially when touching two areas of the same patient.
- Anesthesiologists are not exempt from these recommendations but have been shown to be among the least compliant practitioners.
- Although glove use has been shown to decrease touch sensitivity, the benefits of their use should outweigh this concern.
- Mom was right: Wash your hands! (Even when you don't know that the patient has an infection.)

SUGGESTED READINGS

American Society of Anesthesiologists. Recommendations for infection control for the practice of anesthesiology. 2nd ed. Park Ridge, IL: American Society of Anesthesiologists; 1999. Available at www.asahq.org/publicationsAndServices/infectioncontrol.pdf.

Asai T, Matsumoto S, Shingu K. Incidence of blood-borne infectious micro-organisms: would you still not wear gloves? *Anaesthesia.* 2000;55:591–592.

Asai T, Masuzawa M, Shingu K. Education, in addition to a thin material, encourages anaesthetists to wear gloves. *Acta Anaesthesiol Scand.* 2006;50:260–261.

Boyce JM, Pittet D. Guideline for hand hygiene in health-care settings. Recommendations of the Healthcare Infection Control Practices Advisory Committee and the HICPAC/SHEA/APIC/IDSA Hand Hygiene Task Force. Society for Healthcare Epidemiology of America/Association for Professionals in Infection Control/Infectious Diseases Society of America. *MMWR*. 2002;51:1–45. Available at www.cdc.gov/mmwr/preview/mmwrhtml/rr5116a1.htm.

el Mikatti N, Dillon P, Healy TE. Hygienic practices of consultant anaesthetists: a survey in the north-west region of the UK. *Anaesthesia*. 1999;54:13–18.

Kristensen MS, Sloth E, Jensen TK. Relationship between anesthetic procedure and contact of anesthesia personnel with patient body fluids. *Anesthesiology*. 1990;73:619–624.

Kopka A, Crawford JM, Broome IJ. Anaesthetists should wear gloves—touch sensitivity is improved with a new type of thin gloves. *Acta Anaesthesiol Scand*. 2005;49:459–462.

Pittet D, Simon A, Hugonnet S, et al. Hand hygiene among physicians: performance, beliefs, and perceptions. *Ann Intern Med*. 2004;141(1):1–8.

Pittet D, Stephan F, Hugonnet S, et al. Hand-cleansing during postanesthesia care. *Anesthesiology*. 2003;99:530–535.

Tait AR, Tuttle DB. Preventing perioperative transmission of infection: a survey of anesthesiology practice. *Anesth Analg*. 1995;80:764–769.

Tiefenthaler W, Gimpl S, Wechselberger G, et al. Touch sensitivity with sterile standard surgical gloves and single-use protective gloves. *Anaesthesia*. 2006;61:959–961.

63

NEVER RUSH THROUGH A SIGN-OUT

JOHN T. BRYANT, IV, MD

As symbolized by the seal of the American Society of Anesthesiologists (ASA), the practice of anesthesia is a profession based on vigilance. Attention to detail and continuous situational awareness are essential to anticipate and avoid preventable complications. Similar to other professions requiring constant vigilance, it is generally accepted that periodic relief of anesthesia providers is necessary to promote patient safety. Extrapolating from data in their landmark 1978 study regarding preventable mishaps in the practice of anesthesia, Cooper et al. found that the provision of periodic breaks to anesthesia personnel during long procedures had a favorable effect on preventing critical incidents by allowing their (earlier) detection by the relieving anesthetist. This finding has not been universal, as some evidence shows that continuity of care throughout the course of an anesthetic case decreases the risk of perioperative morbidity and mortality. Though examples have been observed of critical incidents attributed to, or perpetuated by, the exchange of personnel, most of these can be avoided by a detailed and inclusive personnel exchange protocol. This chapter presents a stepwise approach to organizing essential data during personnel exchanges to enhance patient care focusing on three critical categories: patient factors, surgical procedure factors, and key elements of the anesthetic plan.

Effective July 1, 2004, all Joint Commission on Accreditation of Healthcare Organizations (JCAHO)–accredited surgical facilities became required to adopt the Universal Protocol to Prevent Wrong Site, Wrong Procedure, and Wrong Person Surgery. This "time-out" protocol provides a point of embarkation in the initiation of sign-out protocol between anesthesia providers. Confirming demographic information including age, gender, race, and name establishes the context in which all further information can be understood. Included in the introduction is mention of any medical allergies unique to the patient. Furthermore, it is essential that the replacing anesthetist be versed in what surgical procedure is being performed and its indications in order to anticipate anesthetic needs.

Anesthetic technique is dictated not only by surgical requirements but also largely by co-morbid conditions. Consequently, the next logical piece of information to cover deals with the patient's relevant past medical history. The relieving anesthetist should assume care of the patient only after acquiring a thorough grasp of his or her medical problems, concentrating

---

© 2006 Mayo Foundation for Medical Education and Research

on cardiovascular, pulmonary, renal, and neurologic status. Attention should be paid to objective measures of physiologic organ system function such as pertinent laboratory values, radiologic studies, and baseline vital signs. Anticipating and avoiding preventable morbidity hinges on planning around pitfalls inherent to the patient's physiologic state. Knowledge of these comorbidities helps explain the medications that the patient chronically takes that may compliment or complicate anesthetic management. Discovering that a patient is inadequately treated for a certain medical condition may help to modulate the anesthetic plan and thereby avoid morbidity.

The logic of the anesthetic plan should be apparent after establishing what is being done, to whom it is being done, and what special challenges are presented by the patient. To ensure that critical information is not overlooked, it is useful to conduct the discussion of anesthetic technique in chronological order. Beginning with induction, it is essential that the replacing anesthetist have a thorough understanding of what technique was used. Critical items to note include the mode (e.g., mask induction, intravenous induction, or rapid sequence induction) and the medications used.

Airway management is the next critical factor to discuss. If a mask airway was utilized during induction, it is important to note the ease of ventilation and the need for airway adjuncts. The relieving anesthesia provider should be informed of the specifics of the definitive airway plan: The device, its size, depth, and ease of placement are all critical factors. If direct laryngoscopy was conducted, the outgoing anesthetist should highlight what kind of blade was utilized and what his or her view was of the glottic inlet.

The relieving anesthetist will need to have an understanding of the type and indication for the monitors that are utilized. If any indicated monitors were omitted, the original anesthetist should be prepared to articulate the reasoning behind the omission. The relieving anesthetist should be aware of the size and location of invasive devices such as venous access lines, arterial lines, and central venous cannulae. It is incumbent on both anesthetists to confirm that all lines are patent so that fluids, blood products, and medications reach the vasculature as intended. Closely related to the issue of invasive devices is a summary of the amount and type of fluids given, estimated blood loss, and urine output up to the point of personnel exchange.

A thoughtful sign-out should include a summary of important medications administered during the procedure thus far. Important medications to note include premedications given before induction, as these may later have an effect during emergence. Reviewing the dose and timing of antibiotics given may not only be a cue to administer an overlooked medication but also prompts the relieving anesthetist of the possibility that antibiotics may need to be readministered before the close of a lengthy procedure. The relieving anesthetist will need to be aware of the dose and timing of narcotics and antiemetics, as these also have effects at the time of emergence. Viewed in light of the patient's co-morbidities, the administration of any vasoactive medications is of primary importance. Finally, the use and continued need for neuromuscular junction blockers is critical because they can have significant effects on surgical conditions and emergence.

A final topic of discussion pertaining to the anesthetic plan relates to preparing for the end of the procedure. The relieving anesthetist should know the estimated time and major events remaining in the procedure. He or she will need to continue or modify the existing plan for postoperative pain and nausea. Also, he or she will need to plan for disposition of the patient. Whether the patient will be extubated is a key planning factor. If the patient is to be extubated, does the nature of the surgery require a deep extubation, or do patient-specific factors necessitate an awake extubation? Finally, the relieving anesthetist should understand where the patient is to go following the procedure. If the patient is to be admitted, the relieving anesthetist should ensure that a bed in an appropriate ward or unit has been procured.

After gaining a firm understanding of the patient, the procedure, and the anesthetic plan, it is essential that the relieving anesthetist confirm the presence of emergency medications, equipment, and contacts. Inappropriately labeled syringes have been shown to be a common source of preventable error during exchanges of personnel. Such errors have been attributed to the lack of standardization in labels and doses of medications. It is incumbent on the relieving anesthetist to check the identity and concentration of prepared medications and correct any discrepancies. Similarly, the relieving anesthetist will want to confirm the location and functionality of the laryngoscope and accompanying blades. Additional endotracheal tubes of appropriate sizes with stylets should be readily available. If blood products are anticipated to be required, the relieving anesthetist should inquire about their availability. A final essential piece of information is an understanding of who is available for assistance. The relieving anesthetist should not allow his or her predecessor to leave the room without handing down the names and contact numbers for the attending anesthesiologist and anesthesia technician.

TAKE HOME POINTS

- Vigilance is the hallmark of the practice of anesthesia.
- Periodic short breaks during prolonged procedures can enhance patient safety by giving the anesthetist an opportunity to rest and renew focus. They also afford a new perspective on a case and help to discourage complacency.

- To enhance rather than hinder patient care, exchanges in anesthesia personnel must be accompanied by a thorough and thoughtful sign-out. Exchanges of information between providers can be highly variable.
- To promote a thorough, efficient, and retainable exchange, anesthetists should make an effort to give and receive their report free from interruption.
- Other elements that may improve sign-out effectiveness include using a checklist, taking notes, and having the relieving anesthetist read back information to the outgoing anesthetist to ensure comprehension.
- Any successful sign-out protocol must include pertinent discussions of the patient, the procedure, and the plan.
- Approaching the sign-out in a logical manner can assist the anesthetist in assimilating a large body of critical information in an effective, efficient, and safe manner.

SUGGESTED READINGS

Arbous MS, Meursing AE, van Kleef JW, et al. Impact of anesthesia management characteristics on severe morbidity and mortality. *Anesthesiology*. 2005;102(2):257–268.

Cooper JB. Do short breaks increase or decrease anesthetic risk? *J Clin Anesth*. 1989;1(3): 228–231.

Cooper JB, Newbower RS, Long CD, et al. Preventable anesthesia mishaps: a human factors study. *Anesthesiology*. 1978;49:399–406.

Electronic reference by the Joint Commission on Accreditation of Healthcare Organizations. (2004, July 1). Retrieved February 21, 2006, from www.jcaho.org/accredited+organizations/patient+safety/universal+protocol/universal_protocol.pdf.

Patterson ES, Roth EM, Woods DD, et al. Handoff strategies in settings with high consequences for failure: lessons for health care operations. *Int J Qual Health Care*. 2004;16(2):125–132.

64

PREOPERATIVE ANXIOLYSIS: IT'S NOT JUST "TWO OF MIDAZ"

MICHAEL P. HUTCHENS, MD, MA

William Thomas Green Morton did not meet his patient before their encounter in the Ether Dome on October 16, 1846, as he was running late. Robert Hinckley's painting of the scene depicts an anxiety-producing environment—the patient strapped to a chair, the focus of attention in an auditorium full of surgeons. Gilbert Abbott might have benefited from 2 mg of midazolam, had it been available; but perhaps he would then have been unable to tell the audience, as he did immediately postoperatively, that the operation had been painless. As far as history records, his perioperative experience was satisfactory to him, entirely without premedication or a preanesthetic interview. Nonetheless, the preoperative anxiety of Gilbert Abbott and that of modern patients has implications for patient satisfaction and for patient care and physiology. Preoperative anxiety is common—conservatively 25% and up to 80% in some studies. Concerns associated with anxiety include postoperative pain, incapacitation, and death. Preoperative anxiety is correlated with delayed gastric emptying, with increased intraoperative heart rate and anesthetic requirements, and with increased postoperative pain scores.

It remains unclear what preoperative strategy is most effective, in most patients, in reducing perioperative anxiety. Based on a 1997 survey, most U.S. anesthesiologists give anxiolytic medication as part of this therapy, but there are significant geographic, patient age, and hospital size variations. There is no consensus in the literature, and the number of regimens investigated is large and diverse. What is most clear is that patients have increased anxiety before operations, and that interventions performed by anesthesiologists can reduce that anxiety.

An oft-cited study purporting to show that the anesthetic interview is more effective than pentobarbital premedication was performed in 1963, but this study was methodologically flawed. The most anxious patients (those who kept the interviewer past the allotted time) were dropped from the study, but only in the interview arm. There was no assessment of baseline (prehospital) anxiety and no objective measure of anxiety. All patients received intramuscular atropine before assessment, patients were not aware they were part of a study despite being administered study medications, and it is unlikely that it is possible to blind an observer to whether a patient has

© 2006 Mayo Foundation for Medical Education and Research

received pentobarbital, as investigators claimed to have done. The literature on premedication and preoperative anxiolysis is rife with similar methodologic problems (although, thankfully, not the absence of consent). However, at least one well-designed study shows that a visit from an anesthesiologist can play a significant role. In a 1977 study conducted in Britain, Leigh et al. used an objective psychometric questionnaire to assess baseline preoperative anxiety and that after no intervention, a preoperative visit, or viewing a 10-page booklet on anesthesia. All patients had more than normal anxiety preoperatively. The preoperative visit was significantly more effective in reducing anxiety than the booklet or no intervention.

Although the content and tone of the preoperative visit have not been objectively evaluated, several basic principles of physician–patient interaction apply. There is no other physician–patient interaction in which the conscious, competent patient has greater reason for anxiety and is meeting a physician for the very first time. Patient concerns and anxiety must be taken seriously. Although some of these concerns may seem trivial or unusual, they are foremost in the patient's mind and need to be addressed with compassion. An example is fear of intraoperative awareness. Anesthesiologists know that intraoperative awareness is an extremely rare event, that it is almost never complete awareness, and that it is associated with certain situations and kinds of anesthetics. Laypersons do not have access to this knowledge, and the only information to which they may have access (perhaps a television program or a magazine article) will have presented a population in which 100% of subjects are affected ("victims" or "survivors") with the most extreme awareness and are hurt or disabled as a result. It may be a challenge to encourage patients to believe an unknown, new authority rather than one they trust and with whom they are familiar. No pharmacologic agent can substitute for this process; one must simply pay serious attention to patients, gain their trust, and state clearly that it is the anesthesiologist's central concern to assure their safety and comfort. Indeed, amnesia produced by preoperative medication may erode some of the benefit of such a conversation if it is not remembered postoperatively.

The obligation to take patient concerns seriously does not end on leaving the preop area. Patients en route to the operating room often express fears they may have been unwilling to voice in the presence of family or friends. These "corridor concerns" may be trivialized by the setting, but to the patient they may have the gravity of "last wishes," as they know their next experience will be anesthetic induction. If necessary, one should stop patient transportation long enough to confront these fears. In the operating room, in the bustle of activity before induction, patients may again express fear or discomfort resulting from cold, monitoring equipment (tightness of a blood pressure cuff, for example), or claustrophobia from the mask. Patients will express anxiety about "misbehaving under anesthesia" or not having their dentures. Again, these concerns must be taken seriously. Each anesthesia provider eventually develops an individual style, but the fact that the patient's concern is taken seriously may have more effect than alleviating the discomfort that provoked it and probably is not dependent on any one thing the provider says. Tell patients that warm blankets are on the way, allow patients to hold their own mask, let them know that the blood pressure cuff is the cause of their arm discomfort and that the discomfort will go away. Ask if there is anything the staff can do to make them more comfortable before getting started, then tell them you are getting started, and that they are doing well. Children who have access to their parents during induction may have less anxiety, although at least one study has shown no difference between patients given premedicants and those with parental presence at induction. It is most likely that this is a function of population and that some children benefit from parental presence more than others.

Although the presence of the anesthesiologist is a significant factor in reducing preoperative anxiety, many other interventions may be useful. Most commonly, preoperative medication is employed. Midazolam is commonly used because it is relatively short-acting, has amnestic properties, is anxiolytic, and is available in an oral form that can be given to children. Other benzodiazepines are used, but their properties as preoperative medications differ. Lorazepam has the specific disadvantage of producing prolonged (up to 24 hours) cognitive dysfunction, most commonly in the elderly. Two studies show *increased* postoperative pain scores in patients who received preoperative diazepam. Many other classes of medication are employed for preoperative anxiolysis. Clonidine has been shown to reduce postoperative pain scores and intraoperative heart rate and blood pressure. Anticholinergics, butyrophenones, opioids, barbiturates, antihistamines, and antiseizure medications have all been used to reduce preoperative anxiety and have specific roles.

Finally, there are many other preoperative interventions that may reduce patient anxiety. For children, video games and even the presence of a clown-dressed anesthesiologist are reported to reduce anxiety. These interventions, unfortunately, have not been studied in adults. Music, either of the patient's choosing, or of a "soothing" nature, has been shown to reduce preoperative anxiety as reported by the patient, as well as intraoperative bispectral index scores and anesthetic requirements. Physical correlates of anxiety such as plasma catecholamine levels and blood pressure are unchanged by music, but it certainly does not hurt. Hypnosis has also been shown in one study to reduce preoperative anxiety.

It is clear, certainly to patients, that preoperative anxiety is an important component of the perioperative experience. There are many effective interventions that may reduce this anxiety and lead to improved patient satisfaction. Most important of these is the compassionate understanding of a concerned anesthesiologist. Many medication regimens may be employed to augment the anxiolysis of physician counseling, and other interventions such as music, hypnosis, or parental presence for children may be helpful.

TAKE HOME POINTS

- Preoperative anxiety is common and distressing to patients.
- Preoperative anxiety may have deleterious physiologic effects intraoperatively.
- Patient concerns must be taken seriously and assuaged compassionately.
- A visit from an anesthesiologist is an effective way to reduce anxiety.
- Preoperative medication, music, hypnosis, and other interventions may all be effective in reducing preoperative anxiety.

SUGGESTED READINGS

Egbert LD, Battit G, Turndorf H, et al. The value of the preoperative visit by an anesthetist. A study of doctor–patient rapport. *JAMA*. 1963;185(7):553–555.

Ganidagli S, Cengiz M, Yanik M, et al. The effect of music on preoperative sedation and the bispectral index. *Anesth Analg*. 2005;101(1):103–106.

Hidalgo MP, Auzani JA, Rumpel LC, et al. The clinical effect of small oral clonidine doses on perioperative outcomes in patients undergoing abdominal hysterectomy. *Anesth Analg*. 2005;100(3):795–802.

Kain ZN, Mayes LC, Caramico LA, et al. Parental presence during induction of anesthesia. A randomized controlled trial. *Anesthesiology*. 1996;84(5):1060–1067.

Leigh JM, Walker J, Janaganathan P. Effect of preoperative anaesthetic visit on anxiety. *Br Med J*. 1977;2(6093):987–989.

Moyers JR, Vincent CM. Preoperative medication. In: Barash PG, Cullen BF, Stoelting RK, eds. *Clinical Anesthesia*. Philadelphia: Lippincott Williams & Wilkins; 1997:551–565.

Wang SM, Kulkarni L, Dolev J, et al. Music and preoperative anxiety: a randomized, controlled study. *Anesth Analg*. 2002;94(6):1489–1494.

Williams OA. Patient knowledge of operative care. *J R Soc Med*. 1993;86(6):328–331.

65

RECOGNIZE THAT TRANSPORT IS ONE OF THE MOST HAZARDOUS INTERVALS IN THE PERIOPERATIVE PERIOD AND PREPARE ACCORDINGLY

MOHAMMED OJODU, MD AND CHARLES D. BOUCEK, MD

Anesthesiology management includes the transport of patients (from the preanesthesia area or intensive care unit to the operating room, from the operating room to the intensive care unit or recovery room, and from many areas outside of the operating room where anesthesia is administered to the recovery room or the intensive care unit). During transportation, many avoidable pitfalls can arise.

Transportation of patients in the immediate perioperative period carries hazards due to both patient and equipment factors. Human factors and task loading also add to the risk. The anesthesia provider must manage a patient undergoing the transition from the anesthetized to the conscious state while also giving report, charting, removing stationary and applying portable monitors, and physically helping to move the patient. A transportation plan including the destination and route should be established and the patient, the anesthesia personnel, and all necessary equipment should be ready before transportation begins. A telephone call should confirm that the recovery destination is ready to receive the patient. The anticipated distance partially determines the equipment needed. All patients recovering from anesthesia should have supplemental oxygen. Monitoring devices, manual ventilators, intubation equipment, intravenous (IV) poles, portable infusion pumps, and medications may be needed for longer distances or critically ill patients. Useful medications include antiarrhythmics, agents to raise and lower blood pressure, sedation agents, and muscle relaxants. The added equipment and supplies complicate the move and may require more time or additional personnel.

During emergence from anesthesia, patients experience discomfort from both the surgical wound and airway devices. Nausea due to medications or movement, and gagging from pharyngeal stimulation, both can result in emesis and possible aspiration. Teeth clenching may limit the effectiveness of suctioning. Before the full return of situational awareness by the patient, attempts at self-extubation may occur. Self-induced corneal injury may occur when patients who have not yet regained full coordination attempt to rub their eyes. Patients may try to sit up or roll off the table. An

© 2006 Mayo Foundation for Medical Education and Research

individual located at the patient's head is at a mechanical disadvantage in trying to restrain a large patient. Available "safety straps" may also fail.

Residual effects of anesthetics can lead to hypoxia and hypotension. Opioids and muscle relaxants decrease respiratory reserve, whereas antihypertensives, intravenous and inhalational anesthetics decrease blood pressure. The transition from controlled to spontaneous ventilation may be accompanied by heightened airway reflexes. Functional residual capacity and respiratory drives are reduced. Release of dissolved anesthetic gasses, especially nitrous oxide, from the blood may displace oxygen from the alveoli and lead to diffusion hypoxemia. For patients being transported to the intensive care unit while still anesthetized, it is essential that ventilation is controlled and that perfusion is adequate.

One of the most effective ways to avoid hypoxemia is to provide supplemental oxygen. Oxygen delivery systems include nasal cannulae, face masks, manual ventilation bags with face mask, endotracheal tubes or laryngeal mask airways. It has been shown that healthy patients (ASA I and II patients) transported with oxygen after undergoing general anesthesia were less likely to desaturate during transport as compared to healthy patients who did not receive oxygen. For healthy extubated patients, oxygen provided via nasal cannula or face mask may be sufficient. For the transportation of seriously ill, intubated, or pediatric patients (pediatric patients are more prone to desaturate, as they have higher ratios of minute ventilation to functional residual capacity compared to adults), the ability to provide positive-pressure ventilation is important. Before transport begins, the adequacy of the supply of oxygen (usually provided in an e-cylinder) should be checked *personally* by the anesthesia provider because unexpected events may prolong the transport. (Editor's note: Every single anesthesia provider with more than 2 minutes of experience can tell a story of asking the OR nurse to open the oxygen cylinder to 10 L/min, only to realize when the patient starts to desaturate going out the door that an empty tank has been put on the bed.)

Vital signs monitored routinely during the transportation of critically ill intubated patients include invasive or noninvasive blood pressure, pulse oximetry, and the electrocardiogram. Routine end–tidal carbon dioxide level is not essential except in situations in which this value is to be maintained within a narrow range. A portable transport monitor that is adequately charged is needed.

Moving the patient from table to stretcher requires personnel; a minimum of four individuals should be available to help move the patient, one at the patient's side opposite the stretcher, one lifting the feet; the third across the receiving stretcher. The forth supports the patient's head and controls the airway. For large or boisterous patients, additional help may be needed along with rollers or sliding devices. Confirmation that both the table and stretcher wheels are locked is important, but stretcher locks are notoriously unreliable. Safety straps should be removed just before transferring the patient to the stretcher. The move should be called by the person at the head using a "three count" to avoid inadvertent extubation or neck injury. The receiving stretcher should be of appropriate size and the height should be even with the operating table to avoid painful impacts from drops to a lower elevation. Dislodgement of endotracheal tubes, vascular access, and chest, gastric, wound, or bladder drains may occur. Many hospital beds used as stretchers have electric motors and short power cords. Often the most easily available outlet is located on the anesthesia gas machine. The bed may trip the circuit breaker, temporarily inactivating the gas machine's ventilator and monitors.

Hallway obstructions, ramps, and elevators complicate transportation. Supplies should be sufficient to maintain the patient in the event of temporary elevator malfunction. Battery life for monitors and infusion pumps can become an issue. Elevators should be entered patient's feet first so that the patient's head is accessible to the elevator door. This facilitates reintubation, and cardiopulmonary resuscitation without needing to remove the patient from the elevator.

The stretcher is ordinarily pulled by the individual leading from the patient's feet. The speed should permit timely arrival; it should be controlled by the individual at the patient's head so that monitoring and manual ventilation can be provided. Top-heavy IV poles can fall on the patient and may require additional personnel. Portable suction is often inefficient when moving ventilated patient with chest tubes and large air leaks.

On arrival, rapidly depleting battery-powered devices should be connected to wall utilities and oxygen should be changed from tank to stationary supplies. Portable monitors and vasoactive infusions are replaced by those of the receiving unit. Avoid the temptation to remove all monitors simultaneously. The patient remains in the care of the transporting team until report is given and care assumed by the receiving personnel. Report should include identification of the patient and surgeon, the procedure, medications and allergies, complications, fluids, ventilator settings, and analgesic plan.

In anticipation of events that can occur during transport, one needs to have available resources to resolve the situation. In the transport of healthy patients, one may need to provide analgesics for pain. In the transport of critically ill intubated patients, one should be ready to provide for immediate stabilization of anticipated problems.

TAKE HOME POINTS

- Skills to accomplish safe and efficient transport are as critical to an anesthesia provider as airway and access skills.

- Start packing the transport bag or basket well before the end of the procedure. Err on the side of extra equipment and resuscitation drugs. Pack your kit the same way for each type of transport (PACU kit vs. ICU kit).

- Check personally to make sure that a report has been called, ventilator settings have been given, and there is enough oxygen in the tank to get the patient to the destination.

- Transfer from the operating table to the gurney is a prime time for losing lines. For big cases with a lot of invasive lines, one anesthesia provider transfers the head and airway and a second anesthesia provider transfers the lines (somebody else has to do the legs and feet, so call for lifting help if necessary). After transfer onto the gurney, check to make sure that stopcocks, transducers, PA catheter, etc., are intact.

- Sort out the IVs, i.e., "untangle the spaghetti," before leaving the room. Always have ready access to a stopcock in case drugs have to be given during transport or immediately on arrival. Know which IV bag the stopcock is hooked up to and be able to get to the Cair clamp easily. Start the transport with a full fluid bag (you wouldn't start an important car trip with an empty tank of gas, would you?).

- Confirm respiratory effort in the hallways and elevators by whatever is your maneuver of choice. For example, ask the patient to cough or take a deep breath and show you "the fog" in the nonrebreather mask.

- Remember that the surgeons that are helping you transport will probably be walking too fast (especially if they are residents).

- After giving report in the postanesthesia care unit or the intensive care unit, always let the receiving team know you are leaving and ask if they have any issues they would like you to deal with before reporting back to the operating room.

SUGGESTED READINGS

Mathes DD, Conaway MR, Ross WT. Ambulatory surgery; room air versus nasal cannula oxygen during transport after general anesthesia. *Anesth Analg.* 2001;93(4):917–921.

Palmon S, Liu M, Moore LE, et al. Capnography facilitates tight control of ventilation during transport. *Crit Care Med.* 1996;24(4):608–611.

Sarr MG, Felty CL, Hilmer DM, et al. Technical and practical considerations involved in operations on patients weighing more than 270 kg. *Arch Surg.* 1995;130(1):102–105.

Tessler MJ, Mitmaker LW, Covert CR. Patient flow in the post anesthesia care unit: an observational study. *Can J Anaesth.* 1999;46(4):348–351.

Tyler I, Tantisira B, Winter PM, et al. Continuous monitoring of arterial oxygen saturation with pulse oximetry during transfer to the recovery room. *Anesth Analg.* 1985;64:1108–1112.

Warren J, Fromm RE, Orr RA, et al. Guidelines for the inter- and intrahospital transport of critically ill patients. *Crit Care Med.* 2004;32(1):256–262.

66

THE SAME SIMPLE MISTAKES AT INDUCTION (AND EMERGENCE) HAPPEN OVER AND OVER AGAIN—SO DEVELOP A CHECKLIST, AND MAKE IT IRONCLAD

BRANDON C. DIAL, MD AND RANDAL O. DULL, MD, PHD

For the airplane pilot, the most critical moments of a successful flight are takeoff and landing. So it is with anesthesia—the most critical moments occur at induction and emergence of general anesthesia. Like the pilot with a preflight checklist, the successful anesthesiologist has a checklist of important items that are reviewed prior to every induction to avoid many of the common pitfalls that may occur at these crucial times. Preventable anesthetic mishaps are often caused by a lack of familiarity with anesthetic equipment and a failure to check the anesthesia machine for proper function.

INDUCTION

Although there are many such checklists, the following mnemonic has been used at our institution to help ensure that the anesthesia machine and other equipment are ready for use by the prepared practitioner.

S—Suction

O—Oxygen

A—Airway

P—Positive-pressure ventilation

M—Medications

M—Monitors

S is for suction, probably the most easily and hence most commonly overlooked piece of equipment necessary for a successful induction. Although it is not always used, its presence is crucial for patients at risk for emesis and aspiration of gastric contents. It should be turned on and readily available with an appropriate tip and suction strength (-125 to -200 cm H_2O). If you have checked your suction but then left the operating room (OR) for something, you must recheck it again right before induction.

O is for oxygen. The anesthesia machine should be checked to ensure that oxygen is being delivered from the wall outlets and that the flow meters for oxygen and air are working appropriately. A secondary source of oxygen should be available. This is accomplished most commonly by an auxiliary oxygen E-cylinder located at the back of the anesthesia machine. The valve

© 2006 Mayo Foundation for Medical Education and Research

should be opened and the pressure checked to ensure that it is full and ready for emergency use.

A is for airway equipment. Laryngoscope handles should be connected to blades to ensure that the light source is working. If it is not, the batteries or light bulb may need to be replaced. Several sizes of laryngoscope blades should be available, including both straight and curved blades. Despite the thorough preoperative airway exam, many difficult airways are realized *after* induction. Other airway devices such as oral and nasal airways for mask ventilation should be a close reach away. The Eschmann stylet (or Bougie) is a helpful airway tool for the unexpected difficult laryngoscopy. Assorted laryngeal mask airways should be ready for use. Other devices for the difficult airway are noted in the American Society of Anesthesiologists (ASA) emergency airway algorithm. These should be available and the practitioner familiar with their use, including supplies necessary to create a surgical airway. Preparation is paramount in the "can't intubate, can't ventilate" clinical emergency.

P is for positive-pressure ventilation. Failure to check the anesthesia machine for potential malfunction is a significant cause of anesthesia accidents. The anesthesia machine should undergo a leak test to ensure that positive-pressure ventilation can be provided reliably. Many newer machines have automated leak tests that require several minutes but minimal effort. In many older machines, a rapid leak test may be accomplished by turning the ventilator switch to the bag position, closing the APL ("pop-off") valve and occluding the circuit at the Y-piece, then filling the breathing bag and circuit with the oxygen flush button to a level of 30 mm Hg. Maintaining a constant pressure with no leak is a rapid and reliable test that ensures your ability to deliver positive-pressure ventilation.

M is for medications. Induction drugs should be drawn up in sterile syringes. Double doses should be drawn of key induction agents in case they get dropped on the floor, the patient requires more, or a difficult intubation creates a prolonged induction process. *Never use anything that has been dropped on the floor.* Multidose vials should be cleaned with alcohol before needle insertion. Most induction drugs and muscle relaxants are stable in syringes for 24 hours, but use beyond that period should be discouraged because the risk of bacterial contamination increases. Obvious exceptions include propofol, which should be used within 6 hours after accessing the sterile vial. Emergency drugs for unexpected but common events such as hypotension should be drawn up. Ephedrine, phenylephrine, and epinephrine diluted to appropriate concentrations are common examples. Many practitioners consider succinylcholine to be an emergency drug for rapid treatment of laryngospasm.

M is for monitors. Standard ASA monitors including blood pressure, pulse oximetry, capnography, and temperature monitoring are mandatory for every general anesthetic. Another key monitor during induction is the twitch monitor. Its use after administration of a nondepolarizing neuromuscular blocker will ensure optimal intubating conditions.

EMERGENCE

Avoiding common pitfalls during emergence from general anesthesia can be accomplished with a similar checklist.

Once again, having suction at the ready can prevent many problems during extubation. One of the most common causes of laryngospasm during emergence is pooling of secretions on the vocal cords. Patient transport at the end of a general anesthetic should include oxygen, whether or not extubation is planned. Check the oxygen E-cylinder to ensure that it has enough oxygen for the transport. An E-cylinder with 1,000 psig is half-full, and contains about 330 L of oxygen. If it is exhausted at a rate of 6 L/min, this amount will last 55 minutes.

After extubation, airway equipment including a mask and oral airway should be readily available. When transporting an intubated patient to the intensive care unit (ICU), a laryngoscope and endotracheal tube should be brought for emergency reintubation if an unexpected extubation occurs. Positive-pressure ventilation can be given by way of a portable breathing circuit. Common examples used for patient transport include Jackson Rees circuits (Mapleson Class A) and Ambu bags that allow the delivery of positive-pressure ventilation.

Medications, including crystalloid fluids, are especially critical for the transport of an intubated patient to the ICU. Sedation and muscle relaxation may be important. Pressor agents and additional intravenous (IV) fluids should be available for patients with cardiovascular instability. Clinical circumstances may require the need for beta-blockade or other antihypertensive treatment, or narcotics for treatment of surgical pain.

Once again, the twitch monitor can be crucial to avoiding airway compromise from continued neuromuscular blockade if muscle relaxation was administered and extubation is planned. Its use can apprise you of whether reversal agents are needed, and the effectiveness of the reversal agent after it has been given to ensure the patient wakes up without muscular weakness and airway compromise.

One last point for a successful takeoff and landing: know your patient's name. Your safe navigation of these critical tasks requires skill. Knowing your patient's name is part of the professionalism required of a perioperative physician.

- Suction, suction, suction!
- Always have multiple laryngoscopes available.
- Double-draw the crucial induction drugs—including, at a minimum, the induction agent and succinylcholine (if it is not contraindicated).
- Don't pick up anything from the floor and use it on the patient.
- Remember that emergence, in a sense, is induction in reverse. Redundancy of your critical components is just as important during this phase.

SUGGESTED READINGS

Armstrong-Brown A, Devitt JH, Kurrek M, et al. Inadequate preanesthesia equipment checks in a simulator. *Can J Anaesth.* 2000;47(10):974–979.

Hart EM, Owen H. Errors and omissions in anesthesia: a pilot study using a pilot's checklist. *Anesth Analg.* 2005;101:246–250.

67

NEVER FAIL TO REPORT A NEEDLESTICK INJURY

VIDYA K. RAO, MD AND SHAWN T. BEAMAN, MD

According to the World Health Organization (WHO), an estimated 3 million people worldwide suffer from accidental needlestick injuries each year. The Centers for Disease Control (CDC) and the National Institute for Occupational Safety and Health (NIOSH) report that an estimated 600,000 to 800,000 needlestick injuries occur annually among health care workers in the United States. There are limited data regarding specific occupational hazards to anesthesia personnel. However, Greene et al., in a multicenter study, reported 1.35 contaminated needlestick injuries per 1,000 anesthetics administered, or 0.54 per 1,000 hours of anesthesia.

Accidental needlestick injuries in the health care setting have been associated with the transmission of up to 20 blood-borne pathogens, most commonly human immunodeficiency virus (HIV), hepatitis C virus, and hepatitis B virus. Although significant data exist regarding transmission rates based on documented needlestick injuries in the health care setting, exact information is unavailable because of the underreporting of needlestick injuries by health care workers.

Despite well-publicized institutional protocols for reporting needlestick injuries and the ready availability of postexposure prophylaxis and medical follow-up for health care workers, recent research demonstrates that underreporting continues to be a significant problem. In fact, in one report a surprising 60% to 95% of house staff failed to report needlestick injuries! In the United States, only 45% of anesthesia personnel who suffered a needlestick injury sought treatment! Surveys of anesthesiology residents and attending physicians revealed significant underreporting as well. Residents and attending physicians reported only 29% and 19% of needlestick and percutaneous injuries, respectively. Although needlestick injuries may be individually detrimental and potentially life-threatening, the underreporting of these injuries has the secondary effect of preventing precise calculations of disease transmission rates.

COMMON SCENARIOS ASSOCIATED WITH NEEDLESTICK INJURIES

Needlestick injuries may occur any time a needle is exposed. Engineering and technology have dramatically increased the safety of needle use, but

© 2006 Mayo Foundation for Medical Education and Research

these advances represent only one component of accidental needlestick prevention. Examples of safety features include built-in safety devices, such as needle shields, retractable needles, safety catheter encasement devices, and needleless intravenous (IV) delivery systems.

However, accidental needlestick injuries continue to occur despite these advances in technology. These injuries most commonly occur during certain situations:

- During clean-up after use (such as starting an IV, phlebotomy)
- When sharps are disposed of improperly
- When a needle is being recapped
- While manipulating the needle in the patient
- While handling a device or passing a device to another health care worker during or after use
- While handling or transferring specimens
- During collision with a sharp or with a health care worker handling the sharp
- Between steps of a multistep process

Some needlestick injuries are considered to be "high risk." These include injuries from hollow-bore needles, needles that are contaminated with blood, and needles that are blood-filled. Anesthesiology personnel are especially susceptible to the above high-risk situations. Prevention of needlestick injuries involves vigilance on the part of personnel handling sharps. Most injuries have been shown to arise from the use of needles attached to syringes, suture needles, hollow-bore needles, IV catheter-needle stylets, and epidural needles. The majority of contaminated needlestick injuries in anesthesia personnel are preventable. One multicenter study reported that 59% of all injuries, 68% of injuries from the use of hollow-bore needles, and 78% of highrisk contaminated percutaneous injuries were preventable.

HUMAN IMMUNODEFICIENCY VIRUS (HIV)

The risk of HIV transmission to health care workers after percutaneous exposure to HIV-infected blood has been estimated at approximately 0.3% percent, and among anesthesia personnel, an estimated 0.56 HIV infections will occur per year to anesthesia personnel in the United States. The transmission rate varies based on the seroprevalence of the patient population. Projections by Greene et al. cite the 1-year risk of an anesthesia provider contracting HIV from occupational exposure at 0.00013% to 0.3%, and the 30-year risk to be from 0.0038% to 0.94%.

Several factors have been associated with an increased risk of HIV transmission from a patient to a health care worker as a result of a needlestick injury. These factors include an increased quantity of blood transferred during the exposure, use of a larger-bore needle (gauge smaller than 18), deep injury, a device visibly contaminated with the patient's blood, exposure during a procedure that involved placing a needle into a source patient's vasculature, or exposure to a source patient in the terminal stage of acquired immunodeficiency syndrome (AIDS). It is likely that the immunologic status of the injured health care worker also plays a role in determining risk.

Symptoms of primary or acute HIV infection are generally nonspecific, resemble flu-like symptoms, and can occur within days or weeks of the initial exposure. They typically include fever, rash, malaise, pharyngitis, lymphadenopathy, and headache. Some people experience severe symptoms after contracting HIV, whereas others experience no symptoms whatsoever. Given the non-specificity of symptoms, the only reliable method of diagnosing HIV infection is antibody testing, with subsequent confirmation by Western blot. Historically, antibody testing was effective after the "window period," which ranges from 2 weeks to 6 months following exposure. Current enzyme immunoassays, however, are able to detect the HIV antibody within several days.

There are two primary approaches in managing contaminated needle-stick injuries with regard to HIV. One approach involves immediate post-exposure prophylaxis with antiretroviral therapy unless or until the source patient tests HIV-negative or circumstances surrounding the injury indicate a low possibility of transmission. The second approach involves the initiation of antiretroviral therapy if analysis of the exposure indicates a risk of HIV transmission, such as a positive HIV test in the source patient.

There is some evidence to suggest that immediate postexposure prophylaxis is associated with decreased risk of transmission, specifically in animal models. Factors influencing the risk of transmission in those models include viral load, interval between exposure and the start of therapy, duration of therapy, and selection of antiretroviral regimen. The data available on human subjects is far less extensive. A retrospective case-control study conducted by the CDC, specifically on health care workers, indicated an 81% reduction in HIV transmission risk with postexposure treatment with zidovudine. Definitive protection against HIV transmission, however, is not guaranteed with immediate antiretroviral therapy, as limited information exists regarding the optimal treatment regimen, period, or duration.

Current postexposure prophylaxis regimens include two antiretroviral agents or, based on the circumstances of the exposure, an expanded antiretroviral regimen involving a third drug. Although chemoprophylaxis may provide benefit, it is not without risk or side effects. Adverse effects range from mild symptoms such as nausea, diarrhea, and headache to more severe effects such as neutropenia, neuropathy, and hepatotoxicity. Two-drug regimens resulted in increased compliance and fewer adverse effects than expanded three-drug regimens. Additionally, antiretroviral drug resistance has become increasingly problematic, resulting in the use of combination or expanded antiretroviral therapy.

HEPATITIS B VIRUS (HBV)

Hepatitis B virus is much more commonly transmitted via needlestick injuries than HIV, with transmission rates ranging from 2% to 40%, depending on the hepatitis B antigen status of the source patient. Interestingly, the transmission rate has actually experienced a significant decline over the last 20 years, due largely to more widespread hepatitis B immunization among health care workers. There are a number of other factors associated with the risk of transmission, including the patient's hepatitis B surface antigen titers and degree of contact with the patient's blood.

History of previous hepatitis B immunization should not be interpreted as absolute protection against transmission. The duration of immunity conferred by the vaccination has not been determined, and it may not develop after a primary series. Additionally, the effectiveness of the hepatitis B immunization may be reduced by a number of factors, including immunocompromise, obesity, advanced age, smoking history, improper vaccination storage, and location of vaccine administration. Health care workers with a history of vaccination but without measurement of anti-HBsAg titers during the previous 2 years should be evaluated for immunity after a needlestick injury or any other accidental exposure.

Symptoms of acute hepatitis B infection occur in one third to one half of infected people. These symptoms include jaundice, fever, nausea, and abdominal pain. The majority of acute infections resolve, but chronic infection may develop in 5% to 10% of infected people. One in five patients who develop chronic hepatitis B infections has a risk of developing liver cirrhosis, while 6% of chronically infected people may die from liver cancer.

Unlike the questionable effectiveness of postexposure prophylaxis in the prevention of HIV transmission, prophylaxis for hepatitis B virus with hepatitis B hyperimmune globulin and hepatitis B vaccine is >90% effective in preventing HBV transmission. Exposed health care workers should be tested for anti-HBsAg after exposure. Postexposure prophylaxis with HBV hyperimmune globulin and HBV vaccinations are based on the exposed health care worker's vaccination status, response to previous vaccinations, and serum anti-HBsAg titers. HBV hyperimmune globulin, if needed, should be provided within 24 hours of exposure, as efficacy may decline if treatment is postponed. HBV hyperimmune globulin should be followed within 7 days by HBV vaccine.

Health care workers who are vaccinated against HBV should be tested 6 months following primary vaccination to evaluate immunity. If they receive hyperimmune globulin, immunity testing may need to be postponed until

4 to 6 months later. If health care workers follow the recommended regimens following exposure, they are unlikely to become infected and may continue to participate in their normal professional and personal activities.

HEPATITIS C VIRUS (HCV)

The rate of transmission of hepatitis C virus (HCV) has not been well established, but the prevalence of HCV in health care workers is slightly higher than in the general population. The annual incidence of acute infections of HCV is approximately 2% to 4% in health care workers who have a history of occupational exposure to blood, such as with a history of needlestick injuries. The 1-year risk of an anesthesia provider contracting HCV via occupational exposure ranges from 0.00084% to 0.21%, and the 30-year risk ranges from 0.025% to 6.12% based on HCV seroprevalence in the patient population. Among anesthesia personnel in the United States, an estimated 5.18 HCV infections are expected to occur per year. The incidence of anti-HCV seroconversion after accidental percutaneous exposure to HCV is approximately 1.8%, with transmission occurring primarily with the use of hollow-bore needles.

Symptoms of acute hepatitis C infection range from fever, jaundice, and malaise to fulminant hepatic failure. Many patients are asymptomatic during the acute phase. Patients may have elevated liver transaminases. Up to 75% to 85% of acute hepatitis C cases will progress to chronic hepatitis, with a smaller proportion of chronic patients developing cirrhosis or hepatic cancer. Given the nonspecificity of symptoms, HCV antibody testing must be performed to confirm the diagnosis.

Unlike HIV and HBV, there is no vaccine to prevent HCV and no recommended postexposure prophylactic regimens at the present time. There are limited data that support the use of interferon monotherapy early in the course of acute hepatitis C, specifically in the setting of elevated liver transaminases and viremia. This evidence indicates that use of interferon early in the course of acute hepatitis C may increase the rate of resolution of acute infection, potentially preventing progression to chronic infection. Unlike HBV, there is no evidence to support the use of immune globulin as part of postexposure prophylaxis.

If a health care worker is concerned about possible exposure to HCV, he or she should be tested immediately and then again after 6 to 9 months. If HCV is detected, or the individual develops any symptoms of hepatitis, liver function tests should be performed to evaluate for chronic hepatitis. Once the diagnosis of HCV is established, interferon therapy may be considered. Potential side effects of interferon therapy include mild to severe flulike symptoms, tissue damage at the site of injection, depression, diarrhea, pancytopenia, elevated transaminases, skin rash, hair loss, and edema.

Despite the potentially life-threatening consequences of developing HCV infection, at this time, health care workers with accidental exposures need not change their personal or professional activities. However, any health care worker who has experienced a needlestick injury or any percutaneous exposure to the blood of a patient with an uncertain or suspected HCV infection should undergo postexposure surveillance so that seroconversion can be detected early and managed appropriately.

TAKE HOME POINTS

- Needlestick injuries expose health care workers to blood-borne pathogens that can cause potentially fatal diseases. Three of the most pathogens of most concern are HIV, HBV, and HCV.
- Advances in technology and the engineering of safety devices has dramatically reduced the incidence of needlestick injuries.
- Prevention is the best defense against needlestick injuries. Avoid risky behaviors such as needle recapping and transferring of specimens, pay increased attention to proper sharps disposal, and avoid using needles if an alternative is available.
- Needlestick injuries are grossly underreported by physicians, especially house staff. Unreported needlestick injuries could have devastating personal consequences and also prevent the precise calculation of transmission and seroconversion rates.
- *Always* report needlestick injuries! Although postexposure prophylaxis does not provide absolute protection against pathogen transmission, early detection and proper medical follow-up could save your life!

SUGGESTED READINGS

Berry AJ. The use of needles in the practice of anesthesiology and the effect of a needleless intravenous administration system. *Anesth Analg.* 1993;76:1114–1119.

Cardo D. A case-control study of HIV seroconversion in health care workers after percutaneous exposure. *N Engl J Med.* 1997;337(21):1485–1490.

Centers for Disease Control. *Public Health Service Guidelines for the Management of Health-Care Worker Exposures to HIV and Recommendations for Postexposure Prophylaxis.* May 15, 1998.

Centers for Disease Control. *Updated US Public Health Service Guidelines for the Management of Occupational Exposures to HBV, HCV, and HIV and Recommendations for Postexposure Prophylaxis.* June 29, 2001.

Diprose P. Ignorance of post-exposure prophylaxis guidelines following HIV needlestick injury may increase the risk of seroconversion. *Br J Anaesth.* 2000;84(6):767–770.

Gerberding J. Management of occupational exposures to blood-borne viruses. *N Engl J Med.* 1995;332(7):444–451.

Gerberding J. Occupational exposure to HIV in health care settings. *N Engl J Med.* 2003;348(9):826–833.

Greene ES. Multicenter study of contaminated percutaneous injuries in anesthesia personnel. *Anesthesiology.* 1998;89(6):1362–1372.

Greene ES. Percutaneous injuries in anesthesia personnel. *Anesth Analg.* 1996;82:273–278.

National Institute for Occupational Safety and Health. *Preventing Needlestick Injuries in Health Care Settings.* NIOSH Publication 2000-108. November 1999.

68

UNDERSTAND THE UTILITY OF PREOPERATIVE STRESS TESTING IN SUSPECTED HEART DISEASE

MATTHEW V. DeCARO, MD, FACC

Although stress testing is quite useful in preoperative cardiac risk stratification, it is a flawed modality.

There are several serious cardiac complications that can result from noncardiac surgery. These include ischemic events, arrhythmias—both brady- and tachyarrhythmias—and heart failure. Although stress testing can give some insight into an individual's propensity for arrhythmias and heart failure, its role is quite limited. By and large its main use is in the diagnosis of clinically significant coronary artery disease (CAD). Much attention has therefore been focused on stress testing, because the most catastrophic cardiac complication of surgery, myocardial infarction (MI), with the attendant permanent loss of cardiac muscle and thus function, is caused by CAD.

The sensitivity and specificity of exercise stress testing for diagnosing coronary disease varies with the severity of this disease. *Table 68.1* gives average results for various severity subsets across studies.

As can be seen, the test is more useful in severe forms of CAD. It is in these patients that prior intervention (regardless of the proposed surgery) may improve survival. Remember that the greater the sensitivity of a test, the more useful it is for excluding a diagnosis when the test is negative. More specific tests help in establishing a diagnosis when the test is positive. The main utility of the stress test in the context of risk stratification for surgery is in excluding severe CAD in a patient with a negative test. To add to the confusion, many of these statistics are from specialized centers under controlled circumstances. Depending on the population studied, the accuracy of stress testing may be much poorer. In several community hospital studies in a general medical population, the sensitivity was substantially worse ($<50\%$).

The posttest likelihood of CAD is highly dependent on the pretest likelihood. If the pretest probability of CAD is either very low or high, the test provides little additional information. A negative test in a 70-year-old hypertensive diabetic with typical anginal chest pain is not helpful for excluding the diagnosis of CAD. It can be argued that it decreases the statistical chance of severe three-vessel or left main disease, but recall that one of the causes

© 2006 Mayo Foundation for Medical Education and Research

TABLE 68.1	AVERAGE RESULTS FOR VARIOUS SEVERITY SUBSETS	
	SENSITIVITY	SPECIFICITY
Single-vessel CAD	68	77
Multivessel CAD	81	66
Three-vessel/left main CAD	86	53
CAD, coronary artery disease.		

of a false-negative nuclear scan is global ischemia, usually caused by critical left main stenosis.

Unfortunately, although there is a general correlation between severity of CAD and operative morbidity and mortality, it is an imprecise predictor of acute coronary syndromes (ACSs). These include unstable angina, non–ST-segment-elevation MIs (NSTEMI) and ST-segment-elevation MIs (STEMI). It should be recalled that one is just as likely to experience an ACS from a plaque that results in a stenosis ≤50% as it is from a stenosis >50%. This is due to several factors. The primary factor that determines plaque instability is not the severity of the narrowing. Although the physical bulk of the plaque plays a role, other factors such as erosion of the fibrous cap overlying the plaque are more important. Vessel inflammation, of both the humoral and cellular components, are primarily responsible for the thinning, erosion, and ultimately rupture of this cap. This is the proximate cause of the ACSs. Hence, stress testing is an imprecise indicator of an imprecise predictor for ACS! Stress testing can be expected to be much better at predicting what it measures—namely, coronary stenoses of >70% that would produce flow-limiting ischemia, i.e., angina pectoris triggered by physiologic stress.

Pharmacologic testing is only slightly less sensitive and specific than exercise modalities, so the same analysis as above applies here as well. The major disadvantage of these techniques is the loss of clinical information related to the assessment of exercise capacity. This is actually quite meaningful information. The single best prognosticator in some studies on stress testing is the number of minutes the individual can exercise on a symptom-limited test, even more useful in one study than the coronary anatomy at angiography.

TAKE HOME POINTS

- Although stress testing yields some valuable anatomic and physiologic data, it cannot be relied on as the sole, accurate predictor of cardiac risk for noncardiac surgery.

- Many factors need to be factored together to arrive at an individuals risk. The intrinsic risk of the procedure to be performed and the urgency of this procedure are two important issues. In addition, as simple an intervention as the use of beta-blockers in the perioperative period has been shown to reduce morbidity and mortality in certain at-risk patients.
- The risk assessment of an experienced clinician, combining clinical data obtained from a careful history and physical exam, determination of the traditional risk factors for CAD, exercise capacity in daily living, analysis of left ventricular function, supplemented where appropriate by noninvasive and invasive testing for coronary disease, should be considered the "gold standard" for preoperative evaluation.

SUGGESTED READINGS

Boersma E, Poldermans D, Bax JJ, et al. Predictors of cardiac events after major vascular surgery: role of clinical characteristics, dobutamine echocardiography, and beta-blocker therapy. *JAMA*. 2001;285:1865–1873.

Camp AD, Garvin PJ, Hoff J, et al. Prognostic value of intravenous dipyridamole thallium imaging in patients with diabetes mellitus considered for renal transplantation. *Am J Cardiol*. 1990;65:1459–1463.

Eagle KA, Brundage BH, Chaitman BR, et al. Guidelines for perioperative cardiovascular evaluation for noncardiac surgery: report of the American College of Cardiology/American Heart Association Task Force on Practice Guidelines (Committee on Perioperative Cardiovascular Evaluation for Noncardiac Surgery). *J Am Coll Cardiol*. 1996;27:910–948.

Lee TH, Marcantonio ER, Mangione CM, et al. Derivation and prospective validation of a simple index for prediction of cardiac risk of major noncardiac surgery. *Circulation*. 1999;100:1043–1049.

Mark DB, Hlatky MA, Harrell FE Jr, et al. Exercise treadmill score for predicting prognosis in coronary artery disease. *Ann Intern Med*. 1987;106:793–800.

69

PERIOPERATIVE BETA-BLOCKER THERAPY IS INDICATED FOR HIGH-RISK PATIENTS WHO ARE HAVING NONCARDIAC SURGERY, BUT SPECIFIC QUESTIONS REMAIN UNANSWERED

ESTHER SUNG, MD AND RICHARD F. DAVIS, MD, MBA

Perioperative adverse cardiovascular events among patients who are having noncardiac surgery are relatively common, confer additional risk of other serious complications including death, and add significantly to health care costs. Relatively simple methods exist for risk stratification of these patients, including indices such as Goldman's original cardiac risk index and Lee's revised Cardiac Risk Index. However, few effective interventions exist for reducing the incidence of adverse perioperative cardiovascular occurrences and decreasing the associated morbidity and mortality. The risk-stratification schemes mentioned above are based on clinical history and symptoms. In addition to these, noninvasive testing, cardiac catheterization, and, for some subgroups, subsequent myocardial revascularization, together with careful perioperative monitoring, are often cited as reducing the risk of adverse cardiovascular events. In terms of available pharmacologic interventions, the perioperative use of beta-adrenergic-receptor blockers is often advocated as a safe, effective, and relatively inexpensive method of reducing adverse cardiovascular events after noncardiac surgery.

Although the majority of evidence suggests that beta-blockade is effective in reducing cardiovascular events after noncardiac surgery, especially for high-risk surgical patients, many questions currently remain unanswered. For which patients is the perioperative use of beta-blockade actually indicated? Are there patients who could be harmed by such treatment? Does it matter which beta-blocker is used? How early should beta-blockade be started, and how long should therapy continue postoperatively? What is the target heart rate? Is the protective effect mediated by blockade of the beta-adrenergic receptor or is it a heart-rate control effect?

Among the earliest reports of the beneficial effect of perioperative beta-blockade was the randomized trial of atenolol reported by Mangano et al. In this study, a relatively brief exposure to atenolol in the perioperative period was associated with morbidity and mortality improvement measured as late as 2 years after the surgery. Since that publication, numerous studies have been published using various beta-blocking medications in varying doses for varying time intervals in varying patient groups. Most of these show outcome

© 2006 Mayo Foundation for Medical Education and Research

improvements associated with the use of beta-blockade in the perioperative time frame. Another interesting study, with bearing on the heart-rate control versus beta-adrenergic-receptor-blockade question, was carried out by Wallace et al. using clonidine as a heart-rate control intervention in place of beta-blockade. In this study, 190 patients were randomly assigned to either clonidine therapy or placebo; treatment was begun preoperatively and continued for 4 days after surgery. Thirty-day mortality was 6.2% with placebo, compared with just 0.8% with clonidine; 2-year mortalities were 29.2% and 15.2%, respectively. Most recently, Lindenauer published the results of a large-scale retrospective analysis of patients who underwent noncardiac surgery at one of 329 small to mid-size nonteaching hospitals throughout the United States. Among 122,338 patients who received perioperative beta-blockade there was an apparent relationship between underlying health status and benefit or not from the treatment. Using the revised cardiac risk index (rCRI), patients who had no or only minor cardiovascular risk (rCRI score of 0 or 1) had no benefit, and possibly a worsened outcome, associated with beta-blockade. However, patients with an rCRI score of 2, 3, or 4 had benefit (odds ratio for in-hospital death less than 1) associated with beta-blocker treatment. And perhaps more interesting, this risk reduction improved as the rCRI score increased: the higher the risk, the greater the apparent risk reduction from beta-blockade.

There have also been several larger-scale meta-analyses of the individual publications that appear to show clinical outcome advantage to the use of beta-blockers. Auerbach and Goldman, in 2002, assessed five randomized, controlled trials and reached the conclusion that beta-blockade was likely beneficial in preventing cardiac morbidity. Stevens et al. performed a quantitative systematic review in 2003 of pharmacologic myocardial protection for patients undergoing noncardiac surgery and found that the 11 beta-blockade trials reviewed showed decreased ischemic episodes, reduced risk of myocardial infarction, and reduced risk of cardiac death in the beta-blockade group compared to placebo. They also observed that higher-risk patients received greater benefit from beta-blocker therapy. In 2005, McGory et al. performed a formal meta-analysis of six randomized, controlled trials and concluded that beta-blockade therapy was not only associated with reduced perioperative myocardial ischemia, myocardial infarction, and cardiac mortality but also conferred a reduction long-term cardiac mortality and overall mortality.

Meanwhile, the Agency for Healthcare Research and Quality and others have issued statements strongly supportive of the perioperative use of beta-blockers for patients who are having noncardiac surgery, especially those with increased risks of adverse perioperative cardiovascular events. The American College of Cardiology/American Heart Association (ACC/AHA) Task

Force on Practice Guidelines has recently released an updated guideline specific to perioperative beta-blocker usage. According to this statement, beta-blockers should be continued in surgical patients who are already receiving them for angina, arrhythmias, hypertension, or other ACC/AHA Class I guideline indications. Beta-blockers should be given to patients who are undergoing vascular surgery when ischemia has been noted on preoperative testing. Beta-blockers are probably indicated for patients undergoing vascular, high-risk, or intermediate-risk surgeries who have coronary heart disease or multiple clinical risk factors for increased perioperative cardiovascular risk. Beta-blockers may be considered for patients who are undergoing vascular high-risk or intermediate-risk surgeries who have a single clinical risk factor and for patients who are undergoing vascular surgery with low cardiac risk who are not already on beta-blockers. Finally, beta-blockers should not be given to patients undergoing surgery who have absolute contraindication to beta-blockade. The ACC/AHA recommends that beta-blockers be started several days or weeks before elective surgery with a target resting heart rate of 50 to 60 beats/min—an indication that the patient is receiving the benefit of beta-blockade but not yet evidence-based except for one recent study showing that "tight" heart rate control with beta-blockers was beneficial in patients having vascular surgery procedures (Feringa et al.). According to AHA recommendations, therapy should continue intra- and postoperatively to keep heart rates below 80 beats/min.

Some studies and meta-analyses debate the efficacy of beta-blockade in reducing major cardiovascular events or challenge the strength of evidence, but the weight of evidence suggests that perioperative beta-blockade is an inexpensive and effective means of reducing the incidence and associated morbidity and mortality of adverse cardiovascular events. Despite the observations of the current randomized, controlled trials, retrospective studies, and meta-analyses, the current literature is still limited in that several of the trials performed may be inadequately powered and few assess issues such as titration of therapy to effect, optimal beta-blocker type, or ideal target population. Practical matters such as route of administration and length of administration still need to be addressed. Furthermore, there is a lack of data regarding the potential harm of perioperative beta-blockade, especially in low-risk patients, or in patients who experience rebound phenomena after postoperative cessation of beta-blockade. Currently, there are prospective, randomized trials underway or emerging that may shed light on many of these questions.

Lastly, a common and vexing problem for the anesthesia provider is what to do when a patient presents who was intended for preoperative beta-blockade but did not initiate therapy for whatever reason. Or perhaps the patient has had a cardiology consult suggesting a specific heart-rate range but the patient's heart rate is significantly higher, despite being compliant with the medication as ordered. It is the opinion of the senior author of this chapter as well as the cardiology consultant to this book that there are insufficient data to warrant holding the surgery to implement oral beta-blockade before induction. However, for high-risk patients who are having high-risk or moderate-risk surgery (e.g., requiring a general anesthetic with or without planned invasive monitoring), who do not have contraindications, then it is prudent to give some beta-blocker before induction. A reasonable choice is 10 to 50 mg of atenolol PO or intravenous (IV) metoprolol titrated up to 0.1 mg/kg, and then aggressive control of heart rate with an IV agent such as metoprolol or esmolol during the surgery. In addition, it would be prudent to continue the beta-blocker therapy with oral agents (or IV, depending on the circumstances) postoperatively for 72 to 96 hours. This is opinion; it must be stated that there is little or no class 1 or 2 evidence that addresses this specific clinical scenario.

TAKE HOME POINTS

- Perioperative cardiovascular events after noncardiac surgery are common and a source of significant morbidity and mortality.
- The perioperative use of beta-blockade agents is advocated as a safe, effective, and relatively inexpensive method of reducing adverse events.
- The majority of evidence suggests that beta-blockade is effective in reducing cardiovascular events after noncardiac surgery, especially for high-risk surgical patients; however, many questions remain unanswered.
- A reasonable approach for an at-risk patient who has not been beta-blocked is to administer both PO and IV therapy before induction and to control heart rate intraoperatively with IV agents (esmolol or metoprolol).

SUGGESTED READINGS

Auerbach AD, Goldman L. Beta-blockers and reduction of cardiac events in non-cardiac surgery: scientific review. *JAMA*. 2002;87:1435–1444.

Brady AR, Gibbs JS, Greenhalgh RM, et al. Perioperative beta-blockade (POBBLE) for patients undergoing infrarenal vascular surgery: results of a randomized double-blind controlled trial. *J Vasc Surg*. 2005;41:602–609.

Devereaux PJ, Yusuf S, Yang H, et al. How strong is the evidence for the use of perioperative beta-blockers in non-cardiac surgery? Systematic review and meta-analysis of randomized controlled trials. *Br Med J*. 2005;331:313–321.

Feringa HHH, Bax JI, Boersma E, et al. High dose beta-blockade and tight heart rate control reduce myocardial ischemia and troponin T release in vascular surgery patients. *Circulation*. 2006;114(suppl I):I344–I349.

Fleisher LA, Beckman JA, Brown KA, et al. ACC/AHA 2006 guideline update on perioperative cardiovascular evaluation for non-cardiac surgery: focused update on perioperative beta-blocker therapy. *J Am Coll Cardiol*. 2006;47(11):1–13.

Goldman L, Caldera DL, Nussbaum SR, et al. Multifactorial index of cardiac risk in non-cardiac surgical procedures. *N Engl J Med*. 1977;297:845–850.

Lee TH, Marcantonio ER, Mangione CM, et al. Derivation and prospective validation of a simple index for prediction of cardiac risk of major non-cardiac surgery. *Circulation.* 1999;100:1043–1049.

Lindenauer PK, Pekow P, Wang K, et al. Perioperative beta-blocker therapy and mortality after major non-cardiac surgery. *N Engl J Med.* 2005;353:349–361.

Mangano DT, Layug EL, Wallace A, et al. Effect of atenolol on mortality and cardiovascular morbidity after non-cardiac surgery. Multicenter Study of Perioperative Ischemia Research Group. *N Engl J Med.* 1996;335:1713–1720.

McGory ML, Maggard MA, Ko CY. A meta-analysis of perioperative beta-blockade: What is the actual risk reduction? *Surgery.* 2005;138:171–179.

Poldermans D, Boersma E, Bax JJ, et al. The effect of bisoprolol on perioperative mortality and myocardial infarction in high-risk patients undergoing vascular surgery. *N Engl J Med.* 1999;341:1789–1794.

Raby KE, Brull SJ, Timimi F, et al. The effect of heart rate control on myocardial infarction among high-risk patients after vascular surgery. *Anesth Analg.* 1999;88:477–482.

Shojania KG, Duncan BW, McDonald KM, Wachter RM, eds. Making health care safer: a critical analysis of patient safety practices. Evidence report/technology assessment. No. 43. Rockville, MD: Agency for Healthcare Research and Quality; July 2001.

Stevens, RD, Burri H, Tramer MR. Pharmacologic myocardial protection in patients undergoing non-cardiac surgery: a quantitative systematic review. *Anesth Analg.* 2003;7:623–633.

Urban MK, Markowitz SM, Gordon MA, et al. Postoperative prophylactic administration of beta-adrenergic blockers in patients at risk for myocardial infarction. *Anesth Analg.* 2000;90:1257–1261.

Wallace AW, Galindez D, Salahieh A, et al. Effect of clonidine on cardiovascular morbidity and mortality after non-cardiac surgery. *Anesthesiology.* 2004;101:284–293.

Wallace A, Layug B, Tateo I, et al. Prophylactic atenolol reduces postoperative myocardial ischemia. *Anesthesiology.* 1998;88:7–17.

70

A POSITIVE TROPONIN IS NOT NECESSARILY A MYOCARDIAL INFARCTION

MICHAEL P. HUTCHENS, MD, MA AND BRADFORD D. WINTERS, MD, PhD

A common scenario in the preoperative evaluation of an acutely ill patient is the discovery of a positive troponin. Although this is commonly interpreted as a sign of myocardial ischemia, this may or may not be the case. Positive troponins occur without myocardial infarction (MI) in several situations that have implications for perioperative care very different than those of active MI.

Troponins I, T, and C form a complex with actin and myosin and control contraction in cardiac and skeletal muscle. A small amount of cardiac troponin is cytoplasmic, whereas the rest is sarcomeric. Although cardiac and skeletal muscle share isoforms of troponin C, cardiac troponins I and T are distinct from skeletal isoforms.

Since the year 2000, the international consensus definition of MI has included positive troponins with gradual rise and fall, and clinical evidence of MI (characteristic electrocardiogram changes or ischemic symptoms). Within 3 years of the introduction of this definition, the incidence of emergency department–diagnosed acute MI increased nearly 200%. Clearly, troponin values are a sensitive tool with which to diagnose myocardial ischemia, but this sensitivity has posed some problems. The value of this test led to the marketing of a large number of diagnostic assays, which have improved significantly since their introduction; early assays were less specific for cardiac troponins. The variety of assays means that clinical labs at different institutions must promulgate their own norms; values must be interpreted relative to the local reference values. It is not unheard of for neighboring institutions to have upper-limit-of-normal values that differ by an order of magnitude.

The earlier, nonspecific assays created confusion when emergency departments began using them in patients with low pretest probability of MI. What appeared to be spurious positives were found to be quite common. Although the newer assays are more specific, there are still disease states other than acute MI that can elevate blood levels of cardiac troponins T and I. Familiarity with these states can prevent embarrassing mistakes, complications, and unnecessary case cancellations.

© 2006 Mayo Foundation for Medical Education and Research

Chronic renal failure patients represent the largest group of patients who may have elevated troponins in the absence of acute myocardial ischemia or infarction. With newer assays, up to 50% of chronic renal failure patients without acute myocardial ischemia (based on clinical signs and electrocardiogram) have elevated troponin T. Troponin T is more frequently elevated than troponin I in this population, leading to speculation that troponin I is more specific; this speculation is not evidence-vetted, however. The mechanism for this finding is not yet clear. Troponins are large molecules that are cleared by the reticuloendothelial system and not the kidney, and troponin levels are not related to creatinine, blood urea nitrogen (BUN), or calcium phosphate product. Most evidence points to a cardiac source, whether that be clinically silent microinfarction, myocardial strain from heart failure, or alteration in expression of troponin molecules by renal failure. Regardless, what is known is that even in renal failure patients without active MI or coronary artery disease by angiography, positive troponins are a risk factor for intermediate and long-term mortality. The perioperative implications of this finding are not clear but are likely different from those of a patient undergoing surgery in the midst of an acute MI.

Other disease states that have been observed to elevate troponins without other evidence of acute myocardial infarction include congestive heart failure (CHF), left ventricular hypertrophy, supraventricular tachycardia, pulmonary embolism (PE), cardiac surgery, cardiac trauma, defibrillation and cardioversion, sepsis, subarachnoid hemorrhage, cocaine use, methamphetamine use, and endurance running. This is by no means an all-inclusive list. What these things have in common is direct oxidative stress to myocardiocytes or overt necrosis and apoptosis—without occlusion of a large coronary artery. With the exception of marathon running, all of these states are known to have the potential for lasting cardiac effects, and in the case of PE, CHF, and sepsis, studies have shown that elevated troponins portend worse outcome.

So, unless your patient has recently run a marathon or been cardioverted, if the troponin is positive, it's probably a bad sign. Is the patient having an MI though? The diagnosis of MI by troponins requires the characteristic rising and falling of troponins; this usually occurs over a 24-hour period and thus sequential values are needed. They are generally drawn every 8 hours. This definition also requires other evidence of MI: ST changes, new Q wave, or ischemic symptoms. Patients who have positive troponins with appropriate kinetics and electrocardiogram changes or ischemic symptoms are having an acute MI. These patients have very high perioperative risk, and all but the most critical emergency surgical intervention should be postponed. Patients with chronic renal failure and chronically elevated troponins, or critically ill patients with elevated troponins with no new evidence of myocardial ischemia, may not be having an acute MI. Although a positive troponin in this setting has adverse intermediate and long-term prognostic impact, it probably does not carry the same level of perioperative risk as an active, acute myocardial infarction.

TAKE HOME POINTS

- Elevated cardiac troponin is present in acute MI.
- Elevated cardiac troponin is present in disease states other than MI.
- Chronic renal failure patients often have elevated troponin without other evidence of acute MI.
- The diagnosis of MI by troponin requires a rise and fall as well as clinical evidence of ischemia.

SUGGESTED READINGS

Babuin L, Jaffe AS. Troponin: the biomarker of choice for the detection of cardiac injury. *Can Med Assoc J.* 2005;173(10):1191–1202.

Jeremias A, Gibson MC. Narrative review: alternative causes for elevated cardiac troponin levels when acute coronary syndromes are excluded. *Ann Intern Med.* 2005;142:786–791.

Kanderian AS, Francis GS. Cardiac troponins and chronic kidney disease. *Kidney Int.* 2006;69:1112–1114.

71

DO NOT DISREGARD AN ELEVATED PARTIAL THROMBOPLASTIN TIME WHEN THE PROTHROMBIN TIME IS NORMAL

LISA MARCUCCI, MD

The consensus on preoperative laboratory screening in moving toward fewer tests being performed in the perioperative setting. Although the yield is low, preoperative coagulation studies can be vitally important. When they are ordered, these tests must be correctly interpreted for good care. Any abnormality of the partial thromboplastin time (PTT) in the setting of a normal prothrombin time (PT) cannot be dismissed as a lab error, as it can be a marker for an underlying coagulation factor disorder that can cause fatal bleeding.

PTT measures the coagulation ability of the intrinsic pathway, and to a lesser extent, the common pathway in the clotting cascade. Factors in the intrinsic pathway include VIII, IX, XI, XII, and prekallikrein. Factors in the common pathway include fibrinogen, II, V, VII, and X. Anticoagulation with heparin (including the low-molecular-weight heparins if used in sufficiently high doses), hirudins, danaparoid, and argatroban cause a prolonged PTT in the setting of a normal PT. However, a prolonged PTT with normal PT in the absence of these drugs must prompt further laboratory investigation using mixing studies.

Virtually every laboratory has a protocol for performing a PTT mixing study. For PTT mixing studies, the patient's serum is mixed with pooled serum of normal controls and then incubated for 1 to 2 hours at an elevated temperature. The PTT is measured twice after mixing—before and after incubation. There are three possible outcomes of this test:

1) The PTT of the mixture is normal on initial mixing and remains normal after incubation. This suggests that the patient's abnormal PTT is due to a deficiency of factor VIII, IX, XI, XII, or prekallikrein, because the pooled serum provides the missing factor. Specific assays for factors VIII, IX, XI, and XII are performed to find out which factor is deficient. Assays for prekallikrein are not performed, because deficiency of this factor causes an increased PTT but is extremely rare and does not cause abnormal bleeding. Treatment is repletion of the missing factor before a surgery or other invasive procedure.

2) The PTT is immediately prolonged on mixing and remains prolonged after incubation. This suggests the presence of a coagulation inhibitor in

© 2006 Mayo Foundation for Medical Education and Research

the patient's serum. The most common inhibitor that causes this mixing study outcome is lupus anticoagulant, and assays for this can be performed. If this assay is negative, specific assays for inhibitors for factors of IX, XI, and XII are done. Inhibitors are antibodies against the individual factors and are detected by testing for their unique molecular composition. The presence of lupus anticoagulant often causes an increased PTT but is paradoxically associated with thrombosis, not bleeding, and may require preoperative anticoagulation.

3) The PTT of the mixture is initially normal (or significantly shorter than the patient's PTT) and then becomes prolonged after incubation. This strongly suggests the presence of a factor VIII inhibitor. A factor VIII assay should be performed and, if this factor is decreased, then a factor VIII inhibitor assay (Bethesda assay) should be performed. The larger the amount of inhibitor present, the higher is the risk of severe bleeding. Each Bethesda unit connotes reduction in functional factor VIII of 50% (i.e., 3 Bethesda units contain only 12.5% functional factor VIII).

Treatment of acquired factor VIII inhibitor is difficult and is aimed at reversing the coagulopathy and eliminating the inhibitor. Substances used to stop active bleeding include desmopressin acetate (DDAVP), factor VIII bolus/infusion, prothrombin complex concentrates (which bypass factor VIII), recombinant factor VIIa (very expensive), and repletion of ongoing loss of blood components. Treatment protocols aimed at eliminating the underlying inhibitor use corticosteroids, plasmapheresis, intravenous immunoglobulin, and (in resistant cases) cyclophosphamide.

Clinically, acquired factor VIII inhibitor can present as spontaneous muscle and soft tissue hematoma, hematuria, severe epistaxis, or fatal bleeding with even mildly invasive procedures such as cystoscopy or bronchoscopy. As these inhibitors are acquired, lack of a previous bleeding diathesis does not rule out their presence at the time of the prolonged PTT. Most often their etiology is idiopathic, but factor inhibitors are associated with several conditions as listed below:

Autoimmune—systemic lupus erythematosis, rheumatoid arthritis, ulcerative colitis, psoriasis, and pehphigus vulgaris.

Pregnancy—can appear at term or just after delivery, sometimes with spontaneous disappearance 12 to 18 months postpartum; most likely to occur in the first pregnancy.

Malignancy—lymphoproliferative disorders, plasma cell dyscrasias, and solid tumors.

Drugs—sulfa, penicillin, phenytoin, and especially animal-derived, nonautologous fibrin glue. This type of fibrin glue is made from the mixing of several components of bovine serum, of which remnants of bovine factor VIII may survive. Two percent of patients who receive fibrin glue develop acquired factor VIII inhibitor because of this exposure to bovine factor VIII.

TAKE HOME POINTS

- Always obtain mixing studies if the PTT is prolonged.
- Lack of previous bleeding diathesis does not rule out the presence of an **acquired** factor 8 deficiency.

SUGGESTED READINGS

Kleinman MB, Anti-inhibitor coagulant complex for the rescue therapy of acquired inhibitors to factor VIII: case report and review of the literature. *Haemophilia* 2002;8(5):694–697.

Tetrault G. Interpretation of PTT mixing study. *CAP Today* 2005;19(8):8.

Adams JD, Jones S, Brost BC. Development of antibodies to topical bovine thrombin after abdominal hysterectomy. A case report. *J Reprod Med* 2001:46(10):909–912.

72

AVOID A 70% MORTALITY RATE: DO EVERYTHING YOU CAN TO PREVENT PERIOPERATIVE RENAL FAILURE

MICHAEL P. HUTCHENS, MD, MA

Acute renal failure in the postoperative period is appallingly common and has abysmal outcomes. In high-risk populations the incidence may be as high as 25%, and patients who require critical care services and renal replacement therapy have repeatedly been shown to have a mortality rate >70%. Despite this, perioperative resuscitation strategies are frequently formed solely with cardiac and pulmonary outcomes in mind. An early extubation is a pyrrhic victory if it condemns the patient to a slow death or lifetime dialysis. Despite decades of research, the risk factors, etiology, prevention, and treatment of perioperative acute renal failure all remain murky. Numerous interventions have been assessed, with few promising results. There are a few tools at hand, though, and the devastating effect of acute renal failure obligates anesthesiologists to use the tools available with the best possible dexterity.

The most consistent risk factor for perioperative renal failure is preoperative renal dysfunction. Elevated creatinine or decreased creatinine clearance, or a preoperative diagnosis of renal insufficiency, all significantly increase the risk of postoperative renal failure. Preoperative heart failure and diabetes mellitus are also significant predictors, as are the acute comorbidities rhabdomyolysis, fulminant liver failure, abdominal compartment syndrome, and sepsis. Surgical procedures involving cardiopulmonary bypass or aortic cross-clamp (any aortic cross-clamp, not just suprarenal clamping) increase risk as well. Perioperative diagnostic studies involving nephrotoxic radiocontrast and medical management of concurrent nonsurgical disease (chemotherapy, aminoglycosides, nonsteroidal anti-inflammatory drugs [NSAIDs]) can further elevate the risk.

Anesthetic management directed at preventing acute renal failure ranges from banal to complex. If possible, stop nephrotoxic medications preoperatively. Certainly do not give preoperative NSAIDs to improve analgesia in at-risk patients. For procedures that will take 2 hours or more, a Foley catheter should be placed. Ensure that urine enters the Foley catheter when it is placed, as a misplaced Foley and subsequent obstruction can *cause* renal failure. In current practice there is no longer a fixed "goal" for hourly urine output; the objective is to monitor urine output diligently, and if it drops, intervene—increase perfusion pressure, give a fluid challenge, and inform

© 2006 Mayo Foundation for Medical Education and Research

the surgeon. If need be, place a central venous pressure (CVP) monitor to assure adequate intravascular volume. Eschew nephrotoxic agents in your anesthetic plan: ketorolac, dextran, and aminoglycosides should be avoided. It is clear that hypoperfusion contributes to perioperative renal failure; in at-risk patients, maintaining perfusion pressure is a high priority. Have a low threshold for placing an intra-arterial monitoring line, and use vasoactive agents, if necessary, to treat hypotension.

No therapeutic agent has shown broad renal-protective effect in the perioperative setting. Although there is lasting enthusiasm for low-dose dopamine, extensive study has shown it to have no effect on need for dialysis or mortality. Use of dopamine predictably causes tachycardia, which may be deleterious in a patient with concurrent coronary artery disease and increases the incidence of perioperative atrial fibrillation. Mannitol is commonly used in aortic cross-clamp cases; however, evidence to support this use is slim at best. Mannitol has been shown to be effective in preventing acute renal failure when used properly during renal transplant procedures. Although furosemide is popularly used to increase urine output, there is 30 years of evidence that furosemide can cause acute renal failure, and its use in the hypoperfused patient in the operating room (OR) is anathema. Other agents that have been used as putative intraoperative renal protectants include atrial natriuretic peptides, *n*-acetylcysteine, and fenoldopam. All have shown benefits in small studies that have not been replicable in large studies, suggesting that each may have use in a confined population, but what population remains unclear. A tantalizing study by Gandhi et al. in 2005 showed a significant association between intraoperative hyperglycemia and postoperative renal failure (defined as a doubling of creatinine, a creatinine >2, or new requirement for dialysis) in cardiac surgical patients. As intensive insulin therapy in the intensive care unit (ICU) reduces the need for dialysis, and as diabetes mellitus is a known risk factor, this raises the possibility that intraoperative insulin treatment may be renoprotective.

TAKE HOME POINTS

- Although the anesthesiologist may not see it happening in the OR, acute renal failure is an anesthetic outcome with gargantuan impact on patient morbidity and mortality. Remember that we can see only oliguric acute renal failure, because typically we don't check the BUN and creatinine.
- The alert anesthesiologist must consider renal outcome in the anesthetic plan. Recognize the patient who is at risk because of preoperative disease or medical interventions.
- Maintain adequate circulating volume and perfusion pressure, and at all costs avoid doing harm with nephrotoxic agents.

- Consider tight intraoperative glucose control with insulin in diabetic patients.
- Finally, if you are concerned that the patient may be at risk for postoperative renal failure, communicate this to the surgeons, because early recognition and intervention in the postoperative period may improve the outcome.

SUGGESTED READINGS

Jarnberg PO. Renal protection strategies in the perioperative period. *Best Pract Res Clin Anaesthesiol.* 2004;18:645–660.

Levy EM, Viscoli CM, Horwitz RI. The effect of acute renal failure on mortality. A cohort analysis. *JAMA.* 1996;275:1489–1494.

Mahon P, Shorten G. Perioperative acute renal failure. *Curr Opin Anaesthesiol.* 2006;19:332–338.

Metnitz PG, Krenn CG, Steltzer H, et al. Effect of acute renal failure requiring renal replacement therapy on outcome in critically ill patients. *Crit Care Med.* 2002;30:2051–2058.

73

"RENAL DOSE" DOPAMINE MUST DIE

TODD J. SMAKA, MD AND MICHAEL P. HUTCHENS, MD, MA

Dopamine (DA) is an endogenous catecholamine that influences receptors in a concentration-dependent manner. For >20 years, low-dose or "renal-dose" DA (LDD) (1 to 5 mcg/kg/min) has been used in an attempt to preserve renal function in critically ill patients. This use stems from studies that demonstrated increased renal blood flow and diuresis in healthy experimental animals and human volunteers. However, there have never been studies demonstrating benefit in critically ill patients, and recently, several high-quality studies have shown that LDD does not confer meaningful renal protection and indeed may cause harm.

LDD causes renal vasodilatation, predominately by stimulating DA-1 receptors in the renal vasculature. It causes natriuresis by inhibiting Na^+/K^+-ATPase activity in the proximal tubule, thick ascending limb of the loop of Henle, and the cortical collecting ducts. It causes diuresis by stimulating prostaglandin E_2 (PGE_2) production, which antagonizes the effects of antidiuretic hormone. These effects would appear to indicate improved renal function, but consideration of the patient and not the laboratory values suggests otherwise.

In a 1998 study of critically ill patients without renal or hepatic dysfunction, investigators found no correlation between DA infusion rate and DA serum concentration; serum concentrations in patients were significantly higher than in healthy controls. Thus the notion that LDD in healthy volunteers is the same as LDD in critically ill patients is highly questionable. The definitive study of LDD is a large multicenter, randomized, double-blind, placebo-controlled study performed by the Australian and New Zealand Intensive Care Society (ANZICS) Clinical Trials Group and published in 2000. It looked at 328 patients in 23 intensive care units (ICUs) and concluded that LDD does not benefit critically ill patients who are at risk for renal failure. The study demonstrated that LDD did not differ from placebo in resultant peak serum creatinine concentration, creatinine increase from baseline, number of patients requiring renal replacement therapy, duration of ICU stay, duration of hospital stay, and number of deaths. In another large trial, NORASEPT II study investigators performed a retrospective analysis of 395 oliguric patients with sepsis in the placebo arm of a TNF-α antibody sepsis trial and showed that LDD did not reduce the incidence of acute renal failure, the need for dialysis, or the 28-day mortality in patients with oliguria

ⓒ 2006 Mayo Foundation for Medical Education and Research

due to septic shock. These same conclusions have been reached in several meta-analyses. The study data therefore do not support the hypothesis that LDD benefits patients with respect to the meaningful outcomes of death or dialysis.

Although there is physiologic rationale suggesting benefit from LDD, there is also abundant physiologic rationale against it. LDD directly vasodilates vessels in the cortex and indirectly vasodilates vessels in the inner medulla. This causes a redistribution of blood away from the outer medulla, which contains the energy-dependent Na^+/K^+-ATPase channels of the medullary thick ascending limb. Furthermore, the natriuretic effect of LDD causes an increased solute load to the distal tubular cells, which may actually increase oxygen consumption and thereby increase the risk of ischemia. Therefore, although LDD does increase blood flow to the kidney as a whole, it does so at the expense of blood flow to the metabolically active outer medulla, resulting in an increased susceptibility to focal ischemia and eventually acute renal failure.

The increased blood flow and glomerular filtration rate induced by LDD in healthy volunteers has not been demonstrated in patients with early renal failure. Even so, such effects are likely due to LDD's cardiac effects. In fact, there is no evidence that drug-induced diuresis protects renal function in the setting of decreased cardiac output or hypovolemia.

LDD may in fact cause harm. LDD can induce tachycardia, dysrhythmias, and myocardial ischemia. Attenuation of ventilatory response to hypoxia and increased intrapulmonary shunting are known complications. Mesenteric ischemia has been observed in patients receiving LDD. This is particularly harmful in the critical care and intraoperative setting, because it compromises the mucosal lining and reduces perfusion to anastamoses. LDD also causes panhypopituitarisms, including suppression of prolactin, growth hormone, and thyrotropin. Growth-hormone suppression contributes to a negative nitrogen balance in critical illness, and prolactin suppression induces a transient decrease in T-cell function. Other immunologic effects of LDD include inhibition of stimulated lymphocyte proliferation, immunoglobulin synthesis, and cytokine production. It also promotes lymphocyte apoptosis.

Studies showing a renal protective benefit of DA in healthy volunteers either have insufficient power to draw conclusions, are confounded by simultaneous administration of other putative nephroprotective agents, or are associated with doses higher than true LDD. Very strong evidence now shows no meaningful benefit from LDD. At higher doses of DA, the effect on renal physiology is likely due to its cardiac effects, and these effects can be induced with other agents. Although increased blood flow may be advantageous in preventing renal failure, DA should not be used solely for its renal effects. Rather, if renal perfusion is felt to be insufficient, the appropriate drug should be chosen for the clinical situation and should be used in the appropriate *cardiac* dose.

TAKE HOME POINTS

- Renal-dose DA (1 to 5 mcg/kg/min) does not have beneficial effects on the kidney even though urine output may be increased.
- Renal-dose DA does not prevent renal failure.
- Renal-dose DA does not prevent death or the need for dialysis in critically ill patients.
- Renal-dose DA has potential to cause harm.

SUGGESTED READINGS

Bellomo R, Chapman M, Finfer S, et al. Low-dose dopamine in patients with early renal dysfunction: a placebo-controlled randomised trial. Australian and New Zealand Intensive Care Society (ANZICS) Clinical Trials Group. *Lancet.* 2000;356(9248):2139–2143.

Debaveye YA, Van den Berghe GH. Is there still a place for dopamine in the modern intensive care unit? *Anesth Analg.* 2004;98(2):461–468.

Kellum JA, M Decker J. Use of dopamine in acute renal failure: a meta-analysis. *Crit Care Med.* 2001;29(8):1526–1531.

Marik PE. Low-dose dopamine: a systematic review. *Intensive Care Med.* 2002;28(7):877–883.

Marik PE, Iglesias J. Low-dose dopamine does not prevent acute renal failure in patients with septic shock and oliguria. NORASEPT II Study Investigators. *Am J Med.* 1999;107(4): 387–390.

74

REMEMBER THAT THERE ARE AT LEAST SEVEN MODALITIES FOR TREATING HYPERKALEMIA IN THE PERIOPERATIVE PERIOD

GRACE L. CHIEN, MD

Hyperkalemia means that serum potassium levels are elevated beyond normal levels (the upper limit is usually reported as 5 to 5.5 mmol/L). Hyperkalemia has few clinical manifestations. In awake patients, severe muscle weakness beginning with the lower extremities and progressing cephalad, usually sparing cranial nerves and respiratory muscles, is sometimes evident. In patients under general anesthesia, the primary abnormality manifests as electrocardiogram (EKG) changes starting with peaked T waves, shortened QT interval, progressive lengthening of the PR interval, and QRS duration. The P wave may disappear, and ultimately, wide, complex ventricular tachycardia presents, eventually progressing to ventricular standstill. Hyperkalemia may also cause a variety of heart blocks, including bundle branch block and atrioventricular (AV) blocks. The manifestations of hyperkalemia depend on the rate of potassium rise—they are better tolerated by patients with chronic hyperkalemia. EKG changes with hyperkalemia are affected by concomitant hypocalcemia, academia, and hyponatremia.

PATHOGENESIS OF HYPERKALEMIA

Although hyperkalemia has many etiologies (*Table 74.1*), there are three distinct pathways: (i) ineffective elimination of potassium during any interval in the perioperative period, almost always due to renal failure; (ii) acute potassium load from a medication error or massive transfusion of stored blood; (iii) movement of potassium ions from the intracellular space to the extracellular space. This last can occur with the use of succinylcholine, especially for burn patients or paralyzed patients. It can also be seen with changes in ventilation and/or acid–base status in patients on certain drug combinations (spironolactone/beta-blockers) or significant physiologic derangements such as diabetic ketoacidosis. At the cellular level, hyperkalemia interferes with neuromuscular transmission and thus produces skeletal and cardiac muscle abnormalities. Neuromuscular transmission depends on membrane excitability. Increased extracellular potassium depolarizes the cell membrane, making the cell more excitable, and requiring less of a stimulus to generate an action potential. The hyperexcitability eventually

© 2006 Mayo Foundation for Medical Education and Research

TABLE 74.1 DISORDERS THAT CAUSE HYPERKALEMIA	
DISORDERS THAT LEAD TO HYPERKALEMIA CAUSED BY IMPAIRED RENAL EXCRETION OF POTASSIUM	**DISORDERS THAT LEAD TO HYPERKALEMIA CAUSED BY SHIFT OF POTASSIUM INTO THE EXTRACELLULAR SPACE**
Acquired hyporeninemic hypoaldosteronism Addison disease Congenital adrenal hyperplasia (recessive or autosomal dominant) Mineralocorticoid deficiency Primary hypoaldosteronism of hyporeninemia Pseudohypoaldosteronism Renal insufficiency or failure Systemic lupus erythematosus Type IV renal tubular acidosis	Damage to tissue from rhabdomyolysis, burns, or trauma Familial hyperkalemic periodic paralysis Hyperosmolar states (e.g., uncontrolled diabetes, glucose infusions) Insulin deficiency or resistance Tumor lysis syndrome

inactivates sodium channels and leads to cardiac conduction abnormalities and muscle paralysis.

TREATMENT OF HYPERKALEMIA

A valuable resource is the Cochrane Database of Systematic Reviews, which has published recommendations for emergency interventions for hyperkalemia. Current evidence suggests that intravenous (IV) insulin and glucose combined with nebulized beta-adrenergic receptor agonists were more effective than each treatment alone.

Calcium. Calcium stabilizes cardiac muscle and directly antagonizes the hyperexcitability induced by hyperkalemia. Calcium starts acting within minutes and can be used as an infusion over 2 to 3 minutes. The dose is 500 mg to 1 g and may be repeated after 5 minutes. Calcium should not be given with bicarbonate, as calcium carbonate will precipitate. Patients who are taking digitalis are more vulnerable to toxicity with hypercalcemia, so calcium should be used with great caution in these patients.

Insulin and Glucose. Insulin drives potassium ions into the cell by enhancing the sodium/potassium ATPase pump in skeletal muscle. Ten units plus 50 mL of 50% glucose as a bolus, followed by a glucose infusion, had been found to be effective in decreasing serum potassium. Alternatively, 50 mL of 50% glucose may be given to rapidly induce hyperinsulinemia.

Sodium Bicarbonate. Sodium bicarbonate raises the pH of serum and, via the H^+/K^+ exchanger, drives hydrogen-ion release from inside the cell. Potassium in turn moves into the cell to maintain electroneutrality and thus reduces serum potassium levels. Ngugi et al. demonstrated that bicarbonate infusion lowered serum potassium levels by 0.47 ± 0.31 mmol/L at

30 minutes and thereafter. In addition, bicarbonate appears to reduce serum potassium levels by an unknown mechanism. However, the only placebo-controlled study, by Allon, found that bicarbonate did not lower serum potassium levels compared to placebo.

Beta-Adrenergic Agonists. Beta-adrenergic agonists are effective in reducing serum potassium levels by 30 minutes after administration. The effect appears to be dose-responsive. Allon et al. demonstrated that 20 mg of nebulized albuterol reduced serum potassium levels. There does not seem to be a significant difference in effect between IV-administered or inhaled albuterol. With either route of delivery, further reduction in serum potassium levels may be attained by readministration of albuterol at 120 minutes. Of note, epinephrine can be used for its mixed effects if $beta_2$-adrenergic agents are not available. However, α-receptor stimulation causes potassium release from cells, especially in patients with renal failure.

Loop or Thiazide Diuretics. Loop diuretics induce diuresis through sodium excretion, in the process activating the Na/K exchanger and inducing potassium wasting. Loop diuretics may be effective in mild renal impairment because loop diuretics are high-ceiling diuretics, meaning they have dose-dependent effects. Administering Lasix via IV produces effects that depend on the patient's renal function, prior Lasix exposure, and many intraoperative factors such as hydration status. Therapy using diuretics to lower potassium should be guided by frequent serum chemistry, patient symptoms, and expected potassium trend.

Cation-Exchange Resin. Sodium polystyrene sulfonate, administered orally or as a retention enema, binds potassium and releases sodium in the gastrointestinal (GI) tract. The oral dose is 15 to 30 g in 20% sorbitol solution. Enema doses are usually 50 g mixed with 50 mL of 70% sorbitol plus 100 to 150 mL of tap water. One dose can potentially lower plasma potassium by 0.5 to 1 mg/L. Resin seems to be less effective in renal failure patients. The routes of administration and slow onset render resins less effective in the acute rescue of intraoperative hyperkalemia.

Dialysis. Dialysis may be performed in the perioperative period (including in the operating room!) in the event that more conservative treatments fail, if the hyperkalemia is severe, or if the patient has such massive tissue injuries that conservative treatment cannot keep pace with the amount of potassium released from cells. More potassium may be removed with increasing blood flow during dialysis.

Blood Products. Although blood products are not a treatment for hyperkalemia, in cases in which massive transfusion is ongoing, especially if there is a degree of renal insufficiency, the anesthesia provider should request that the blood bank send recently donated blood and/or "washed" packed red blood cells to try to reduce the levels of exogenously administered potassium.

TAKE HOME POINTS

- Be aware of the situations in which hyperkalemia commonly occurs—succinylcholine "mishaps", crush injuries, reperfusion of transplanted organs or ischemic limbs, and patients on spironolactone and beta-blockers.
- Consider hyperkalemia if the patient develops a new bundle branch or atrioventricular block in the perioperative period.
- Calcium stabilizes cardiac muscle membranes, but it must be used cautiously in patients on digitalis.
- Other therapies use the Na^+/K^+ and H^+/K^+ exchangers to move potassium intracellularly.
- Ask the blood bank to send packed red cells <5 days "old" or washed units.
- For severe or refractory cases, dialysis may be warranted.

SUGGESTED READINGS

Allon M, Dunlay R, Copkney C. Nebulized albuterol for acute hyperkalemia in patients on hemodialysis. *Ann Intern Med.* 1989;110(6):426–429.

Allon M, Shanklin N. Effect of albuterol treatment on subsequent dialytic potassium removal. *Am J Kidney Dis.* 1995;26(4):607–613.

Allon M, Shanklin N. Effect of bicarbonate administration on plasma potassium in dialysis patients: interactions with insulin and albuterol. *Am J Kidney Dis.* 1996;28(4):508–514.

Bashour T, Hsu I, Gorfinkel HJ, et al. Atrioventricular and intraventricular conduction in hyperkalemia. *Am J Cardiol.* 1975;35(2):199–203.

Berne RM, Levy MN. *Cardiovascular Physiology.* 4th ed. St. Louis: Mosby; 1981.

Costello-Boerrigter LC, Boerrigter G, Burnett JC, Jr. Revisiting salt and water retention: new diuretics, aquaretics, and natriuretics. *Med Clin North Am.* 2003;87(2):475–491.

Ferrannini E, Taddei S, Santoro D, et al. Independent stimulation of glucose metabolism and Na^+-K^+ exchange by insulin in the human forearm. *Am J Physiol.* 1988;255(6 pt 1):E953–E958.

Fraley DS, Adler S. Correction of hyperkalemia by bicarbonate despite constant blood pH. *Kidney Int.* 1977;12(5):354–360.

Freeman SJ, Fale AD. Muscular paralysis and ventilatory failure caused by hyperkalaemia. *Br J Anaesth.* 1993;70(2):226–227.

Gruy-Kapral C, Emmett M, Santa Ana CA, et al. Effect of single dose resin-cathartic therapy on serum potassium concentration in patients with end-stage renal disease. *J Am Soc Nephrol.* 1998;9(10):1924–1930.

Gutzwiller JP, Schneditz D, Huber AR, et al. Increasing blood flow increases kt/V(urea) and potassium removal but fails to improve phosphate removal. *Clin Nephrol.* 2003;59(2):130–136.

Livingstone IR, Cumming WJ. Hyperkalaemic paralysis resembling Guillain-Barre syndrome. *Lancet.* 1979;2(8149):963–964.

Mahoney BA, Smith WA, Lo DS, et al. Emergency interventions for hyperkalaemia. *Cochrane Database Syst Rev.* 2005(2):CD003235.

McClure RJ, Prasad VK, Brocklebank JT. Treatment of hyperkalaemia using intravenous and nebulised salbutamol. *Arch Dis Child.* 1994;70(2):126–128.

Ngugi NN, McLigeyo SO, Kayima JK. Treatment of hyperkalaemia by altering the transcellular gradient in patients with renal failure: effect of various therapeutic approaches. *East Afr Med J.* 1997;74(8):503–509.

Weiner ID, Wingo CS. Hyperkalemia: a potential silent killer. *J Am Soc Nephrol.* 1998;9(8):1535–1543.

Zehnder C, Gutzwiller JP, Huber A, et al. Low-potassium and glucose-free dialysis maintains urea but enhances potassium removal. *Nephrol Dial Transplant.* 2001;16(1):78–84.

75

MANAGE OBSTRUCTIVE SLEEP APNEA PATIENTS CONSERVATIVELY

DANIELA DAMIAN, MD AND
IBTESAM A. HILMI, MB, CHB, FRCA

Obstructive sleep apnea (OSA) is defined as air flow cessation during sleep for at least 10 seconds, caused by the collapse of the airway. Hypopnea is defined as a moderate reduction in air flow that is associated with arousal diagnosed by electroencephalogram. Hypopnea represents a $>50\%$ reduction in air flow or a $<50\%$ reduction in air flow that is associated with a desaturation of $>3\%$ from the baseline reading.

EPIDEMIOLOGY

The exact incidence of OSA in the adult population is unknown. It was previously thought to be between 5% and 10%, but a recent study showed that one in four U.S. adults appears to be at high risk for OSA. This fact underscores the increased chance of having a patient with undiagnosed OSA as a candidate for general anesthesia.

RISK FACTORS

The most clearly recognized risk factor for OSA is a narrow upper airway. The most common etiologies involve congenital abnormalities of the airway (e.g., Pierre-Robin syndrome, midface hypoplasia), hypertrophy of the adenoids and tonsils (especially in children), macroglossia (e.g., Down syndrome), and increased uvula size. Other important risk factors are obesity (body mass index >30 kg/m^2), nasal polyps, deviated nasal septum, and chronic rhinitis. Neck circumference of >17 in for men and >16 in for women also represents an additional risk for OSA. Obesity by itself can lead to OSA or can worsen a pre-existing OSA. In the adult population the male-to-female ratio is 2:1, but this ratio does not apply to children or post-menopausal females. In women over the age of 65 years, the risk for OSA increases threefold. Other predisposing factors for OSA include a family history of OSA, smoking, and use of alcohol, tranquilizers, or sedatives.

PATHOLOGY

The patient with OSA has a smaller and more easily collapsible upper airway. The risk of complete collapse of the airway is accentuated at the end of expiration, when the tissue pressure overcomes intraluminal pressure. The critical collapsible area is usually seen in the velopharynx, as evidenced

© 2006 Mayo Foundation for Medical Education and Research

by imaging studies (computerized tomography, magnetic resonance, or fluoroscopy). Recurrent apnea will lead to intermittent hypoxemia, hypercapnia, and sleep fragmentation, with secondary increase of the sympathetic tone. OSA represents an independent risk factor for cardiovascular morbidity and mortality. A plausible explanation seems to be the increased oxidative stress secondary to alternate hypoxia/reoxygenation. The oxidative stress causes systemic inflammatory response with activation of endothelial cells, leukocytes, and platelets that culminates in early signs of atherosclerosis. OSA is one of the leading causes of systemic hypertension, left ventricular hypertrophy, pulmonary hypertension with right ventricular failure and congestive heart failure, cardiac dysrhythmias, ischemic heart disease, and stroke.

Sleep fragmentation leads to chronic fatigue, excessive daytime somnolence that markedly increases the risk of motor vehicle accidents, memory problems, anxiety, and depression.

DIAGNOSIS

The diagnosis of OSA is based on patient history, clinical presentation, physical examination, and sleep study (polysomnography). The classical symptoms of OSA are snoring, excessive daytime sleepiness, and witnessed episodes of breathing cessation during sleep. Usually, the patient with OSA is a man, over age 60 years, obese, with a short and thick neck. The "gold standard" for diagnosing OSA remains the polysomnography or sleep study performed overnight in a sleep laboratory. An accurate measurement requires 12 physiologic signals (*Table 75.1*) with a computer-based automated sleep analysis.

The final result of the analysis is the apnea–hypopnea index (AHI), which is the total number of apnea and hypopnea events per hour of total sleep time. According to the AHI, the severity of OSA can be stratified as shown in *Table 75.2*.

TREATMENT

The mainstay of treatment for OSA is continuous positive airway pressure (CPAP) applied during sleep via a tight nasal or facial mask. Indications for CPAP therapy are an AHI >10 accompanied by symptoms or an AHI >30 regardless of symptoms. This technique has been proven to be efficient in preventing the collapse of the airway and improving breathing during sleep. CPAP therapy improves concentration, alertness, neurocognitive function, and mood. The CPAP has favorable effects on cardiovascular outcome but necessitates a strict commitment from the patient. The addition of humidification, bi-level positive airway pressure (BiPAP), and auto-titration of positive airway pressure has been tried to improve compliance and patient comfort. Mandibular repositioning appliances represent a simple and noninvasive alternative method of treatment for mild OSA (AHI 5 to 15) and are used in

TABLE 75.1	SIGNALS REQUIRED FOR POLYSOMNOGRAPHY (HYPOPNEIC AND APNEIC EVENTS ARE ASSOCIATED WITH AROUSAL FROM REM SLEEP, OXYHEMOGLOBIN DESATURATION, POSSIBLE ARRHYTHMIAS AND HIGH BLOOD PRESSURE.)	
FUNCTION	**SIGNAL**	**RESPONSE IN OBSTRUCTIVE SLEEP APNEA**
Sleep	Electroencephalogram (EEG)	Arousal episodes
	Electrooculogram (EOG)	Rapid eye movements (REM)
	Electromyography submentalis (EMG)	Decrease of chin muscle tone
Respiration	Oronasal air flow	Decrease or cessation of air flow
	Ribcage and abdominal movement	Increased respiratory effort
	Oxygen saturation	Desaturation
	End-tidal CO_2	Increased value after apnea
Cardiovascular	Electrocardiogram (EKG)	Cyclical variation of bradycardia episode associated to apnea followed by tachycardia Other arrhythmias
	Blood pressure	Possible elevated values linking to cardiovascular consequences of OSA
Movement	Electromyography tibialis	Limb movement
Position	Body position	Correlation with occurrence of OSA
Behavior	Video, audio	Snoring, sleep talking, sleep apnea events, movement disorder, seizures

patients who are unable to tolerate CPAP. The mechanism of action is similar to the jaw-thrust technique. Surgery is reserved for severe OSA or lack of response to CPAP. The main objective of any surgical technique is to enlarge the upper airway. Adenoidectomy, tonsillectomy, nasal polypectomy, septoplasty, uvulopalatopharyngoplasty, maxillomandibular advancement and hyoid expansion are all procedures used to alleviate the symptoms of OSA

TABLE 75.2	APNEA–HYPOPNEA INDEX (AHI) AND SEVERITY OF OBSTRUCTIVE SLEEP APNEA (OSA)	
SEVERITY OF OSA	**ADULT AHI**	**PEDIATRIC AHI**
None	0–5	0
Mild OSA	6–20	1–5
Moderate OSA	21–40	6–10
Severe OSA	>40	>10

surgically. If these are unsuccessful and the obstruction is severe, the last option is tracheostomy. As adjuvant therapy, the following may be helpful: losing weight, position therapy, topical application of soft tissue lubricant, and the use of acetazolamide to increase respiratory drive to compensate for the metabolic acidosis caused by hypoxia.

OUTCOME

The natural history of sleep apnea is not yet fully described, but the mortality is increased with the development of cardiovascular complications, especially in the middle-aged population. CPAP, surgery, and dieting can improve the outcome and lower the risk of death from cardiovascular complications.

IMPLICATIONS FOR ANESTHESIA

In October 2005 the American Society of Anesthesiologists (ASA) developed practice guidelines for perioperative management of patients with obstructive sleep apnea. This document should be considered required reading for every anesthesia provider.

Preoperative Evaluation. Patients with an established diagnosis of OSA with the severity of the OSA graded from the results of the sleep study (AHI) (*Table 75.1*) should be managed according to certain practice guidelines that are recommended by the ASA. Otherwise, all surgical patients should be evaluated for OSA risk factors. Multiple screening methods are available, such as the Berlin Questionnaire, which has been proven to be specific and sensitive for OSA screening. The Berlin Questionnaire focuses primarily on symptoms of snoring, apnea, fatigue, hypertension, and body mass index (BMI).

The ASA has come up with two models, one for identification and assessment of OSA and a second to be used as a scoring system (*Tables 75.3* and *75.4*) to predicate the possibility of OSA from the presence of various risk factors. The ASA modules need clinical validation and proof of their usefulness in the perioperative management of OSA.

In patients who are evaluated as being at high risk for OSA and/or who are undergoing a major surgical procedure with a possible requirement for high doses of opioids for postoperative pain, it is advisable to postpone an elective surgery until further evaluation and proper management of their OSA can be undertaken.

During the preoperative evaluation of surgical patients with OSA, it is vital to perform a comprehensive history and physical examination to learn of any comorbidities or previous anesthesia-related complications and to document the settings of the patient's CPAP/BiPAP. One should also make sure that the patient's equipment will be available for postoperative use.

The use of sedatives and analgesics should be avoided in the preoperative setting because of the increased sensitivity to any respiratory depression.

TABLE 75.3   ASA PROPOSED EXAMPLE FOR IDENTIFICATION AND ASSESSMENT OF OSA

Clinical signs and symptoms suggesting the possibility of OSA

1) Predisposing physical characteristics	BMI >35 kg/m^2 (95th percentile for age and gender) Neck circumference >17 in (men); >16 in (women) Craniofacial abnormalities affecting the airway Anatomical nasal obstruction Tonsils touching or nearly touching in the midline
2) History of apparent airway obstruction during sleep	Snoring (loud enough to be heard through closed door) Frequent snoring Observed pauses in breathing during sleep Awakens from sleep with choking sensation Frequent arousals from sleep Intermittent vocalization during sleep Parental report of restless sleep, difficult breathing, or struggling respiratory efforts during sleep
3) Somnolence	Frequent somnolence or fatigue despite adequate "sleep" Falls asleep easily in a nonstimulating environment Parent or teacher comments that the child appears sleepy during the day, is easily distracted, overly aggressive, or has difficulty concentrating Child often difficult to arouse at usual awaking time

If patient has signs or symptoms in two or more of the above categories, there is a significant probability that OSA is present.

Sleep study done

SEVERITY OF OSA	ADULT AHI	PEDIATRIC AHI
None	0–5	0
Mild OSA	6–20	1–5
Moderate OSA	21–40	6–10
Severe OSA	>40	>10

ASA, American Society of Anesthesiologists; OSA, obstructive sleep apnea; BMI, body mass index; AHI, apnea–hypopnea index.

TABLE 75.4	ASA PROPOSED EXAMPLE FOR OSA SCORING SYSTEM	
a) Severity of sleep apnea based on sleep study or clinical indicators if sleep study not available; point score (0–3)	None	0
	Mild	1
	Moderate	2
	Severe	3
b) Invasiveness of surgery and anesthesia; point score (0–3)	Superficial surgery under local or peripheral nerve block anesthesia without sedation	0
	Superficial surgery with moderate sedation or general anesthesia	1
	Peripheral surgery with spinal/ epidural anesthesia (no more than moderate sedation)	1
	Peripheral surgery with general anesthesia	2
	Airway surgery with moderate sedation	2
	Major surgery with general anesthesia	3
	Airway surgery with general anesthesia	3
c) Requirement for postoperative opioids; point score (0–3)	None	0
	Low-dose oral opioids	1
	High-dose oral opioids, parenteral or neuraxial opioids	3

Estimation of perioperative risk: overall score = score from A plus the greater of the score for either B or C; point score (0–6)

ASA, American Society of Anesthesiologists; OSA, obstructive sleep apnea

The consequences of upper-airway muscle tone relaxation could lead to devastating effects before the start of surgery and anesthesia. It is important not to underestimate the challenge of mask ventilation and/or intubation in these patients and to remember to have a clear plan for airway management before going ahead with a general anesthetic.

Intraoperative Management. OSA patients should be considered potential difficult airway management patients, and the anesthesia team should be prepared in advance for this possibility.

As a general rule, whenever it is possible, a regional anesthesia technique should be used instead of general anesthesia. General anesthesia with a secured airway is a better choice than monitored anesthesia care (MAC) with spontaneous breathing and an unsecured airway. Short-acting anesthetic drugs represent an attractive choice for general anesthesia.

For monitoring, standard noninvasive monitoring such as pulse oximeter, capnography, electrocardiography (EKG), and blood pressure are critical, especially for patients who are breathing spontaneously under MAC.

Extubation should be done in the semiupright position when the patient is fully awake and completely recovered after muscular blockade.

Postoperative Care. The main objectives in postoperative care are oxygenation and maintenance of a patent airway using supplemental oxygen and CPAP/BiPAP support. This is especially true for patients who are already on these treatments or high-risk patients.

Adequate analgesia with minimal depression of respiratory drive provided by continuous analgesia through regional techniques such as continuous nerve blocks, paravertebral blocks, or epidurals are the best choice for postoperative pain control. When appropriate, regional techniques should be used, preferably without opioids. Nonsteroidal anti-inflammatory drugs or other adjuvants should be used whenever possible to decrease opioid requirements. The use of patient-controlled analgesia (PCA) without the continuous-infusion mode represents a better alternative than opioids administered on a regular or as-required basis. The antidote for opioid overdose should be readily available to rescue the OSA patient with respiratory compromise. Supine position should be avoided, and lateral, prone, or sitting position should be used.

Continuous monitoring of oxygenation, breathing, blood pressure, and heart rhythm is required because of the possibility of serious complications such as hypertension, dysrhythmias, hypoxia, and airway obstruction, the latter potentially requiring urgent reintubation.

Discharge Criteria. In addition to the standard discharge criteria used routinely in the postanesthesia care unit (PACU), patients with OSA should be able to maintain adequate oxygenation on room air with no hypoxemia or critical airway obstruction when they are asleep. OSA patients should stay at least 3 hours longer than non-OSA patients to ensure the required discharge criteria. OSA patients who develop an episode of hypoxemia or critical airway obstruction while in the PACU require an extended monitoring period of 7 hours (median time recommended by ASA guidelines in this circumstance) and the most careful evaluation thereafter (many anesthesia providers simply secure a postoperative bed in this instance). Patients with mild OSA who have undergone minor surgery (superficial plastic surgery, eye procedures, and superficial orthopedics) under local or regional anesthesia can be discharged home on the same day. Patients with moderate OSA and intermediate co-morbidities who have undergone intermediate-risk surgery (does not include abdominal, faciomaxillary, thoracic, or intracranial) should be hospitalized in a standard surgical unit. Patients with severe OSA, necessitating CPAP at home and/or who have had major surgical procedures, should be admitted to a step-down unit or intensive care unit until the threat of respiratory complications is no longer present.

TABLE 75.5	CONSULTANT OPINIONS REGARDING PROCEDURES THAT MAY BE PERFORMED SAFELY ON AN OUTPATIENT BASIS FOR PATIENTS AT INCREASED PERIOPERATIVE RISK FOR OBSTRUCTIVE SLEEP APNEA
TYPE OF SURGERY/ANESTHESIA	**CONSULTANT OPINION**
Superficial surgery/local or regional anesthesia	Agree
Superficial surgery/general anesthesia	Equivocal
Airway surgery (e.g., UPPP)	Disagree
Tonsillectomy in children <3 years old	Disagree
Tonsillectomy in children >3 years old	Equivocal
Minor orthopedic surgery/local or regional anesthesia	Agree
Minor orthopedic surgery/general anesthesia	Equivocal
Gynecologic laparoscopy	Equivocal
Laparoscopic surgery, abdominal surgery	Disagree
Lithotripsy	Agree

UPPP, uvulopalatopharyngoplasty.
Source: American Society of Anesthesiologists. Practice guidelines for the perioperative management of patients with obstructive sleep apnea. *Anesthesiology.* 2006;104(5):1087.

Outpatient Surgery. Outpatient surgery for OSA patients remains controversial. According to Sabers et al., the presence of OSA does not increase the risk of readmission to the hospital after ambulatory surgery. However, this view is not shared by many same-day surgery anesthesia providers, and it is the practice in some ambulatory surgery centers to refuse care to sleep apnea patients (and sometimes even suspected sleep apnea patients). Risk must be assessed for each individual patient, because there are a large number of undiagnosed cases of OSA (*Table 75.5*).

OSA CHARACTERISTICS FOR CHILDREN

The peak period for OSA in the pediatric population is preschool age, with equal boy/girl distribution. The common causes are adenotonsillar hypertrophy, obesity, and craniofacial anomalies. Usually, children with OSA suffer growth retardation, hyperactivity disorders, developmental delay, or attention deficit disorders. Excessive daytime somnolence is uncommon in children with OSA. Sleep studies show normal sleep architecture and a <50% cortical arousal with apnea, but results should be interpreted according to the age of the child (*Table 75.1*). The treatment is primarily surgical (adenotonsillectomy), and CPAP is used as required.

Anesthetic management of children with OSA should not include premedication with sedatives and respiratory depressant medication, and a difficult airway should always be anticipated. Induction of general anesthesia is achieved by inhalational agents. The application of an artificial oral airway and CPAP will improve airway patency and mask ventilation. Administration of antisialagogue (anticholinergic) medications can be beneficial during both the intraoperative and postoperative periods. Neuromuscular blockade should either be avoided or full recovery from its effects ensured before extubation. Doses of opioids should be decreased, and it is preferable to use short-acting, noncumulative agents. The incidence of airway obstruction in the immediate postoperative period is higher in children with OSA, especially in those who undergo adenotonsillectomy. Because of the increased risk for postobstructive negative-pressure pulmonary edema that necessitates reintubation and mechanical ventilation, children with moderate to severe OSA should always be hospitalized overnight after surgery.

TAKE HOME POINTS

- Snoring, excessive daytime somnolence, and witnessed apnea episodes together with an AHI >5 are positive for OSA diagnosis.
- In the absence of sleep study, have a high index of suspicion to the diagnosis of OSA in the presence of risk factors.
- Avoid preoperative benzodiazepines or opioids.
- Use regional anesthesia whenever appropriate or general anesthesia with secured airway (an endotracheal tube or, controversially, a laryngeal mask airway).
- Extubate in semiupright position, when the patient is awake and fully recovered from neuromuscular blockade.
- Use supplemental oxygen with or without CPAP and monitor oxygen saturation.
- Avoid the supine position.
- Use adjuncts to decrease opioid requirement.
- Discharge adult patients when they reach their baseline room-air oxygen saturation and have no hypoxemia or critical airway obstruction when not stimulated.
- Pediatric patients with moderate to severe OSA should be hospitalized overnight after surgery.

SUGGESTED READINGS

American Academy of Sleep Medicine Task Force. Sleep related breathing disorders in adults: recommendations for syndrome definition and measurement techniques in clinical research. *Sleep*. 1999;22:667–689.
American Society of Anesthesiologists. Practice guidelines for the perioperative management of patients with obstructive sleep apnea. *Anesthesiology*. 2006;104(5):1081–1093.
Bandla P, Brooks LJ, Trimarchi T, et al. Obstructive sleep apnea syndrome in children. *Anesthesiol Clin North Am*. 2005;23:535–549.

Hiestand MD, Britz P, Goldman M, et al. Prevalence of symptoms and risk of sleep apnea in the US population. Results from the National Sleep Foundation *Sleep in America* 2005 Poll. *Chest.* 2006;130(3):780–786.

Netzer NC, Stoohs RA, Netzer CM, et al. Using the Berlin Questionnaire to identify patients at risk for the sleep apnea syndrome. *Ann Intern Med.* 1999;131:485–491.

Sabers C, Plevak DJ, Schroeder DR, et al. The diagnosis of obstructive sleep apnea as a risk factor for unanticipated admissions in outpatient surgery. *Anesth Analg.* 2003;96:1328.

Suzuki YJ, Jain V, Park AM, et al. Oxidative stress and oxidant signaling in obstructive sleep apnea and associated cardiovascular diseases. *Free Radic Biol Med.* 2006;40(10):1683–1692.

76

HAVE A HIGH INDEX OF SUSPICION FOR PERIOPERATIVE PULMONARY EMBOLISM IN PATIENTS WHO HAVE TRAVELED TO YOUR HOSPITAL BY AIR[*]

ABRAM H. BURGHER, MD AND JURAJ SPRUNG, MD, PhD

Prolonged immobility associated with long-distance air travel predisposes patients to deep vein thrombosis (DVT) and venous thromboembolism (VTE). A recent systematic review found that long-haul flights of 8 hours or more increased the risk of thrombosis, with asymptomatic DVT developing in up to 10% of such travelers. The prolonged immobility and hypercoagulable state associated with major surgery (especially lower-extremity orthopedic or pelvic surgery) may add to this risk. Therefore, patients who travel long distances to have surgery may be at high risk for perioperative venothrombotic events. Indeed, in a large retrospective review at Mayo Clinic, patients traveling more than 5,000 km had a higher rate ($\approx$30×) of perioperative VTE than those traveling a shorter distance before surgery. In that study, those in whom VTE developed also were younger, had VTE development significantly earlier in the postoperative course, had a higher American Society of Anesthesiologists (ASA) physical status classification, and were more likely to be smokers. Therefore, all perioperative physicians should be aware of this risk and must be ready to recognize even the subtle signs and symptoms of DVT and pulmonary embolism (PE) to avoid catastrophic perioperative complications of PE.

Several mechanisms have been proposed by which long-haul air travel may contribute to the risk of VTE. Long periods of relative immobility (also called "economy class syndrome"), especially in patients sitting in nonaisle seats; obstruction of venous return as a result of compression of popliteal veins at the edge of the seat; exposure to hypobaric, low-humidity air; the stress of travel; hypercoagulability (seen even in healthy volunteers exposed to a simulated airplane cabin environment); and possibly dehydration resulting from decreased fluid intake or excessive use of alcohol during the trip all may be additive risk factors.

Morbidity and mortality from VTE is attributable primarily to PE, which is sometimes difficult to diagnose in the perioperative period because

---

[*] Portions of this chapter were previously published in Gajic D, Warner DO, Decker PA, Rana R, Bourke DL, Sprung J. Long-haul air travel before major surgery: a prescription for thromboembolism? *Mayo Clin Proc.* 2005;80:728–731. Used with permission of Mayo Foundation for Medical Education and Research.

clinical manifestations are often nonspecific. Manifestations include dyspnea, substernal chest pain, syncope, tachycardia or even cardiac dysrhythmias, and worsening of pre-existing congestive heart failure. Pleuritic chest pain and hemoptysis are seen only when pulmonary infarction has occurred. Physical examination may indicate lower-extremity swelling resulting from obstruction of venous outflow by thrombus in large vessels.

Results of electrocardiography are altered in most cases, although abnormalities are often subtle and nonspecific. T-wave inversion in the precordial leads ("anterior ischemic pattern") is the most common finding in massive PE. Tachycardia and signs of right ventricular strain (right-axis deviation, peaked P waves, and ST–T-segment abnormalities) may be observed. When seen together, an S wave in lead I, a Q wave in lead III, and an inverted T wave in lead III are suggestive of PE. This "S1, Q3, T3" pattern has a sensitivity of about 50% for both massive and nonmassive PE.

Arterial blood gas analysis generally shows arterial hypoxemia with a widened alveolar-to-arterial O_2 gradient and respiratory alkalosis. Because of its high sensitivity (>95%), testing for elevated D-dimers may potentially be a useful preoperative screen for patients suspected of having VTE. However, because D-dimer levels can fluctuate widely in the postoperative period, this test is not likely to be of great utility immediately after surgery without corroborative evidence. Definitive testing for DVT or VTE can only be accomplished with venous angiography, computed tomography, or pulmonary angiography (for PE only). Definitive testing may be merited in patients presenting with any of the above signs or symptoms, especially in long-distance travelers, a group known to have a higher probability of VTE.

Patients traveling long distances (especially overseas) before surgery should be made aware of the potential for increased risk of perioperative thrombotic complications. Preoperative in-flight prevention could include maintaining hydration, exercise, and elastic compression stockings. In addition, high-risk patients may benefit from perioperative pharmacologic prophylaxis for DVT and VTE. Because VTE is sometimes a difficult diagnosis to make in the perioperative period and its potential morbidity is so high, these patients should have careful perioperative surveillance. Unexplained hypoxemia, leg swelling, and electrocardiographic abnormalities are all alarming findings in a patient traveling a long distance for surgery.

TAKE HOME POINTS

- Venous thromboembolism is not rare in long-haul air travelers—ask your patients how they traveled to the hospital, especially if you are at a tertiary referral center.

- VTE is more common in patients who are younger, have higher ASA status, and who are smokers.
- Consider examining your patients specifically for signs of VTE in the immediate preoperative period. Also consider a repeat electrocardiogram to look for new changes that might be indicative of PE.
- One final note—many referral hospitals in the Midwest and Western states (including those in the public health system) draw patients long distance by car or bus. Patients traveling more than 500 miles by car on the day before surgery may warrant similar consideration.

SUGGESTED READINGS

Adi Y, Bayliss S, Rouse A, et al. The association between air travel and deep vein thrombosis: systematic review & meta-analysis. *BMC Cardiovasc Disord.* 2004;4:7.

Barash PG, Cullen BF, Stoelting RK, eds. *Clinical Anesthesia.* 4th ed. Philadelphia: Lippincott Williams & Wilkins; 2001.

Belcaro G, Cesarone MR, Shah SS, et al. Prevention of edema, flight microangiopathy and venous thrombosis in long flights with elastic stockings: a randomized trial: the LONFLIT 4 Concorde Edema-SSL Study. *Angiology.* 2002;53:635–645.

Bendz B, Rostrup M, Sevre K, et al. Association between acute hypobaric hypoxia and activation of coagulation in human beings. *Lancet.* 2000;356:1657–1658.

Ferrari E, Imbert A, Chevalier T, et al. The ECG in pulmonary embolism: predictive value of negative T waves in precordial leads: 80 case reports. *Chest.* 1997;111:537–543.

Gajic O, Sprung J, Hall BA, et al. Fatal acute pulmonary embolism in a patient with pelvic lipomatosis after surgery performed after transatlantic airplane travel. *Anesth Analg.* 2004;99:1032–1034.

Gajic O, Warner DO, Decker PA, et al. Long-haul air travel before major surgery: a prescription for thromboembolism? *Mayo Clin Proc.* 2005;80:728–731.

Lippi G, Veraldi GF, Fraccaroli M, et al. Variation of plasma D-dimer following surgery: implications for prediction of postoperative venous thromboembolism. *Clin Exp Med.* 2001;1:161–164.

Stein PD, Hull RD, Patel KC, et al. D-dimer for the exclusion of acute venous thrombosis and pulmonary embolism: a systematic review. *Ann Intern Med.* 2004;140:589–602.

77

BE AWARE THAT SCHIZOPHRENIC PATIENTS HAVE GREATER PERIOPERATIVE RISKS THAN AGE-MATCHED CONTROLS

NEIL B. SANDSON, MD

A large body of evidence has demonstrated that schizophrenic individuals are afflicted with a wide array of medical problems. Some of these issues are likely due to genetic abnormalities that are associated with schizophrenia. Other medical concerns develop as a result of poor attention to self-care and inconsistent medical follow-up that arise from the hypofrontality/ negative symptoms that actually generate most of the longitudinal morbidity of schizophrenia. Schizophrenic patients are also more likely to engage in lifestyle behaviors that affect their health status adversely, such as poor compliance with medications and/or perioperative instructions, smoking, poor dietary intake, and use of drugs and alcohol. It is also likely that antipsychotic medications contribute to this greater prevalence of medical co-morbidities. Taken together, these medical issues significantly increase operative risk in schizophrenic patients.

It has been estimated that schizophrenic patients have a 20% shorter life expectancy than age-matched controls. Another study found that schizophrenia is associated with a greater prevalence of heart disease, chronic obstructive pulmonary disease, hypertension, and diabetes. Some research suggests that there are increased rates of hyperglycemia and diabetes, hyperlipidemia, hypercholesterolemia, and obesity that occur as intrinsic, associated features of this illness. Obstructive sleep apnea is especially prevalent among schizophrenic patients. The operative risks posed by these problems are only exacerbated by the tendency for schizophrenic patients to neglect their own care. These metabolic abnormalities are allowed to persist without medical intervention far more frequently than is the case in the general population. Thus, progression to significant cardiac, pulmonary, and renal pathology is more frequent, leading to greater operative risk.

Although antipsychotic drugs are essential in the management of schizophrenia, the vast majority of these agents have been implicated in generating all of these metabolic abnormalities. Thus, these drugs can exacerbate the risks that already arise from the illness itself. Additionally, antipsychotic agents often increase the length of the QT interval, yielding a greater risk of malignant arrhythmias. One drug in particular, clozapine, has

© 2006 Mayo Foundation for Medical Education and Research

been associated with myocarditis as well as significant lowering of the seizure threshold.

Although it may seem counterintuitive or irrelevant to the core symptoms that define schizophrenia, it is important to keep the greater prevalence of medical co-morbidities in mind when assessing operative risk in this patient population.

TAKE HOME POINTS

- Besides the obvious mental health issues, schizophrenic patients warrant careful attention to their medical status.
- The increase in perioperative risk is multifactorial.
- *Be aware that sleep apnea is especially prevalent in schizophrenic patients.* An anecdote from the author: It was a great relief for everybody (patients and staff alike) when the "dorm rooms" housing six patients were eliminated from the modern psychiatric hospital layout. "In the old days," it was not unheard of to have six large, male, schizophrenic patients, all of whom had gained 30 pounds from their atypical antipsychotic medications, all suffering from a degree of sleep apnea, disrupting each others' sleep, and making it difficult for anyone to get rested and/or well.

SUGGESTED READINGS

Allison DB, Casey DE. Antipsychotic-induced weight gain: a review of the literature. *J Clin Psychiatry* 2001;62(suppl 7):22–31.

Covell NH, Jackson CT, Weissman EM. Health monitoring for patients who have schizophrenia. Summary of the Mount Sinai Conference recommendations. *Postgrad Med (Special Report)*. September 2006:20–26.

Glassman AH, Bigger JT Jr. Antipsychotic drugs: prolonged QTc interval, torsade de pointes, and sudden death. *Am J Psychiatry.* 2001;158(11):1774–1782.

Lambert TJ, Velakoulis D, Pantelis C. Medical comorbidity in schizophrenia. *Med J Aust.* 2003;178(suppl):S67–S70.

Winkelman JW. Schizophrenia, obesity, and obstructive sleep apnea. *J Clin Psychiatry.* 2001;62(1):8–11.

78

USE EXTRA CARE IN POSITIONING PATIENTS WHO HAVE HAD AMPUTATIONS

CAROL F. BODENHEIMER, MD AND CATHERINE MARCUCCI, MD

All anesthesia providers must take extra care with patients with amputations to avoid positioning injuries. Be aware that limbs that have sustained partial amputation have undergone subtle but very real changes in musculoskeletal structure, skin integrity, and somatic and autonomic innervation.

The joints proximal to an amputation are often affected on both the contralateral and ipsilateral sides. For example, because of increased weight bearing in the contralateral leg, it is very common after lower-limb amputation for the contralateral hip to develop significant osteoarthritis. This is true even for patients who use a prosthesis. On the ipsilateral side in above-knee amputations, a hip flexure contracture results from immobility (more time sitting) and a hip abduction contracture from loss of the insertions of the adductors to the distal femur. On the ipsilateral side in below-knee amputations, a knee flexion contracture develops as a result of impaired mobility and loss of quadriceps extension strength. This is very common even in relatively young and active patients and will predispose a patient to injury in any position involving extension at the knee, such as the simple supine position. A pad below the distal thigh allows mild knee flexion and protects the integrity of the skin at the end of the stump.

In all types of amputation, there can be subcutaneous fibrosis at the amputation site that puts the overlying skin at risk because of increased tension and decreased blood flow. In many patients with amputations, the underlying medical reason for the amputation (diabetes or vascular disease) may mean that the skin of the residual limb is at high risk for skin breakdown independent of amputation. Even in patients whose limb loss was due to trauma, there is a higher risk of skin breakdown because of concomitant skin disorders such as contact dermatitis and verrucous hyperplasia. Patients who show skin breakdown or ulceration on a residual limb should be positioned so that there is minimal chance of further pressure injuries. Perturbations in both the somatic and autonomic nervous systems can cause patients who have had amputations to experience a variety of hypersensivity and chronic pain syndromes, including causalgia and phantom limb pain. Positioning injuries therefore can also cause an acute-on-chronic pain syndrome that can be especially distressing to the patient.

© 2006 Mayo Foundation for Medical Education and Research

It is now understood that the perception of pain involves cortical processing of afferent input to the nervous system. There is also a tremendously complex interplay among all types of pain and psychologic and emotional resilience. Amputation patients have an array of psychological "defenses" pertaining to their amputations, ranging from World War II veterans who say simply, "I got my leg shot off in Germany," as if they were ordering coffee, to patients who carefully guard their residual limbs. Patients who have had recent amputations may also be prone to depression. Ask if there is pain in the limb and discuss the plan for careful positioning with the patient. This can lessen anxiety, which is a good start to preventing pain. It is also appropriate to check for changes in the usual pain pattern during the postoperative check.

TAKE HOME POINTS

- A new generation of war-wounded patients will be entering care in both civilian and veterans hospital—a significant percentage of whom will have had one or more amputations.
- Be attentive to changes in musculoskeletal structure, skin, and innervation.
- Above-knee amputees can have hip flexion and abduction contractures requiring positioning that must account for this.
- Below-knee amputations can result in knee flexion contractures.
- Subcutaneous fibrosis can put the overlying skin at increased tension with decreased underlying blood flow.
- Positioning injuries can result in acute-on-chronic pain in amputated limbs.
- If possible, involve the patient in the positioning before induction of anesthesia.

SUGGESTED READINGS

Bryant PR, Pandian G. Acquired limb deficiencies in children and young adults. *Arch Phys Med Rehab*. 2001;82:3(suppl 1):S3–S8.

McAnelly RD, Faulkner VW. Lower limb prostheses. In: Braddom, RL, ed. *Physical Medicine and Rehabilitation*, Philadelphia: WB Saunders; 1996:289–320.

Pandian G, Huang ME, Duffy DA. Perioperative mangement in acquired limb deficiencies. *Arch Phys Med Rehab*. 2001;82:3(suppl 1):S9–S16.

Wikoff, EK. Preprosthetic management. *Phys Med Rehab: State Art Rev.* 1994;(8)1:61–72.

79

POSITIONING PATIENTS FOR SPINE SURGERY: HOW TO MINIMIZE THE RISKS

IHAB R. KAMEL, MD, DAVID Y. KIM, MD, AND
RODGER BARNETTE, MD, FCCM

The obligatory positions required for spine surgery subject patients to significant risk above and beyond the inherent risk of the procedure itself. These risks include, but are not limited to, injury to the eyes, ears, nose, breasts, penis, extremities, and peripheral nerves. Peripheral nerve injury is a well-recognized anesthetic complication and is the second largest cause of malpractice actions in anesthesiology, accounting for 16% of claims. Minimizing potential injury to peripheral nerves through proper positioning and monitoring is extremely important.

Monitoring of somatosensory evoked potentials (SSEP) is frequently utilized during spine surgery (75%) and is available in most institutions in the United States (94%). In addition to monitoring spinal cord function, SSEP can detect peripheral nerve injury during spine surgery. Conduction changes, such as a decrease in amplitude or an increase in latency of the signal, are believed to indicate impending upper-extremity nerve injury. Modification of the arm position by the anesthesiologist often improves the SSEP signal and may return it to baseline. Reversal of position-related SSEP changes can influence impending nerve injury and prevent postoperative peripheral nerve injury.

The prone position is a dangerous position for patients. Attention to securing the airway is very important, as it is difficult to re-establish an airway in the prone position. Though we must always be cautious regarding protection of the eyes, this position raises additional concerns. Both ophthalmic ointment and occlusive eye tape may be appropriate if the procedure involves the cervical spine; prep solution that comes into direct contact with the eyes can lead to corneal injury. Additionally, we must assure that there is no direct pressure on the eye, ears, or nose. Pressure could lead to loss of function and/or a disfiguring ischemic injury. For the same reason, it is important when positioning chest rolls to assure yourself that the breasts in women and the genitalia in men are free from compression of any sort.

With regard to the patients' extremities, the mechanisms of nerve injury associated with surgical positioning and anesthesia are not completely understood. Peripheral nerve injury may be due to direct trauma or more commonly due to ischemia of the intraneural capillaries. Compression of

© 2006 Mayo Foundation for Medical Education and Research

peripheral nerves or stretch beyond 15% of original length may also cause peripheral nerve injury. Diabetes, hypertension, and uremia are known to affect peripheral nerves and predispose them to injury; intraoperative conditions such as prolonged hypotension and anemia are believed to facilitate ischemic injury. Finally, certain operative positions are known to place patients at increased risk for nerve damage. During spine surgery the overall incidence of impending upper-extremity peripheral nerve injury, as defined by changes in the SSEP, is >6%.

The ulnar nerve and the brachial plexus are the most commonly injured neural structures during this type of surgery. Risk factors for ulnar nerve injury include male gender, very thin or very obese patients, and prolonged hospitalization for >14 days. Risk factors for brachial plexus injury include the use of shoulder braces, the prone head-down position, and some regional anesthetic techniques such as interscalene and axillary blocks.

There are five positions commonly employed during spine surgery: supine, arms out; supine, arms tucked; lateral decubitus; prone "Superman" position; and prone, arms tucked. The prone "Superman" position and the lateral decubitus position have been identified as high-risk positions for upper-extremity nerve injury; especially if the surgical procedure is prolonged. Techniques for minimizing injury in these positions are reviewed below.

The incidence of impending upper-extremity nerve injury during spine surgery in the supine arms-out position is 3.2%. Overstretch of the brachial plexus can occur as a result of abduction of the shoulder >90 degrees and should be consistently avoided. Direct compression of the ulnar nerve against the medial epicondyle may occur, especially if the forearm is in the prone position. Placing the forearm in the supine or neutral position decreases pressure over the ulnar nerve at the elbow. Elbows should be padded to further protect the nerve from compression. Direct compression of the radial nerve in the spiral groove of the humerus can be avoided with proper padding. Overextension of the elbow should be avoided because it may stretch the median nerve. The patient's head and neck should ideally be maintained in a midline position. Tilting the head and neck laterally may stretch the contralateral brachial plexus.

The incidence of impending upper-extremity nerve injury during spine surgery in the supine arms-tucked position during spine surgery is 1.8%. The tucked arms should be placed in neutral positions to decrease the pressure over the ulnar nerve. The ulnar nerve should be padded at the elbow for additional protection. Shoulder tape, which is often applied by the surgeon to pull the shoulders down and maximize the lateral radiographic view of the spine, may compress the brachial plexus. The duration of application of this shoulder tape should be minimized. The head and neck should be maintained in midline position. Placement of the patient's forearms on the lower abdomen should be avoided, as excessive flexion at the elbow joint can simultaneously stretch and compress the ulnar nerve.

The lateral decubitus position is a challenging position for the anesthesiologist. The incidence of impending upper-extremity peripheral nerve injury during spine surgery in the lateral decubitus position is 7.5%. Compression of the brachial plexus is the most common mechanism of injury. The dependent brachial plexus can be compressed between the clavicle and first rib as well as against the humeral head. Obese patients and patients placed in a head-down position are at higher risk, as compressive forces are augmented. A chest roll should be placed to elevate the dependent chest and decrease the likelihood of compression. The chest roll should not be placed in the axilla, but under the lateral, superior chest; the goal is to prevent compression of the contents of the axillae. The dependent arm should be padded at the elbow and maintained in the supinated position to avoid compression of the ulnar nerve. To minimize the likelihood of brachial plexus stretch, abduction of the dependent and nondependent arm should be less than 90 degrees. Excessive flexion or extension at the elbow should be avoided. The elbow in the nondependent forearm should be padded, and lateral rotation of the shoulder should be avoided. The patient's head and neck should be maintained in a midline neutral position without excessive flexion or extension.

The prone "Superman" position is another challenging position with a relatively higher incidence of impending upper-extremity nerve injury (7%). Stretching forces on the brachial plexus is the commonest mechanism of injury. Again shoulder abduction beyond 90 degrees should be avoided, and the patient's head and neck should be in a neutral midline position. Elbows should be padded and the forearm and hand placed in a neutral position. Placing patients in steep head-down position should be avoided or limited if possible. Pressure from chest rolls should not be directly on the shoulders and the clavicle, as they may compress the brachial plexus, especially in obese patients. In women, the position of the chest rolls should be checked to ensure that there is no possibility of ischemic injury to the breasts. In men, the position of the lower roll should be checked to confirm that the genitalia are free from direct compression.

The prone arms-tucked position is relatively lower-risk compared to the prone "Superman" and the lateral decubitus positions. The incidence of impending nerve injury in the prone arms-tucked position during spine surgery is 2.1%. Special attention should be given to positioning the head and neck as described in the previous paragraph. The forearms should be in neutral positions. Shoulder tape, applied to maximize the lateral radiographic view of the neck, should be minimized. The elbows should be padded to avoid compression by arm sleds. Direct compression by the chest rolls is of concern as in the prone "Superman" position.

Attention to detail is one of the reasons for our specialty's superior safety record. When caring for patients undergoing spinal surgery, we must assume an integral role in positioning, monitoring, and interceding as appropriate.

TAKE HOME POINTS

- The prone position can be dangerous for patients. Attention must be given to preventing injury to eyes, ears, nose, breasts, penis, extremities, and peripheral nerves.
- Somatosensory evoked potential monitoring can be used to detect and prevent peripheral nerve injury during spine surgery.
- The lateral decubitus position and the prone "Superman" position are high-risk positions for nerve injury during spine surgery.
- Abduction of the shoulder beyond 90 degrees should be avoided because it stretches and may injure the brachial plexus.
- Excessive flexion of the elbow should be avoided; it stretches and compresses the ulnar nerve.
- Excessive extension of the elbow should be avoided because it stretches the median nerve.
- The forearm in the supinated position may be safest because of the decreased pressure on the ulnar nerve; the neutral position is a good second choice.
- Appropriate padding can minimize excessive pressure on the radial nerve in the spiral groove.

SUGGESTED READINGS

Caplan RA. Will we ever understand perioperative neuropathy? *Anesthesiology*. 1999;91:345–354.

Kamel IR, Drum ET, Koch SA, et al. The use of somatosensory evoked potentials to determine the relationship between patient positioning and impending upper extremity nerve injury during spine surgery: a retrospective analysis. *Anesth Analg*. 2006;102:1538–1542.

Kroll DA, Caplan RA, Posner K, et al. Nerve injury associated with anesthesia. *Anesthesiology*. 1990;73:202–207.

Lawson NW, Meyer DJ Jr. Lateral positions. In: Martin JT, Warner MA, eds. *Positioning in Anesthesiology and Surgery*. 3rd ed. Philadelphia: WB Saunders; 1997:127–152.

Mahla M, Black S, Cucchiara R. Neurologic monitoring. In: Miller RD, ed. *Miller's Anesthesia*. 6th ed. Philadelphia: Churchill Livingstone; 2005:1511–1550.

Martin JT. The ventral decubitus (prone) positions. In: Martin JT, Warner MA, eds. *Positioning in Anesthesiology and Surgery*. Philadelphia: WB Saunders; 1997:155–195.

Prielipp RC, Morell RC, Walker FO, et al. Influence of arm position and relationship to somatosensory evoked potentials. *Anesthesiology*. 1999;91:345–354.

Schwartz DM, Drummond DS, Hahn M, et al. Prevention of positional brachial plexopathy during surgical correction of scoliosis. *J Spinal Disord*. 2000;13:178–182.

80

BE VIGILANT DURING PLACEMENT OF THE CAMERA IN LAPAROSCOPIC PROCEDURES AND ALWAYS WATCH CAREFULLY FOR THE PHYSIOLOGIC EFFECTS OF CARBON DIOXIDE (CO_2) INSUFFLATION

JENNIFER A. DECOU, MD AND RANDAL O. DULL, MD, PHD

Laparoscopic surgery presents challenging issues for the anesthesiologist. It is one of the few procedures in which the surgical "incision" has resulted in life-threatening events. It is also in the category of surgical procedures (much like the methylmethacrylate cases in orthopedic surgery) in which the *surgeons* administer a substance with wide-ranging physiologic sequelae.

The first task for the anesthesiologist is to ascertain by query or observation the planned technique for initial entry into the abdomen. Surgical practice has tended to evolve away from the Veress needle technique, which involves picking up the skin on either side of the umbilicus and using a "blind" technique to first pass a needle followed by a trochar. This technique has resulted in the uncommon but devastating complications of aorta and bowel injury. Much more common today is the Hassan cannula technique, which involves a microlaparotomy and placement of the initial intra-abdominal instrument (which is blunt-tipped) under direct observation. Subsequent trochars are then placed under camera visualization after insufflation.

Try to observe the placement of the trochars personally. It is not necessarily true that several attempts to place trochars and/or failure to initially insufflate to a proper pressure means trouble, especially with the Hassan technique. The trochars have a "cocking" mechanism that allows the sharp point to protrude out of the sheath, and this may need to be reset if activated when the surgeon attempts to place the trochar through the layers of the abdominal wall. Also, there may be leakage around the Hassan cannula, and the surgeon may ask for Xeroform to wrap around the cannula to get a seal. In general, however, placement of the trochars should go fairly smoothly without an excessive number of attempts.

Of course, it is the insufflation of the abdomen or pelvis with gas (usually CO_2) to improve visualization of the surgical field that results in the physiologic changes that are of interest to us. The high solubility of CO_2 allows rapid diffusion into the blood compartment and causes predictable changes in blood gas chemistries and hypercapnia. It must be remembered at all times

© 2006 Mayo Foundation for Medical Education and Research

that the physiologic effects of insufflation and the resulting hypercapnia are multisystemic and quite complex.

CARDIOVASCULAR EFFECTS

The potential cardiovascular effects are the ones most pronounced at the time of and just after insufflation. They require that a range of resuscitative drugs be available. Hypercarbia and the associated acidosis cause direct cardiac depression and peripheral vasodilatation, which can lead to hypotension. However, hypercarbia also promotes a strong sympathetic reflex and increases in plasma catecholamine levels may offset this depressant activity. The result is a hyperkinetic circulation with hypercarbia causing a tachycardia, increased cardiac output, increased contractility, and increased systemic blood pressure. These changes may increase myocardial O_2 demand, and patients with known or suspected coronary artery disease will require appropriate interventions. In addition, arrhythmias are a commonly encountered problem during laparoscopic procedures. Hypercarbia, acidosis, and the associated increase in catecholamines may sensitize the myocardium and induce a variety of arrhythmias. Vagally mediated reflexes caused by insufflation can induce a variety of bradyarrhythmias, including asystole. Lastly, increases in intra-abdominal pressure can inhibit venous return, resulting in decreased cardiac output and hypotension; adjustments to intravascular volume may be required to normalize venous return and maintain cardiac output.

INTRACRANIAL EFFECTS

The intracranial effects of insufflation are the easiest to overlook, as it is extremely rare to have direct measurement of intracranial pressure (ICP) during laparoscopic surgery.

CO$_2$ is the primary regulator of cerebral blood flow through its effect of inducing cerebral vasodilatation. Cerebral blood flow increases linearly with changes in P_{CO_2} between 20 and 100 mm Hg. ICP is a function of brain mass, cerebrospinal fluid volume, and blood volume. Although the relationship between cerebral blood flow and ICP is complex, a general assumption should be that increases in P_{CO_2} will increase ICP. In the absence of direct ICP monitoring, prudence suggests that any change in CO_2 above normal may increase ICP. It is not uncommon for a senior practitioner to hear the question, "How high can we let the CO_2 go?" A reasonable answer is that acceptable limits to the increase in P_{CO_2} during laparoscopic procedures should be directly related to concerns regarding elevated ICP. Thus a patient who should be exposed to only moderate increases in ICP should undergo only moderate increases in P_{CO_2}.

PULMONARY EFFECTS

Insufflation of the abdomen is generally considered among the stronger indications for endotracheal intubation because the pulmonary changes that occur during CO_2 insufflation are usually related to increased intra-abdominal pressure. The upward displacement of the diaphragm can predispose to passive or active regurgitation, cause atelectasis, reduce functional residual capacity (FRC), create an intrapulmonary shunt, and produce ventilation/perfusion (V/Q) mismatching and hypoxemia. Higher P_{CO2} levels as the case progresses may also cause the resumption of spontaneous ventilation. To offset these changes, administration of higher doses of neuromuscular blockade, adjustments to the rate of mechanical ventilation, tidal volume, inspiratory flow rate, and the implementation of lung volume recruitment efforts are all part of intraoperative management during laparoscopic procedures. In addition, the anesthesiologist must always be vigilant for increases in airway pressure caused by a pneumothorax, which can occur when laparoscopic procedures are performed close to the diaphragm (e.g., gastric fundoplication).

SOFT TISSUE EFFECTS

It is common for patients to develop subcutaneous emphysema during long laparoscopic procedures. Because of the high solubility of CO_2, considerable quantities can accumulate within body tissues during long procedures. Consider carefully and on an individual basis before extubating patients who have undergone extended laparoscopic procedures. The large majority of patients can be and are extubated at the end of the procedure, but there are several issues complicating extubation. Subcutaneous emphysema involving the head and neck can be ascertained by visual inspection or by palpation—the patient may have a "crackling" under the skin. This may require postoperative intubation to prevent airway obstruction and while tissue stores are removed. Also, always be aware that subcutaneous emphysema can be a sign of pneumothorax. Additionally, elderly patients and/or those with pre-existing pulmonary disease may be unable to sustain the P_{CO2}-induced high minute ventilation following extubation and are at higher risk for reintubation.

One final note regarding the management of the sequelae of insufflation and hypercapnia is that in patients with comorbidities, those with impaired CO_2 excretion capacity (e.g., patients with chronic obstructive pulmonary disease), and patients with acute cardiopulmonary disturbances, strongly consider an arterial line for hemodynamic and blood gas monitoring.

TAKE HOME POINTS

■ Personally observe placement of the trochar—make sure the surgeons are using the Hassan technique.

- The physiologic effects of insufflation and hypercapnia are complex and can result in significant sequelae in cardiovascular, intracranial, and pulmonary status.
- Check every patient for significant subcutaneous emphysema in the chest and neck—look for "crackling" under the skin. Subcutaneous emphysema can indicate a clinically significant pneumothorax or predict a failed extubation.

SUGGESTED READINGS

Gutt CN, Mehrabi A, Schemmer P, et al. Circulatory and respiratory complications of carbon dioxide insufflation. *Digestive Surg.* 2004;21:95–105.

Miller R, ed. *Miller's Anesthesia.* 6th ed. Philadelphia: Elsevier Churchill Livingstone; 2004:2286–2299.

81

DO NOT USE URINE OUTPUT AS AN INDICATOR OF VOLUME STATUS IN HYPOTHERMIC PATIENTS

JUAN N. PULIDO, MD AND DANIEL R. BROWN, MD, PhD

Hypothermia is a clinical entity defined as a core body temperature less than 35°C (95°F) and is classified in four stages depending on the temperature, symptomatology, and effect on specific organ physiology (*Table 81.1*).

All organs are ultimately affected by hypothermia, including the kidneys. The renal response to cold is rapid and varies with the different stages of hypothermia. Initially, peripheral vasoconstriction results in relative central hypervolemia producing an increase in urine output. This response, termed "cold diuresis," has been described even in patients with mild to moderate hypothermia. The etiology of this phenomenon is multifactorial and includes an initial increase in cardiac output and renal blood flow resulting from hypothermia-induced changes in vascular capacitance. Other important contributors are nonosmotic suppression of antidiuretic hormone (ADH) release by the hypothalamus and subsequent decreased renal tubular reabsorption. These responses usually begin as soon as the core body temperature reaches 35°C and become more pronounced until moderate hypothermia, when decreased renal blood flow and glomerular filtration rate (reduced 50% at 27°C to 30°C) may lead to renal failure.

Even in the setting of a large diuresis (the urine is usually dilute, with osmolarity <300 mOsm/L and specific gravity <1.003), the kidneys are unable to handle nitrogenous waste because of tubular dysfunction. Although they are uncommon, electrolyte disturbances including hypernatremia, hyperchloremia, and hyperkalemia can occur and are more frequent as hypothermia progresses in duration and/or severity. "Cold diuresis" is exacerbated by ethanol ingestion and water submersion, which may coexist with hypothermia and can potentiate inappropriate diuresis by inhibiting ADH secretion.

It is important to understand the pathophysiology of this phenomenon when making clinical decisions regarding fluid management in hypothermic patients. The "cold diuresis" can be massive and generally creates a hypovolemic state that worsens with rewarming because of the reverse changes in vascular tone as core body temperature is raised. If it is overlooked or underappreciated, this phenomenon can exacerbate electrolyte disturbances, contribute to hypotension, and result in prerenal stress.

© 2006 Mayo Foundation for Medical Education and Research

TABLE 81.1

STAGE	CORE TEMPERATURE, °C (°F)	CHARACTERISTICS
Mild	32 (89.6) to 35 (95)	Increased metabolic rate, hypertension, tachycardia, shivering, *cold diuresis*, CNS hyperexcitability, coagulopathy
Moderate	28 (82.4) to 32 (89.6)	Decreased cardiac output, hypoventilation, CNS depression, atrial arrhythmias, ↓ O_2 consumption (~25–50%)
Severe	22 (71.6) to 28 (82.4)	Progressive hypotension and bradycardia, ventricular arrhythmias, VF, decreased CBF, areflexia, loss of bulbar reflexes, decreased O_2 consumption (<50% of baseline)
Profound	<22 (71.6)	Asystole, EEG burst suppression

CNS, central nervous system; VF, ventricular fibrillation; CBF, cerebral blood flow; EEG, electroencephalogram.

Intravascular volume status should be closely monitored to avoid complications of this "physiologically inappropriate" renal response. Initially, it should be assumed that the patient is significantly dehydrated. Frequent measurements of electrolytes and hematocrit will help guide fluid therapy and electrolyte replacement, and help monitor for dehydration. Central venous access should be considered to allow for safer electrolyte replacement and rapid-volume administration, though electrolyte abnormalities may increase cardiac irritability and arrhythmia risk during catheter placement. Invasive arterial blood pressure monitoring should also be considered to facilitate laboratory determinations and to evaluate fluid responsiveness.

TAKE HOME POINTS

- The kidneys respond rapidly to hypothermia.
- Cold diuresis will occur even in patients with mild to moderate hypothermia.
- The etiology is multifactorial, including changes in cardiac output, organ perfusion, and suppression of ADH.
- Cold diuresis is exacerbated by ethanol ingestion and water submersion.

■ Assume that cold patients are significantly dehydrated—consider central venous access and invasive arterial blood pressure monitoring.

SUGGESTED READINGS

Auerbach PS. *Wilderness Medicine*. 4th ed. Philadelphia: Mosby; 2001:135–155.

Irwin RS, Rippe JM, eds. *Irwin and Rippe's Intensive Care Medicine*. 5th ed. Philadelphia: Lippincott Williams & Wilkins; 2003:751–755.

Morgan ML. Mechanism of cold diuresis in the rat. *Am J Physiol*. 1983;244(2):F210–F216.

82

ANESTHESIA FOR EYE SURGERY—THE INNATE CULTURE OF "1-N-1"

AMIT SHARMA, MD AND SAJEEV S. KATHURIA, MD, FACS

"Indolence is a delightful but distressing state; we must be doing something to be happy"—Mahatma Gandhi

"What are your concerns during an eye surgery?" we asked the resident. "My attending might walk into the room and catch me snoozing!" was his reply. "What about your anesthesia?" we tried challenging him. "Oh! I will just use my one-and-one," he said cautiously.

This benign scenario is disturbingly common across the anesthesia community. With the advancement and increasing acceptance of topical and regional techniques, general anesthesia is uncommonly needed for ophthalmic surgeries. Even with regional techniques, the onus of block performance has shifted toward the surgeons, further impeding our involvement in patient care. Under these circumstances, it is not surprising that more and more anesthesia providers dislike working on the "eye surgery" cases, because they all "enjoy" doing the "stuff" and hate *just sitting there*. Interestingly, there is a lot more to anesthetic care for eye surgeries than just providing 1 mL of midazolam and fentanyl. The purpose of this chapter is to highlight some of these vital issues.

Topical and regional anesthesia seems to be adequate for the majority of eye cases. Most ophthalmic surgeons prefer the quicker recovery with these techniques and do not request "general anesthesia" unless it is necessary. For some cases, however, it is necessary (*Table 82.1*). It is also occasionally necessary to convert to a general anesthetic in the middle of the procedure. When faced with a request for general anesthesia, junior anesthesia providers sometimes have a tendency to both "oversedate" and "overdebate" before complying with the request. There are several ways to avoid this.

The first step is to make sure that a complete set of intubating and resuscitative drugs is available and readily accessible as well as laryngoscopes and endotracheal tubes.

After that, a little understanding about ocular anatomy helps in predicting cases that may not be effectively covered by available regional techniques. For most ocular surgeries, blocking five cranial nerves (CN II through CN VI) is usually sufficient. CN II (optic nerve) conveys vision; CN III

© 2006 Mayo Foundation for Medical Education and Research

TABLE 82.1   INDICATIONS FOR GENERAL ANESTHESIA IN OCULAR SURGERIES

Absolute
1) Pediatric patients
2) Uncooperative patients (e.g., those with altered mental status, anxiety, or severe claustrophobia)
3) Lengthy procedures (>3 hours)
4) Surgical procedures not adequately covered by regional anesthetic techniques

Relative
1) Patients with penetrating eye injuries
2) Patients on anticoagulant therapy
3) Surgical cases requiring complete ocular akinesia
4) Patients with a history of nystagmus
5) Anatomic abnormalities making regional techniques challenging or unsafe
6) Patient's or surgeon's preference

Source: Navaleza JS, Pendse SJ, Blecher MH. Choosing anesthesia for cataract surgery. *Ophthalmol Clin North Am.* 2006;19(2):233–237.

(oculomotor), IV (trochlear) and VI (abducens) supply the extra-ocular muscles; while the sensory supply of the globe (or eyeball) is mainly from the ophthalmic division of CN V (trigeminal). The periorbital skin (eyelids, eyebrow, forehead, and nose) is supplied by branches of the ophthalmic division of trigeminal nerve and the intraorbital nerve (a division of V_2). Most of the extraocular muscles arise from the annulus of Zinn at the orbital apex and insert onto the globe near the corneal limbus. Together they form a conical potential space (annulus or muscle cone) behind the globe that encases the ophthalmic artery, cranial nerves II, III, and the nasociliary branch of the trigeminal nerve. CN IV (the trochlear nerve), which supplies the superior oblique muscle, lies outside the muscle cone.

As expected, injection of local anesthetic solution within or around the muscle cone reliably anesthetizes the globe. Anesthetizing the orbit (the eye socket and all its contents), in contrast, can be more challenging due to anatomical consideration its conspicuous sensory nerve supply (*Fig. 82.1*). Thus, oculoplastic cases involving surgical manipulation of the orbit are less well tolerated under regional anesthesia. For instance, the senior author of this chapter estimates that up to 40% of his oculoplastics cases require general anesthesia (similarly, expect that enucleation of a blind, painful eye will often require general anesthesia for patients' psychological welfare). Frequently employed ocular regional techniques for most other cases include retrobulbar, peribulbar, and subtenon block. When the block needle is inserted within the muscle cone, the regional technique is called a retrobulbar block. To reduce the complication rates associated with this technique, peribulbar block was later described, whereby anesthetic solution is injected around

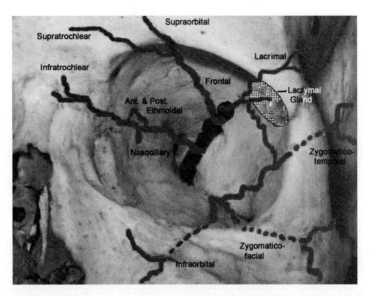

FIGURE 82.1. Sensory nerve supply to the orbit. [Modified from Rene C. Update on orbital anatomy. *Eye.* 2006;20(10):1119–1129.]

(but not within) the muscle cone. Pertinent differences between these techniques are outlined in *Table 82.2*. Despite providing adequate anesthesia to the globe, these techniques fail to provide complete akinesia of the eyelids. The muscles involved in eyelid movements are the orbicularis oculi (innervated by the facial nerve, CN VII) and the levator palpebrae (innervated by the oculomotor nerve). For prolonged surgeries, squeezing by the eyelids is prevented by separate facial nerve blocks by Van Lint, O'Brien, Atkinson, or Nadbath technique. Various other regional anesthetic techniques such as subtenon, infraorbital, supraorbital, infratrochlear, and supratrochlear nerve blocks are often utilized by ophthalmic surgeons, but their discussion is beyond the scope of this chapter.

In this changing era, most ocular regional techniques are performed by the surgeons. Each technique comes with its own set of complications (*Table 82.3*). It is important for anesthesiologists to know how to detect and manage these problems. Communication with the surgeon will help in knowing the specific technique(s) planned and the anticipated issues. Retrobulbar block is often known to be associated with more frequent and worrisome problems that require close monitoring during and after the block. Retrobulbar hemorrhage is the most common ocular complication (incidence ~1% to 2%) and presents clinically as increasing proptosis, and subcutaneous and/or subconjunctival ecchymosis. Depending on the severity, treatment

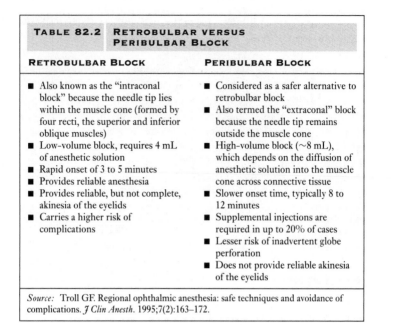

TABLE 82.2	RETROBULBAR VERSUS PERIBULBAR BLOCK	
RETROBULBAR BLOCK	**PERIBULBAR BLOCK**	
■ Also known as the "intraconal block" because the needle tip lies within the muscle cone (formed by four recti, the superior and inferior oblique muscles) ■ Low-volume block, requires 4 mL of anesthetic solution ■ Rapid onset of 3 to 5 minutes ■ Provides reliable anesthesia ■ Provides reliable, but not complete, akinesia of the eyelids ■ Carries a higher risk of complications	■ Considered as a safer alternative to retrobulbar block ■ Also termed the "extraconal" block because the needle tip remains outside the muscle cone ■ High-volume block ($\sim$8 mL), which depends on the diffusion of anesthetic solution into the muscle cone across connective tissue ■ Slower onset time, typically 8 to 12 minutes ■ Supplemental injections are required in up to 20% of cases ■ Lesser risk of inadvertent globe perforation ■ Does not provide reliable akinesia of the eyelids	

Source: Troll GF. Regional ophthalmic anesthesia: safe techniques and avoidance of complications. *J Clin Anesth.* 1995;7(2):163–172.

may vary from intermittent digital pressure application to immediate decompressive lateral canthotomy by the ophthalmologist.

Systemic complications are often quicker to present and normally require intubation and/or full cardiopulmonary resuscitation. It is recommended to prepare airway equipment and emergency drugs before initiation of any periocular block. Two of the systemic complications, retrobulbar apnea

TABLE 82.3	COMPLICATIONS OF PERIOCULAR REGIONAL TECHNIQUES RELEVANT TO ANESTHESIOLOGISTS	
OCULAR COMPLICATIONS	**SYSTEMIC COMPLICATIONS**	
1) Retrobulbar hemorrhage 2) Perforation of globe 3) Penetration of optic nerve 4) Optic atrophy and retinal vascular occlusion 5) Postoperative ptosis	1) Allergic reaction to local anesthetics 2) Local anesthetic toxicity 3) Arterial injection 4) Retrobulbar apnea syndrome (secondary to optic nerve sheath injection) 5) Oculocardiac reflex	

Sources: Troll GF. Regional ophthalmic anesthesia: safe techniques and avoidance of complications. *J Clin Anesth.* 1995;7(2):163–172. Ben-David B. Complications of regional anesthesia: an overview. *Anesthesiol Clin North Am.* 2002;20(3):665–667, ix.

syndrome and oculocardiac reflex, are worth mentioning. Retrobulbar apnea syndrome (RAS) occurs as a result of inadvertent injection of local anesthetic solution into the optic nerve sheath. The anesthetic solution presumably spreads along the nerve sheath to subdural or subarachnoid areas, leading to brainstem anesthesia. Signs and symptoms include initial drowsiness, mild agitation, or confusion, progressing to respiratory depression or arrest within a few minutes of injection. The presence of ptosis, mydriasis, loss of vision, and contralateral ophthalmoplegia often help in formulating an early diagnosis. Treatment is often supportive, but requires cardiopulmonary resuscitation. The oculocardiac reflex (OCR), frequently seen in the context of strabismus cases in children, has also been described following retrobulbar block. It often manifests as cardiac arrhythmia, such as sinus bradycardia, nodal rhythm, ectopies, or even asystole. Treatment is mainly supportive.

Given the facts, it is evident that anesthesia for eye surgery requires a fair amount of preparation and constant vigilance during and after the regional block. Any indolence on the part of the anesthesia provider could potentially turn out to be a life-threatening situation for the patient.

TAKE HOME POINTS

- Anesthesia for eye surgery requires fair understanding of periocular regional techniques, especially the complications associated with them.
- Constant watchfulness is crucial in early detection and treatment of complications associated with these techniques.
- General anesthesia is not infrequently required for ocular surgeries.

SUGGESTED READINGS

Ben-David B. Complications of regional anesthesia: an overview. *Anesthesiol Clin North Am.* 2002;20(3):665–667, ix.

Navaleza JS, Pendse SJ, Blecher MH. Choosing anesthesia for cataract surgery. *Ophthalmol Clin North Am.* 2006;19(2):233–237.

Rene C. Update on orbital anatomy. *Eye.* 2006;20(10):1119–1129.

Troll GF. Regional ophthalmic anesthesia: safe techniques and avoidance of complications. *J Clin Anesth.* 1995;7(2):163–172.

83

REMEMBER THAT FIRES IN THE OPERATING ROOM CAN BE PREVENTED BY MINIMIZING JUST ONE COMPONENT OF THE FIRE TRIAD

ANNE B. HAUPT, RN, BSN, CNOR AND
CATHERINE MARCUCCI, MD

You are on call and are notified that a patient is coming to the operating room (OR) urgently for a stab wound to the neck. You make your way to the room that has been set up for cases from the emergency room, the standard OR table is already made up with a draw sheet. You know that this is actually a polyurethane foam mattress, covered with a synthetic fabric, covered with a cotton sheet, but of course, you are not really thinking about that right now. The patient arrives shortly in a cloth hospital gown and a paper hat. She is a young woman who ran into trouble while out clubbing; she is wearing both hair gel and perfume. After induction, the patient's skin is quickly cleaned with an alcohol-based prep solution, with little or no time to place pads to catch drips. Her head and neck are draped as quickly as possible with four cotton towels and a clear incise drape. Dry sponges are placed on the field. The patient is breathing high-concentration oxygen or perhaps a combination of oxygen and nitrous oxide. Of course, there was not time to check for frayed power cords or current inspection stickers, and that's not something the anesthesia provider typically does anyway. You notice there are multiple foot pedals at the surgeon's feet and wonder what the cases had been in that room during the day. The surgical case starts and you notice several times that the electrosurgical unit (ESU) pencil is not holstered when not in use; instead it is allowed to rest on the drapes. You see the ESU spark a bit the next time the surgeon picks it up, then suddenly, it "flashes" on you—this is the perfect setup for an OR fire.

Fire is the result of a chemical reaction between a fuel and oxygen. It will occur in any setting where the three elements that form the fire triad (fuel, oxygen, and heat) come together. Approximately 100 surgical fires are reported each year, resulting in about 20 serious injuries and one to two patient deaths, although these numbers may represent only a fraction of actual fires. Besides the devastating consequences of physical injury and death, OR fires can cause great psychological trauma to patients, family members, and staff. Unfortunately, there are also unfavorable public relations as well as potential legal ramifications.

© 2006 Mayo Foundation for Medical Education and Research

The vast majority of fires ignite on or in the patient—34% in the airway (see Chapter 12), 28% on the head or face, and 38% elsewhere on or inside the patient. Thus, the most common injuries are airway burns, skin or internal burns, and burns to the patient's unprotected eyes during laser surgery. Also, the volatile gases and toxic fumes and by-products that are produced as synthetic materials melt are caustic to both the skin and eyes and can be lethal if inhaled. Most flames have a temperature that is approximately 1,200°C, with ambient temperatures ranging from 90°F near the floor to 600°F. Smoke from an uncontrolled fire can fill a room in approximately 3 minutes.

A fuel is anything that will burn. Remember that the OR environment has abundant fuel sources. These include bone cement, cloth and paper items (drapes, dressings, sponges, patient gowns), plastic and rubber items (anesthesia circuit, blood pressure cuffs, endotracheal tubes, mattresses, masks, positioning devices, and tourniquets), solutions and ointments (petroleum-based ointments, prep solutions, suture pack solutions, tincture of benzoin), and the patient (head, facial, and body hair, gastrointestinal methane gas, hairspray, and perfume). Items that would not normally burn in room air (21% oxygen) most likely will burn in an oxygen-enriched environment. The higher the oxygen concentration, the less energy is required to ignite the materials. It has been found that an oxygen-enriched environment was present during 74% of fires. Nitrous oxide is also an oxidizer and is capable of supporting combustion.

High-energy ignition sources are also plentiful in today's ORs, including ESUs, lasers, and fiber-optic light cords. Other heat sources include high-speed burrs and drills, embers from charred tissue, and sparks produced from activating the ESU pencil on the end of a hemostat.

Prevention of OR fires is widely recognized to be based on the team concept. It is the responsibility of *all* OR team members to be cognizant of the factors that predispose to fire (including human complacency!) and to understand how the various OR team members will function in the event of a fire. Communication and cooperation are vital. The Joint Commission on Accreditation of Healthcare Organizations (JCAHO) recommends a number of steps to reduce the risk of fire and fire injuries, including staff education; developing, implementing, and testing procedures; understanding laser basics, principles of electricity, and mode of operation of the ESU; the location of emergency equipment; and the location of gas shut-off valves and who is authorized to turn them off.

In the event of a "surgical" fire (i.e., other than an airway fire), the goal is to remove the drapes from the patient as quickly as possible to protect against burns and inhalation of toxic gases and then stabilize and treat the patient as necessary. In some cases, it will be necessary to first douse and then remove the drapes. The scrub nurse will assist with wet towels and water. Drapes should be removed horizontally to prevent spread of the fire up the drapes. Remember that paper drapes are water-repellant, so a fire burning under these drapes still may not be completely extinguished. The scrub nurse will also help pack open incisions with saline-soaked laps, and then move away from the table to assemble the instruments necessary to close the patient. The circulating nurse will call for help, notify the charge nurse, activate the alarm, and assist the anesthesia provider in preparing to move the patient to another room if required.

The anesthesia provider must replace wall anesthetic gases with tank gases (in case the charge nurse or fire chief gives the order to discontinue wall gases) and get ready to move patient elsewhere so the procedure can be completed. OR personnel should *not* try to contain fires that extend beyond the patient—the building and sprinkler systems are designed to do this. Rather, the goal is to "put the patient out" and then get him or her moved as quickly as possible to safety. Keep in mind that hospital sprinkler systems are flushed regularly, but the 300 gallons of water that will be dumped in the OR are far from sterile, so the patient should be covered as much as possible.

Every modern OR will have a fire and fire evacuation plan. The authors strongly encourage anesthesia providers who are new to an operating room theater to obtain a copy and review it thoroughly. This is truly an area of clinical practice that deserves the utmost vigilance.

TAKE HOME POINTS

- The fire triad is oxygen, fuel, and heat.
- All are plentiful in the OR, so instead of viewing OR fires as unlikely or rare events, consider that OR conditions are actually very favorable for the creation of fires.
- Develop a method to maintain vigilance with respect to fires. One of the authors used to keep an empty matchbook cover in her tackle box with her airway equipment as a "reminder."
- If the fire is not an airway fire, the anesthesia provider must be ready to switch from wall gases to tank gases and immediately prepare to transport the patient to safety.
- Actively seek out the fire and fire evacuation plan when joining a new OR staff. Attend all fire drills given by your operating room department.

SUGGESTED READINGS

AORN guidance statement: fire prevention in the operating room. *AORN J.* 2005;81(5):1067–1075.

Daane SP, Toth BA. Fire in the operating room: principles and prevention. *Plast Reconstr Surg.* 2005;115(5):73e–75e.

Lypson ML, Stephens S, Colletti L. Preventing surgical fires: who needs to be educated? *Jt Comm J Qual Patient Saf.* 2005;31(9):522–527.

Meeting JCAHO's goal on surgical fires. *OR Manager.* 2004;20(11):26–28.

Pollock GS. Eliminating surgical fires: a team approach. *AANA J.* 2004;72(4):293–298.

Prasad R, Quezado Z, St Andre A, et al. Fires in the operating room and intensive care unit: awareness is the key to prevention. *Anesth Analg.* 2006;102(1):172–174.

Salmon L. Fire in the OR—prevention and preparedness. *AORN J.* 2004;80(1):42–48, 51–54; quiz 57–60.

Smith C. Surgical fires—learn not to burn. *AORN J.* 2004;80(1):24–36;quiz 37–40.

84

REMEMBER THAT ELEVATED TEMPERATURE IS A LATE FINDING IN MALIGNANT HYPERTHERMIA

JAMES C. OPTON, MD

Malignant hyperthermia (MH) is a clinical syndrome characterized by un-controlled skeletal muscle metabolism. First defined in 1960 by Denborough and Lovell, it is classically "triggered" by volatile anesthetics and the depolar-izing muscle relaxant succinylcholine in genetically susceptible individuals. MH is caused by uncontrolled calcium release in skeletal muscle cells as a result of abnormal function of the ryanodine receptor (RYR1). Diagnosis can be made clinically, by caffeine–halothane contracture testing of a muscle biopsy specimen, or by genetic testing. The caffeine–halothane test is very sensitive. However, it is invasive and expensive (about $800). Genetic testing for one of several known mutations of the RYR-1 genes is done via a simple blood test. Although it is not very sensitive, it is very specific and much less costly (about $200).

The overall incidence of MH-susceptible patients in the general pop-ulation is hard to estimate, because it is a "cluster" disease. However, in 2005, there were 12 confirmed cases and an additional 10 probable cases in the United States, according to an official at the Malignant Hyperthermia Association of the United States (MHAUS).

MH can occur at any time during anesthesia or in the immediate post-operative period. It is the standard of care to ask every patient exposed to a triggering agent if he or she has a family history suspicious for MH ("Has a family member ever had a dangerous or unusual reaction to anesthesia? etc."). Although it is a rare disease, it is an important one in terms of anesthetic practice—anesthesiologists are expected from a medical/legal standpoint to be able to recognize and treat MH even if they are seeing it for the first time.

The most consistent indicator of potential MH is a large increase in end-tidal carbon dioxide. End tidal CO_2 can double or triple in minutes (al-though it may increase over hours). Masseter rigidity is another early sign, and tachycardia, arrhythmias, unstable or rising blood pressure, cyanosis and mottling, myoglobinuria, and tachypnea follow. Whole-body rigidity is a specific sign of MH and is seen in the limbs, abdomen, and chest if muscle relaxants have not been used. Respiratory and metabolic acidosis indicate ful-minant MH and are typically followed by temperature elevation, a late sign. The temperature rise can be rapid and may exceed 43°C. Rhabdomyolysis

© 2006 Mayo Foundation for Medical Education and Research

and disseminated intravascular coagulation (DIC) may also occur. Death is usually from cardiac arrest secondary to acidosis or hyperkalemia. In the dantrolene era, mortality from MH is less than 10%.

TREATMENT OF ACUTE MH

- Call for help! Get dantrolene!
- Discontinue volatile anesthetics and succinylcholine.
- Hyperventilate with 100% oxygen at high fresh gas flows.
- Give dantrolene 2.5 mg/kg by intravenous (IV) bolus. Repeat dose as needed until signs of MH are controlled.
- Place two large-bore peripheral IV lines and an arterial line.
- Treat acidosis with bicarbonate as guided by blood gas analysis.
- Actively cool patient with IV cold saline, nasogastric lavage, rectal lavage, and surface cooling. Discontinue cooling when temperature has fallen to 38°C.
- Treat hyperkalemia with hyperventilation, bicarbonate, insulin with glucose. Life-threatening hyperkalemia should be treated with calcium.
- Dysrhythmias usually respond to treatment of acidosis and hyperkalemia. If not, use appropriate antiarrhythmics with the exception of calcium-channel blockers.
- Serially monitor end-tidal CO_2, arterial blood gases (ABG), serum potassium and other electrolytes, urine output, and international normalized ratio (INR)/prothrombin time (PTT).
- Ensure urine output of at least 2 mL/kg/h by hydration and/or diuretics. Consider central venous or pulmonary artery monitoring to guide fluid management.
- Call the MH Hotline.

TREATMENT OF POSTACUTE MH

- Observe in intensive care unit (ICU) for at least 24 hours, as recrudescence may occur.
- Give dantrolene 1 mg/kg IV every 4 to 6 hours for 24 to 48 hours after the episode.
- Follow arterial blood gases, creatine kinase (CK), potassium, coagulation factors, urine myoglobin, and temperature until they return to normal. CK may stay elevated for up to 2 weeks.
- Report patients to the North American MH Registry of MHAUS and refer patients to MHAUS for information.

WHAT TO STOCK IN THE MALIGNANT HYPERTHERMIA CART

The MHAUS is very specific about what needs to be stocked in the MH cart. In addition to the standard American Society of Anesthesiologists (ASA) monitors, all locations where general anesthesia is administered should have a posted plan to treat MH; a means to continuously monitor end-tidal CO_2, blood oxygen saturation, and core body temperature; and a means to actively cool a patient. A malignant hyperthermia cart stocked with the following should be immediately available wherever general anesthesia is administered:

Drugs
1) Dantrolene sodium for injection: 36 vials (each able to be diluted at the time of use with 60 mL sterile water).
2) Sterile water for injection USP (without a bacteriostatic agent) to reconstitute dantrolene: 1,000 mL $\times$ 2.
3) Sodium bicarbonate (8.4%): 50 mL $\times$ 5.
4) Furosemide 40 mg/ampule $\times$ 4 ampules.
5) Dextrose 50%: 50-mL vial $\times$ 2.
6) Calcium chloride (10%): 10-mL vial $\times$ 2.
7) Regular insulin 100 U/mL $\times$ 1 (refrigerated).
8) Lidocaine for injection, 100 mg/5 mL or 100 mg/10 mL in preloaded syringes ($\times$ 3). Amiodarone is also acceptable. Advanced cardiac life support (ACLS) protocols, as proscribed by the American Heart Association (AHA), should be followed when treating all cardiac derangements caused by MH.

General Equipment
1) Syringes (60 mL $\times$ 5) to dilute dantrolene.
2) Mini-spike IV additive pins $\times$ 2 and Multi-Ad fluid transfer sets $\times$ 2 (to reconstitute dantrolene). Call MHAUS for ordering info.
3) Angiocaths: 16G, 18G, 20G, 2-in; 22G, 1-in; 24G, $3/4$-in (4 each) for IV access and arterial line.
4) Nasogastric (NG) tubes: sizes appropriate for your patient population.
5) Blood pump.
6) Irrigation tray with piston syringe ($\times$ 1) for NG irrigation.
7) Toomey irrigation syringes (60 mL $\times$ 2) for NG irrigation.
8) Microdrip IV set ($\times$ 1).

Monitoring Equipment
1) Esophageal or other core temperature probes.
2) Central venous pressure (CVP) kits (sizes appropriate for your patient population).
3) Transducer kits for arterial and central venous cannulation.

Nursing Supplies
1) A minimum of 3,000 mL of refrigerated cold saline solution.
2) Large sterile Steri-Drape (for rapid drape of wound).
3) Three-way irrigating Foley catheters (sizes appropriate for your patient population).

4) Urine meter × 1.
5) Irrigation tray with piston syringe.
6) Large clear plastic bags for ice × 4.
7) Small plastic bags for ice × 4.
8) Bucket for ice.

Laboratory Testing Supplies
1) Syringes (3-mL) for blood gas analysis for ABG kits × 6.
2) Blood specimen tubes (each test should have 2 pediatric and 2 large tubes): (A) for CK, myoglobin, SMA 19 (LDH, electrolytes, thyroid studies); (B) for PT/PTT, fibrinogen, fibrin split products; (C) complete blood count (CBC), platelets; (D) blood gas syringe (lactic acid level).
3) Urine-collection container for myoglobin level. Pigmenturia indicates that renal protection is mandated; unless the centrifuged or settled sample shows supernatant, i.e., the coloration is due to ret cells in the sample.
4) Urine dipstick: hemoglobin.

Forms
1) Laboratory request forms: ABG form × 6; hematology form × 2; chemistry form × 2; coagulation form × 2; urinalysis form × 2; physician order form × 2.
2) Adverse Metabolic Reaction to Anesthesia (AMRA) Report form (obtained from MH Registry).
3) Consult form, if needed, for requesting a consultation from another physician.

PREPARING THE ANESTHESIA MACHINE FOR MH-SUSCEPTIBLE PATIENTS

- Ensure that vaporizers are disabled by removing, draining, or taping in the "OFF" position.
- Some consultants recommend changing the CO_2 absorbent.
- Flow 10 L/min O_2 through circuits via ventilator for at least 20 minutes.
- Place new, disposable breathing circuit and breathing bag.
- Use expired-gas analyzer to confirm absence of volatile gases.

CONTACT INFORMATION

- MH Hotline: 1-800-644-9737 or 1-315-464-7079 (outside U.S.).
- North American MH Registry of MHAUS registers information about specific families and patients. Registry is located at Children's Hospital at the University of Pittsburgh. See www.mhreg.org or call 1-888-274-7899.

■ MHAUS provides educational and technical information to patients and health care providers at www.mhaus.org. They generally do not register cases in other countries, but do field calls from all over the world.

SUGGESTED READINGS

American Society of Anesthesiologists website. www.asahq.org.

Coté A. *Practice of Anesthesia for Infants and Children.* 3rd ed. Philadelphia: WB Saunders; 2001.

Denborough MA, Lovell RRH. Anaesthetic deaths in a family. *Lancet.* 1960;2:45–46.

Malignant Hyperthermia Association of the United States website. www.mhaus.org.

85

CONSIDER METHEMOGLOBINEMIA AFTER RULING OUT THE COMMON CAUSES FOR A LOW PULSE OXIMETER READING

LEENA MATHEW, MD, PHILIP SHIN, MD, AND WALTER L. CHANG, MD

A morbidly obese 39-year-old man presented for open gastric bypass surgery. He had a history of obstructive sleep apnea, requiring continuous positive airway pressure (CPAP) at night. He had no known allergies to medications. The anesthetic plan was to proceed with an awake fiber-optic intubation for general endotracheal anesthesia. He was given a treatment of aerosolized 4% lidocaine for 20 minutes before entering the operating room (OR). In the OR, Cetacaine (benzocaine 14%, tetracaine 2%, and butyl amino benzoate 2%) spray was applied to the posterior oropharynx.

A transtracheal block was performed using 3 mL of 2% lidocaine. An awake nasal fiber-optic intubation was completed without difficulty. Within 15 minutes of intubation, the patient's pulse oximetry registered a progressive decline to 90% on a FiO_2 of 100%. As the surgeon made the incision he commented that the blood on the field looked "dark like chocolate." When an arterial blood sample was taken, it was also noted to be dark chocolate-colored. A presumptive diagnosis of methemoglobinemia was entertained. The arterial blood sample was sent for blood gas analysis and methemoglobin (MHb) levels. Because of technical difficulties in the laboratory, there was a delay in processing the blood gas sample. At this point the decision was made to treat empirically with methylene blue; accordingly, 70 mg of methylene blue diluted in 50 mL of normal saline was given intravenously over 10 minutes. After an initial drop in the pulse oximetry reading to 88%, the reading rose progressively to the high 90s. Ten minutes after the entire dose, pulse oximetry read steadily at 99% on 100% oxygen. The patient was extubated without difficulty at the end of the procedure and discharged to home several days later. The result of the MHb level, available on postoperative day 1, was 24.6%.

Anesthesiologists commonly use local anesthetics to anesthetize the airway and pharynx in preparation for awake fiber-optic intubations or endoscopies. A rare though potentially serious toxicity associated with the use of local anesthetics is methemoglobinemia (MHbemia). Anesthesiologists should understand the pathophysiology, presentation, diagnosis, and treatment of MHbemia to prevent and/or manage potential problems.

© 2006 Mayo Foundation for Medical Education and Research

In the case above, the patient experienced arterial desaturation to 90% on a FiO_2 of 100% oxygen. The differential diagnosis for a low pulse oximetry measurement (SpO_2) included: pulse oximetry artifact, hypoxemia, abnormal hemoglobin variants, sulfhemoglobinemia, and MHbemia. Pulse oximetry relies on measurement of absorbed light from two diodes, one emitting light at 660 nm (red) and another emitting light at 940 nm (near-infrared). It is well known that pulse oximetry is distorted by artifacts arising from motion, ambient light, poor perfusion, and injected dyes including indigo carmine and methylene blue.

Hypoxemia is the most critical cause for low SpO_2 and must be investigated urgently. Hypoxemia may result from hypoxia, hypoventilation, shunting, ventilation/perfusion mismatching, decreased partial pressure of oxygen in mixed venous blood, and rarely, diffusion abnormalities. Quickly ruling out these causes of a low SpO_2 is paramount to caring for any patient. In this case, the patient was ventilated manually with 100% FiO_2. The tube placement was verified to be correct with a fiber-optic scope; auscultation, and presence of end-tidal CO_2. The nasotracheal endotracheal tube was suctioned and the breathing circuit checked for kinks. New-onset diffusion abnormality was highly unlikely.

METHEMOGLOBINEMIA

Only after ruling out the most common and critical causes for a low SpO_2 should one consider the possibility of MHbemia as the cause. Methemoglobin is the oxidized form of hemoglobin in which the iron moiety of MHb is in a trivalent (Fe^{3+}) ferric state rather than a divalent (Fe^{2+}) ferrous state. MHb is unable to bind oxygen and thus reduces the oxygen-carrying capacity of blood. In addition, MHb shifts the oxygen dissociation curve to the left, thus impairing release of oxygen from the heme molecule to tissue. Significant levels of MHbemia can place patients in a state of functional anemia.

METHEMOGLOBIN FORMATION AND REDUCTION

Normally there is a steady-state equilibrium between the levels of hemoglobin and MHb. The auto-oxidation of hemoglobin to MHb occurs at a rate of 0.5% to 3% per day. Levels of MHb remain below 2% by a mechanism of constant reduction (addition of an electron). The primary mechanism of MHb reduction to ferrous hemoglobin is through the nicotinamide adenine dinucleotide (NADH)–cytochrome b5 reductase pathway. An alternate enzymatic pathway for the reduction of MHb is mediated by NADPH MHb reductase. This pathway generates electrons from glucose-6-phosphate dehydrogenase in the hexose monophosphate shunt, which requires methylene blue and/or flavin to function. Other minor pathways that reduce MHb include ascorbic acid, reduced glutathione, reduced flavin, tetrahydropterin, cysteine, cysteamine, 3-hydroxyanthranilic acid, and 3-hydroxykynurenine.

CAUSES OF METHEMOGLOBINEMIA

Significant MHbemia occurs when there is an imbalance between hemoglobin oxidation and reduction. The causes of MHbemia may be categorized as congenital or acquired. The rare congenital causes include hemoglobin M and cytochrome b5 deficiency.

Hemoglobin M is a variant of hemoglobin that has an amino acid substitution rendering it resistant to reduction. It is inherited in an autosomal dominant pattern. Patients with this form of hemoglobin usually present with a long-standing history of cyanosis and a positive family history.

NADH–cytochrome b5 reductase deficiency is the other congenital cause of MHbemia. Inheritance of this deficiency occurs following an autosomal recessive pattern. This deficiency is subdivided into types 1 and 2. Type 1 NADH–cytochrome b5 reductase deficiency is limited to the soluble form in erythrocytes. Cyanosis is often the only symptom, and patients with this deficiency are not usually treated. Type 2 deficiency involves both the soluble and bound isoforms of the enzyme. As opposed to the type 1 deficiency, patients with type 2 deficiency may have severe progressive neurologic symptoms which are untreatable.

The acquired causes of MHbemia are more common than the congenital causes. Acquired causes mostly involve medication/drug administration. Drugs known to cause MHbemia include antimalarials (chloroquine, primaquine), nitrites or nitrates, nitroprusside, inhaled nitric oxide, sulfonamides, acetanilide, metoclopromide, phenacetin, phenytoin, probenecid, chlorates, phenazopyridine hydrochloride, and local anesthetics including prilocaine, benzocaine, and lidocaine.

SIGNS AND SYMPTOMS

The most common sign of MHb is cyanosis. In addition, patients with MHbenemia have been noted to have chocolate-brownish-colored blood. Our patient's blood was described as being such by the surgeon, and the anesthesia team observed "chocolate"-colored blood on obtaining the arterial blood gas.

DIAGNOSIS

The diagnosis of MHbemia requires co-oximetry. Co-oximeters are spectrophotometers able to emit at least four different wavelengths of light, thus allowing for the measurement of four hemoglobin species: hemoglobin, oxyhemoglobin, carboxyhemoglobin, and MHb. An arterial blood gas sample should be drawn and sent to the laboratory specifically requesting co-oximetry for methemoglobin levels.

TREATMENT

Not everyone with MHbemia requires treatment. MHb levels <30% usually resolve spontaneously over 15 to 20 hours without serious consequences.

Those patients with higher MHb levels or patients limited by symptoms of MHb may be treated with methylene blue. The recommended dosage of methylene blue is 1 mg/kg over 5 minutes, and the dose may be repeated in 1 hour if the first dose is not ineffective. Methylene blue accelerates the action of the NADPH–MHb reductase, which is the body's alternate pathway for MHb reduction.

Methylene blue acts as an electron acceptor of NADPH-dependent MHbemia reduction, which under normal circumstances does not have an electron acceptor. Because treatment with methylene blue depends on NADPH as an electron donator, there must be adequate levels of NADPH available via the glucose-6-phosphate dehydrogenase (G-6-P-D) pathway. Therefore, methylene blue needs an intact pentose phosphate pathway to regenerate NADPH for effectiveness.

For this reason, methylene blue would not be the treatment of choice in patients with G-6-P-D deficiency. In fact, giving these patients methylene blue may increase levels of MHbemia and cause hemolysis, because high concentrations of methylene blue can act as an oxidant. In patients with a G-6-P-D deficiency, treatment is available through the administration of ascorbic acid and riboflavin. Finally, in refractory or life-threatening cases, exchange transfusion and the use of a hyperbaric oxygen chamber may be necessary to treat MHb.

TAKE HOME POINTS

- Anesthesia providers should be aware of the complication of acquired methemoglobinemia resulting from the use of local anesthetics.
- The topicalization of a patient's airway for fiber-optic intubation is an especially vulnerable time for both the development of local anesthetic toxicity and MHbemia. This has been corroborated by multiple case reports in the gastrointestinal literature of MHbemia secondary to Cetacaine spray topicalization of oral mucosa for endoscopic gastroduodenoscopies.
- In addition, there have been case reports in the cardiology literature of MHbemia from Cetacaine spray preparation of the oral mucosa for trans-esophageal echocardiogram.
- The early recognition and treatment of methemoglobinemia in patients can prevent adverse outcomes in these patients and avoid unnecessary interventions that may contribute to morbidity.

SUGGESTED READINGS

Barker SJ, Tremper KK, Hyatt J. Effects of methemoglobinemia on pulse oximetry and mixed venous oximetry. *Anesthesiology*. 1989;70:112–117.
Collins JF. Methemoglobinemia as a complication of 20% benzocaine spray for endoscopy. *Gastroenterology*. 1990;98:211–213.

Douglas WW, Fairbanks VF. Methemoglobinemia induced by a topical anesthetic spray (Ceta-caine). *Chest.* 1977;71:587–591.

Fincher ME, Campbell HT. Methemoglobinemia and hemolytic anemia after phenazopyri-dine hydrochloride (Pyridium) administration in end-stage renal disease. *South Med J.* 1989;82:372–374.

Hurford WE, Kratz A. Case records of the Massachusetts General Hospital. Weekly clinico-pathological exercises. Case 23-2004. A 50-year-old woman with low oxygen saturation. *N Engl J Med.* 2004;351:380–387.

Jaffe ER. Enzymopenic hereditary methemoglobinemia: a clinical/biochemical classification. *Blood Cells.* 1986;12:81–90.

Kahn NA, Kruse JA. Methemoglobinemia induced by topical anesthesia: a case report and review. *Am J Med Sci.* 1999;318:415–418.

Sandza JG Jr, Roberts RW, Shaw RC, et al. Symptomatic methemoglobinemia with a commonly used topical anesthetic, Cetocaine. *Ann Thorac Surg.* 1980;30:187–190.

Vessely MB, Zitsch RP 3rd. Topical anesthetic-induced methemoglobinemia: a case report and review of the literature. *Otolaryngol Head Neck Surg.* 1993;108:763–767.

Wright RO, Lewander WJ, Woolf AD. Methemoglobinemia: etiology, pharmacology, and clinical management. [See comment]. *Ann Emerg Med.* 1999;34:646–656.

Yubisui T. [Methemoglobin reductases in erythrocytes]. *Seikagaku—J Jpn Biochem Soc.* 1982;54:1233–1254.

EQUIPMENT

86

Pulse Oximetry: Even a Simple Device Requires User Understanding

JORGE PINEDA, JR, MD AND
STEPHEN T. ROBINSON, MD

Pulse oximetry has become an invaluable tool in the current practice of perioperative medicine. It offers dynamic assessment of oxygenation status, which allows for rapid recognition and evaluation of interventions in cases during times of hypoxia on a nearly moment-to-moment basis. Advantages of this monitor include its noninvasiveness, wide availability, and simplicity. However, studies have shown a lack of knowledge concerning the limitations and interpretation of pulse oximetry saturation among both physicians and medical staff.

Pulse oximetry is based on three principles. First, every substance has a unique absorbance spectrum. Different types of hemoglobin have different absorption spectra. The two light-emitting diodes (LEDs) of the pulse oximeter each emit a different, specific wavelength of light within the red to near-infrared range, and a photo detector measures the amount of light transmitted through the tissue. The second principle is based on the Beer-Lambert Law which states that the absorption of light as it passes through a clear nonabsorbing solvent is proportional to the concentration of the solute and the length of the path along which the light travels in that solvent. Finally, the third principle states that the presence of a pulsatile signal generated by arterial blood is relatively independent of the nonpulsatile venous blood in the tissues. By measuring transmitted light several hundred times per second, the pulse oximeter can distinguish the variable, pulsatile component of arterial blood from the unchanging component of the signal made up of the tissue, venous blood, and nonpulsatile arterial blood. The pulsatile or alternating component, which generally comprises 1% to 5% of the total signal, can then be isolated by canceling out the static component.

Accuracy

Pulse oximetry, or the determination of SpO_2 level, is derived from calibration curves of oxygen saturation that were experimentally measured in healthy volunteers. Values obtained with coincident determination of oxygen saturation by the pulse oximeter were compared with values obtained in *in vitro* laboratory co-oximetry during normal oxygenation and induced hypoxia. Researchers were limited in the degree of hypoxemia inducible

© 2006 Mayo Foundation for Medical Education and Research

in these volunteers to an arterial saturation (SaO_2) of approximately 75% to 80%. Thus, the shape of the curve below these levels must be extrapolated. For peripheral arterial saturation, most manufacturers report accuracy to within ±2% for SpO_2 of 70% to 100% and ±3% for SpO_2 of 50% to 70%. There is no reported accuracy below 50% saturation. These claims are largely supported by several review studies addressing accuracy by correlating SaO_2 with SpO_2. As an SaO_2 level of 75% represents a PaO_2 level of 40 mmHg, reduced accuracy in this low range does not have any meaningful clinical implications.

There is a delay between when alveolar oxygen delivery changes and when the SpO_2 level shows a change. In general, finger probes are slower (24 to 35 seconds) when compared with earlobe probes (10 to 20 seconds). Changing ventilator management to improve oxygenation requires allowing time for the alveolar oxygen concentration to rise, for the blood with higher oxygen content to reach the site of the pulse oximeter probe, for signal processing to occur, and then for display of the processed signal on the monitor as an SpO_2 value. Sufficient time should be allowed when interventions are made based on pulse oximetry readings.

SIGNAL ARTIFACTS

The major limitations of pulse oximetry can be divided into two major categories: those arising from optical signal artifact and those resulting from optical interference. Most problems with pulse oximetry arise from signal artifact. Signal artifact can result from false sources of signal or from a low signal-to-noise ratio. The presence of a sharp pulsatile waveform on the oximeter does not guarantee no signal artifact.

Sources of false signal include detection of nontransmitted light (ambient light or optical shunt) and nonarterial sources of alternating or pulsatile signal. Because light can be a potentially major source of interference, designers divided the LED and photo detector activities into three sensing periods, which can cycle at hundreds of times per second. Of these three periods, two use light emitted by the LEDs at each of the two incident wavelengths. During the third period, neither LED is activated and the photo detector measures only ambient light. This measurement is then eliminated from the LED-illuminated sensing periods. Despite this, ambient light still interferes, and implicated sources include fluorescent lights, surgical lamps, fiberoptic instruments, and sunlight. A simple solution is covering the probe with an opaque shield.

Optical shunt occurs when light emitted from an LED reaches the photo detector without passing through an arterial bed. This typically occurs when the probe is positioned poorly or when an inappropriate probe is used (for example, a finger probe placed on the ear). Nonarterial sources of alternating signal are typically produced by patient movement and resulting motion artifact. Shivering, movement during cardiopulmonary resuscitation, repetitive cough, and the cycling of ventilators are common potential sources of motion artifact.

OPTICAL INTERFERENCE

Optical interference can limit the value of pulse oximetry. Several substances in the blood can interfere optically with pulse oximetry. These substances absorb light within the red and near-infrared wavelengths used in pulse oximetry. Carboxyhemoglobin (COHb) and methemoglobin (MetHb) are the most significant potential false absorbers. By conventional two-wavelength pulse oximetry, COHb will appear much like O_2Hb in the red range, with virtually no effect in the infrared range. The net effect on SpO_2 is an overestimation of true oxygen saturation. What occurs in the instance of elevated MetHb level is that the MetHb contributes greatly to the perceived absorption of both deoxyHb and oxyHb, driving the ratio of relative absorbances calculated by the pulse oximeter to one. When this ratio is one, the calibrated saturation is approximately 85% leading to an underestimation of true oxygen saturation.

Intravenous dyes can produce falsely low pulse oximetry readings. Changes begin 30 to 45 seconds after dye injection, and recovery to baseline occurs within 3 minutes. Methylene blue causes a profound false decrease in SpO_2. Five mL of methylene blue was reported to decrease oxygen saturation in one patient to as little as 1%. Oxygen saturation can decrease less significantly after intravenous administration of indocyanine green and indigo carmine. False desaturations with these dyes are also noted on the multiwavelength cooximeter.

Skin pigmentation has been shown to affect pulse oximetry. Signal detection failures are more common in patients with dark skin. Darker skin appears to make light penetration more difficult. Nail polish may also affect accuracy of readings and, when problems occur, they appear to arise more commonly from blue or black polish.

CLINICAL APPLICATION

In most cases, a normal SPO_2 is a reassuring result, whereas a low SPO_2 is an indication for further investigation. Unfortunately, a low SpO_2 is a very non-specific finding. Assuming the value is accurate, all aspects of oxygen delivery, including the basic aspects of resuscitation, must be addressed. The clinician must ensure that the airway is patent; airway obstruction, esophageal intubation, or even endobronchial intubation can cause significant hypoxia or anoxia. The clinician must ensure that the patient has adequate ventilation, oxygen concentration, circulation, and tissue perfusion, and, in many cases, can do so by quickly inspecting the patient, the anesthesia machine, and the patient monitors. In other cases, determining the cause of the low SpO_2 value can be difficult. Depending on the clinical circumstances, the clinician may consider, among other things, atelectasis, pneumothorax, low cardiac output, and anemia. The clinician must consider auscultation, and a chest x-ray may be indicated. Occasionally, measuring arterial blood gas levels to determine the partial pressure of carbon dioxide ($PaCO_2$) and checking the acid-base status to validate the partial pressure of oxygen (PaO_2) may be appropriate.

Pulse oximetry is a measure of arterial oxygen concentration at the site being measured. A normal value obtained at the finger tip does not always permit conclusions to be drawn regarding adequate oxygen delivery to tissues. Adequate organ and tissue perfusion requires both an adequate perfusion pressure and blood flow to achieve sufficient oxygen delivery. Tissues or organs distal to tourniquets or other arterial obstruction can suffer significant ischemic injury.

SaO_2 and PaO_2 have a curvilinear relationship. For SpO_2 values in the mid 90s and lower, SpO_2 is a reasonable predictor of PaO_2. At the highest SpO_2 values (99% or 100%), predicting PaO_2 is not possible. At PaO_2 values from 150 to 600 mmHg, the SpO_2 should be 100%. SpO_2 values can be unreliable in predicting PaO_2 values when PaO_2 is high but dropping or is simply lower than expected. For example, during an episode of apnea, PaO_2 levels decline; however, a corresponding change in SpO_2 level may not show until response time is limited. Other monitors, such as capnography or apnea alarms, generally provide an earlier warning.

Healthy patients receiving 100% inspired oxygen with an endobronchial intubation or lobar atelectasis often have SpO_2 values of 100%. A stable but lower PaO_2 value could be a symptom of an underlying problem that a normal SpO_2 value is masking.

In cases in which the oximeter cannot find a pulse, potential underlying cardiopulmonary problems should be addressed first. If use of a finger probe is causing the problem, changing the probe location may prove successful. Earlobe probes have been shown to produce better signal than do digit probes in some cases. Studies have shown that the earlobe is less vasoactive than the finger pad or nail bed and, so, is less susceptible to vasoconstrictive effects. Forehead probes also exist. Other solutions include using topical nitroglycerin, local heat, or massage. Even digital blocks and intra-arterial vasodilators via ipsilateral radial artery lines have proven successful without much systemic effect, although many would regard them as extreme interventions. Placement of the sensor on the same extremity as a blood pressure cuff can also cause erroneously low readings while the cuff is inflating and should be avoided when possible.

Most currently used pulse oximeters use complex algorithms to distinguish signal artifact (noise) from actual signal and will only accept a certain signal-to-noise ratio. However, sometimes noise is processed and presented as signal. A low signal-to-noise ratio results from absent or low amplitude pulses. Causes include hypotension; hypovolemia; hypothermia; peripheral vascular disease; and iatrogenic causes, such as noninvasive blood pressure cuff inflation and vasoconstrictor administration. A low-pulse state would cause a drop out of signal in older models, whereas newer, more sensitive models can detect low signals but may display a false low saturation.

TAKE HOME POINTS

- Pulse oximetry is a widely available, noninvasive, and reliable monitor that provides an early warning of hypoxemia that frequently is not detected upon subjective observation.
- Pulse oximetry uses the differential absorbance of light by oxyhemoglobin and deoxyhemoglobin to estimate oxygen saturation.
- Pulse oximetry monitors oxygenation, not ventilation.
- Understanding both the physiologic and technical limitations of pulse oximetry is necessary to use it appropriately. Major aspects to be considered include accuracy, response time, the issue of hypoperfusion or "the low-pulse problem," and problems caused by motion artifact.

SUGGESTED READINGS

Aoyagi T. Pulse oximetry: its invention, theory, and future. *J Anesth*. 2003;17(4):259–266.

Costarino AT, Davis DA, Keon TO. Falsely normal saturation reading with pulse oximeter. *Anesthesiology*. 1987;67:830–831.

Hinkelbein J, Genzwuerker HV, Fiedler F. Detection of a systolic pressure threshold for reliable readings in pulse oximetry. *Resuscitation*. 2005;64:315.

Kelleher JF. Pulse oximetry. *J Clin Monitoring*. 1989;5:37–62.

Scheller MS, Unger RJ, Kelner MJ. Effects of intravenously administered dyes on pulse oximetry readings. *Anesthesiology*. 1986;65:550–552.

Sinex JE. Pulse oximetry: principles and limitations. *Am J Emerg Med*. 1999;17(1):59–66.

Soubani AO. Noninvasive monitoring of oxygen and carbon dioxide. *Am J Emerg Med*. 2001;19(2):141–146.

Tremper KK, Barker SJ. Pulse oximetry. *Anesthesiology*. 1989;70:98–108.

Volgyesi GA, Spahr-Schopfer I. Does skin pigmentation affect the accuracy of pulse oximetry? An in vitro study. *Anesthesiology*. 1991;75:A406.

87

THE END-TIDAL CO$_2$ MONITOR IS MORE THAN JUST A "THE TUBE IS THE AIRWAY" DEVICE

BRIAN WOODCOCK, MB, CHB, MRCP, FRCA, FCCM

Anesthesia providers most commonly use a capnogram to confirm tracheal intubation and to exclude the possibility of esophageal intubation. However, the ETCO$_2$ level shown by the capnogram and the pattern of the capnogram can also indicate many hemodynamic and respiratory conditions. Anesthesia providers should recognize that many conditions may lead to an increased arterial–end-tidal CO$_2$ gradient.

REVIEW OF CAPNOGRAPHY

The most commonly used capnometers are of the infrared (IR) light absorption type. The analysis can occur at the machine or in the ventilator circuit. In the first instance, airway gases can be sampled along a narrow tube to the machine. Alternatively, an adaptor placed in the airway circuit uses IR light absorption to measure the CO$_2$ concentration directly in the gas stream. This second method provides a very fast response time and avoids problems with clogged tubing and water vapor condensation. It has fallen out of favor because of the extra weight near the endotracheal tube, a concern about reusing a device within the circuit, and the fact that the externalization of the sensor makes it more prone to damage during usage.

CAPNOMETRY VERSUS CAPNOGRAPHY

Capnometry is the determination of the end-tidal partial pressure of CO$_2$. Capnography is the graphic display of instantaneous CO$_2$ partial pressure versus time during the respiratory cycle. This relation is displayed as a CO$_2$ waveform or capnogram. The simplest use of measured end-tidal CO$_2$ (ETCO$_2$) is to follow changes in PaCO$_2$ level. Although the ETCO$_2$ level may be lower than the actual PaCO$_2$ level, in the absence of severe dead-space effects, alterations in PaCO$_2$ level will be mirrored by changes in ETCO$_2$ level, and these changes can be continuously monitored. This may be particularly useful when changes in minute ventilation are made and PaCO$_2$ levels are changing.

The waveform produced by the monitor as a capnogram gives further information in addition to the numeric value of the ETCO$_2$.

© 2006 Mayo Foundation for Medical Education and Research

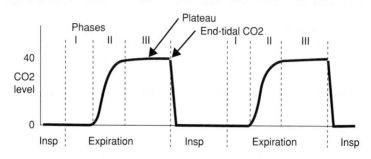

FIGURE 87.1. The normal capnogram. Insp, inspiration.

NORMAL CAPNOGRAM

Dead space (ventilated but unperfused airway) can be divided into apparatus and anatomic (or conductive) dead space, which is in series with the alveoli, and alveolar (or physiologic) dead space, which is in parallel with the alveoli.

Apparatus and anatomic dead space causes the initial expired gas to have a CO_2 level of zero (phase I, *Fig 87.1.*). As expiration continues, alveolar gas is detected and the capnogram rises rapidly (phase II). In phase III, known as the alveolar plateau, the apparatus and anatomic dead-space gases have been expired and the gas sampled is from alveoli. If all these alveoli were perfused, then the CO_2 level would be that of "ideal" alveolar gas, i.e., very close to the $PaCO_2$ level. However, the CO_2 level is lower than the $PaCO_2$ level during the plateau because of admixture of gas from unperfused alveoli with a CO_2 level of zero (alveolar dead space). This means that the $ETCO_2$ level will be close to the $PaCO_2$ level in patients with low alveolar dead space; however, if alveolar dead space increases (e.g., as in emphysema), then the $ETCO_2$ will be reduced, compared to $PaCO_2$. The difference between end-tidal and arterial CO_2 level depends on alveolar dead space and is not altered by changes in apparatus or anatomic dead space.

FACTORS INFLUENCING ALVEOLAR DEAD SPACE

Table 87.1. lists the factors influencing alveolar dead space.

Ventilation-perfusion mismatch increases the arterial–end-tidal CO_2 gradient, and studies have shown this increase to be significantly higher in patients with morbid obesity (body mass index >40 kg/m^2) and in patients receiving anesthesia in the lateral position. Increased gradients have also been reported in older patients; in patients with a high American Society of Anesthesiologists' physical status classification system (ASA) score; and in patients having episodes of hemodynamic instability, during such episodes.

TABLE 87.1	FACTORS INFLUENCING ALVEOLAR DEAD SPACE
FACTOR	**EFFECT**
Hydrostatic failure of alveolar perfusion	Gravity increases perfusion to the lowermost portions of the lung. Uppermost portions have a higher V/Q ratio, i.e., dead space
Pulmonary embolism	Clot, air, fat, or amniotic fluid reduces perfusion to ventilated alveoli and causes dead space.
Ventilation of unperfused airspace	Alveolar destruction occurs in emphysema. Bullae
Precapillary obstruction to blood flow	Hypoxic pulmonary vasoconstriction results.
Tidal volume and PEEP	Alveolar dead space increases if tidal volume and PEEP increase excessively.

V/Q, ventilation/perfusion; PEEP, positive end-expiratory pressure.

DECREASED CAPNOGRAM

Gas exchange requires both ventilation and circulation. A markedly depressed or absent capnograph tracing may be due to ventilator circuit disconnection or ventilator malfunction; cardiac arrest or decreased cardiac output; massive pulmonary embolus; or a dislodged, misplaced, or obstructed endotracheal tube. Capnography may thus be the first warning of catastrophic events or complications. The Closed Claims Project review of adverse anesthetic outcomes suggests that there has been a decrease in severity of injury in anesthesia malpractice claims and that anesthesia safety has improved since the establishment of monitoring standards using pulse oximetry and end-tidal capnography.

End-tidal CO_2 monitoring may provide clinically useful information that can be used to guide therapy during cardiopulmonary resuscitation (CPR). The level of the $ETCO_2$ may indicate the adequacy of CPR and can also provide the first evidence of the return of spontaneous circulation.

During the application of a limb tourniquet, the amount of tissue releasing CO_2 into the circulation is decreased and $ETCO_2$ level will fall. Decreases in CO_2 level may also occur with hypothermia.

INCREASES IN ETCO₂ LEVEL

The earliest warning of a serious hypermetabolic condition, such as malignant hyperthermia, thyroid storm, or severe sepsis, may be a rise $ETCO_2$ level, reflecting the increase in $PaCO_2$ level. Administration of intravenous bicarbonate leads to generation of CO_2 and this is reflected in the tracing within minutes. Other causes of an elevated $ETCO_2$ level include the release of a limb tourniquet; the restoration of blood flow, resulting from unclamping a large artery or vein; and the development of venous CO_2 embolism during laparoscopy.

EFFECT OF PEEP

The Pa-ET CO_2 gradient may be an indicator of optimal levels of (PEEP) for ventilated patients. As PEEP increases and there is maximal recruitment of gas exchange units, then lung ventilation should be more even, phase II of the capnogram will be shorter and the Pa-ET CO_2 gradient will be reduced. An excess of PEEP can distend alveoli excessively and redistribute blood flow, causing an increase in alveolar dead space, increasing the Pa-ET CO_2 gradient.

BRONCHOSPASM

Phase II of the capnogram reflects the emptying of bronchopulmonary units; as more units empty into anatomic dead-space gas, the waveform rises. If lung units have differing time constants, due to uneven lung ventilation, then this will be reflected by a slower rise in the phase II of the capnogram (*Fig. 87.2.*). Phase II may be so prolonged that the alveolar plateau, or phase III, is never reached, resulting in a larger Pa-ET CO_2 gradient. This situation may occur with obstructive airway disease, such as asthma or chronic obstructive pulmonary disease. A change in the capnogram pattern to this shape could indicate that the $ETCO_2$ level is no longer a reliable indicator of the $PaCO_2$ level.

NEGATIVE ARTERIAL—END-TIDAL GRADIENT

$ETCO_2$ levels that exceed $PaCO_2$ levels have been reported in the following circumstances:

- Healthy patients during low-frequency, high-tidal-volume ventilation
- Pregnant patients
- Infants and children
- Patients that recently have had cardiopulmonary bypass
- Patients that are or recently were exercising

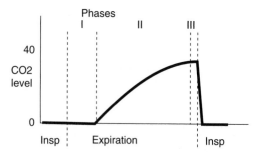

FIGURE 87.2. Capnogram in the presence of bronchospasm. Insp, inspiration.

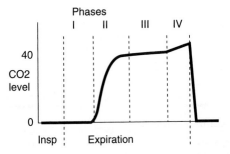

FIGURE 87.3. Phase-IV secondary elevation in plateau PCO_2 level. Insp, inspiration.

Alveolar PCO_2 level varies during the respiratory cycle, being lowest at end-inspiration and highest at end-expiration. Opening of alveoli with long time constants towards the end of expiration allows the addition of gas with a higher PCO_2 level, particularly if the alveoli have a low V/Q ratio. This may be seen as a phase IV in the curve of the capnogram, in which there is a secondary rise in the alveolar phase of expiration (*Fig. 87.3.*). This secondary rise may be to a higher level than the $PaCO_2$ level, which is an averaged level due to mixing in the circulation and syringe.

ALTERATIONS IN INSPIRATORY CO₂

Elevation of the baseline above zero may indicate rebreathing of expired gas, possibly resulting from exhaustion of the soda lime; malfunction of valves in the anesthesia circuit; or use of a rebreathing system (such as Mapleson A, B, C, or D (Bain), or an E circuit) without adequate fresh-gas flow.

OTHER VARIATIONS IN WAVEFORM

Waning neuromuscular blockade may allow small respiratory efforts, causing a dip in the plateau waveform; this is known as a "curare cleft" (*Fig. 87.4*).

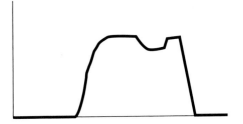

FIGURE 87.4. Curare cleft.

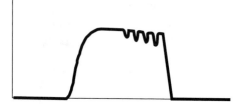

FIGURE 87.5. Cardiac oscillations.

Towards the end of expiration, as expiratory flow decreases to a low level, cardiac contraction may change intrathoracic volume enough to draw gas into the airway from the anesthetic machine circuit. These cardiac oscillations are seen as regular dips at the end of the plateau matching the heart rate (*Fig. 87.5*). These oscillations may continue into the descending limb of the curve if expiration is prolonged.

TAKE HOME POINTS

- Capnography is a standard of care for every general anesthetic because it monitors the adequacy of ventilation.
- Production of $ETCO_2$ requires both ventilation and circulation.
- Capnography can noninvasively detect many of the catastrophic problems that occur during anesthesia.
- There are many circumstances in which $ETCO_2$ level does not accurately represent $PaCO_2$ level.
- Analysis of the shape of the waveform may give useful information on changes in the patient's condition, the anesthesia circuit, or the effects of surgery.

SUGGESTED READINGS

American Society of Anesthesiologists. *Standards for Basic Anesthetic Monitoring.* 2005. http://www.asahq.org/publicationsAndServices/standards/02.pdf.

Barton CW, Wang ES. Correlation of end-tidal CO_2 measurements to arterial $PaCO_2$ in non-intubated patients. *Ann Emerg Med.* 1994;23(3):560–563.

Bhavani-Shankar K, Moseley H, Kumar AY, et al. Capnometry and anaesthesia. *Can J Anaesth.* 1992;39:617–632.

Garnett AR, Ornato JP, Gonzalez ER, et al. End-tidal carbon dioxide monitoring during cardiopulmonary resuscitation. *JAMA.* 1987;257:512–515.

Lee LA. The closed claims project: has it influenced anesthetic practice and outcome? *Anesthesiol Clin North America.* 2002;20(3):485–501.

Wahba RJM, Tessler MJ. Misleading end-tidal CO_2 tensions. *Can J Anaesth.* 1996;43(8): 862–866.

88

NONINVASIVE BLOOD PRESSURE MANAGEMENT—IT'S NOT JUST A PIECE OF NYLON AROUND THE ARM

JORGE PINEDA, JR, MD AND STEPHEN T. ROBINSON, MD

The automated, noninvasive, blood-pressure cuff is a safe, commonly used monitoring device. It provides consistent, reliable values for systolic, diastolic, and mean arterial pressure (MAP). One great advantage of such a monitor is that it frees the anesthesiologist for other tasks. Blood-pressure–cuff cycling intervals can be set and the machine can store data to provide trends. Automated devices also provide alarm systems to draw attention to extremes in blood-pressure values. Disadvantages include frequent failure with profoundly hypotensive patients, patients with arrhythmias, and during periods of movement artifact (resulting, for instance, from shivering or tremors).

OSCILLOMETRY

Most noninvasive devices used in current practice measure blood pressure by oscillometry. In this method, variations in cuff pressure resulting from arterial pulsations during cuff deflation are sensed by the monitor and used to determine pulsations corresponding closely to true mean arterial pressure. The cuff is inflated to a pressure above the previous systolic pressure and then it is deflated incrementally. A transducer senses the pressure changes, which are then processed by the microprocessor. This technique has an accuracy of $\pm 2\%$. The mean arterial pressure corresponds to the maximum oscillation (maximum amplitude $= A_{max}$) at the lowest cuff pressure (*Fig. 88.1*).

Systolic and diastolic pressure readings are derived indirectly from formulas that examine the rate of change of the pressure pulsations. It has been determined that systolic and diastolic pressure occur when the amplitudes of oscillation ($A_{systolic}$ and $A_{diastolic}$) are a certain fraction of A_{max}. The systolic pressure corresponds to the onset of rapidly increasing oscillations. Algorithms used by different manufacturers vary and are never publicly disclosed, making it impossible for investigators to verify the accuracy of their underlying physiologic principals. In general, the systolic pressure is chosen as the pressure above the mean pressure at which oscillations are increasing in amplitude and are at 25% to 50% of the maximum ($A_{systolic}/A_{max} = 0.25$ to 0.5). Diastolic pressure corresponds to the onset of rapidly decreasing oscillations and is more difficult to determine. It is commonly labeled as the

ⓒ 2006 Mayo Foundation for Medical Education and Research

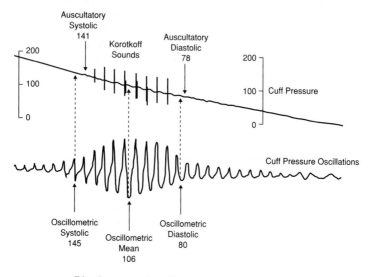

FIGURE 88.1. Blood pressure from Karotkoff sounds (*top*) compared to oscillometry (*bottom*).
From Geddes LA. *Cardiovascular Devices and their Applications.* New York: John Wiley; 1984: *Fig. 34.2.*

point below the mean pressure at which the pulse amplitude has declined to 60% of A_{max} ($A_{diastolic}/A_{max} = 0.6$), or it is calculated from the systolic and mean arterial pressure, using the following formula: MAP = diastolic + one-third pulse pressure. main problem with this technique is that the amplitude of the oscillations depends on several factors other than blood pressure, such as the stiffness of the arteries. Elderly subjects and patients with "stiff," atherosclerotic arteries have a loss of arterial wall compliance, which is associated with higher systolic and diastolic blood pressure readings using blood-pressure cuffs as compared with values obtained from direct arterial measurements.

PROPER USE

Appropriate sizing and positioning of the blood-pressure cuff are important in measuring pressure accurately. Cuff width should be 20% greater than arm diameter, and the cuff should be applied snugly after any residual air has been squeezed out. The pneumatic bladder inside the cuff should span at least half the circumference of the arm and should be centered over the artery. In general, a cuff that is too large works well and produces little error; however, a cuffs that is too narrow yields falsely elevated values for blood pressure because the pressure within the cuff is incompletely transmitted to the underlying artery.

In certain situations, noninvasive blood-pressure cuffs may be used on one extremity but not on another. Noninvasive blood-pressure cuffs should not be used on an extremity with deep-vein thrombosis, ischemic changes, arteriovenous fistula, or arteriovenous graft. In addition, such cuffs should not be applied directly over a peripherally inserted central catheter. If a patient has had a mastectomy or lumpectomy, avoid using noninvasive blood-pressure cuffs on the involved arm or arms to avoid worsening lymphedema. Use this monitor cautiously in patients with depressed consciousness or pre-existing peripheral neuropathies. Arrhythmias may lead to unreliable measurements from oscillometric devices.

In some situations, noninvasive blood-pressure monitoring is inadequate, and placement of an arterial line is indicated. Situations that require beat-to-beat, blood-pressure monitoring; frequent cuff cycling for prolonged periods; titration of vasoactive infusions; or frequent laboratory draws of arterial blood gas are better suited to invasive monitoring with an arterial line. Keep in mind that the peripheral arterial line is not without its limitations. For example, in a patient with substantial vasodilation during the period immediately after a cardiopulmonary bypass procedure, blood-pressure measurements obtained using a noninvasive blood-pressure cuff on the arm may be more accurate than a radial-artery invasive line secondary to the cuff's more central location.

ERRORS OF MEASUREMENT

Atherosclerotic lesions in the subclavian or axillary arteries, causing obstruction of flow, may lead to misleadingly low pressure distally in the affected arm. Thus, elderly patients or patients with known peripheral atherosclerosis should have blood pressure verified in both arms, and the arm with the higher blood pressure should be monitored to avoid this "pseudohypotension." If both arms are diseased, resulting in bilateral falsely low pressures, the femoral artery may be the best option for monitoring. Alternatively, if the risks of invasive monitoring are too substantial, relative to its benefit, the noninvasive pressure may be followed as a trend relative to its baseline.

Besides cuff size and bladder placement, other potential sources of error include arrhythmias causing pulse irregularities; small wrinkles or folds in the cuff expanding and changing the cuff's volume suddenly during data collection; and small movements of the patient, which may create excessive artifact. When the heart rate is irregular, the cardiac output and blood pressure vary greatly from beat to beat. Performance of the oscillatory cuff depends on all measurements made during a cycle. Cuff bladders are set to deflate at a manufacturer-specific "bleed rate," which assumes a regular pulse between bleed steps as part of the algorithms used to determine systolic and diastolic pressure. Therefore, any error caused by irregular beats or by motion of the patient may affect the accuracy of the blood-pressure device.

Data that include significant artifacts should be identified and discarded. The source of the artifact, such as poor positioning of the cuff, tubing occlusion, patient movement, and intermittent compression by the surgeon, should be removed and the affected data should be discarded. The entire cycle should be repeated if measurements are determined to be unreliable. If it is not possible to remove the source of the artifact, consider moving the cuff to an alternative site.

COMPLICATIONS

Complications with use of the noninvasive blood-pressure cuff may occur on rare occasions despite its being noninvasive and relatively safe. These complications include skin irritation and bruising, infection, neuropathy, thrombophlebitis, venous stasis, petechiae, ecchymoses, and even compartment syndrome and skin necrosis. Compartment syndrome is a serious complication and requires prompt surgical intervention. Patients taking anticoagulants are at an increased risk for formation of hematoma and development of compartment syndrome with use of noninvasive blood-pressure cuffs. These events typically occur during prolonged periods of use with excessively frequent cuff cycling, which results in local trauma or impaired distal limb perfusion. Other contributing factors include poor positioning of the cuff across a joint, the continuous pressure of a firmly applied deflated cuff, or repeated attempts to determine blood pressure in the presence of a malfunctioning cuff or an artifact-producing condition, such as involuntary tremors.

TAKE HOME POINTS

- Automated noninvasive blood-pressure devices are reliable and sufficient in most clinical settings.
- The blood-pressure cuff should be properly sized and placed to be effective.
- Problems with accuracy of noninvasive readings may arise in those patients with severe hypotension, arrhythmias, or severe atherosclerosis.
- Use an arterial line when beat-to-beat monitoring of blood pressure, use of vasoactive infusions to control blood pressure, or frequent laboratory draws of arterial blood gas are anticipated.
- Although relatively safe, this device has been associated with development of complications, including skin irritation, bruising, infection, neuropathy, thrombophlebitis, venous stasis, petechiae, ecchymoses, compartment syndrome, and skin necrosis.

SUGGESTED READINGS

Alford JW, Palumbo MA, Barnum MJ. Compartment syndrome of the arm: a complication of noninvasive blood pressure monitoring during thrombolytic therapy for myocardial infarction. *J Clin Monit Comput.* 2002;17:163–166.

Butani L, Morgenstern BZ. Are pitfalls of oxcillometric blood pressure measurements preventable in children? *Pediatr Nephrol.* 2003;18(4):313–318.

Hensley FA Jr, Martin DE, Gravelee GP, eds. *A Practical Approach to Cardiac Anesthesia.* 3rd ed. Philadelphia: Lippincott Williams & Wilkins; 2003;103–114.

Lin CC, Jawan B, de Villa MV, et al. Blood pressure cuff compression injury of the radial nerve. *J Clin Anesth.* 2001;13:306–308.

Miller RD, ed. *Miller's Anesthesia.* 5th ed. New York: Churchill Livingstone; 2000:1121–1123, 1860.

Sutin KM, Longaker MT, Wahlander S, et al. Acute biceps compartment syndrome associated with the use of a noninvasive blood pressure monitor. *Anesth Analg.* 1996;83:1345–1346.

Van Montfrans GA. Oscillometric blood pressure measurement: progress and problems. *Blood Press Monit.* 2001;6:287–290.

Vidal P, Sykes PJ, Saughnessy OM, et al. Compartment syndrome after use of an automatic arterial pressure monitoring device. *Br J Anaesth.* 1993;73:902–904.

89

DON'T LET THE TOURNIQUET TIME RUN LONG

BYRON D. FERGERSON, MD AND RANDAL O. DULL, MD, PHD

A senior anesthesiologist once facetiously remarked to the authors that tourniquet use requires its own little anesthetic plan—discussion of risks and benefits, inflation (equals induction?), maintenance, deflation (equals emergence?), and post-tourniquet (equals postoperative?) pain management. There is a kernel of truth in this.

Tourniquets are used by surgeons during surgery on extremities to decrease overall blood loss and to facilitate operating conditions by keeping the surgical field clear of blood. To deliver effective care to patients, anesthesia providers must carefully maintain a state of vigilance over all aspects of tourniquet use. Surgeons inform patients of plans to use a tourniquet during the procedure, and plans for tourniquet use may be noted in consents as well. However, planned tourniquet use may necessitate a separate discussion between the anesthesia provider and the patient, especially if a regional block is planned to counteract pain resulting from tourniquet use.

Application of the tourniquet is often preceded by exsanguination of the limb by circumferential wrapping of the limb in an Esmarch bandage. An alternative to using an Esmarch bandage is elevating the limb for 5 minutes (at 90°- and 45°-angles for upper and lower extremities, respectively). The cuff should be from 7 to 15 cm greater that the circumference of the limb and should be placed at the site of maximal circumference. The padding placed under the cuff should have no obvious folds. It is recommended that the cuff be inflated to a level 50 mmHg above the level at which distal pulse is lost, as assessed by Doppler, or to a level 50 mmHg above the patient's systolic-pressure level for upper-limb procedures and 100 mmHg above the patient's systolic-pressure level for lower-limb procedures. Most authors agree that from 1.5 to 2 hours is the outer limit for safe use of a tourniquet. This period can be extended by cooling the limb or allowing for 10 minutes of reperfusion for every hour of cuff inflation. Paying vigilant attention to the length of tourniquet use, inflation pressure, and proper cuff fit is important in preventing complications. Communicating with the surgeons also helps; do not be shy about asking questions and expressing concerns, especially if the length of tourniquet use is running long. Establishing open communication before a crisis arises will facilitate resolution of any problem, so discuss plans

© 2006 Mayo Foundation for Medical Education and Research

and target goals for the length of tourniquet use with the surgeons before beginning the procedure.

Tourniquets are among the oldest medical devices in history. There is a considerable body of literature on the consequences of tourniquet application, and the physiologic effects are protean.

MUSCLE

Predictably, tourniquet use affects muscle tissue. During tourniquet inflation, the combination of acute ischemia and pressure may cause increased microvascular permeability. Cellular hypoxia occurs within minutes of inflation. Ischemic cells release lactic acid, lysozymes, myoglobin, proteolytic enzymes, and inflammatory mediators, including histamine, leukotrienes, platelet-activating factors, and oxygen radicals. All of these substances are redistributed into the systemic circulation immediately after tourniquet deflation and may cause significant vasodilatation and hypotension. In addition, venous stasis distal to tourniquets allows the accumulation of high levels of CO_2 and metabolic byproducts, including potassium, which may cause arrhythmias. After tourniquet deflation, reperfusion hyperemia can lead to compartment syndrome, rhabdomyolysis, and the post-tourniquet syndrome of stiffness, pallor, and weakness without paralysis or numbness.

NERVES

Nerve conduction stops approximately 30 minutes after inflation of the tourniquet, possibly due to axonal hypoxia. Nerve injuries, from simple paresthesia to paralysis, have been reported following tourniquet use. Nerves are most commonly injured at the edges of the tourniquet where the applied pressure is greatest. The radial nerve is the nerve most commonly injured by tourniquets, followed by the ulnar and median nerves. The overall incidence of tourniquet-induced nerve injury in the upper extremity is 1 in 11,000 procedures. In the lower extremity, the sciatic nerve is the most susceptible, with injuries occurring in approximately 1 in 250,000 procedures. The use of Esmarch bandages to exsanguinate the upper limb increases the risk of injury, because it can generate pressures of as much as 1000 mmHg.

Tourniquet use is frequently painful and patients who are awake during tourniquet use often show signs of increasing distress. The patient may deny incisional or operative pain but complain bitterly of an aching or burning pain in the distal extremity. Slow, unmyelinated, C-nerve fibers are thought to be responsible. Under normal circumstances, pain impulses from fast, myelinated A fibers inhibit C-fiber conduction, but these fast fibers are more susceptible to compression and are thus blocked earlier, leaving C-fiber conduction uninhibited.

The anesthesia provider must manage pain from tourniquet use on an ongoing intraoperative basis. Because pain may be experienced as soon as

30 minutes after inflation, the patient may say that "the block is not working." Sedation is often called for, but, unfortunately, pain from tourniquet use does not respond to narcotics or sedation in a predictable manner. Most experienced anesthesia providers, however, have and are willing to use an informal algorithm for the intravenous treatment of pain from tourniquet use. Some feel that ketamine, given in sedation doses with an appropriate benzodiazepine, may provide help; others initiate a low-dose propofol infusion.

Using a very dense sensory block with a long-acting anesthetic as the primary technique may provide the best chance of avoiding pain from tourniquet use. For the upper extremity, an adjunctive "ring" or musculocutaneous nerve block may also be done with 10 cc of local anesthetic, often an equal-parts mixture of lidocaine and bupivacaine. Remember that, in the limb bearing the tourniquet, epidural and intrathecal sensory levels must be assessed by touch instead of pinprick. Blockade of the nerve fibers associated with touch occurs more slowly and regresses more quickly than blockade of those associated with pinprick sensation. Use of epinephrine, morphine, and clonidine should be considered, because these drugs increase the intensity of the neuraxial sensory block.

Occasionally, asking the surgeons to consider deflation after 120 minutes of tourniquet use or at some other point during surgery is necessary. This request can cause considerable contention in the operating room, as surgeons rarely plan for premature tourniquet deflation. The final option is to begin using a general anesthetic at that point.

CARDIOVASCULAR

Significant blood volume shifts can be associated with inflation and deflation of the cuff. Exsanguination of and inflation of the cuff on a lower limb can lead to a 15% increase in circulating blood volume, thus increasing the pulmonary-artery, central-venous, and systemic arterial pressures. These effects can be exaggerated in patients with severe varicose veins or poor left ventricular compliance. Patients under general anesthesia will show an increase in blood pressure and heart rate about 30 minutes after cuff inflation. Deepening the level of anesthesia does not always effectively resolve this problem, and use of vasoactive substances may be necessary. Caution is advised, however, because the hemodynamic effects of inflation are reversed at deflation and reperfusion. Anesthesia practitioners at all levels are usually prepared for an initial decrease in the hemodynamic state; what sometimes surprises less-experienced practitioners is how persistent it can be. Previous administration of a significant dose of hydralazine can compound the problem.

HEMATOLOGIC

The major hematologic concern is the incidence of thrombosis, although study results regarding whether tourniquet use actually increases the incidence of deep-vein thrombosis and subsequent pulmonary embolism are inconclusive. Several studies using transesophageal echocardiography have documented emboli in the right atrium following cuff deflation in up to 100% of patients having total-knee arthroplasty. Emboli tend to form in a large portion of lower-extremity surgeries, regardless of whether a tourniquet is used, but tourniquets are associated with larger, more hemodynamically significant emboli. Sickle-cell disease is a relative contraindication to tourniquet use as there is a theoretical risk that the hypoxic and acidotic environment distal to the cuff may induce a vaso-occlusive crisis. However, several studies suggest that if normothermia, normocarbia, and normoxia are maintained and the limb is properly exsanguinated, tourniquets can be used safely in these patients.

PHARMACOKINETICS

Tourniquet inflation and deflation also alter drug kinetics. Drugs given before inflation may be sequestered in the limb, although this is of uncertain clinical significance. Antibiotics should be given at least 5 minutes before inflation to ensure adequate concentrations at the surgical site. Drugs with large volumes of distribution, such as fentanyl and midazolam, have prolonged durations of action when given after inflation, particularly in the elderly.

TAKE HOME POINTS

- Watch the tourniquet time.
- Tourniquets have predictable physiological effects.
- Tourniquets cause pain in awake patients and elicit sympathetic activation in patients under general anesthesia.

SUGGESTED READINGS

Blaisdell FW. The pathophysiology of skeletal muscle ischemia and the reperfusion syndrome: a review. *Cardiovasc Surg.* 2002;10(6):620–630.

Gielen MJ, Stienstra R. Tourniquet hypertension and its prevention: a review. *Reg Anesth Pain Med.* 1991;16(4):191–194.

Kam PC, Kavanagh R, Young FE, et al. The arterial tourniquet: pathophysiological consequences and anaesthetic implications. *Anaesthesia.* 2001;56(6):534–545.

Wakai A, Winter DC, Street JT, et al. Pneumatic tourniquets in extremity surgery. *J Am Acad Orthop Surg.* 2001;9(5):345–351.

90

BRAIN FUNCTION MONITORS ATTEMPT TO LINK AN INTRAOPERATIVE MEASUREMENT WITH POSTOPERATIVE RECALL—MUCH IS KNOWN AND MORE IS UNKNOWN AS DEFINITIVE PRACTICE PARAMETERS AND "BEST USE" GUIDELINES FOR THESE MONITORS

STEPHEN T. ROBINSON, MD AND
CATHERINE MARCUCCI, MD

BACKGROUND

In October, 2005, the American Society of Anesthesiologists (ASA) published a Practice Advisory for Intraoperative Awareness and Brain Function Monitoring (Practice Advisory). A task force composed of anesthesiologists, methodologists, and consultants, some of whom disclosed financial relationships with the brain-monitoring device companies, prepared the Practice Advisory. The primary issue addressed in the Practice Advisory is whether use of clinical techniques, conventional monitoring systems, or brain-function monitors to assess the depth of anesthesia will reduce the occurrence of intraoperative awareness. The Practice Advisory summarizes the most pertinent information on brain-function monitoring and provides an in-depth review of the literature. We recommend that all anesthesia providers review this document in its entirety.

One of the key points of the Practice Advisory is that "intraoperative awareness cannot be measured during the intraoperative phase of general anesthesia, since the recall component of awareness can only be determined postoperatively by obtaining information directly from the patient." Essentially, the term "intraoperative awareness" is commonly used to mean explicit recall. Brain-function monitors attempt only to monitor depth of anesthesia, defined by the ASA as "a continuum of progressive central nervous system depression and decreased responsiveness to stimulation." Calling such monitors, which monitor brain function or brain activity, "awareness monitors" is misleading.

AWARENESS MATTERS

Published studies have indicated that the incidence of intraoperative recall may be as high as 1 to 2 per 1,000 patients receiving general anesthetics. One

© 2006 Mayo Foundation for Medical Education and Research

study concluded that the use of brain-function monitors could reduce this incidence by as much as 80%.

Intraoperative recall is an important event. Some patients who have had unplanned intraoperative awareness have suffered from posttraumatic stress disorder, primarily relating to the circumstance of being aware during surgery, and possibly in pain, without the ability, because of paralysis, to convey their predicament. Unfortunately, the ability to measure the presence and impact of implicit memory is beyond our current technology.

TRADITIONAL SIGNS OF ANESTHETIC DEPTH

Traditionally, anesthesia providers evaluated heart rate, blood pressure, purposeful movement, papillary responses, lid reflex, sweating, and tearing and monitored the patient with an end-tidal analyzer to assess whether anesthesia depth was adequate. At present, no clinical trials or other comparative studies have examined the effect of clinical assessment or conventional monitoring on the incidence of intraoperative awareness; however, some cases have been documented in which patients had intraoperative awareness in the absence of observed increases in heart rate and blood pressure. In a consensus opinion, the Practice Advisory recommends continued use of these physiologic parameters to assess anesthetic depth in all patients.

CURRENT TECHNOLOGY AND APPLICATION

The major devices currently being marketed to assess anesthetic depth use forehead electrodes to record electroencephalographic (EEG) activity with or without electromyographic (EMG) information, or they use auditory evoked potentials (AEP). An analog EEG signal is processed via various public or proprietary algorithms applied to one or more of the following categories of data: frequency, amplitude, latency, and phase-relationship. A unitless number, often referred to as an "index," is generated. It typically is scaled from 0 to 100, and it represents the spectrum of states of consciousness. Zero corresponds with an isoelectric EEG or absent middle-latency AEP, and 100 corresponds with a state of complete wakefulness.

The bispectral (BIS) monitor (made by Aspect Medical Systems, Inc.) is the best known device and is the device most frequently cited in published studies. It uses a BIS-analysis approach to a single channel of frontal-lobe EEG signal processing. A linearly decreasing BIS number is generated from the nonlinear EEG changes as plasma concentrations of anesthetics increase. The manufacturer posits that a BIS monitor number of from 40 to 60 reflects a low probability of consciousness under anesthesia, and the literature supports this to an extent. One randomized controlled clinical trial found lower explicit recall rates when BIS monitors were used than when they were not used. Other studies have shown shorter periods for emergence from anesthesia, first response, and eye opening as well as lower consumption of anesthetic drugs and shorter post anesthesia care unit (PACU) times with use of BIS monitors.

LIMITATIONS AND CAVEATS

Several caveats govern use of BIS and other brain-activity monitors, and anesthesia providers using these devices must be aware of these limitations. First, the index values generated by individual devices are not standardized across the various monitoring technologies. Second, the measured values do not have uniform sensitivity across a cross-section of patients. For example, mean preinduction values for the BIS monitor have been reported to range from 80 to 98. Third, although the monitors provide numeric values that *generally* correlate with depth of anesthesia, equipotent doses of drugs may produce different values, depending on the use of opioids and nitrous oxide. Fourth, the monitors require time to collect and process sufficient information to provide accurate results. If there is a rapid change in the dosage of anesthetics or the level of surgical stimulation, other signs of inadequate anesthesia may precede indication of a change by the brain-activity monitor.

Some case reports describe additional difficulties with brain-activity monitors. Both routine and untoward intraoperative events may interfere with monitor function. These events include administration of muscle relaxants, use of the electrocautery, patient warming or cooling, hemorrhage, and cerebral ischemia. Of great interest to the clinical anesthesiologist, several reports have been made of patient awareness despite a generated BIS index value consistent with a depth of anesthesia sufficient to produce minimal risk of recall. These cases serve as an important reminder that, even with a low BIS number, all conversation near the patient should be conducted as if the patient were awake.

WHEN TO USE

Practice standards for brain-function monitors are far from complete. Except for situations in which anesthesia providers cannot place the electrodes, there are no situations in which brain-function monitoring is absolutely indicated or contraindicated. In the Practice Advisory, the ASA task force distinguishes among situations in which such monitoring likely would have differing degrees of clinical usefulness. The circumstances that tended to increase support for monitoring were those in which the patient was likely to have very light general anesthesia as a result of patient condition or surgical procedure.

The ASA task force does *not* agree with the statement that a brain–electrical-activity monitor should be used to assess intraoperative depth of anesthesia for all patients. They agree that an electrical activity monitor may or should be used to gauge depth of anesthesia for patients with certain conditions requiring smaller doses of anesthetics, but they also state that "there is insufficient evidence to justify a standard, guideline, or absolute requirement that these devices be used to reduce the occurrence of intraoperative awareness in high-risk patients undergoing general anesthesia." Further, the ASA task force is equivocal about basing use of brain-activity monitors on the type of surgery (Cesarean section, cardiac surgery, trauma surgery, etc.).

In an editorial accompanying the release of the Practice Advisory, ASA president Eugene Sinclair, MD, writes that the entire area of brain-function monitoring likely will require continuing and frequent review, both by the ASA and the individual anesthesia provider. He suggests that, much like pulse-oximetry monitoring, the clinical-practice issues pertaining to the use of the BIS monitor (and other monitors) eventually may not be driven by outcome studies, but by an evolving legal climate. One can hope that good science will ultimately determine the use of these monitors.

TAKE HOME POINTS

- Explicit memory is the only reliable end point that can be used to determine whether intraoperative awareness has occurred.
- Awareness monitors are more accurately characterized as brain-activity or brain-function monitors.
- The primary goal of using such monitors is providing intraoperative values that reflect the likelihood of explicit recall.
- Several devices, of which the best known and most commonly used is the BIS monitor, are used to measure anesthetic depth. The BIS monitor uses a bispectral-analysis (or BIS-analysis) approach to a single channel of frontal-lobe EEG signal processing.
- In October, 2005, the American Society of Anesthesiologists (ASA) published a Practice Advisory for Intraoperative Awareness and Brain Function Monitoring, which contains an overview of the subject of brain-function monitoring and elucidates several clinical situations in which brain-function monitoring may be sufficiently useful to recommend its use.
- Using a brain-function monitor is not a substitute for using traditional techniques to determine depth of anesthesia; nor does it guarantee that the patient will not have explicit or implicit memory. Maintaining proper decorum in the presence of patients is a must.
- Many anesthesia providers use brain-function monitors regularly and feel that such monitors are an important tool in clinical care; however, practice parameters are still evolving.

SUGGESTED READINGS

Ekman A, Lindholm ML, Lennmarken C, et al. Reduction in the incidence of awareness using BIS monitoring. *Acta Anaesthesiol Scand.* 2004;48(1):20–26.

Gan TJ, Glass PS, Windsor A, et al. Bispectral index monitoring allows faster emergence and improved recovery from propofol, alfentanil, and nitrous oxide anesthesia. *Anesthesiology.* 1997;87:808–815.

Monk TG, Saini V, Weldon BC, et al. Anesthetic management and one-year mortality after noncardiac surgery. *Anesth Analg.* 2005;100:4–10.

Mychaskiw G, Horowitz M, Sachdev V, et al. Explicit intraoperative recall at a bispectral index of 47. *Anesth Analg.* 2005;100:1363–1364.

Myles PS, Leslie K. Bispectral index monitoring to prevent awareness during anaesthesia: The b-aware randomised controlled trial. *Lancet.* 2004;363:1757–1763.

Practice Advisory for Intraoperative Awareness and Brain Function Monitoring; A report by the American Society of Anesthesiologists Task Force on intraoperative awareness. *Anesthesiology.* 2006;104:847–864.

91

DO NOT IMPROVISE TECHNIQUES TO WARM PATIENTS—USE WARMING DEVICES *ONLY* AS PER MANUFACTURERS' RECOMMENDATIONS

JEFF T. MUELLER, MD

NORMAL THERMOREGULATION AND MONITORING STANDARDS

In human beings, thermoregulatory mechanisms maintain a core body temperature of approximately 37°C, with a "normal" range of only 0.2°C. (circadian and menstrual influences also cause up to a 1.0°C variation of the core temperature). The body-temperature control system operates via an elegant feedback loop. Widely distributed, distinct heat and cold receptors send afferent thermal input via nerve fibers to the central nervous system and more specifically to the hypothalamus, which is the primary thermoregulatory control center. Hyperthermia results in efferent hypothalamic output that causes cutaneous vasodilation and sweating. Hypothermia generates hypothalamic outputs leading to vasoconstriction, shivering, and, in infants, nonshivering thermogenesis. *Overall*, the most important mechanism for maintaining normal human body temperature is behavior. The obvious inability of anesthetized patients to add clothing and blankets or adjust the thermostat removes their most important defense against hypothermia.

It has long been recognized that metabolic functions deteriorate when internal temperatures are abnormal and also that both regional and general anesthesia impair thermoregulatory mechanisms. This knowledge is reflected in the American Society of Anesthesiologists' Standards for Basic Anesthetic Monitoring, which state that "during all anesthetics, the patient's oxygenation, ventilation, circulation, and *temperature* should be continually evaluated" and that "every patient receiving anesthesia shall have temperature monitored when clinically significant changes in body temperature are intended, anticipated or suspected."

Core-temperature monitoring sites include the tympanic membrane, pulmonary artery, nasopharynx, and the distal portion of the esophagus. Whether the bladder is a site permitting accurate measurement of core temperature depends upon urine flow. Core temperature may be measured in the bladder if urine flow is high; however, if urine flow is low, the measurement made may reflect peripheral temperature.

© 2006 Mayo Foundation for Medical Education and Research

COMPLICATIONS OF HYPOTHERMIA

Evidence suggests that perioperative hypothermia contributes to increases in surgical-wound infections, intraoperative blood loss, transfusion requirements, myocardial ischemia, and arrhythmias. The cardiac risks are highlighted in perioperative guidelines published by the American College of Cardiology and American Heart Association. Hypothermia has also been shown to slow the metabolism of anesthetic drugs and to increase the duration of postanesthetic recovery. The postoperative sensation of cold and shivering is unpleasant for patients and is recalled by some as causing more discomfort than was caused by surgery.

THE PATHOPHYSIOLOGY AND PHYSICS OF HYPOTHERMIA

Perioperative hypothermia is caused when a patient is in a relatively hypothermic environment while simultaneously experiencing a loss of thermoregulatory control.

The difference between the patient temperature and the operating room ambient temperature drives heat transfer from the patient to the surrounding environment. There are four modes of heat transfer: radiation, convection, evaporation, and conduction. All play some role in heat loss in surgical patients; the greatest amount occurs by radiation.

Both general anesthesia and regional anesthesia impair thermoregulation. General anesthesia inhibits thermoregulation in a dose-dependent manner. Cold-response thresholds are significantly reduced, and warm-response thresholds are slightly elevated. Anesthesia increases the above-mentioned threshold range from $0.2°C$ to $2°$ to $4°C$. The initial phase of anesthesia is dominated by a rapid redistribution of heat from the core to the periphery due to vasodilation. During the next 2 to 4 hours, core temperature decreases, albeit at a slower rate, primarily because heat loss exceeds metabolic heat production. Neuraxial anesthesia disrupts thermoregulatory mechanisms by blocking sensation and neural transmission, causing vasodilation without inducing any compensatory mechanisms. Thus, a combination of anesthesia-induced thermoregulatory dysfunction and an unfavorable thermal environment result in heat loss and hypothermia in surgical patients.

PREVENTING HYPOTHERMIA

All members of the patient's surgical care team are responsible for preventing perioperative hypothermia, beginning with care in the preoperative area and extending into the operating room by maintaining the ambient room temperature at a reasonable level. A normal and comfortable room temperature is required during patient transport into and out of the operating room. For the comfort of the care team, it may be reasonable to lower the ambient temperature once the patient is covered, the surgical site is prepped, and warming devices have been applied. The operating room ambient temperature is the most important determining factor of heat loss. In addition to ambient temperature management, warming devices can be used to prevent hypothermia. Less than 10% of metabolic heat is lost through the respiratory tract. Therefore, active heating and humidification of ventilator gases has minimal impact on core-temperature maintenance. The temperature of intravenous fluids is also a consideration. Since the temperature of intravenous fluids and blood products cannot significantly exceed body temperature, actively heating patients with fluid warmers is not possible. However, heating of fluids is required to prevent heat loss when large volumes are administered. Preventing cutaneous heat loss is also necessary. Passive insulation, such as using blankets, may be adequate for small operations. More extensive operations require active cutaneous warming, using forced-air or circulating-water devices.

PREVENTING PATIENT INJURY WHILE PREVENTING HYPOTHERMIA

Warming devices should always be operated according to the manufacturer's instructions. Improper use can result in excessive heat and burns. The use of forced-air blankets should be avoided in areas affected by peripheral vascular disease or other causes of significantly impaired circulation, especially vascular cross clamping. These warming devices should be used only with the appropriate, specified blanket. The heated forced-air output should not be used in any other way since improper use has been documented to cause thermal injury to the patient. In addition, operating-room warming cabinets must be operated at a safe temperature. Burns can also occur when heated intravenous fluid bags or blankets are used as positioning aids. Items pressed against the patient may reduce perfusion in the contact area and cause burns at temperatures that would otherwise be safe. All operating rooms should follow a rigorous plan for monitoring and maintaining safe temperatures in warming cabinets. An analysis of the American Society of Anesthesiologists closed claims database revealed that intravenous fluid bags or bottles were the most common cause of claims related to operating-room burns; the second most common cause was warming devices, such as heating pads and blankets. Remember that any warming device can potentially harm anesthetized patients, who cannot sense excessive heat.

TAKE HOME POINTS

- Regional and general anesthesia impair thermoregulation.
- Hypothermia can harm patients by impairing coagulation, increasing infection rates, and contributing to myocardial stress.

- Patients can be kept normothermic when appropriate measures are instituted throughout the perioperative period.
- Misuse of warming devices can cause thermal injury.
- Do *not* use heated bags of crystalloid solution to warm patients!

SUGGESTED READINGS

American Society of Anesthesiologists. *Standards for Basic Anesthetic Monitoring*. Amended October 25, 2005. www.asahq.org.

Eagle KA, Berger PB, Calkins H, et al. ACC/AHA guideline update for perioperative cardiovascular evaluation for noncardiac surgery update: a report of the American College of Cardiology/American Heart Association Task Force on Practice Guidelines (Committee to Update the 1996 Guidelines on Perioperative Cardiovascular Evaluation for Noncardiac Surgery). 2002. Available at the American College of Cardiology web site: http://www.acc.org/clinical/guidelines/perio/ update/periupdate_index.htm.

Kressin KA, Posner KL, Lee LA, et al. Burn injury in the OR: a closed claims analysis. *Anesthesiology*. 2004;101:A-1282.

Sessler DI. Mild perioperative hypothermia. *N Eng J Med*. 1997;339(24):1730–1737.

Wass CT. Thermoregulation and perioperative hypothermia. In: Faust RJ, Cucchiara RF, Wedel DJ, et al, eds. *Anesthesiology Review*. 3rd ed. Churchill Livingstone; 2001;91–92.

Sessler, DI. Temperature monitoring. In: Miller RD, ed. *Miller's Anesthesia*. 6th ed. Elsevier Churchill Livingstone, 2005;1571–1597.

92

REMEMBER THAT THE EFFECTS OF PRONE POSITIONING DEPEND ON FRAMES

LAURA H. FERGUSON, MD AND SHAWN T. BEAMAN, MD

Prone positioning is necessary for surgical access to the posterior spine, the posterior fossa, and the posterior aspect of the lower extremities. Spine procedures commonly using the prone position are discectomy, laminectomy, and spinal fusion. Recent studies have shown that the cardiopulmonary effects of prone positioning depend on which surgical frame is used, rather than on patient body mass index. Knowing the various frames therefore will greatly assist anesthesiologists as they care for patients in the prone position.

Many surgical frames are used for posterior spine procedures, and the differences between them can confuse the anesthesiologist. Keep in mind that the surgical frame selected should help expose the surgical field and decrease blood loss, which commonly results from prone positioning. Spine surgeons choose surgical frames based on whether the procedure requires preserving or decreasing lordosis of the cervical and lumbar spines. Preserving lordosis maintains alignment of the spine for fusion procedures. Decreasing lordosis allows better access to the intervertebral space and is commonly used for discectomy after herniation. Understanding the commonly used surgical frames will help the anesthesiologist understand the cardiopulmonary physiology encountered during procedures done on patients in the prone position.

The two frames that maintain lordosis involve using longitudinal bolsters or the Jackson table. Longitudinal bolsters, consisting of two parallel chest rolls commonly made from foam or rolled sheets, are inexpensive and effective. The bolsters extend from just caudad to the clavicle to just beyond the inguinal area, bilaterally, and are used on a conventional surgical table. The Jackson table is an elaborate, free-standing surgical table with 360-degree rotational capabilities and pads to support the thighs, pelvis, and chest, which allows the abdomen to hang freely. Using the Jackson table has been shown to affect ventilatory mechanics and hemodynamics less than does using longitudinal bolsters.

The frames that decrease lordosis are the Wilson frame, the Relton-Hall frame, and various kneeling frames. The Wilson frame involves using two longitudinal, curved pads to provide continuous support to the chest

© 2006 Mayo Foundation for Medical Education and Research

and pelvis. This frame is used on a conventional surgical table. With space between the two pads, the abdomen is not fully compressed using this frame. The curve in the Wilson frame pads can also be decreased to restore lordosis to permit a fusion to be done. The Relton-Hall frame, consisting of two pairs of V-shaped pads, one pair in the upper thoracic region and one pair along the pelvis, leaves the abdomen hanging free. Kneeling frames come in many varieties including the knee-chest, the modified knee-chest (Andrews), the tuck, and the modified tuck frames. Use of these frames optimizes pulmonary physiology, especially in obese patients, but increases the risk for nerve palsies and hypotension, because these frames cause blood to pool in the lower extremities. Use of the kneeling frames is also contraindicated in patients whose vertebral columns are unstable.

Prone positioning alters pulmonary mechanics and hemodynamics no matter which frame is used. Specifically, prone positioning decreases pulmonary compliance. The magnitude of this decrease varies with the frame used. The main cause of such reduced pulmonary compliance is elevated intra-abdominal pressure resulting from the surgical table or frame compressing the abdominal wall and abdominal viscera. This increased pressure is referred to the diaphragm and, in turn, to the lungs, resulting in a decrease in pulmonary compliance. These changes are manifested clinically as high peak airway pressures during positive pressure ventilation. Pressure control ventilation can be used to limit the high airway pressures. Palmon et al. demonstrated that pulmonary mechanics in the prone position depend on which frame is used and not on body habitus. This study concluded that use of the Jackson table disturbed ventilatory mechanics, as measured by peak airway pressure, less than did use of the Wilson frame or longitudinal bolsters. Several studies have assessed the efficacy of different surgical frames for prone positioning. Use of a surgical frame that allows the abdomen to hang freely in the prone position has repeatedly been shown to decrease pulmonary compliance less than does use of other surgical frames.

Hemodynamic changes in patients in the prone position also stem from elevated pressure on the abdominal wall, which exerts increased pressure on the abdominal viscera. The pressure is transmitted throughout the abdomen and can compress blood vessels, specifically the inferior vena cava (IVC). Venous return is forced to follow collateral pathways to the right heart. One such pathway is the epidural plexus, and engorgement of epidural veins can significantly increase blood loss during and otherwise complicate spine procedures. In addition to increasing blood loss, compression of the IVC can also decrease preload, which, in turn, decreases cardiac output and systemic blood pressure. Use of an appropriate surgical frame is intended to decrease abdominal compression and, consequently, to decrease surgical blood loss and systemic hypotension. Dharmavaram et al. studied hemodynamic and cardiac function in prone patients using transesophageal echocardiogram. The changes in hemodynamics noted in this study with use of various frames were not statistically significant. Despite the lack of statistical significance, the data reflected that prone positioning affects hemodynamic function. A trend in the data suggested that the Jackson table may produce the least amount of hemodynamic variation with prone positioning. Note that the patients in this study were healthy; hemodynamic changes may become clinically and statistically significant in patients with decreased cardiac reserve.

Prone positioning poses other unique risks to the patient, and the anesthesia provider must consider these risks in the preoperative assessment and discuss them with the patient. Before the procedure, patients should be informed of the possibility of vision loss, neuropathies, and need for blood transfusion due to surgical blood loss. Perioperative vision loss, according to The American Society of Anesthesiologists (ASA) Closed Claims Database, is becoming more frequent in spine surgery. The Post Operative Vision Loss (POVL) Registry was formed to permit study of these relatively rare complications. A recent retrospective case analysis of cases involving POVL demonstrated that 83% of cases of POVL resulted from ischemic optic neuropathy (ION) and were not related to pressure on the globe during prone positioning. The development of ION positively correlates with intraoperative blood loss of more than 1 liter or anesthesia lasting more than 6 hours; the etiology of this correlation is unknown. Central retinal artery occlusion (CRAO), a less frequent cause of POVL, however, is thought to be related to pressure on the globe, is usually unilateral, and typically is accompanied by ipsilateral periorbital erythema, corneal abrasion, ptosis, or decreased supraorbital sensation. Development of POVL can devastate patients, and informing patients in advance of this rare risk is prudent.

Any surgery may result in development of neuropathies; however, brachial plexus injury and lateral femoral cutaneous nerve palsy are specific risks in procedures done on patients in the prone position. Lateral femoral cutaneous nerve palsy is thought to result in as many as 20% of patients who have spine surgery while in the prone position. It is manifested by decreased sensation over the lateral thigh and has been shown to resolve in as many as 90% of patients. Brachial plexus injury, although rarer, is thought to result from turning the patient's neck and overstretching the nerves of the brachial plexus while the patient is in the prone position. The patient's head must be left in a neutral position, using a foam prone positioning pillow or cradle.

TAKE HOME POINTS

- Increased intra-abdominal pressure decreases pulmonary compliance in patients in the prone position.

- Using a surgical frame that allows the abdomen to hang freely disturbs pulmonary compliance less than does use of other frames.
- Prone positioning can also decrease systemic blood pressure and increase blood loss.
- Use of particular frames in surgery on healthy patients has not been shown to change hemodynamic variables significantly; however, it may do so in patients with decreased cardiac reserve.
- Use of the Jackson table affects ventilatory mechanics and hemodynamics less than does use of other frames.
- Prone positioning also increases the risk for development of peripheral neuropathies and postoperative vision loss (POVL). Discussing these complications with patients before surgery is important.

SUGGESTED READINGS

Barash PG, Cullen BF, Stoelting RK, eds. *Clinical Anesthesia*. 5th ed. Philadelphia: Lippincott Williams & Wilkins, 2006;643–644, 657–661.

Dharmavaram S, Jellish WS, Nockels RP, et al. Effect of prone positioning systems on hemodynamic and cardiac function during lumbar spine surgery: an echocardiographic study. *Spine*. 2006;31(12):1388–1893; discussion 1394.

Lee LA, Roth S, Posner KL, et al. The American Society of Anesthesiologists Postoperative Visual Loss Registry. *Anesthesiology*. 2006;105:652–659.

Miller RD, ed. *Miller's Anesthesia*. 6th ed. Philadelphia: Elsevier Churchill Livingstone, 2004;1151–1166.

Palmon SC, Kirsch JR, Depper JA, et al. The effect of the prone position on pulmonary mechanics is frame-dependent. *Anesthesia and Analgesia*. 1998;87(5):1175–1180.

Schonauer C, Bocchetti A, Barbagallo G, et al. Positioning on surgical table. *European Spine Journal*. 2004; Oct 13 (suppl 1):S50–S55. Epub: 2004 Jun 22. Review.

93

CARDIAC OUTPUT MEASUREMENT: DO YOU REALLY UNDERSTAND THE UNDERLYING PRINCIPLES?

VALERIE SERA, DDS, MD AND
MATTHEW CALDWELL, MD

Fegler introduced the thermodilution method for measuring blood flow in 1954. The introduction of the flow-directed pulmonary artery catheter (PAC) in the 1970s permitted clinicians to measure intracardiac pressures directly. Hemodynamic data gathered from PAC use are widely used to diagnose and to help guide medical therapy in critically ill patients in the operating room, cardiac catheterization laboratory, and intensive care unit. Such data can be helpful in differentiating between cardiogenic and noncardiogenic shock and in guiding decision-making about fluid, vasoactive, and inotropic drug therapy over time. For the patient to benefit from PAC use, the clinician must thoroughly understand the interpretation and use of hemodynamic data and must be well aware of the limitations of data obtained from PAC use. Although pulmonary artery catheterization has not been proven to improve outcome, expert opinion continues to support its judicious use after evaluation of the potential risks and benefits for each patient (Pulmonary Artery Catheter Consensus Conference 1997).

HOW PAC TECHNOLOGY WORKS

The PAC is 100 cm long, with proximal and distal ports that enable the measurement of intravascular and intracardiac pressures and the sampling of blood as well as the infusion of vasoactive and inotropic drugs and fluids. At the very tip of the PAC lies the thermistor. The thermistor, when appropriately positioned in the pulmonary artery, continuously measures the temperature of the blood passing by the tip of the PAC in the pulmonary artery. Relatively cold (iced or room-temperature) fluid is injected into the right atrium via the proximal port of the PAC and decreases the temperature of the blood passing distally by the thermistor into the pulmonary circulation. A thermodilution curve is generated by plotting the decline in the pulmonary artery temperature against time in seconds. The area under the curve is integrated and then incorporated into the Stewart-Hamilton equation to yield the cardiac output (CO):

$$CO = [V \times (T_b - T_i) \times K_1 \times K_2]/[\int \Delta T_b(t)dt]$$

© 2006 Mayo Foundation for Medical Education and Research

where V = volume of injectate, T_b = temperature of blood, T_i = temperature of injectate, K_1 = density factor, K_2 = computation constant, and $\int \Delta T_b(t)dt$ = integral of blood temperature over time. The computation constant is specific to the brand of catheter, and it incorporates specific variations in catheter dead space, approximate injection temperature, injection rate, heat exchange, and unit conversion. The greater the cardiac output the smaller the temperature change over time. Matching the constant with the correct volume (5 or 10 cc) and temperature (iced or room temperature) of injectate to be used is imperative. Dissection of this equation exposes a number of data points that, if inaccurately obtained, will result in a miscalculated CO, which may lead to an inaccurate diagnosis and a misguided therapy.

PLACEMENT AND RISK

Assessing the overall risks and benefits of placing a PAC is important. Placing a PAC not only permits calculation of CO but also permits direct measurement of pulmonary-artery systolic, diastolic, and mean pressures and right heart filling pressures as well as indirect measurement of left ventricular filling pressures. *Figure 93.1* depicts the correct path of the PAC through the right heart. An extra port in the PAC permits direct infusion of vasoactive and inotropic drugs into the central venous circulation.

Placing the large bore catheter that allows the introduction of the PAC into the central venous circulation poses risks for infection, pneumothorax, hemothorax, and bleeding at the puncture site or from disconnection of a line. Placing the PAC itself increases the risk for arrhythmia while the PAC floats through the right atrium and ventricle to the pulmonary artery. The most devastating complication associated with PAC use is pulmonary artery rupture. Although pulmonary artery rupture with hemorrhage is infrequent, with an incidence of 0.2%, it is associated with a mortality rate of up to 50%. The right pulmonary artery is involved in 93% of such cases, which usually affect the right lower or middle lobe branches.

ERRORS OF MANAGEMENT

Keep in mind that the thermodilution method measures pulmonary blood flow. Under normal circumstances, pulmonary blood flow equals systemic blood flow. The presence of intracardiac shunts, tricuspid regurgitation (TR), and cardiac arrhythmias, and rapid infusion of intravascular fluid can affect the accuracy of thermodilution CO measurements. The presence of a left-to-right shunt will yield a falsely high CO, because the pulmonary blood flow exceeds the systemic blood flow by an amount equal to the shunt from left to right. The presence of significant TR makes the CO calculations unreliable; it invalidates the thermodilution method, because a portion of the cold indicator continues to stay in the right atrium and right ventricle, therefore not producing a significant change in blood temperature. The

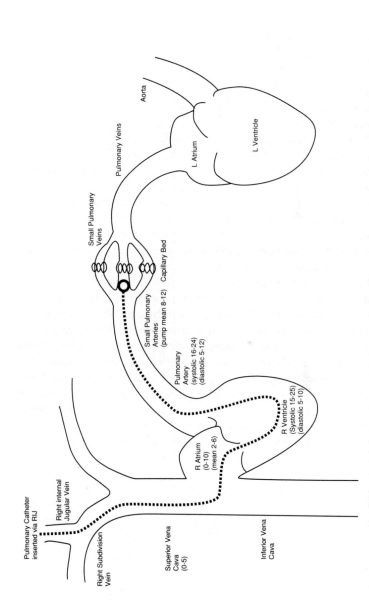

FIGURE 93.1. The path of a PAC through the right heart chambers to the pulmonary artery and the relation of PCWP to left atrium pressure. Normal pressures are given in mmHg. RIJ, right internal jugular vein.

presence of cardiac dysrhythmias alters the beat-to-beat cardiac ejection, thereby yielding an inaccurate CO.

The accuracy of the CO calculation depends highly on operator consistency. Averaging at least three measurements made by the same operator yields the most reliable results, eliminating interoperator inconsistency and improving the precision of the CO calculation. The number of measurements averaged for each determination greatly affects the standard error of the mean (SEM), which is the basis for predicting reproducibility. There is a 2% to 5% variance in SEM when three measurements are averaged to calculate a single CO, and there is a 3% to 9% variance in SEM when only one measurement is used. When comparing CO over time and using three measurements per CO determination, a difference of 15% or more is needed to indicate that the results are actually different. If only one measurement per CO determination is used, then a difference of 26% or more is needed to indicate that the results are actually different. Therefore, at least three measurements should be done by the same operator and the average should be used to calculate CO.

Five or 10 cc of room-temperature or colder injectate should be selected. The volume and temperature must remain consistent. Use of room-temperature and use of colder injectate both have produced accurate and reproducible results. Variations in injectate volume alter results. Excess volume yields falsely low CO calculations, whereas inadequate volume yields falsely high CO calculations. Injectate should be administered steadily over 2 to 4 seconds. Deviation from this rate may alter heat transfer with the surrounding tissues, reducing the accuracy of the computation constant. A faster rate of injection may affect filling volume for the cardiac cycles being measured. Measurements used to calculate CO should be done at end expiration because, at that time, the baseline pulmonary artery blood temperature varies less.

ERRORS OF INTERPRETATION

Whether the risk-to-benefit ratio favors use of the PAC in critically ill patients remains unclear; however, it remains one of the procedures most commonly done on critically ill patients around the world. For more than three decades, the PAC has been used primarily to monitor cardiac function via the thermodilution method, and it also is used to indicate left-ventricular end-diastolic pressure (LVEDP) and left-ventricular end-diastolic volume (LVEDV) status by measuring pulmonary artery occlusion pressure (PAOP). Measuring PAOP and thereby indicating LVEDP in a critically ill patient permits more accurate prediction of the change in cardiac output in response to a fluid challenge. To use PAOP as an accurate surrogate for LVEDP or LVEDV, the PAOP tracing must be valid, accurate, and correctly interpreted; the PAOP must reflect accurately left-ventricular end-diastolic pressure; and, most importantly, the relation between LVEDP and LVEDV must be predictable.

Normally the relation between LVEDP and LVEDV depends on ventricular compliance and, when graphed, has a characteristic curvilinear appearance. The criteria noted in the previous paragraph for use of PAOP as an accurate surrogate for LVEDP or LVEDV are not likely to be met simultaneously in a clinical setting; in addition, the presence of other clinical factors, such as mechanical ventilation or positive end-expiratory pressure, may reduce accuracy. The change in PAOP after a fluid challenge appears to indicate better left-ventricular compliance than it does left-ventricular filling. However, the change in CO may indicate the position of the left ventricle on the Frank-Starling curve. Many studies have shown that PAOP does not indicate LVEDP reliably and predicts recruitable CO poorly.

ALTERNATIVE OR SUPPLEMENTAL TECHNIQUES

Assessing patients using data derived from the PAC may no longer be the gold standard. In critically ill patients, clinician assessment of left-ventricular dysfunction and ventricular preload status showed lower predictive probability than did assessment by transesophageal echocardiography (TEE). Unfortunately, extensive training in and experience with TEE are necessary for its use in assessing ventricular function, volume status, and cardiac output, and such training and experience are not universal among intensive care unit and operating room personnel. Physicians have been shown to acquire skill rapidly in using transthoracic echocardiography (TTE) to assess volume only. Potential use of TTE to estimate LVEDV directly, using CO, is quite promising.

Additional ways to measure cardiac output exist and have limitations of their own. Esophageal Doppler has been used to guide fluid therapy by optimizing stroke volume in cases in which the patient has lost a large amount of blood, and its use has been shown to reduce the length of hospital stay. By integrating the velocity of blood flow through the aorta over time and multiplying it by the cross-sectional area of the aorta, a stroke volume is determined, conferring information on contractility, preload, and vascular resistance. This method has technical limitations. Frequent adjustment of the Doppler probe is necessary for accurate measurements, and calculation of stroke volume depends on the cross-sectional area of the aorta being cylindrical and not changing over time. The Doppler method's advantage is that it is much less invasive than other methods; however; the learning curve associated with its use is steep. Its use is limited to intubated patients.

Pulse contour analysis assumes that the elasticity and impedance of the aorta remain constant and that the shape of arterial pulsation is proportional to stroke volume. To determine the elasticity and impedance of the aorta,

TABLE 93.1	CERTAIN VARIABLES' EFFECT ON CARDIAC OUTPUT	
TECHNICAL ERRORS	**MEASUREMENT ERROR CONSEQUENCE**	**COMMENT**
Rate of injection too slow >4 seconds	Inaccurate CO	
Rate of injection too fast <2 seconds	Inaccurate CO	
Falsely high computation constant	Falsely high CO	May occur if entered constant for room-temperature injection when using iced injection
Falsely low computation constant	Falsely low CO	May occur if entered constant for iced injection when using room-temperature injection
Excess volume injected	Falsely low CO	Will cause larger temperature change at catheter tip
Inadequate volume injected	Falsely high CO	Will cause smaller temperature change at catheter tip
L → R shunt	Falsely elevated CO	Pulmonary CO > systemic CO
Tricuspid regurgitation	Falsely elevated CO	
Cardiac dysrhythmias	Less precise result	Greater beat-to-beat variability

an independent cardiac output determination by indicator dilution must be made. Some systems for doing so exist, have been validated, and are slowly emerging in the market place. The most reliable systems tend to be the most invasive. For example, one reliable system requires use of a central line and a femoral arterial line for optimal calibration. Thoracic bioimpedance, carbon dioxide rebreathing, and perfusion surrogates are other methods, but are clumsy and clinically impractical.

Table 93.1 illustrates certain variables' effects on cardiac output accuracy.

TAKE HOME POINTS

- The risks of inserting a PAC should be weighed carefully against the value of the data that will be obtained.
- Operator knowledge and experience influence the reliability of cardiac output measurements.
- Taking at least three measurements and using the average is important because of the variability among measurements.
- Inputting the correct catheter constant is essential to obtaining a valid cardiac output measurement.

- Operator consistency increases the accuracy of the cardiac output measurement.
- Understanding the limitations of PAOP as a surrogate of LVEDV is important.
- Using TEE or TTE along with CO may provide the most complete picture of a patient's cardiovascular status.

SUGGESTED READINGS

American Society of Anesthesiologists Task Force on Pulomonary Artery Catheterization. An Updated Report by the ASA Task Force on Pulmonary Artery Catheterization. *Anesthesiology.* 2003;99(4):988–1014.

Beaulieu Y, Marik PE. Bedside ultrasonography in the ICU: part 1. *Chest.* 2005;128(2):881–895.

Boyd KD, Thomas SJ, Gold J, et al. A prospective study of complications of pulmonary artery catheterizations in 500 consecutive patients. *Chest.* 1983;84(3):245–249.

Cholley BP, Payen D. Noninvasive techniques for measurements of cardiac output. [Review] [67 refs]. *Current Opinion in Critical Care.* 2005;11(5):424–429.

Cigarroa RG, Lange RA, Williams RH, et al. Underestimation of cardiac output by thermodilution in patients with tricuspid regurgitation. *American Journal of Medicine.* 1989;86(4): 417–420.

Elkayam U, Berkley R, Azen S, et al. Cardiac output by thermodilution technique. Effect of injectate's volume and temperature on accuracy and reproducibility in the critically Ill patient. *Chest.* 1983;84(4):418–422.

Fegler G. Measurement of cardiac output in anaesthetized animals by a thermodilution method. *Quarterly Journal of Experimental Physiology & Cognate Medical Sciences.* 1954;39(3): 153–164.

Fontes ML, Bellows W, Ngo L, et al. Assessment of ventricular function in critically ill patients: limitations of pulmonary artery catheterization. Institutions of the McSPI Research Group. *Journal of Cardiothoracic & Vascular Anesthesia.* 1999;13(5):521–527.

Ganz W, Donoso R, Marcus HS, et al. A new technique for measurement of cardiac output by thermodilution in man. *American Journal of Cardiology.* 1971;27(4):392–396.

Marik PE. Pulmonary artery catheterization and esophageal doppler monitoring in the ICU. *Chest.* 1999;116(4):1085–1091.

Nadeau S, Noble WH. Limitations of cardiac output measurements by thermodilution. *Canadian Anaesthetists' Society Journal.* 1986;33(6):780–784.

Pulmonary Artery Catheter Consensus Conference: Consensus Statement. *Critical Care Medicine.* 1997;25(6):910–925.

Shah KB, Rao TL, Laughlin S, et al. A review of pulmonary artery catheterization in 6,245 patients. *Anesthesiology.* 1984;61(3):271–275.

Stetz CW, Miller RG, Kelly GE, et al. Reliability of the thermodilution method in the determination of cardiac output in clinical practice. *American Review of Respiratory Disease.* 1982;126(6):1001–1004.

Summerhill EM, Baram M. Principles of Pulmonary Artery Catheterization in the Critically Ill. *Lung.* 2005;183:209–219.

Swan HJ, Ganz W, Forrester J, et al. Catheterization of the heart in man with use of a flow-directed balloon-tipped catheter. *New England Journal of Medicine.* 1970;283(9):447–451.

Vender JS, Franklin M. Hemodynamic assessment of the critically ill patient. [Review] [72 refs]. *International Anesthesiology Clinics.* 2004;42(1):31–58.

94

INFUSION PUMPS: GREAT TECHNOLOGY WHEN IT WORKS

STEPHEN T. ROBINSON, MD AND
RICHARD BOTNEY, MD

Infusion pumps are invaluable devices for delivering drugs and fluids at reliable and controlled rates. They are especially valuable for establishing stable blood levels of short-acting drugs. The three basic infusion delivery methods are gravity, peristalsis or metered delivery, and piston (syringe pump).

GRAVITY

Before infusion devices were widely used, infusion rates were regulated manually, and the rate was estimated by counting drops (gtts) in the intravenous (IV) drip chamber (*Fig. 94.1*). Adjustments were made by moving the roller ball on the IV tubing. Typical chambers delivered an estimated 10 to 60 gtts/ml. Depending on the chamber design, 10 to 60 gtts/min were required to deliver 60 ml/hr. Although manual regulation is still used for simple IV fluid infusions, it is generally not appropriate for most drug administration unless there is a wide tolerance for error, close user observation and regulation, or an emergency situation.

Relying on gravity poses many challenges. No alarms or other safety features alert the user of problems or prevent errors in flow rate. Since the flow rate depends on gravity and on the patency of the IV line, the flow rate may change as the hydrostatic pressure from the bag decreases as the fluid is consumed. IV bags commonly empty unnoticed, requiring flushing of air from the IV line before continuation of infusion. Adjusting the wrong line can cause delivery of an inadequate amount of drug or cause inadvertent delivery of a bolus of a high-risk medication, such as potassium, with disastrous results. Labeling each line near the regulator and taping the roller ball may help reduce this risk.

Gravity devices are essentially manual systems that use a calibrated constrictor on the IV tubing. Using these devices, when they are working as intended, provides a more reliable infusion rate than does using the roller ball. Using gravity devices also reduces the risk for inadvertent delivery of a bolus of drugs, but poses the same risks as do standard gravity setups for obstruction and reduced delivery. In short, gravity devices are easy to set up and simple to use, but require close user monitoring.

© 2006 Mayo Foundation for Medical Education and Research

d = desired infusion rate in mcg/kg/min

w = weight in kg

c = concentration in mg/ml

g = drops per milliliter (gtts/ml) for that tubing

$k_1 = 1000$ mcg/1mg

$k_2 = 60$ min/hr

$$\text{gtts/min} = \frac{d \cdot w \cdot g}{c \cdot k_1}$$

$$\text{ml/hr} = \frac{d \cdot w \cdot k_2}{c \cdot k_1}$$

FIGURE 94.1. Calculating infusion rates in gtts/min (a) or ml/hr (b) for doses in mcg/kg/min.

EARLY ELECTRONIC INFUSION DEVICES

There were many early infusion devices, all of them crude by today's standards and prone to substantial errors. One early device counted drops and adjusted the flow to match the desired count per minute. It was critical that the operator knew the volume/gtt. Converting the desired dose to the corresponding rate was a nontrivial exercise. If the sensor was partially dislodged, the device was prone to administer a large bolus because of the faulty feedback. Another device used special tubing that was tightly wound around three occluding rollers. Based on the bore of the selected tubing and the revolutions per minute of the device, one could estimate the delivery rate from a table provided by the manufacturer. Different models had different rate profiles. Of course, the wrong tubing or confusion of units (for instance, ml/min vs. ml/hr) posed some threat to the patient. Both of these systems could deliver wide-open flow when disconnected from the device without first manually occluding the IV tubing.

Early syringe pumps used a screw and piston to advance the plunger into the barrel of the syringe. The rate was determined from a table that calculated the rate in ml/min or ml/hr, based on syringe bore and screw revolutions per minute. All of the complications described below with current devices as well as additional risks existed. These pumps had no high pressure alarm, and the risk of error in calculating the rate was substantial.

When using any early infusion system, infusing drugs in some forms, such as mcg/kg/min, required using a relatively complex formula, and the potential for error was great.

COMMON PRINCIPLES

Current devices primarily provide peristaltic or similar, metered delivery or are syringe pumps. They can be programmed to deliver fluids or drugs in a wide array of units, such as ml/hr or mcg/kg/min. Many allow the entry of a drug name to provide default settings, including concentration, rate parameters, bolus permission with parameters, and even differing protocols, for that drug.

Infusion devices must be set up and operated properly. Fluid connection must be done appropriately and aseptically. The drug and its concentration must be checked carefully to ensure that they correspond to the values entered on the pump. Carefully inspecting the fluid path, including all connections, can help prevent obstruction of flow and inadvertent infusion of fluid into the atmosphere as well as inadvertent administration of air into the vein. Labeling each set of tubing at both the site of rate regulation and the site of insertion into the common carrier can avoid trouble downstream.

When administering drugs, a carrier should be used. To ensure reliable delivery, the carrier should be placed on a pump. Lines with drugs should be placed close to the distal end of the carrier tubing to limit dead space, to reduce the risk for inadvertent delivery of a bolus, and to reduce changing flow rates' effect on the rate of drug administration.

Newer pumps have safety features, which usually make the device safer. These features may include dosing recommendations, alarms, and automated stopping features. Standardized protocols, especially for drug concentration, are useful to avoid large errors of drug administration. Never assume that a drug has been prepared with the recommended concentration because a protocol exists. Each use requires doing the appropriate checks.

Alarms alert the user that a device has failed and assist in troubleshooting the cause. An obstruction-to-flow alarm is probably the most useful type of alarm. Some alarms, like high-pressure alarms, sound unnecessarily when set too sensitively and thus distract the user. However, setting such alarms too permissively may delay recognition of an obstruction for a prolonged period, especially when a lower flow rate is used. Automated stopping is most typically for volume regulation or air identification. Proper de-airing of the line is critical to avoid pump failure. When clearing air or when decompressing an obstruction, avoid inadvertent delivery of a bolus of drug by ensuring that the tubing is disconnected from the patient or that the drug has an alternative pathway for elimination from the system.

Multiple infusions pose special problems. One must ensure reasonable drug compatibility if using a common carrier line. Spaghetti tangles can cause obstruction, disconnects, and administration errors. Neatness counts.

PERISTALTIC AND METERED DEVICES

Peristaltic devices are the most commonly used infusion devices in hospitals and are primarily used to administer drugs and fluids from a bottle or bag. They have been manufactured to handle from one to four simultaneous infusions. The portion of tubing that passes through the device must be matched to the device. Although some devices can be modified to accommodate syringes, the higher resistance associated with pulling the plunger into the barrel tends to limit such use. Inadvertent delivery of a bolus of fluid is possible when connecting or disconnecting these devices. To prevent this, the manufacturers routinely provide a device that automatically obstructs flow when removing the tubing from the device. They also, wisely, recommend that a manual regulator on the IV tubing be fully closed when loading or unloading tubing.

SYRINGE PUMPS

Syringe pumps tend to be smaller and lighter than standard peristaltic pumps. They work by loading a syringe into an array of clamps and plungers. A rotating screw functions as a piston to push the syringe plunger at the desired rate. The faster the screw spins, the faster the plunger is advanced into the barrel of the syringe. To match the actual flow rate of the syringe with the programmed rate of flow, the correct brand and size of syringe must be entered into the pump. If the syringe's actual bore is larger than the size programmed into the pump, the rate of fluid administration will be greater than expected. Most devices have sensors attached to the barrel fastener to prevent large errors in bore size from being entered. Such sensors would prevent, for example, a 10 cc syringe from being programmed as a 20 cc syringe. However, differences in bore size among syringes of a given size produced by different manufacturers are too small for these devices to distinguish accurately yet are large enough to create errors in the range of 5% to 10% if there is a mismatch between the actual and programmed brands.

Syringe pumps can fail in several ways to deliver fluids. Obvious causes include programming the device erroneously, triggering safety features and preventing activation; failing to turn on the device; clamping the tubing; and depleting the battery instead of using AC power. Improperly loading the syringe can cause problems. Failing to secure properly the barrel of the syringe can cause the whole syringe to advance rather than advance the plunger into the barrel. Even when a user follows the loading process reasonably well, additional sometimes more minor loading errors may prevent the system from working. Improper priming of the system may cause delays in delivering fluids at very low rates (<10ml/hr), because the entire screw, piston, plunger axis has not been fully engaged. Manually advancing the piston is not priming, because some slack may remain in the screw–piston connection. At higher rates, this is less of a concern. Use the purge function to prime the pump, but do not purge into the patient's IV.

TAKE HOME POINTS

- Be properly trained on the device before you use it on a patient.
- Generally, peristaltic pumps are more versatile, but syringe pumps can be simpler to use in some locations.
- Carefully load, program, and label each drug and fluid.
- When initiating the administration of a drug, ensure that the device is properly connected and that flow is not obstructed.
- Use a carrier that is also on a pump.
- Use standardized concentrations where possible to avoid errors when changing bags or syringes.

SUGGESTED READING

Zarmsky RF, Parker AJ, Sinatra RS. Infusion pumps. In: Ehrenwerth J, Eisenkraft JB, eds. *Anesthesia Equipment: Principles and Applications.* St. Louis: Mosby; 1993:647–673.

95

SCAVENGING WASTE GASES BENEFITS THE STAFF BUT MAY HARM THE PATIENT

TERRENCE L. TRENTMAN, MD

Why scavenge waste anesthetic gases? Since the early days of anesthesia, anesthesia providers have been both concerned with and challenged by minimizing the risks associated with volatile anesthetics. Ether and cyclopropane were known to cause explosions, and, by the 1960s, serious questions had also arisen with regard to possible mutagenicity, carcinogenicity, and teratogenicity of the volatile anesthetics. Because the volatile anesthetics are likely to remain ubiquitous in clinical practice, the anesthesia provider must be aware of the following issues: the history behind current anesthetic waste gas scavenging practice; the recommended limits for trace gas levels issued by the National Institute for Occupational Safety and Health (NIOSH); the real risks of teratogenicity; the mechanics of scavenging systems, including open versus closed interfaces and active versus passive gas–disposal assemblies; sources of exposure to waste gas; and the risk of obstructions in the scavenging system.

CHRONIC EXPOSURE TO WASTE GASES

Studies done in the 1960s on the risks of chronic exposure to waste anesthetic gases yielded conflicting results. A human study suggested an increased incidence of spontaneous abortion among female anesthesiologists, and an animal study showed that high concentrations of nitrous oxide could cause skeletal deformities in offspring. Subsequent publications supported the idea that waste anesthetic gases put anesthesia providers at risk for adverse health effects. In the 1970s, NIOSH recommended that waste anesthetic gases be scavenged and set recommended acceptable waste gas levels (*Table 95.1*). However, both prospective and epidemiologic studies conducted in the 1980s and 1990s have shown that, when scavenging is used to reduce amounts of volatile anesthetics to trace amounts, the waste gases pose no risk of adverse health effects. Also, health risks are not associated with short-term clinical (or unscavenged) exposure to potent volatile agents, such as isoflurane or sevoflurane. Experimental nitrous oxide exposure has been associated with animal reproductive abnormalities; however, these conditions do not exist for workers in the clinical environment in which scavenging is present. Of note, NIOSH transmitted its recommendation to the Occupational Safety and Health Administration (OSHA) in 1977. Since that time,

© 2006 Mayo Foundation for Medical Education and Research

TABLE 95.1	NATIONAL INSTITUTE FOR OCCUPATIONAL SAFETY AND HEALTH TRACE GAS RECOMMENDATIONS, 1977	
ANESTHETIC GAS		MAXIMUM CONCENTRATION (PPM)
Agent alone		
Halogenated		2
Nitrous oxide		25
Combined halogenated and nitrous oxide		
Halogenated agent		0.5
Nitrous oxide		25

Adapted from US Department of Health, Education, and Welfare: Criteria for a Recommended Standard: Occupational Exposure to Waste Anesthetic Gases and Vapors. Washington, DC, US Department of Health, Education, and Welfare, March, 1977.

OSHA has not taken the necessary steps to promulgate the standards, but it has published technical instructions regarding waste gases. The Joint Commission on Accreditation of Healthcare Organizations has recommended that each anesthesia machine be equipped with a scavenging system and that monitoring be carried out.

SCAVENGING SYSTEMS

An anesthesia provider can use several methods to minimize the concentrations of anesthetic gases in the operating room environment. These methods include ensuring a tight mask fit, flushing into the waste gas system rather than the room, turning gas flow off at the end of each case, carefully filling vaporizers using a keyed filler rather than a funnel, and using a cuffed endotracheal tube when possible. In addition, a leak test should be done routinely on both the high- and low-pressure components of the anesthesia machine. *Most important is the presence of a properly functioning waste-gas-scavenging system.*

A waste-gas-scavenging system has five components (*Figure 95.1*), including the gas-collecting assembly, the transfer means, the scavenging interface (open versus closed), the gas-disposal assembly tubing, and the gas-disposal assembly (active versus passive). Excess gas from the patient is collected via the ventilator relief valve or the adjustable pressure limiting (APL) valve. Collected gas is transferred to the scavenging interface via short, rigid (nonkinking) tubing. If the transfer causes obstruction of the tubing, *patient barotrauma can result as this portion of the scavenging system is proximal to the pressure relief capability of the scavenging interface.*

The scavenging interface can be of two types, open or closed. An open system is valveless and is essentially a canister open to the atmosphere. Gas

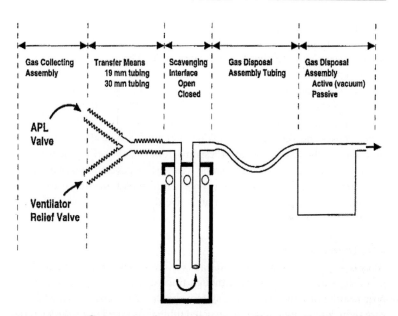

FIGURE 95.1. Components of a scavenging system. (Reproduced with permission from Barash PG, Cullen BF, Stoelting RK, eds. *Clinical Anesthesia.* 5th ed. Philadelphia: Lippincott Williams & Wilkins; 2006:589.) APL, adjustable pressure limiting valve.

from the transfer tubing is delivered to the bottom of the canister which serves as a reservoir. This arrangement prevents excessive negative- and positive-pressure build-up within the system; however, an active gas-disposal assembly (central vacuum) is necessary to ensure that waste gases stored in the reservoir (canister) do not escape into the room. The reservoir should be large enough to handle a variety of gas flow rates and gas surges. Some open systems rely upon the user to regulate the vacuum by adjusting a vacuum control valve.

Closed scavenging interfaces use valves to communicate with the atmosphere. A positive-pressure relief valve is necessary to protect the system from excess downstream pressure. The positive-pressure relief valve will open to room air if an obstruction occurs between the scavenging interface and the gas-disposal assembly. If the closed scavenging interface uses a passive gas-disposal assembly, only a positive-pressure relief valve is necessary. In this arrangement, the pressure from the waste gas itself moves the gas toward the disposal assembly, and neither a reservoir bag nor a negative-pressure relief valve is required.

When an active (e.g., central-vacuum) gas-disposal assembly is in place, a negative-pressure relief valve is necessary in the closed scavenging interface.

This prevents excessive negative-pressure build-up within the system by entraining room air as needed. A reservoir bag is also necessary to store, briefly, excess gases during the ventilator cycle. The vacuum control valve is adjusted so that the bag is neither under- nor over-inflated. The bag will be seen to expand during expiration and deflate during inspiration.

The gas-disposal tubing transfers waste gases to the disposal assembly. The appearance of such tubing should differ from that of the breathing system hoses and should resist kinking. The tubing is ideally run overhead to minimize the risk of the anesthesia machine or other equipment rolling on top of it. The gas-disposal assembly vents waste gases to a point outdoors that is remote from air intakes and people. The disposal assembly can employ a piped central-vacuum system or an active-duct system, in which fans or blowers move gases outside.

AVOIDING MISHAPS

Anesthesia providers can avoid mishaps by first understanding the mechanics of the scavenging system. Although trace waste anesthetic gases do not pose health risks, the scavenging system should be visually inspected to ensure tight connections and unobstructed tubing. As noted in *Figure 95.1*, the scavenging system uses 19- or 30-mm tubing that can be distinguished from the 15- and 22-mm tubing of the breathing system. Unfortunately, misconnections are still possible. The use of adapters or tape to make connections should warn the anesthesia provider of a possible misconnection.

One-hundred percent oxygen should be administered at the end of each case to wash excess gases into the disposal system. The vaporizers should be filled using a keyed filler, and the connections should be securely tightened. Use of low gas flows also reduces waste gas, as does use of regional and intravenous anesthetic techniques. However, minimizing waste gas should not supersede clinical considerations in choice of anesthetic technique.

Invariably, all anesthesia machines leak somewhat. Testing machines daily for leakage and servicing machines regularly minimizes leakage. Room ventilation systems should also be inspected and serviced by the institution's facilities department. Scavenged gases should be vented to the outside and not to other rooms in the hospital in which personnel may be exposed or the gases may contribute to fire risk (e.g., machine rooms).

TAKE HOME POINTS

- Short-term clinical (unscavenged) or long-term trace (scavenged) exposure to potent volatile agents does not cause adverse health effects.
- When scavenging systems are in place, nitrous oxide exposure has not been shown to increase reproductive risks.

- The anesthesia provider can use various techniques to minimize exposure to trace anesthetic gases, including inspecting the components of the scavenging system to ensure proper connections and absence of obstruction.
- The scavenging system protects health care workers, but malfunction of the system can lead to patient injury, including barotrauma or negative-pressure injury.

SUGGESTED READINGS

Dorsch JA, Dorsch SE. *Understanding Anesthesia Equipment.* 4th ed. Baltimore: Williams & Wilkins; 1999.

Barash PG, Cullen BF, Stoelting RK, eds. *Clinical Anesthesia.* 5th ed. Philadelphia: Lippincott Williams & Wilkins; 2006.

Fink BR, Shepard TH, Blandau RJ. Tertogenic activity of nitrous oxide. *Nature.* 1967;214: 146–148.

McGregor D. Occupational exposure to trace concentrations of waste anesthetic gases. *Mayo Clin Proc.* 2000;75:273–277.

National Institute for Occupational Safety and Health. *Occupational Exposure to Waste Anesthetic Gases and Vapors: Criteria for a Recommended Standard.* Cincinnati, Ohio: US Dept of Health, Education, and Welfare, Public Health Service, Center for Disease Control, National Institute for Occupational Safety and Health; 1977. Publication DHEW (NIOSH);77–140.

Vaisman AI. Working conditions in the operating room and their effects on the health of anesthetists [in Russian]. *Eksp Klin Anesteziol.* 1967;12:44–49.

www.osha.gov/dts/osta/anestheticgases/index.html

96

CARBON DIOXIDE ABSORBERS SAVE GAS AND MOISTURE BUT CREATE THE POTENTIAL FOR MECHANICAL HAZARDS, CHEMICAL SOUP, OR A THERMAL DISASTER

MICHAEL AXLEY, MD, MS AND STEPHEN T. ROBINSON, MD

The purpose of anesthesia circuits is to provide an efficient configuration to deliver oxygen and anesthetic gases and vapors to the patient. If only fresh gas is going to be delivered, the required gas flows may need to be as high as two and one half times the patient's minute ventilation (MV) to avoid rebreathing of carbon dioxide (CO_2). A patient with an MV of 6 L/min would require a fresh gas flow of 15 L/min. Using a CO_2 absorber, fresh gas flows of 500 ml/min or lower can be achieved.

BASIC MANAGEMENT OF ABSORBERS

Currently available CO_2 absorbents consist of soda lime (sodium hydroxide lime), barium hydroxide lime, potassium-hydroxide-free lime, calcium hydroxide lime, and non-caustic lime. These absorbents all contain hydroxide bases as their active component. The main reactant in these absorbents (except for in barium hydroxide lime) is calcium hydroxide. Since it is a slow reactant, other constituents are needed to allow the conversion to occur at a sufficient rate in vivo.

Soda Lime Reaction:

1) $CO_2 + H_2O \rightarrow H_2CO_3$ (fast)

2) $H_2CO_3 + 2NaOH \text{ (or KOH)} \rightarrow Na_2CO_3 \text{ (or } K_2CO_3) + 2H_2O$
$+ \text{ Energy (fast)}$

3) $Na_2CO_3 \text{ (or } K_2CO_3) + Ca(OH)_2 \rightarrow CaCO_3 + 2NaOH$
(or KOH) (slow)

The CO_2 absorbent is typically stored in two containers that operate in sequence on the expiratory limb of the anesthetic circuit. They lie distal to the ventilator relief valve and the adjusting pressure limiting (APL) valve. Hence, exhaled gas is preferentially routed to the scavenging system before it is cleared of CO_2. The lower the fresh gas flow, the more rapid the consumption of absorbent.

Because the flow of expired gas is unidirectional, most of the reaction occurs in the proximal chamber. As the reactant is consumed, the pH changes and the indicator in the white granules turns blue. Generally, the first

© 2006 Mayo Foundation for Medical Education and Research

chamber shows substantial change in color before the second chamber shows any change in color. The second chamber begins to change in color when the amount of available reactant becomes insufficient to eliminate fully the CO_2 at lower flows. It is then necessary to change the reactant or to use higher fresh gas flows.

Caustic water and residue can build up at the base of the absorber and along the distal tubing. To avoid inadvertent obstruction to gas flow, draining the fluid periodically and following routine maintenance recommendations, as provided by the anesthesia machine manufacturer, are necessary.

MECHANICAL COMPLICATIONS

Channeling is a condition that occurs when the gas flow through the absorbent is diverted through areas of low resistance, causing a 'channel' to be formed. Gas flowing through a channel does not undergo the reaction clearing CO_2—hence, absorbents that form channels are less effective. More ominously, absorbent that is exhausted or in which channeling has occurred may permit rebreathing of CO_2 through the circuit, with subsequent patient morbidity.

The issue of channeling is related to that of absorbent pellet size. Air flow through a mass of pellets varies inversely with pellet size; that is, larger pellets generate less resistance through the circuit. At the same time, large pellets expose less total surface area to air flow, decreasing the total surface area available to participate in the reaction that removes CO_2. The most commonly available pellet size for CO_2 absorbents is 4 to 8 mesh. "Mesh" indicates the number of openings per linear inch in a sieve used to measure the pellet particles.

Not all CO_2 rebreathing is related to consumption of CO_2 absorbent. Inspiratory and expiratory valves stuck in the open position can cause rebreathing. Kinked anesthesia hoses can also play a role.

Improperly sealing the CO_2 canister can cause a leak. The leak may be caused by failing to close the canister or by a loose granule obstructing the seal. Prepackaged granules, although more expensive, may reduce this risk. Improperly placed soda lime can also obstruct flow. This has been reported to occur with prepackaged granules when the packaging was not removed before insertion into the circuit.

ADVERSE CHEMICAL REACTIONS

The hydroxide bases in CO_2 absorbents are caustic and can cause tissue damage with skin exposure or inhalation. Persons handling these materials must take care to avoid splashing or spilling the new or used chemical. Gloves and eyewear should be worn when the canisters are moved or replaced.

In addition to removing CO_2 from the gas-and-vapor mixture, these strong bases break down or degrade the potent inhaled anesthetic agents.

The breakdown products differ among the various agents. Sevoflurane, upon degradation, generates a potentially nephrotoxic product called Compound A (2,2-difluoro-1-(trifluoromethyl)vinyl ether). Using fresh gas flows of 2 L/min or greater can prevent this reaction. Lower flow rates are acceptable for moderate periods of time. Isoflurane, desflurane and enflurane, under circumstances in which the CO_2 absorbent is dehydrated, can be broken down into carbon monoxide (CO), with subsequent reported cases of CO poisoning.

Dehydration is an important component of breakdown—the reaction of anesthetics increases as the water content of the CO_2 absorbent decreases. Complete desiccation of absorbent requires exposure to dry gas at room temperature for a number of hours, i.e., a fresh gas flow of 5 L/minute for 24 hours.

In addition to CO or Compound A, the reaction of inhalational anesthetics with desiccated CO_2 absorbent can produce flammable organic compounds. In the case of sevoflurane, these by-products include methanol and formaldehyde. Further, these breakdown reactions are exothermic. The combination of exothermic reaction and flammable breakdown products can accelerate the overall cycle to the point where spontaneous combustion may occur. Use of sevoflurane, in particular, has been reported to cause acute respiratory distress syndrome and spontaneous ignition and fire when combined with barium hydroxide lime absorbent. The combustion reaction may also consume sufficient anesthetic gas as to make maintenance of anesthesia problematic.

The desiccation of absorbent and the subsequent production of CO cannot be detected with routine anesthetic monitors. Traditional absorbents typically turn a blue-violet color when approaching exhaustion—this does not occur with desiccation. Diagnosing CO toxicity can be quite difficult when a general anesthetic has been used; symptoms such as confusion, nausea, shortness of breath, and dizziness might also be attributed to emergence from anesthesia. A pulse oximeter can measure arterial saturation of CO, but its efficacy in the operating room setting has not been well demonstrated.

Some experts have advocated monitoring the temperature of absorbents as a way to avoid potentially lethal outcomes. Such monitoring can be done, for example, by placing a temperature probe in the center of each canister of absorbent and sealing the edge of the canister with foam tape. Yet what temperature cut-off signals an impending event is unclear, as the temperature of the absorbent is elevated during normal use.

Although the capnogram is not a foolproof method of determining absorbent exhaustion, the presence of an elevated inspired CO_2 baseline may indicate absorbent exhaustion and or desiccation.

Of note, not all CO_2 absorbents are equal in terms of their propensity to react with anesthetic agents. Barium hydroxide lime appears to be significantly more reactive than soda lime, which is more reactive than potassium hydroxide-free lime, which is more reactive than calcium hydroxide lime and non-caustic lime.

Absorbent manufacturers have developed products, some moist and some desiccated, that produce an insignificant amount of or no compound A or CO. These products also produce minimal heat and minimally adsorb volatile agents.

The Anesthesia Patient Safety Foundation has issued recommendations for the use of absorbents, including use of CO_2 absorbents "whose composition is such that exposure to volatile anesthetics does not result in significant degradation of the volatile anesthetic." The foundation also recommends implementing policies at the institutional and departmental level "regarding steps to prevent desiccation of the carbon dioxide absorbent should they choose conventional carbon dioxide absorbents that may degrade volatile anesthetics when absorbent desiccation occurs." It further recommends adopting some simple approaches, including turning off gas flow when the machine is not in use, changing the absorbent at regular intervals, changing both canisters, and changing the canisters if they have been exposed to long-term fresh gas flow.

TAKE HOME POINTS

- CO_2 absorbers allow for safe, economical use of anesthetic gases.
- Anesthesia machines must be maintained to avoid leaks and obstruction of flow.
- The breakdown of anesthetic gases, particularly of sevoflurane, can lead to production of toxic byproducts and of CO.
- Desiccated CO_2 absorbent tends to promote adverse reactions.
- Breakdown reactions produce heat, and operating room fires can ensue under the right conditions.
- Use of more reactive formulations, such as barium hydroxide and those using potassium hydroxide, is being replaced by use of less reactive formulations. Note: Baralyme (Allied Health Care/Chemtron) brand of barium hydroxide lime has been removed from the market.

SUGGESTED READINGS

Barash PG, Cullen BF, Stoelting RK, eds. *Clinical Anesthesia*. 4th ed. Philadelphia: Lippincott Williams & Wilkins; 2001.

Baum, JA, Woehlck, HJ. Interaction of inhalational anesthetics with CO2 absorbents. *Best Pract Res Clin Anaesthesiol*. 2003;17(1):63–76.

Berry PD, Sessler DL, Larson MD. Severe carbon monoxide poisoning during desflurane anesthesia. *Anesthesiology*. 1999;90(2):613–616.

Fatheree, RS, Leighton, BL. Acute respiratory distress syndrome after an exothermic baralyme-sevoflurane reaction. *Anesthesiology*. 2004;101(2):521–533.

Woehlck, H. Sleeping with uncertainty: anesthetics and desiccated absorbent. *Anesthesiology*. 2004;101(2):276–278.

Wu J, Previte J, Adler E, et al. Spontaneous ignition, explosion and fire with sevoflurane and barium hydroxide lime. *Anesthesiology*. 2004;101(2):534–537.

97

Do not use your cell phone in the operating room

GRANT T. CRAVENS, MD AND JURAJ SPRUNG, MD, PHD

Electronic medical devices have become a mainstay of modern health care, and their complexity and usefulness continue to grow. Similarly, cellular telephones and other wireless communications devices have become commonplace in the United States and around the world, and their use also continues to increase with time. As part of this trend, many hospitals now use cellular telephones (cell phones), two-way pagers, and other wireless communications devices to assist with health-care delivery. Since the advent of cell phone technology, numerous and reproducible reports have documented cell phone use interfering with the operation of medical devices. These reports have prompted hospitals to enact various restrictions on cell phone use within hospital grounds, and they raise the question of whether cell phones can be safely used in proximity to medical devices. This question is of particular importance to anesthesia providers, who work with complex medical devices daily.

MECHANISMS OF INTERFERENCE

Radio waves can induce currents within electrical circuits. Some electrical circuits are designed for this purpose (e.g., an antenna), which is the basis for the use of radio waves as communication signals. Unfortunately, radio waves can sometimes induce unwanted electrical currents within the circuitry of medical devices, thereby causing interference. This phenomenon is known as electromagnetic interference (EMI). Cell phones operate on radio frequencies that are reserved for their use, so even medical devices that are designed to receive data via radio waves are unlikely to have interference by mistaking a cell phone transmission for an appropriate incoming signal. Rather, cell phone radio waves can induce currents in circuits that were not designed to receive radio waves at all. Other wireless communications devices, such as some personal digital assistants (PDAs) and two-way pagers, transmit data in the same way that cell phones do and are theoretically capable of producing EMI.

The risk of cell phone use causing EMI with a medical device depends on the distance between the devices, telephone transmission power, and device construction. Risk decreases with distance, and increases with higher transmission power. A cell phone's transmission power varies inversely with the strength of the signal it receives from its telephone tower. A cell phone receiving a strong signal will decrease its output to conserve battery life; a phone receiving a weak signal will increase its output to ensure more reliable reception. However, power output is always at a maximum when the cell phone is ringing. Characteristics of the medical device, such as outer metal shielding, can decrease vulnerability to EMI.

EFFECTS OF ELECTROMAGNETIC INTERFERENCE ON MEDICAL DEVICES

The devices most commonly affected by EMI are electrocardiographic (ECG) monitors, which often display signal noise and baseline movement as a result of EMI. Interference with ECG monitors is worrisome because of possible effects on defibrillator function. One European study tested automated external defibrillator response to nearby cell phone use and demonstrated that monitor display and voice commands were often distorted; however, at no time did an automated external defibrillator fail to deliver or incorrectly deliver a defibrillator shock because of EMI. Loss of synchronization with QRS complexes has been demonstrated in a defibrillator as a result of nearby cell phone use.

Mechanical ventilators have also shown vulnerability to EMI. Effects include change of readouts, variation of operation (including changes in rate, tidal volume, and positive end-expiratory pressure), inappropriate sounding of alarms, and shutdown. Death has even occurred because of ventilator shutdown resulting from EMI caused by nearby cell phone use.

Implantable cardiac devices seem relatively immune to EMI effects. Permanent pacemakers have demonstrated overpacing and underpacing but never at a distance greater than 2 cm between the cell phone and the pacemaker pocket. Also, newer pacemakers that include electromagnetic filters have not shown any vulnerability to EMI. Implantable cardioverter-defibrillators also have shown no vulnerability to EMI resulting from nearby cell phone use; however, one report documented an incident in which an antitheft scanner in a bookstore produced EMI that caused an implantable cardioverter-defibrillator to deliver inappropriate shocks.

Many other devices, including dialysis machines, drug infusion pumps, ultrasonographic probes, anesthesia machines, and heart-lung bypass machines, have shown vulnerability to EMI.

RISK OF ELECTROMAGNETIC INTERFERENCE

The probability of EMI with medical devices resulting from nearby cell phone use is difficult to quantify. Many studies have examined EMI but without rigorous standardization of testing protocols or of devices tested. A recent study indicated that 44% of medical devices showed at least some form of EMI from nearby cell phone use, whereas other studies have found that as few as 15% and as many as 60% show such EMI. Sending or receiving a cell phone call may cause EMI. All cellular telephone transmission technologies in use in the United States have been shown to cause EMI. In general, newer medical devices are less vulnerable to EMI. EMI has been shown at distances of as much as 4 m between the phone and the device, but most EMI occurs when this distance is 30 cm or less.

Although the number of medical devices vulnerable to EMI is substantial, clinically relevant EMI is less common. For example, many of the interference effects noted in studies (such as ECG signal noise and inappropriate sounding of ventilator alarms) are a nuisance but do not ultimately alter patient care. When defined as EMI that hinders data interpretation or alters patient treatment, clinically relevant interference has been shown in 10% or fewer of devices. One review found this proportion to be less than 1% when the distance between the phone and the device is 1 m or more. A recent report of the use of cell phones in the hospital environment reported no clinically important interference in 300 testings performed. Cell phones were used in a "typical manner," but the authors did not specify proximity of the cell phone to the medical device tested. Finally, this report is from a single institution (Mayo Clinic) with relatively new medical equipment that may be less prone to interference.

REGULATION AND STANDARDIZATION

At present, the US Food and Drug Administration uses EMI vulnerability standards set by the International Electrotechnical Commission when it evaluates medical devices for approval. Devices compliant with these standards should be vulnerable to EMI only at distances of 50 cm or less. This practice has been in place since 1998 and helps explain why newer devices seem to be more resistant to EMI. However, a device is not legally required to meet these or any other standards to attain approval.

TAKE HOME POINTS

- EMI with medical devices resulting from nearby cell phone use is a documented problem and has harmed patients.
- The exact incidence of EMI resulting from nearby cell phone use is difficult to quantify; however, the risk increases as the distance between the cell phone and the device decreases.
- Likewise, the risk of EMI resulting from nearby cell phone use increases as the phone's power output increases; a phone's power output is always greatest when it is ringing.
- To provide the safest possible care, anesthesia providers should be aware of EMI, especially with older medical devices, resulting from nearby cell phone use and should consider it as a possible cause in cases of equipment malfunction.

SUGGESTED READINGS

Fung HT, Kam CW, Yau HH. A follow-up study of electromagnetic interference of cellular phones on electronic medical equipment in the emergency department. *Emerg Med J.* 2002;14:315–319.

Kanz KG, Kay MV, Biberthaler P, et al. Effect of digital cellular phones on tachyarrhythmia analysis of automated external defibrillators. *Eur J Emerg Med.* 2004;11:75–80.

Klein AA, Djaiani GN. Mobile phones in the hospital: past, present, and future. *Anaesthesia.* 2003;58:353–357.

Lawrentschuk N, Bolton DM. Mobile phone interference with medical equipment and its clinical relevance: a systematic review. *Med J Aust.* 2004;181:145–149.

Morrissey JJ. Mobile phones in the hospital: improved mobile communication and mitigation of EMI concerns can lead to an overall benefit to healthcare. *Health Phys.* 2004;87:82–88.

Morrissey JJ, Swicord M, Balzano Q. Characterization of electromagnetic interference of medical devices in the hospital due to cell phones. *Health Phys.* 2002;82:45–51.

Shaw CI, Kacmarek RM, Hampton RL, et al. Cellular phone interference with the operation of mechanical ventilators. *Crit Care Med.* 2004;32:928–931.

Tri JL, Severson RP, Firl AR, et al. Cellular telephone interference with medical equipment. *Mayo Clin Proc.* 2005;80:1286–1290.

Tri JL, Severson RP, Hyberger LK, et al. Use of cellular telephones in the hospital environment. *Mayo Clin Proc.* 2007;82:282–285.

Trigano A, Blandeau O, Dale C, et al. Reliability of electromagnetic filters of cardiac pacemakers tested by cellular telephone ringing. *Heart Rhythm.* 2005;2:837–841.

Wallin MK, Marve T, Hakansson PK. Modern wireless telecommunication technologies and their electromagnetic compatibility with life-supporting equipment. *Anesth Analg.* 2005;101:1393–1400.

98

REMEMBER THAT THE LINE ISOLATION MONITOR IS BASED ON A SIMPLE PRINCIPLE OF ELECTRICAL SAFETY: MAKE SURE THE PATIENT DOES NOT BECOME PART OF A GROUNDED CIRCUIT

JEFFREY D. DILLON, MD, RICHARD BOTNEY, MD, AND RANDAL O. DULL, MD, PHD

The issue of electrical safety in the operating room has several factors. Anesthesiologists must manage the risk for patient injury caused by electrical currents several orders of magnitude apart in amperage, and they must use complex equipment-laden electrical setups. In addition, the monitor primarily used by anesthesiologists to indicate electrical issues, the line isolation monitor, rarely sounds an alarm and, in reality, does not guarantee electrical safety. This subject can provoke anxiety in anesthesiologists and merits frequent review.

The presence of any electrical device in the operating room creates the possibility of an unintended completed current pathway or circuit. Basically, the goal is to prevent the patient (or staff member) from becoming part of that circuit. An analogy to household electrical circuits is helpful—the safety features used in operating rooms do not differ in purpose from those used in houses (ground fault circuit interrupters) and appliances (three-pronged cords).

Electrical current involves the flow of electrons down a potential (i.e., *voltage*) gradient, following the path of least *resistance*. Ohm's Law defines the relationship between voltage (V), current (I), and resistance (R):

$$V = I R$$

For a shock to occur, the flow of electrons must complete a circuit. In most cases of shock, in both household and operating room situations, the circuit is completed by the flow of electrons from a source (usually an energized power line or faulty equipment), through the affected person, who is in contact with the *ground*, and then back to the original power source.

Electrical current harms a person at several current levels and in several ways. In general, electricity alters the electrochemical activity of the body and the organs and cells that it flows through. Exogenous electrical current causes nerve excitation and muscle contraction (exploited for clinical use with the nerve stimulator). Exogenous current also induces cardiac dysrhythmias

ⓒ 2006 Mayo Foundation for Medical Education and Research

when it flows through the heart (exploited for clinical use with defibrillators). As electrical current encounters resistance as it flows through the tissues of the body, the electrical current loses energy in the form of heat, which can cause both external and internal burns. The amount of tissue damage relates to the amount of current, the duration of the exposure, the current's frequency (i.e., frequencies that exceed roughly 10 kHz do not cause ventricular fibrillation), and the area over which the current is delivered (current density). Which specific injury occurs depends on the amount of current and the resistance in the electrical pathway. Microshock results when a current is applied internally in the body and bypasses the high resistance of the skin. Central venous catheters, pulmonary artery catheters, and pacemakers have all been known to conduct electricity internally and cause microshock. Currents as low as $100 \ \mu A$ have been reported to induce ventricular fibrillation. The second category of electrical injury is called macroshock, in which a large amount of current is applied externally to the skin; the patient usually perceives such shock. The amount of current, applied externally to dry skin, required to produce ventricular fibrillation is about 100 mA. Sensation of electrical current will occur around 1 mA and electrical burns occur at about 6 A.

Modern operating rooms are designed to lessen the probability of completing a circuit through a patient. Keeping the patient ungrounded in a grounded operating room, which contains metal tables, fluid pathways, etc., is not practical; accordingly, keeping the entire operating room electrically isolated or ungrounded is the goal. Using a transformer to create an isolated power system accomplishes this goal. One side of the transformer is grounded and receives a direct source of power. This current flow creates an electromagnetic field that induces current flow in two separate lines (Line 1 and Line 2) that provide current to the operating room. Since Line 1 and Line 2 are not grounded, they theoretically cannot complete a circuit, thus eliminating the risk of shock.

However, in reality, the isolated power system does not completely prevent the risk of shock. If a person were to come in contact with both Line 1 and Line 2, the circuit could be completed and a shock could occur. In addition, the isolated power system could become grounded accidentally if faulty equipment that permits a current leak to ground is connected to the power system. Then, if a person were to come in contact with one of the power lines, a circuit could be completed through the grounding created by the faulty equipment. Capacitive coupling can also result in leakage currents to ground. If enough equipment is plugged into an isolated power supply, the resultant cumulative leakage current can also transform an isolated power supply to a grounded system.

Because a faulty piece of equipment that converts the isolated power supply back to a grounded system may continue to function normally, a line isolation monitor is used to identify when the isolated power system has become accidentally grounded. The line isolation monitor assesses the resistance from Line 1 to ground and Line 2 to ground. Should the resistance from either line of the isolated power system to ground become sufficiently reduced, an audible and visual alarm activates to alert operating room staff to a fault and the power system's loss of isolation, or connection to ground. Activation of the line isolation monitor's alarm does *not* mean that a shock has occurred; rather, it indicates that the power system in the operating room has become grounded in some way and that a second fault in the system could harm a patient or a staff member. To identify the cause of the ground fault, the last piece of equipment that was plugged in should be unplugged, and then the second to last, and so on, until the alarm turns off. The magnitude of the current change shown on the line isolation monitor indicates whether a piece of equipment is faulty or too many pieces of equipment were plugged in. If a piece of equipment is faulty, the displayed leakage current would show a large change. Alternatively, if too many pieces of equipment were plugged in, the displayed leakage current would show a much smaller change. However, there may be circumstances in which the magnitude of the leakage current cannot be quantified (e.g., if the line isolation monitor does not have a meter). In that case, if the equipment may be moved (i.e., if it is not necessary for life support), it can be taken to a different location and plugged in. In the new location, if the equipment is faulty, the line isolation monitor's alarm should activate; however, if too many pieces of equipment being plugged in activated the alarm, the line isolation monitor's alarm should not activate. If an item is found to have a ground fault, then it should be removed from service and should not be used again until it can be properly inspected and repaired.

Like the isolated power system, the line isolation monitor does not completely protect the patient or staff from electrical hazards in the operating room. Line isolation monitors cannot detect all faults. For instance, they do not protect against the capacitance between two wires in proximity, which can cause microshock.

To reduce the risk posed by faulty equipment, the casing ("chassis") is connected to ground via the third prong on a standard plug, which is known as the grounding prong. If the equipment's casing connects accidentally to the internal electrical circuitry (fault), a low-resistance pathway is provided along which current may flow to ground, rather than through a person. Hence the adage that the equipment, not the person, should be grounded.

Finally, although sometimes referred to as the "grounding pad," the gel-coated blue pad that nurses often put on the patient's thigh is *not* a grounding pad. It could more correctly be called the "dispersive electrode." It provides a large area, low-resistance pathway along which applied current may leave the body, and it prevents current from a cautery from leaving the body via pacemaker wires, electrocardiogram electrodes, or contact points between the patient and the metal table.

TAKE HOME POINTS

- Current, voltage, and resistance are related by Ohm's Law:

$$V = IR.$$

- The magnitude of macroshock current required to induce ventricular fibrillation is 100 mA.
- Activation of the line isolation monitor's alarm does *not* mean that a shock has occurred; rather, it means that the power system in the operating room has become grounded in some way and that a second fault in the system could harm a person.
- Upon such activation, unplug pieces of equipment sequentially, starting with the last piece of equipment that was plugged in before activation of the alarm, and, if it has a ground fault, do not use it until it can be repaired.

SUGGESTED READINGS

Bernstein MS. Isolated power and line isolation monitors. *Biomed Instrum Technol.* 1990;24(3):221–223.

Bruner JMR, Leonard PF. *Electricity, Safety and the Patient.* Chicago: Year Book Medical Publishers; 1989.

Helfman SM, Berry AJ. Review of electrical safety and electrosurgery in the operating room. *Am J of Anes.* 1999;26:313–320.

Hopps JA. Shock hazards in operating rooms and patient-care areas. *Anesthesiology.* 1969;31:142.

Litt L, Ehrenwerth J. Electrical safety in the operating room: important old wine, disguised new bottles. *Anesth Analg.* 1994;78:417–419.

Nielsen R. Possible causes of alarming... Line isolation monitors. *Biomed Instrum Technol.* 2004;38(4):288–289.

REGIONAL ANESTHESIA

99

COMPLICATIONS OF REGIONAL ANESTHESIA: DON'T TOUCH THE NEEDLE UNTIL YOU KNOW THEM

DAVID A. BURNS, MD

INTRODUCTION

With the ever-growing number of older persons that need joint replacements and the never-ending orthopedic trauma of the entire population, the practice of regional anesthesia is a growing wave of the future. Regional anesthesia, however, is not without risks or complications. This chapter discusses these risks and and how to manage them.

INFECTION

Whenever the integrity of the integument is violated, the risk of introducing infection is present, and, when a foreign body (like a peripheral nerve catheter) is left in situ, that increases the risk by maintaining a conduit for skin flora to bypass the protective barriers of the skin. Further, the location of the regional technique is important as an epidural abscess or spinal meningitis can cause significant morbidity or mortality. Infection localized to the insertion site would contaminate the needle as it passes through, allowing direct access of the microorganisms to the nerve plexus. Finally, systemic infection or bacteremia can allow infection to be spread hematogenously to the foreign body.

- Factors predisposing toward infection:
  - Immunocompromised state
    - Immunosuppression
    - Steroid use
    - Diabetes
    - Sepsis or concurrent infection
  - Extended duration of use
  - Sterile technique not employed
- Techniques for avoiding infection:
  - Sterile preparation of the site
  - Aseptic technique
  - Sterile occlusive dressings
- Techniques for avoiding or limiting gross contamination:
  - Limit duration or tunnel the catheter (or both).
  - Avoid placement through sites of infection.

© 2006 Mayo Foundation for Medical Education and Research

- Administer a dose of antibiotics before placement of invasive lines or nerve-block catheters in patients with sepsis. Studies of placement of such lines and catheters have shown the risk of infection with bacteremia is reduced to baseline if administration of antibiotics has been started before placement. Therefore, you should carefully weigh the risks and benefits of the technique and make sure an appropriate antibiotic has been given at least 1 hour before the procedure.
- Limit breaks in tubing for bag changes. Every time the integrity of the tubing system is violated by reservoir changes, contamination of the local anesthetic solution is possible–limit such opportunities for contamination.
- Follow the patient daily and inspect the patient for signs of infection, including erythema, pus, tenderness at the site, and fever.
- Treatments for infection:
  - If infection is suspected, remove the catheter. Usually such removal leads to avoidance or resolution of infection, unless the patient is immunocompromised.
  - Ensure that the patient is receiving appropriate antibiotics.
  - Continue to follow the patient's case to ensure resolution of infection.
  - In the case of suspected epidural abscess, speed of diagnosis and treatment is of the essence to avoid permanent neurologic injury.

BLEEDING

The anatomic locations where many peripheral nerves are blocked contain major blood vessels (for example, axillary, infraclavicular, supraclavicular, femoral, popliteal fossa, and sciatic). Many are deep locations at which applying direct pressure would be difficult or impossible (for example, epidural, spinal, classic paravertebral, infraclavicular, supraclavicular, lumbar plexus). Because the epidural space has an extensive venous plexus, bleeding can easily be caused by epidural or spinal anesthesia, inducing an expanding hematoma in a fixed and enclosed space that would cause spinal cord compression and paralysis.

- Techniques for avoiding bleeding:
  - While placing the block, maintain continuous aspiration for blood.
  - If you are proficient in ultrasound techniques, use visualization of the vessels in real-time with the passage of the needle to avoid vascular puncture and to place the local anesthetic more precisely.
  - If anticoagulant drugs are being used before or during surgery (the incidence of such use has grown tremendously), understand the drugs being used, know their duration of effect, and closely monitor the patient during their use. In addition, know which anticoagulant drugs the patient received before surgery and which the patient is receiving

---

TABLE 99.1   ASRA GUIDELINES IN A NUTSHELL

- Warfarin:
  - Avoid patients taking coumadin if the International Normalized Ratio (INR) is greater than 1.5. Also, the INR should be <1.5 for removal of an epidural.
- Heparins:
  - Use of subcutaneous, unfractionated heparin at a prophylactic dosage presents no contraindication.
  - For patients receiving heparin infusions, the infusion needs to be stopped 4 hours before the block and the Partial Thromboplastin Time (PTT) drawn showing return to <1.5 times normal. The catheter may be removed after heparin administration has been discontinued for 2 to 4 hours. Heparin should not be re-administered until 1 hour after placement or after catheter removal.
  - For patients taking subcutaneous heparin or Low Molecular Weight Heparins (LMWH) at therapeutic (bid) dosages for Deep Venous Thrombosis/Pulmonary Embolus (DVT/PE) or Acute Myocardial Infarction (AMI), if the patient has received one dose, wait 12 hours before doing the block. If the patient has received more than one dose, wait 24 hours.
  - For patients taking LMWH at a prophylactic (q day) dosage, wait 12 hours after the last administration of a dose to place and to remove the catheter, and wait 2 hours after removal before administering the next dose.
- Antiplatelet medications:
  - Use of aspirin, nonsteroidal anti-inflammatory drugs, or COX-2 inhibitors presents no contraindication.
  - Patients taking clopidogrel (Plavix) should discontinue use for 7 days.
  - Patients taking ticlopidine (Ticlid) should discontinue use for 14 days.
  - Patients taking GP IIb/IIIa inhibitors (abciximab [ReoPro]) should discontinue use for 48 hours, and patients taking eptifibatide (Integrilin) or tirofiban (Aggrastat) should discontinue use for 8 hours.
- Co-morbid conditions:
  - Thrombocytopenic patients with platelet counts of less than 80K, or 100K if platelets are impaired as in uremia.
  - Hemophiliac patients should not receive a block unless they have had their factor concentrates infused to provide adequate levels for surgery.

Horlocker TT, Wedel DJ, Benzon H, et al. Regional anesthesia in the anticoagulated patient: defining the risks (The Second ASRA Consensus Conference on Neuraxial Anesthesia and Anticoagulation). *Reg Anesth Pain Med.* 2003;28:172–197.
This table is my own summary of the recommendations from this reference.

---

upon placement of the block and upon removal of the continuous catheter.

- American Society of Regional Anesthesia (ASRA) guidelines for anticoagulants are followed for all neuraxial anesthetics and for placement of deep peripheral-nerve blocks at our institution (*Table 99.1*).
- In the patient with normal coagulation, bleeding complications rarely cause clinical morbidity.

NERVE DAMAGE

The incidence of nerve damage after use of a regional block is reported to be between 0.04% and 5%. The vast majority of these are dysesthesias that last less than a week. It is more common to damage a nerve by many means that are unrelated to the regional anesthetic but are coincidental in their timing. Nerve damage may result from surgical trauma, retractor use, excessive pressure from tourniquet use, or excessively long tourniquet use. Poor positioning, leading to tension, stretch, or compression, not only in the operating room but also elsewhere, caused by casts, bandages, bed rails, or failure to protected pressure points, may damage nerves. Although use of a regional anesthetic often is initially blamed for nerve damage, only careful investigation will lead to the true cause.

Theoretically, use of a regional block can damage the nerve in the following ways: the needle may cut the nerve; an intraneural injection may mechanically disrupt the nerve; an intraneural injection with high pressure may cause ischemia; additives like epinephrine may cause intense vasoconstriction; and, finally, neurotoxicity of the solutions may damage the nerve.

Techniques for avoiding nerve damage:

- Avoid using deep sedation and general anesthesia during placement. If the patient cannot tell you reliably whether he has pain upon injection or has a paresthesia, you have lost that safety monitor.
  - Stop if the patient has pain upon injection. Intraneural injection may cause pain in the distribution of that nerve.
    - By the same logic, consider avoiding "rescue" or supplemental blocks because the patient's ability to feel pain of paresthesia is diminished.
  - Avoid paresthesias. The majority of cases of nerve damage also coincided with a paresthesia upon placement.
- Avoid using currents of less than 0.2 mA. Because current density is proportional to the distance squared, avoiding needle placement that results in a motor response with a current of less than 0.2 mA is widely believed to prevent intraneural injection. However, this belief is currently being widely challenged as ultrasound techniques have shown intraneural needle placement without any motor response.
- Use short-beveled needles. Such use is widely thought to reduce the likelihood of cutting the nerve.
- Use low pressure to inject. If there is resistance to injection, the needle may be placed intraneurally. In fact, a group of anesthesia providers located in New York uses a pressure manometer in doing injections.
- Remember that the neurotoxicity of all local anesthetics increases with increasing concentration. Such increases are nominal at clinically used concentrations unless injected intraneurally.
- Use ultrasound guidance. Ultrasonographic visualization of the nerves and the needle allows you to avoid poor positioning.

ALLERGIC REACTIONS

Allergic reactions to regional anesthetics are extremely rare and are often misdiagnosed as an iatrogenic reaction or an immunologic response to a different antigen, like the preservatives methylparaben or metabisulfite. The ester local anesthetics are hydrolyzed to PABA (para-aminobenzoic acid), which can be allergenic.

BLOCKADE OF OTHER NERVES

Examples of such blockades include blockade of the ipsilateral phrenic nerve with nearly every interscalene block as well as blockade of the recurrent laryngeal nerve. It sounds like the recurrent laryngeal nerve is also blocked every time so I clarified. Such blockades may cause significant reduction in respiratory function and hoarseness and therefore may be contraindicated in patients with poor respiratory reserve or contralateral, recurrent laryngeal-nerve palsy. Other examples include epidural spread from paraneuraxial techniques like the interscalene, paravertebral, or lumbar plexus blocks. In addition, the femoral nerve can become blocked with a field block for an inguinal hernia.

INTRAVASCULAR INJECTION AND LOCAL ANESTHETIC TOXICITY

This complication and its treatment are addressed in Chapter 110.

SUPPLIES AND EQUIPMENT THAT SHOULD BE AVAILABLE WHEN DOING REGIONAL ANESTHESIA

- Airway equipment:
  - Laryngoscope blades, endotracheal tubes, a suction device, a self-inflating bag, a mask, and a source of oxygen.
- Emergency drugs:
  - Epinephrine, atropine, propofol, succinylcholine, benzodiazepines.
- Cardiopulmonary bypass capabilities and 100 ml of 20% Intralipid, especially if using bupivacaine.

SUGGESTED READINGS

Ben-David B. Complications of peripheral blockade. *Anesthesiol Clin North America.* 2002;20:457–469.

Hadzic A, Vloka JD. *Peripheral Nerve Blocks: Principles and Practice.* McGraw-Hill; 2004.

Finucane BT. *Complications of Regional Anesthesia.* Churchill Livingstone; 1999.

Hahn MB, McQuillan PM, Sheplock GJ. *Regional Anesthesia: An Atlas of Anatomy and Techniques.* Mosby; 1996.

Horlocker TT, Wedel DJ, Benzon H, et al. Regional anesthesia in the anticoagulated patient: defining the risks (The Second ASRA Consensus Conference on Neuraxial Anesthesia and Anticoagulation). *Reg Anesth Pain Med.* 2003;28:172–197.

100

KNOW THE FACTS AND BE READY WITH AN ANSWER WHEN A PATIENT WHO WILL RECEIVE SPINAL ANESTHESIA ASKS "CAN THIS PARALYZE ME?"

ANGELA M. PENNELL, MD

Despite ongoing efforts to educate patients, reluctance to accept spinal anesthesia is still fairly common. Patients in all demographic groups ask about the toxicity of spinal anesthetic agents, the possibility of paralysis, or both, even when they have already consented to neuraxial blockade. Patients also commonly refer to troubles experienced by a family member or acquaintance after spinal anesthesia. "My buddy had the needle in his back and it messed him up good" has been heard by just about every practicing anesthesiologist. Periodically reviewing both the basic knowledge base and the recent literature on the neurotoxicity of spinal agents and other general risks is helpful as new reports on the incidence of the adverse effects of spinal and epidural anesthesia continue to be published.

CAUDA EQUINA SYNDROME
The incidence of cauda equine syndrome is 32 in 1.2 million subarachnoid blocks and 32 in 450,000 epidurals. The syndrome is a combination of bowel and bladder dysfunction with paresis of the lower extremities and sensory dysfunction in a patchy distribution. It is often associated with hyperbaric lidocaine (lidocaine combined with dextrose) or highly concentrated lidocaine (5%) and suggests neurotoxicity caused by the agent itself. However, this syndrome has also been observed with other local anesthetics, such as 0.5% hyperbaric bupivacaine. Therefore, the etiology *may* be related to insufficient mixing of local anesthetic with cerebrospinal fluid, with resulting neurotoxicity. Cauda equina syndrome has also been linked to the use of microcatheters for repeated or continuous dosing where concentrated, local anesthetic pools around the sacral nerve roots (microcatheters are now prohibited by the FDA).

TRANSIENT NEUROLOGIC SYMPTOMS (TNS)
Transient neurologic symptoms consist of back pain radiating to the lower extremities, without sensory or motor deficits, occurring after resolution of the spinal block and subsiding after several days. These symptoms are

© 2006 Mayo Foundation for Medical Education and Research

most commonly seen with lidocaine use and in outpatients having surgery in the lithotomy position and are thought to be secondary to neurotoxicity (probably not related to concentrations of <5%). Whether the true etiology is neurotoxicity or soreness from muscle strain is unclear.

OTHER NEUROLOGIC DEFICITS

The incidence of other neurologic deficits is 20 in 1.2 million subarachnoid blocks and 20 in 450,000 epidurals. Permanent or transient neurologic deficits probably represent direct damage to the nerve roots. These deficits are commonly associated with multiple attempts at accessing the intrathecal space. Paraplegia can result if there has been direct contact between spinal cord and needle. Frequently observed are loss of bowel and bladder function; paralysis of the biceps femoris muscles; and sensory loss in the dorsal thigh, saddle region, or great toes as often seen with damage to the conus medullaris. Deficits may also be due to neurotoxicity of the local anesthetic agent.

MENINGITIS AND ARACHNOIDITIS

The incidence of meningitis or arachnoiditis is 29 in 1.2 million subarachnoid blocks and 29 in 450,000 epidurals. Meningitis and arachnoiditis may be infectious or noninfectious; present as pain coupled with other neurologic symptoms; and are identified using radiography, which shows clumped nerve roots. Meningitis and arachnoiditis have been previously attributed to detergents used in procaine or solutions used to clean reusable spinal needles.

SPINAL HEMATOMA

The incidence of spinal hematoma is 33 in 1.2 million subarachnoid blocks and 32 in 450,000 epidurals. It is secondary to trauma to an epidural vein caused by a needle or catheter and is most often seen in patients with abnormal coagulation or bleeding disorders. It is also associated with technically difficult or bloody blocks. In addition, a spinal hematoma may occur immediately after removal of an epidural catheter. The hematoma behaves as a mass directing pressure to the neural tissue of the spinal cord. Symptoms initiate as sharp back and leg pain that progress to numbness and motor dysfunction (including loss of bowel and bladder control).

BUPIVACAINE

Bupivacaine is an amide local anesthetic commonly used for spinal anesthesia. Having a higher pKa of 8.1, it has a slower onset but a longer duration of action than some other amide anesthetics. Concentrations range from 0.25% to 0.75%. Hyperbaric formulations in 8.25% dextrose are available. It affects sensory-nerve fibers more readily than motor-nerve fibers. The central nervous system toxicity of bupivacaine is relatively low compared with its cardiac toxicity. However, cauda equina syndrome has been associated with intrathecal bupivacaine use (although not as frequently as with lidocaine use). The toxic intravenous dose of bupivacaine is considered to be 1.6 mg/kg. At this dosage, cardiac complications, including dysrhythmias, hypotension, and depression of cardiac output, have been observed. The maximum total dose of bupivacaine is 3 mg/kg.

LIDOCAINE

Lidocaine is an amide local anesthetic. Concentrations range from 0.5% to 5%. Compared with other amide anesthetics, lidocaine has a more rapid onset and a shorter duration of action, due to its lower pKa (7.7), and lower lipid solubility. Its maximum dosage is 4.5 mg/kg without epinephrine and 7 mg/kg with epinephrine. Cauda equina syndrome and TNS are consistently linked to intrathecal lidocaine (especially 5% lidocaine and hyperbaric lidocaine). Therefore, lidocaine concentration should not exceed 2.5%, a lidocaine dose should not exceed 60 mg, and combining lidocaine use with epinephrine use should be avoided.

ROPIVACAINE

Ropivacaine is an ester local anesthetic with a pKa of 8.1, a long duration of action, and high lipid solubility. Ropivacaine has been used less than some other local anesthetics in spinal anesthesia, and it does not seem to have an advantage over bupivacaine for intrathecal use. The maximum recommended dose is 3 mg/kg.

TETRACAINE

Tetracaine is an ester local anesthetic with a pKa of 8.2, a long duration of action, and high lipid solubility. Tetracaine use provides a higher degree of motor blockade than does bupivicaine use. Combined use of epinephrine and tetracaine may prolong tetracaine's duration of action by 50%. Tetracaine use, at a concentration of 0.5%, with repeated doses or via small-bore catheters (or both), has been associated with cauda equina syndrome. Of note, tetracaine is the only local anesthetic that does not contain epinephrine or glucose but also does not carry the "Not for Spinal Anesthesia" warning on its label. It requires reconstitution of its crystals with sterile, normal saline to result in an isobaric solution. The maximum recommended total dose is 3 mg/kg.

CHLOROPROCAINE

Chloroprocaine is an ester local anesthetic with a pKa of 9.0, higher than those of other local anesthetics. Chloroprocaine use is associated with prolonged neurologic deficit attributed to neurotoxicity. This neurotoxicity is presumed to result from chloroprocaine's low pH when it is combined with preservative. The former preparation used sodium bisulfate as a preservative; the current preparation uses EDTA as a preservative. A preservative-free formulation also is available. Another etiology of neurotoxicity may be the use of large volumes (>40 ml) of chloroprocaine. The maximum recommended dose is 12 mg/kg.

TAKE HOME POINTS

- Know the complications that can result from spinal anesthesia.
- Know the incidence of each complication:
  - Cauda equina syndrome: 32 in 1.2 million intrathecal injections or 450,000 epidurals;
  - Transient neurologic symptoms: the incidence is unclear and these symptoms resolve by themselves;
  - Other neurologic injury: 20 in 1.2 million intrathecal injections or 450,000 epidurals;
  - Meningitis: 29 in 1.2 million intrathecal injections or 450,000 epidurals; and
  - Hematoma: 33 in 1.2 million intrathecal injections or 450,000 epidurals.

Know the maximum allowable dose of each local anesthetic.

SUGGESTED READINGS

Auroy Y, Benhamou D, Bargues L, et al. Major complications of regional anesthesia in France: the SOS Regional Anesthesia Hotline Service. *Anesthesiology.* 2002;97(5):1274–1280.

Chabbouh T, Lentschener C, Zuber M. Persistent cauda equina syndrome with no identifiable facilitating condition after an uneventful single spinal administration of 0.5% hyperbaric bupivacaine. *Anesth Analg.* 2005;101:1847–1848.

Ganem EM, Vianna PT, Marques M, et al. Neurotoxicity of subarachnoid hyperbaric bupivacaine in dogs. *Reg Anesth Pain Med.* 1996;21(3):234–238.

Hodgson PS, Neal JM, Pollock JE, et al. The neurotoxicity of drugs given intrathecally (spinal). *Anesth Analg.* 1999; 88(4):797–809.

Johnson ME. Neurotoxicity of lidocaine: implications for spinal anesthesia and neuroprotection. *J Neurosurg Anesthesiol.* 2004;16(1):80–83.

Levsky ME, Miller MA. Cardiovascular collapse from low dose bupivacaine. *Can J Clin Pharmacol.* 2005;12(3):e240–5. Epub 2005 Oct 24.

Moen V, Dahlgren N, Irestedt L. Severe neurological complications after central neuraxial blockades in Sweden 1990–1999. *Anesthesiology.* 2004;101(4):950–959.

Morgan GE Jr, Mikhail MS, Murray MJ. *Clinical Anesthesiology.* New York, NY: Lange Medical Books/McGraw-Hill Medical Publishing Division; 2002:266–280.

101

REMEMBER THE LOW-RISK AND HIGH-YIELD BLOCKS

JENNIFER VOOKLES, MD, MA

You are in the midst of a busy day in the orthopedic operating rooms. You dash through the postanesthesia care unit (PACU) and happen to notice a patient reading the paper. The next day, you notice another patient in the PACU reading the paper. The PACU nurse tells you that Dr. Doe's patients are so comfortable, they usually ask to read or watch TV while waiting for their floor beds. The following day, when you take your total-knee arthroplasty patient to the PACU, the nurse asks if you did a femoral-nerve block. When you reply that there wasn't time, she frowns a little and says, "Well, I guess we won't be needing any newspapers today."

Peripheral nerve blocks provide a variety of perioperative benefits. The most obvious benefit is analgesia extending for many hours postoperatively, both from direct action of the local anesthetic but also potentially from pre-emptive analgesic mechanisms if the block is established prior to incision. In addition, they can help reduce the need for intraoperative doses of volatile agents and opioids; this may reduce recovery times by decreasing postoperative sedation and nausea. Finally, peripheral-nerve blocks can also reduce the need for muscle relaxants by blocking motor as well as sensory fibers.

Despite these benefits, peripheral-nerve blocks are often omitted when a general anesthetic or spinal is planned, because they can be time consuming to perform and carry their own procedural risks. However, even recognizing these limitations, there are a few "low-risk and high-yield" blocks that are relatively quick to perform and should always be considered as an adjunct to primary anesthetic. These blocks include the superficial-cervical-plexus block, femoral-nerve block, and obturator-nerve block.

SUPERFICIAL-CERVICAL-PLEXUS BLOCK

The cervical plexus has both superficial and deep components. The superficial plexus contains cutaneous branches from the ventral rami of C2-4 providing innervation from the posterior cranium to the shoulder via the lesser occipital, greater auricular, transverse cervical, and supraclavicular nerves. The superficial plexus can be very easily blocked and utilized as supplementary analgesia for carotid endarterectomy (CEA) and other neck surgeries. As the sole anesthetic, one study even found equivalent benefits of the superficial-cervical-plexus block compared to combined superficial- and

© 2006 Mayo Foundation for Medical Education and Research

deep-cervical-plexus blocks for CEA. It can also be used to ensure cutaneous coverage of the shoulder following interscalene block.

Infiltration of local anesthetic deep to the posterior border of the sternocleidomastoid muscle will block the superficial cervical plexus. At the midpoint of the muscle's posterior border, a 22G 4-cm needle is inserted just below to the muscle and 5 mL of local anesthetic is injected. The needle is then redirected cephalad and caudad along the muscle border, with a total of 10 mL injected along these paths. The external jugular vein often overlies this area and should be avoided. When this block is properly performed, deeper structures should not be affected; however, one should be aware of the proximity of the phrenic nerve, the internal jugular vein, and the carotid artery if the needle is inserted too deeply.

FEMORAL NERVE BLOCK

The femoral nerve is formed from branches of L2-L4; it crosses the pelvis in a groove between the psoas and iliacus muscles to emerge beneath the inguinal ligament lateral to the femoral artery. The femoral nerve can begin to divide into its branches at or above the inguinal ligament. This nerve provides both deep and superficial innervation of the anterior thigh extending to the knee with a distal branch, the saphenous nerve, continuing along the anteromedial shin to the ankle and occasionally into the dorsum of the foot.

Although a femoral-nerve block must usually be combined with a sciatic nerve block or a lateral-femoral-cutaneous-nerve block (or both) to provide adequate anesthesia for surgery on the leg and foot, a femoral-nerve block on its own can provide significant postoperative analgesia for surgery involving the anterior thigh, femur, and knee. The patient may still have some discomfort in the posterior knee, but this is usually easily managed.

Landmarks for the femoral-nerve block are the pubic tubercle and anterior superior iliac spine. A line is drawn connecting these points, and the femoral artery is palpated along this line. The needle insertion site is on this line immediately lateral to the femoral artery. Using a nerve-stimulation technique, the injection site can be determined by observing quadriceps twitch; do not be misled by stimulation of the sartorius muscle.

A femoral-nerve block can often be completed as a field block. Beginning at the same entry site, the needle is initially inserted perpendicular to the artery and then redirected laterally in a progressive, fan-like manner. Approximately 20 mL of local anesthetic should be injected incrementally in this process. It can also be helpful to displace the needle site 1 cm lateral and, aiming medially, place 2 to 5 mL of local anesthetic posterior to the femoral artery. If available, ultrasound can be useful in better localizing the artery; in experienced hands, the nerves themselves can also be visualized.

OBTURATOR NERVE BLOCK

The obturator nerve is formed by the ventral branches of the L2–L4 anterior primary rami and emerges from the medial border of the psoas at the pelvic brim. It follows the lateral wall of the pelvis to exit via the obturator foramen, emerging into the anteromedial thigh. The anterior branch supplies the hip joint and anterior adductor muscles and sends sensory branches to the skin over the medial thigh. The posterior branch supplies the deep adductor muscles and a sensory branch, which extend to the posterior knee joint.

The obturator-nerve block can be used in combination with the sciatic, femoral, and lateral-femoral-cutaneous blocks to allow complete surgical anesthesia for the lower extremity. It can also be useful in treating hip–joint pain and in relieving adductor-muscle spasticity. The obturator-nerve block can also be used to suppress a reflex-adductor contraction not uncommonly seen during transurethral resection of the lateral bladder wall lesion; this reflex is often not abolished by spinal anesthesia.

There are several approaches to performing this block. For the "classic" approach, the patient is supine with legs slightly adducted. The entry site is 1.5 cm both caudal and lateral to the pubic tubercle. A needle is inserted perpendicular to the skin and advanced 2 to 4 cm until the inferior edge of the superior pubic ramus is contacted. The needle is then withdrawn slightly and redirected laterally about 45% to a depth 2 to 3 cm deeper. Fifteen mL of local anesthetic should be injected while advancing and withdrawing slightly. If a nerve stimulator is utilized, thigh adductor contractions should be observed.

The newer "inguinal" approach is simpler and less uncomfortable for the patient; but it usually does not block the articular branches to the hip. A nerve stimulator must be used for this approach. With the hip abducted, the insertion site is found by marking the midpoint between the pubic tubercle and pulsation of the femoral artery, as it emerges beneath the inguinal ligament. The needle is directed roughly 30% cephalad. Once stimulation of the gracilis and adductor longus muscles are obtained, the needle is directed slightly lateral and advanced another 0.5 to 1.5 cm. After the adductor magnus is stimulated, 5 to 7 mL of local anesthetic is injected.

TAKE HOME POINTS

- These three blocks can be performed relatively quickly and have relatively low risk associated with them.
- As with any peripheral-nerve blocks, care should be taken to avoid local-anesthetic toxicity. Always inject slowly and incrementally, attempting to aspirate after every 3 to 5 mL to detect intravascular needle placement.

■ Consider adding low-dose epinephrine to the local anesthetic to further aid detection of intravascular injection and to slow absorption.

■ A more precise description of the techniques for performing these blocks can be found in many regional anesthesia texts or in online resources.

SUGGESTED READINGS

Alvez de Sousa A, Filho MAD, Faglione W, et al. Superficial vs combined cervical plexus block for carotid endarterectomy: a prospective randomized study. *Surg Neurol.* 2005;63(s1): S22–S25.

Brown D. *Atlas of Regional Anesthesia.* Philadelphia: WB Saunders; 1992; 91–95,105–107, 167–171.

Choquet O, Capdevila X, Bennourine K, et al. A new inguinal approach for the obturator nerve block: anatomical and randomized clinical studies. *Anesthesiology.* 2005;103(6):1238–1245.

Hadzic A, Vloka J, eds. *New York School of Regional Anesthesia – Peripheral Nerve Blocks.* http://www.nysora.com. Accessed Oct 23 2006.

102

Consider the Paramedian Approach for Spinal Anesthetic Placement if the Patient is in the Lateral Position

Catherine Marcucci, MD and Moustafa M. Ahmed, MD, MBBCh

A spinal anesthetic may be placed on a patient in the lateral position for several reasons: The patient may require significant sedation; be at risk for a vasovagal reaction; have pain in the sitting position due to trauma or disease process, such as a fractured hip or perirectal abscess; or may be difficult to turn quickly after placement of the spinal due to morbid obesity. The lateral position is also very typically used if a hyperbaric or hypobaric one-sided spinal is planned. However, the advantages of having a patient in the lateral position are often offset by increased difficulty in correctly placing the spinal needle, especially if a midline approach is attempted. The issues to be aware of are the loss of visual anatomic landmarks, particularly the longitudinal midline bony landmarks, and the relative inability of patients to curl into the correct position to open the interspinous spaces.

Gravity can be blamed for increasing the chances of unintended deviation from the interspinous spaces in patients who are in the lateral position. Typically, less experienced anesthesia providers correctly palpate and appreciate the bony structures and spaces of the spinal column during the preparatory and draping phases but then use the visual cue of the longitudinal "dimple" in the soft tissue and skin in placing the introducer and spinal needles. Particularly in older or overweight patients, there can be as much as 1 to 2 cm of "sag" of the soft tissues towards the dependent side and it is extremely easy to get off the midline. A resident who is consistently contacting bone during a midline approach is usually tapping the dependent lamina. On repeated palpation of the bony structures and redirection of the needle, the true midline of these patients is almost always found to be "more towards the ceiling."

Patients in the lateral position may have difficulty in flexing both the knees and hips actively to assume and maintain a kyphotic position. Psychological and muscular relaxation due to sedation or a startle reflex will cause the patient to extend at both joints, narrowing the interspinous spaces. Patients who aggressively curl up will also tend to roll anteriorly, which shifts

© 2006 Mayo Foundation for Medical Education and Research

the midline axis away from the perpendicular plane of the operating room table or floor.

The paramedian approach, which does not depend on maintaining an open interspinous space and is much more forgiving of unintended deviations in the lateral traverse of the needle, should be considered if the midline approach on a patient in the lateral position is unsuccessful after one or two attempts. To review briefly, first establish the deviation of the patient's back from the plane perpendicular to the bed by lightly resting your palm flat against the patient's back–it is easier for you to determine whether your hand is off that plane than to gauge visually whether the patient is off that plane. Second, place the spinal needle about 1 to 2 cm lateral to the interspace. Most practitioners choose the dependent side of the spinal column and place the needle slightly towards the "bottom" of the interspace. Then, direct the needle 15° medial and cephalad to the plane of the back and advance until the ligamentum flavum is transversed and the spinal fluid is entered. An alternative technique is to place the needle 1 cm lateral to the midline, but first to advance perpendicular to the back, expecting to contact the lamina. The needle is then partially withdrawn and the medial and cephalad angle is increased in increments until the needle is "walked off" the edge of the lamina and the spinal canal is entered.

TAKE HOME POINTS

- Spinal anesthetics are frequently done in the lateral position due to disease process or need for deeper sedation.
- The lateral position can make it difficult for patients to curl into the fetal position and for anesthesia providers to appreciate the bony landmarks.
- It is very common for practitioners attempting the midline approach to be as much as one centimeter off the midline.
- Placement of intrathecal anesthetics can usually be easily and safely accomplished using the paramedian approach.

SUGGESTED READINGS

Barash PG, Cullen BF, Stoelting RK. Clinical anesthesia. 4th ed. Lippincott Williams & Wilkins, Philadelphia, PA. 2001;694.
Black SM, Chambers WA, Essential anatomy for anesthesia, Livingstone, New York, 1997, 91.

103

CONSIDER THE PARAMEDIAN APPROACH FOR THORACIC EPIDURAL PLACEMENT, ESPECIALLY AT THE MIDTHORACIC LEVEL

AMIT SHARMA, MD

You are scheduled to do the anesthesia for a lung resection for a 68-year-old man with severe chronic obstructive pulmonary disease. You usually use intrathecal preservative-free morphine for this type of case. Today, however, you hear from the surgical resident, surgical fellow, and surgical attending, all within a 15-minute interval and all requesting a thoracic epidural. It isn't your favorite type of catheter to place, but you decide to give it a try. Unfortunately, all you and your junior resident seem to hit is "bone everywhere." You and your patient are both getting a bit uncomfortable and discouraged. You call your favorite senior pain attending, who is doing cases in the outpatient center and, fortunately, he can come within 5 minutes. He arrives and does one of the "Mr. Miyagi" moves he is famous for—and the catheter is in, taped, and test dosed within 2 minutes. You wonder to yourself, "How the heck does he do that?"

Neuraxial (spinal and epidural) techniques are a vital component of anesthesia and pain-management practice. Since August Bier first described spinal anesthesia in 1898, neuraxial techniques have been in constant use and have been the subject of a vast amount of clinical research and inquiry directed at maximizing both safety and efficacy. Today, epidural analgesia is widely used for postoperative pain control after thoracoadominal and lower-extremity procedures. Insertion of a thoracic epidural catheter is often considered more challenging than placement of its lumbar counterpart. Fortunately, a thorough understanding of the anatomy of the thoracic spine and adherence to a few simple principles will alleviate trepidation and facilitate placement.

The spinal cord is divided into eight cervical (C), twelve thoracic (T), five lumbar (L), five sacral (S), and a few coccygeal (Co) segments. Each spinal segment (except C1) involves a dorsal (sensory) and a ventral (motor) nerve root on either side that join to form a spinal nerve. Each spinal nerve subsequently exits through an intervertebral foramen of the vertebral column. The bony vertebral column surrounds and protects the spinal cord and the spinal nerves encased by arachnoid membrane filled with cerebrospinal fluid. The epidural space is a potential area just outside the dura mater,

© 2006 Mayo Foundation for Medical Education and Research

bound anteriorly by the posterior longitudinal ligament; posteriorly by the vertebral laminae and the ligamentum flavum; and laterally by the vertebral pedicles and intervertebral foramina. At the thoracic level, the epidural space is around 3 to 5 mm in width and contains fat, veins, arteries, lymphatics, and connective tissue. Local anesthetic solution administered in the epidural space bathes the spinal nerves, leading to sensory and motor blockade. Similarly, opioid medications are either absorbed by the venous plexus and act systemically or they cross the dura mater and bind to the opioid receptors on the spinal cord.

Thoracic dermatomes are organized in circumferential bands from axilla to iliac crest. The T4 dermatome (sensory distribution of T4 spinal nerve) is often located at the level of nipples and T10 at the level of umbilicus (these are universally used reference points). There is a degree of dermatomal overlap, which can cause difficulties with insufficient block for all areas of the surgical site. This problem has been overcome by introduction of newer multibore epidural catheters that enhance the local anesthetic spread and therefore are expected to cover a wider dermatomal distribution.

Technically, both the upper (T1-T2) and the lower thoracic (T10-T12) vertebral interspaces are functionally equivalent to lumbar area since spinous processes at these levels are almost angled horizontally. In contrast, placing epidural catheters at the T3 to T9 level is challenging because of the acute downward angulation of these respective spinous processes (*Fig. 103.1*). Since successive spinous processes are angled less acutely, the interspinous space is narrower at the distal end (superficial), making the needle entrance harder.

Most anesthesia providers who do not have experience in treating pain start with the midline approach, even in the midthoracic region and that is perhaps why they often have such difficulty in placing the catheter. A senior pain anesthesiologist or an experienced regional anesthesia provider would probably suggest using the paramedian approach to facilitate placing the thoracic epidural catheter at these middle thoracic interspaces. With this approach, the needle is entered slightly inferolateral to the spinous process and angled cephalomedial, thus avoiding the crowded interspinous space. With this technique, the needle tip travels through the skin, subcutaneous tissue, and ligamentum flavum before entering the epidural space, unlike the classic *interspinous* technique in which supraspinous and interspinous ligaments are also encountered in needle trajectory.

The epidural catheter should be placed on the unilateral side, approximately at the mid-dermatomal level to the corresponding surgical incision. For instance, if the intended thoracotomy incision is planned at the right T5-T7 dermatomes, the epidural catheter should be inserted at the right T5-T6 interspace. The unilateral catheter placement is perhaps necessary

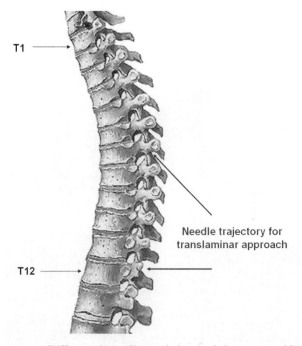

T1 ⟶

Needle trajectory for
translaminar approach

T12 ⟶

FIGURE 103.1. Difference in needle angulation needed to access epidural space at midthoracic level.
Modified from Netter FH. *Atlas of Human Anatomy.* 3rd ed., 2003. *Icon Learning Systems*, Teterboro, NJ. Plate 146.

since Blomberg described midline epidural septa or dorsomedian connective tissue bands in 1986 and are believed to be one of the causes of unilateral anesthesia after an adequate catheter placement.

Midthoracic epidural technique using the paramedian approach is optimally carried out with the patient in the sitting position. The patient is asked to flex at the thoracic spine by bending forward, and his (or her) forehead is placed on a padded bedside table. A commercially available epidural positioning device (EPD) can make this process simple and can also obviate the need for an assistant to hold the patient (*Fig. 103.2*). Before beginning the procedure, adequate landmarks should be identified and marked on the patient's skin. The most important landmark is the spinous process of C7 vertebral body, which is very prominent at the midline of the posterior and inferior margin of neck. Subsequent spinous processes can be identified by palpating downwards along the spine. This method is recommended even for the inferior thoracic epidural placement, since a parallel line connecting the superior borders of the iliac crest is an unreliable method of identifying the

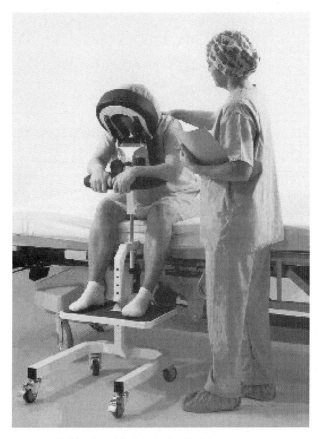

FIGURE 103.2. Epidural positioning device (EPD).
From Valley Technology, Inc., with permission. (http://www.valleytechnology.
com/).

L4–5 inter-laminar space. After the target inter-laminar space is identified,
the inferior tip of the superior spinous process is marked. The site of needle
entry is 1 cm inferior and 1 cm lateral from this point.

After adequate skin preparation and draping, the skin is anesthetized
using 1% lidocaine. After raising a skin wheal, local anesthesia should be
infiltrated along the path of probable needle trajectory (30° to 45° cephalomedian). The 17-gauge, 3½-inch Hustead or Tuohy needle is then inserted
perpendicular to the skin into the subcutaneous tissues and advanced until
it touches the lamina of inferior vertebral body. This step gives the anesthesia provider an estimation of the depth of epidural space. The needle is
now withdrawn to the skin and redirected 30° to 45° cephalomedian almost

TABLE 103.1	TROUBLESHOOTING STEPS FOR THORACIC EPIDURAL TECHNIQUE		
RESPONSE OBTAINED	**INTERPRETATION**	**PROBLEM**	**ACTION**
Bony contact is made after the initial needle pass.	Contact with lamina of interior vertebral body or articular process of facet joint is made.	None; needle depth should be noted.	Needle should be withdrawn to skin and redirected 30° to 45° cephalomedial.
Bony contact is made after the second needle pass.	Contact with lamina of interior or superior vertebral body or articular process of facet joint is made.	Needle is angled excessively in either direction.	Needle should be withdrawn to skin and redirected 5° to 10° cephalomedial. If similar response is encountered, a 5° to 10° change should be made in either direction and needle should be advanced until loss of resistance is observed.
Clear fluid is observed to drip from the needle hub after epidural space is entered and glass syringe is removed.	If the flow stops after few drops, it is probably the saline used with loss-of-resistance technique. If the flow is constant, it is indeed cerebrospinal fluid.	Dura is penetrated.	The needle should be withdrawn and the epidural technique may be repeated at a different interspace. Drug dosages should be adjusted since subarachnoid migration of drugs through the dural rent can occur.
Blood is observed to drip from the needle hub after epidural space is entered and glass syringe is removed.	Needle tip is positioned in the lumen of an epidural blood vessel.	Needle penetrated the dense epidural venous plexus.	The needle bevel is rotated slightly until blood flow stops. If this maneuver fails, the needle tip be withdrawn 1 to 2 centimeters and redirected into the epidural space using loss-of-resistance technique.
Resistance is encountered during advancement of epidural catheter.	False loss of resistance or catheter tip is stuck against dura.	Improper needle tip position.	Loss of resistance should be rechecked after withdrawing the catheter. If present, needle bevel is rotated 30° to 45° and catheter is reinserted.

to the initial depth, as noted in the previous step. Once the needle is positioned at the specified angulation and depth, the stylet is removed and further advances are cautiously made, using the loss-of-resistance technique with either the saline or the dual-chamber (air-saline) method. The mean depth of thoracic epidural space using the paramedian technique is $5.11+/-0.94$ cm and varies with body weight, body mass index, and anatomic levels. The greater the patient's weight and the higher the puncture level, the deeper the thoracic epidural space from the body surface.

After the epidural space is identified, the syringe is gently removed and the epidural catheter is inserted approximately 3 to 5 cm into the epidural space. There should be very little resistance to passage of the catheter, once it has exited the needle. The catheter should be tested for intrathecal or intravascular placement, using 3 mL of 1.5% lidocaine mixed with 1:200,000 epinephrine and tunneled, taped, or both, as planned. The correct epidural placement of the catheter can also be confirmed using fluoroscopy, a low-current, electrical-stimulation test, or a Tsui test. The needle should be withdrawn immediately if the patient reports sudden pain in a radicular fashion at any time during the procedure. The troubleshooting process for each step of this procedure is described in *Table 103.1.*

TAKE HOME POINTS

- Neuraxial techniques are valuable tools in the hands of anesthesiologists and pain physicians.
- Thoracic epidural placement is often difficult and time consuming. Understanding spinal anatomy well and using the paramedian technique can facilitate such placement.
- This chapter briefly describes certain important technical steps as basic principles. Consistently following these guidelines can make thoracic epidural placement a pleasant and an organized venture.

SUGGESTED READINGS

Blomberg R. The dorsomedian connective tissue band in the lumbar epidural space of humans: an anatomical study using epiduroscopy in autopsy cases. *Anesth Analg.* 1986;65(7):747–752.

Lai HC, Liu TJ, Peng SK, et al. Depth of the thoracic epidural space in paramedian approach. *J Clin Anesth.* 2005;17(5):339–343.

Tsui BC, Gupta S, Finucane B. Confirmation of epidural catheter placement using nerve stimulation. *Can J Anaesth.* 1998;45(7):640–644.

Waldman SD. Thoracic epidural nerve block: paramedian approach. In: Waldman SD, ed. *Atlas of Interventional Pain Management.* 2nd ed. Philadelphia: WB Saunders Company; 2004:216–221.

104

INCORPORATE ULTRASOUND GUIDANCE FOR PERIPHERAL NERVE BLOCKADE INTO YOUR PRACTICE

MICHAEL AZIZ, MD AND JEAN-LOUIS HORN, MD

Use of ultrasound-guided, peripheral-nerve blockade has become more popular in the last 5 years. Historically, peripheral-nerve blockade was facilitated by contacting the nerve with the block needle to elicit a parasthesia or by feeling a "pop" with fascial perforation (or both). In the 1970s, nerve stimulation allowed for more precise location of peripheral nerves based on motor-stimulation patterns. Despite the growing popularity of regional anesthesia, it remains burdened with failures and occasional complications, including nerve injury and parasthesia, local anesthetic toxicity, pneumothorax, painful muscle stimulation, and neuroaxial anesthesia. With the decrease in cost and improved portability of high-resolution ultrasound devices, we now have access to devices that visualize peripheral nerves and surrounding structures to guide needle and catheter placement for peripheral-nerve blockade. Using ultrasound-guided, peripheral-nerve block decreases the length of procedures and the period during which the block takes effect; improves the quality of the block; improves the success rate; and reduces the risk for complications.

Understanding the basic physics of ultrasound is necessary to safely master its clinical uses. The echo is a sound wave generated by the vibration of piezoelectric crystals aligned at the tip of a probe. The received sound wave vibrates the piezoelectric crystals to generate an electric current. Structures are visualized depending on their specific acoustic impedance or echogenicity. Depth is measured by the delay of the echo wave's return to the probe, assuming a speed of sound of 1540 m/sec in human soft tissue. The echo pulse can be absorbed, reflected, refracted, or scattered, creating artifacts. Image resolution and echo penetration relates to the frequency of the sent signal. High frequency signals (from 8 MHz to 15 MHz) produces high-resolution images at the expense of penetration and is suited for superficial structures only. As the frequency decreases (from 2MHz to 8 MHz), penetration increases, but resolution decreases. To maintain proper orientation, each probe has a mark on its side that corresponds to a mark on the screen.

Simultaneous use of a nerve stimulator is valuable to those learning to use ultrasound guidance. Attention to sterility is crucial as adding a probe

© 2006 Mayo Foundation for Medical Education and Research

to the field complicates sterile technique. The identification of nerves requires detailed knowledge of trans-sectional anatomy and the characteristic echogenicity of the adjacent structures and nerves in question. Scanning a nerve in a transverse plane, as opposed to a longitudinal plan, facilitates its identification. Neurons appear to be hypoechoic or black, and connective tissue appears to be hyperechoic or grey or white. Each nerve has its own characteristic pattern of echogenicity, depending on its location: The trunks of the brachial plexus appear to be hypoechoic, whereas distal nerves are relatively hyperechoic. Nerves are anisotropic meaning their echogenicity changes depending on the angle of incidence of the echo beam, a property that can be utilized to differentiate peripheral nerves from other structures less anisotropic (tendons) or not anisotropic (muscle, fat, bone), which do not change echogenicity. Standardizing the approach by developing a specific pattern of recognition for each peripheral nerve is useful. First, specific surrounding structures are identified (bones, vessels, muscles), and then nerves are located. When learning the technique, the nerve, the needle shaft, and the tip of the needle should be visualized using the long axis of the probe to maintain constant visualization of the needle. A motor pattern can be elicited and the practitioner can observe appropriate local anesthetic spread in the tissue or the advancement of a catheter for continuous perineural infusion. Some authors have identified preferable patterns of local anesthetic spread along the nerve. Ideally, the local anesthetic should be seen bathing the entire nerve as the local anesthetic is injected to ensure reliable anesthesia of the nerve (donut sign). When dealing with separated nerves, as in the axillary approach of the brachial plexus, local anesthetic should be seen bathing all desirable nerves or the needle can be moved appropriately if only partial local anesthetic spread is visualized.

Using ultrasound guidance presents several important potential advantages. It takes much of the guessing out of the regional technique and relieves the anxiety of not being able to find a nerve, as anatomic variations are frequent. It minimizes the number of needle passes, with a subsequent decrease in procedural pain and trauma. Preblock scanning precisely maps the topography of the targeted area, including the depth of structures, and defines the best angle of approach (*Fig. 104.1*). Real-time tracking of the needle can avoid injury to vascular structures, pleura, and spinal cord. Visualizing local anesthetic spread and adjusting the needle to bathe the targeted nerves thoroughly with local anesthetic can improve success rate and efficiency (*Fig. 104.2*). Using a nerve-stimulator technique alone, current is dispersed immediately after an initial injection of local anesthetic and nerve relocalization becomes difficult with subsequent needle repositioning. Experienced users of ultrasound guidance may not need to use a nerve stimulator, because they have better control of needle positioning near the nerve. Using

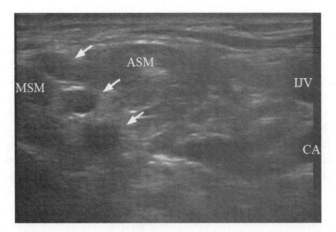

FIGURE 104.1. Interscalene brachial plexus. Arrows indicate nerve roots; ASM, anterior scalene muscle; MSM, middle scalene muscle; IJV, internal jugular vein; CA, carotid artery.

ultrasound guidance may reduce the incidence of neuropathy by avoiding direct nerve puncture and nerve injury.

Ultrasound guidance has some limitations. Ultrasound machines with high resolution are costly and complicated to use. Mastering the techniques and learning the detailed trans-sectional anatomy takes months of education

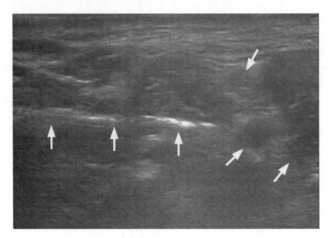

FIGURE 104.2. Interscalene brachial plexus with local anesthetic. Local anesthetic fills the interscalene groove. Arrows indicate needle with tip in close proximity to nerve.

and practice. Needle guidance under ultrasound represents another challenge, because the beam is very narrow (about 1 mm thick) and a sharp angle of approach limits needle visualization. To date, no formal education program with certification exists to facilitate training. Those well trained in regional anesthesia have a strong understanding of the involved anatomy and can perform fast and efficient nerve blocks without ultrasound. For those clinicians, the extra time required to learn this new approach seems like a burden on an already-efficient practice; however, no technique is free from failure or complication, and we should always look for ways to improve patient care. The literature is beginning to show the benefits of using ultrasound guidance. Several prospective, randomized, controlled trials have shown use of ultrasound guidance to reduce the length of procedures and the period during which the block takes effect; to extend the duration of the block; and to reduce the amount of local anesthetic needed to obtain a complete block. The literature is beginning to demonstrate increased success rates and reduced complication rates. Most of those anesthesiologists who provide regional anesthesia and who have embraced ultrasound in their practice believe that the literature will ultimately support its widespread use for improved patient care and safety.

TAKE HOME POINTS

- Ultrasound technology has become a useful adjunct to peripheral-nerve blockade.
- Becoming familiar with the trans-sectional anatomy and appearance of nerves on ultrasound takes time and practice.
- Ultrasound guidance adds certainty and comfort to needle placement and visualizes nearby structures to be avoided.
- Visualization of local anesthetic spread around nerves assures a reliable block and can be used to guide relocation of a needle.
- Look for future evidence to validate that using ultrasound guidance in placing nerve blockades increases the success rate and reduces the complication rate more than does using nerve-stimulation technique alone.

SUGGESTED READINGS

Dabu A, Chan V. *A Practical Guide to Ultrasound Imaging for Peripheral Nerve Blocks.* Toronto: University of Toronto Press; 2004.

Marhofer P, Greher M, Kapral S. Ultrasound guidance in regional anesthesia. Review. *J Anaesth.* 2005;94(1):7–17.

Williams SR, Chouinard P, Arcand G, et al. Ultrasound guidance speeds execution and improves the quality of supraclavicular block. *Anesth Analg.* 2003;97:1518–1523.

www.usra.ca.

105

DO NOT OVERLOOK THE "OLD-FASHIONED" BIER BLOCK, BUT BEWARE OF THE SPEEDY SURGEON!

SURJYA SEN, MD AND
MICHAEL W. BARTS, CRNA, BSANESTH, AAAPM

A 26-year-old woman with no significant past medical history presents for removal of a ganglion cyst on the dorsum of her wrist. The surgeon predicts a quick procedure, and an intravenous regional anesthetic with lidocaine is chosen. As promised, from incision to closure, the operation is completed within 12 minutes. Planning for a rapid turnover and quick recovery, the tourniquet is released and the patient is taken to the postanesthesia recovery unit. Within seconds after arriving, the patient begins to complain of severe pain in her arm, then dizziness, and, ultimately, she begins to seize. What happened? Could such an outcome have been predicted? If so, what could have been done to prevent it?

INTRODUCTION AND HISTORY

Described by August Bier in 1908, "vein anesthesia" was originally proposed for surgery of the elbow and amputations of the feet. It was noted to use a "new avenue" for getting the anesthetic agent "to the end apparatus of the nerves as well to the nerve trunks": the blood vessel. Though Bier reported his method in at least five journals over the course of 2 years, the technique did not rapidly gain popularity. It involved special equipment (Esmarch bandages were not widely available at the time), meticulous exsanguinations of the limb, and a cutdown to locate the vein. With the introduction of brachial plexus blocks in 1911, interest in "vein anesthesia" quickly faded.

Nearly three decades after its introduction, use of the technique surged when it became particularly useful on the battlefields of World War II. The introduction of safer amide local anesthetics (i.e., lidocaine), the use of percutaneous needles to cannulate veins, and the introduction of a commercially available double-cuff tourniquet helped what was then known as the Bier block gain popularity.

ADVANTAGES AND DISADVANTAGES

With some of the initial disadvantages being overcome by advancements in the field of anesthesia, the advantages of the block are more apparent. From a technical standpoint, all that is needed is successful cannulation of a vein in the involved extremity. Anesthesia can be set up quickly and easily, the

© 2006 Mayo Foundation for Medical Education and Research

length of anesthesia is predictable, recovery is rapid, and the block itself is extremely reliable.

Any clinician planning to use the block technique must also be aware of the disadvantages of the procedure. As originally described by Bier himself, upon release of the tourniquet, the local anesthetic may cause systemic toxicity. Second, pain from tourniquet use is the primary limitation on the duration of anesthesia. To combat this, double tourniquets and subcutaneous infiltration anesthesia have been proposed but have not yet eliminated this limitation. It is also important to note that postoperative pain relief is virtually nonexistent with this method. Unlike brachial and lumbar plexus blocks, once the tourniquet is released, surgical anesthesia quickly dissipates and the patient is left without the benefit of residual analgesia.

Two other limitations involve patient selection. First, the block cannot be used for a patient in whom movement of the operative extremity causes pain. The process of exsanguination with an Esmarch bandage can generate significant pressures that can be quite painful. Second, the venous system of the involved extremity must be intact. Traumatic hematomas, open fractures, and the like are contraindications to performing the block.

TECHNIQUE

1) Place a small-gauge intravenous catheter in the distal portion of the extremity to be blocked. A smaller gauge helps decrease the area through which the injected local anesthetic can ooze out after exsanguination and tourniquet inflation

2) Wrap soft cloth over the proximal portion of the extremity to be blocked. This wrap should be free of wrinkles and have a smooth circumferential fit, since the tourniquet will compress it.

3) Place the tourniquet over the cloth padding. Raise the limb to allow venous drainage via gravity. To exsanguinate the forearm and particularly the hand for the purpose of finger, hand or wrist short procedures, one of the authors (MWB) has the patient squeeze a tennis ball in his hand. The ball has the correct shape, size, and degree of hardness to force the palmar blood out during Esmarch exsanguination. The structures of the hand remain in anatomic alignment, so there is less discomfort with compression. If cross contamination of the ball is a concern, first place the ball in a disposable glove for protection.

4) Next, exsanguinate the extremity by wrapping an Esmarch bandage in a distal to proximal manner.

5) Inflate the tourniquet to 300 mmHg. If using a double tourniquet, inflate the distal cuff first. Then, inflate the proximal cuff and deflate the distal cuff.

6) Inject local anesthetic into the vein, and raise the extremity to allow "downward" flow via gravity.

7) The block is significantly better tolerated with concomitant intravenous sedation (via an intravenous catheter in the other arm, of course!). Sedation can specifically help a patient tolerate pain from tourniquet use for longer durations and may raise the patient's seizure threshold. If a double tourniquet is used, inflation of the distal cuff followed by deflation of the painful proximal cuff can add 15 to 30 minutes of operative time. Alerting the surgeon of this "window" of time when the cuff is changed is important.

AGENTS AND ADJUNCTS

Most commonly, the local anesthetic agent of choice is lidocaine. Large volume, dilute concentrations (i.e., 50 mL of 0.5% lidocaine) have been advocated, but smaller, more concentrated amounts (12 to 15 mL of 2% lidocaine) can also serve the same purpose. Mepivacaine provides a well-tolerated alternative to lidocaine, one that has some longer anesthetic and analgesic effects after the tourniquet is released. Typical dosing involves 1.5% 30 cc diluted with 20 cc of NaCl (preservative free). This renders a final concentration of 0.9% in 50 cc, which can be used in 35-cc to 50-cc aliquots for small to large arms. Other local anesthetics, such as ropivacaine (0.2%) and even bupivacaine (0.25%), have been described for use in the Bier block. However, since the block is usually limited by pain from tourniquet use and not by local anesthetic duration, these choices do not offer major advantages. Use of ropivacaine or bupivacaine poses higher risks for significant cardiac toxicity in the event of inadvertent tourniquet failure and resulting release of drug, which sometimes leads to resuscitative difficulty. Most anesthesia providers feel that the benefits of using these anesthetics do not justify the risks of using them.

Various adjuncts to the use of local anesthetics have also been studied. In a systematic review, Choyce et al. noted minimal positive benefits for most adjuncts. Opiates, such as meperidine and morphine, showed slightly faster onset and somewhat slower recovery. Fentanyl, however, did not provide any detectable advantage.

The primary benefit of using nonsteroidal anti-inflammatory drugs as an adjunct to use of local anesthetics is prolonged postoperative analgesia. Alkalinization helped to decrease the discomfort of injection but failed to provide a statistically significant advantage in terms of anesthesia or postoperative pain relief. Additionally, neuromuscular blockers, such as atracurium, were noted to help with muscle relaxation (particularly helpful for fracture reduction) but carried the additional risk of residual blockade.

Overall, nonsteroidal anti-inflammatory drugs and clonidine were the adjunctive agents noted to supplement the primary properties of the local anesthetic best.

CAUTIONS

The most common complication of the use of intravenous regional anesthesia is that of systemic toxicity of local anesthetic. The clinician should be aware of both central nervous system and cardiac symptoms of toxicity–especially premonitory ones, such as circumoral numbness, dizziness, and tinnitus. To avoid this complication, the tourniquet should always be deflated in a gradual, step-wise fashion. Most texts recommend that tourniquets be left inflated for a minimum of 20 minutes, even for procedures that are shorter in duration.

Other complications include hematomas (especially at the site of intravenous catheter insertion), ecchymoses, and subcutaneous hemorrhage—all of which require vigilance and careful padding with prolonged direct pressure for treatment.

Lastly, insufficient tourniquet pressure can be of significant concern with this method of regional anesthesia. If the tourniquet pressure is not carefully maintained above systolic pressure, arterial inflow with lack of venous outflow can cause engorgement of the extremity. This can be particularly common with lower-extremity procedures in which arteries can be harder to compress (either due to calcifications or location deep within the leg musculature).

TAKE HOME POINTS

- Wrap the extremity in soft cloth before placing the tourniquet.
- Use a small intravenous catheter for introducing the local anesthetic.
- Keep an eye on the pressure gauge of the pneumatic tourniquet (or use a constant-pressure automated tourniquet).
- When deflating the proximal cuff and inflating the distal cuff, double check the valves and lines of each cuff to make sure that the proper one is being deflated or inflated. An error in this part of the procedure can introduce a bolus of the local anesthetic into the patient's system with potential risk for toxicity.
- Have a plan for postoperative pain control in place before terminating the block. Peri-incisional infiltration, intravenous opiates, and appropriate amounts of anxiolytics and amnestics can be very useful adjuncts.
- Pay attention to postprocedure tourniquet deflation. If the operation is completed quickly (i.e., in less than 45 minutes when lidocaine is used),

multi-stage deflation to allow gradual washout of the local anesthetic is recommended.

SUGGESTED READINGS

Brill S, Middleton W, Brill G, et al. Bier's block; 100 years old and still going strong! *Acta Anaesthesiol Scand.* 2004;48(1):117–122.

Brown DL. *Atlas of Regional Anesthesia.* 2nd ed. Philadelphia: WB Saunders; 1999:57–61.

Choyce A, Peng P. A systematic review of adjuncts for intravenous regional anesthesia for surgical procedures. *Can J Anaesth.* 2002;49(1):32–45.

Miller RD. *Anesthesia.* 5th ed. Churchill Livingstone; 2000:1529–1530.

106

CONSIDER EPIDURAL ANESTHETIC AS AN ADJUNCTIVE OR PRIMARY TECHNIQUE FOR PATIENTS HAVING MASTECTOMY

JENNIFER VOOKLES, MD, MA

Mastectomies are commonly performed under general anesthesia; however, various regional anesthetic techniques for breast surgery have been evaluated to serve as the primary anesthetic, the adjunctive anesthesia, or the postoperative analgesia, or to serve as a combination of these roles. Examples of these techniques include field local infiltration, brachial-plexus blocks, paravertebral blocks, intercostal nerve blocks, and thoracic epidural anesthesia.

These different approaches have a wide range of utility. At one extreme, local infiltration is very limited and could only be used as the sole anesthetic choice for more confined surgeries. Also, the benefits of local anesthesia as well as of some of the peripheral nerve blocks cannot be extended beyond the duration of the local anesthetic effect. At the other extreme, thoracic epidural analgesia (TEA) can be used as the sole anesthetic for extensive breast procedures and can provide prolonged postoperative pain control via continuous infusion. Use of TEA obviates the need for using volatile anesthetics and opioid analgesics, and, as a result, less postoperative nausea and vomiting and shorter recovery times have been reported with TEA use. Even using TEA as an adjunct to a general anesthetic can provide substantial benefits. Using TEA and a local anesthetic selectively blocks cardiac sympathetic fibers, resulting in greater hemodynamic stability, improved myocardial oxygen balance, and an attenuated stress response. Pre-emptive analgesia may also play a role in decreasing postoperative pain and opioid requirements. Greater patient satisfaction has been reported.

Yeh and Doss both used TEA for their primary anesthetic plus sedation. They placed catheters at a T5-6 or T6-7 level and threaded catheters 3 to 5 cm into the epidural space. One reports maintaining a block between C5-T6 with 2% lidocaine; the other reports maintaining a block from roughly 2 cm below the clavicle and to the costal arch inferiorly with 0.2% ropivacaine. Both approaches were successful, although, in some patients, the surgeons needed to supplement with local anesthetic during the axillary-node dissection.

Using various epidural infusions can maintain postoperative analgesia. Doss recommends infusing 0.2% ropivacaine, beginning with 4 to 6 mL/hr. Systemic opioids may be needed if the patient experiences inadequate analgesia. At my institution, an infusion containing a lower concentration of

ⓒ 2006 Mayo Foundation for Medical Education and Research

local anesthetic in combination with a low dose of opioid is more commonly used (usually 0.1% ropivacaine, hydromorphone 10 mcg/mL); our initial infusion rate is 10 mL/hr, but this can titrate as indicated by either pain or side effects.

Either technique can be effective, but each has unique precautions. With higher doses of local anesthetic, upper-extremity weakness and subjective shortness of breath should be monitored. Subjective shortness of breath generally results from chest-wall numbness, and patients generally tolerate this well with education. Diaphragmatic weakness would not be expected in the absence of proximal upper-extremity weakness. Such weakness is less common using lower concentrations of local anesthetic; however, patients receiving such lower doses usually need some opioid for adequate analgesia. The opioid can be provided as part of the epidural infusion, as is done at my institution, or systemically. The usual side effects from opioid use can occur with either approach.

TAKE HOME POINTS

- Epidural anesthesia is a well-described and efficacious technique for patients having mastectomy.
- Greater patient satisfaction has been reported with use of epidural anesthesia in patients having mastectomy.
- Various strategies for catheter management and dosing give satisfactory results. Also, if you are using epidural anesthesia as your primary anesthetic, ask the surgeons to supplement with local anesthesia for axillary-node dissection.
- This author uses a low-dose local anesthetic and a low-dose opioid infusion for postoperative analgesia.

SUGGESTED READINGS

Atansoff PG, Alon E, Weiss BM. Intercostal nerve block for lumpectomy: superior postoperative pain relief with bupivacaine. *J Clin Anesth*. 1994;4:47.

Doss N, Ipe J, Crimi T, et al. Continuous thoracic epidural anesthesia with 0.2% ropivacaine vs general anesthesia for perioperative management of modified radical mastectomy. *Anesth Analg*. 2001;92(6):1552–1557.

Fassoulaki A. Brachial plexus block for pain relief after modified radical mastectomy. *Anesth Analg*. 1982;61:986.

Klein SM, Bergh A, Steel SM, et al. Thoracic paravertebral block for breast surgery. *Anesth Analg*. 2000;90:1402–1405.

Liu S, Carpenter RL, Neal JM. Epidural anesthesia and analgesia. *Anesthesiology*. 1995;82:1474–1506.

Lynch EP, Welch KJ, Carabuena JM, et al. Thoracic epidural anesthesia improves outcome after breast surgery. *Ann Surg*. 1995;222:663.

Oakley N, Dennison A, Shorthouse A. A prospective audit of simple mastectomy under local anesthesia. *Eur J Surg Oncol*. 1996;2:131–136.

Yeh C, Yu J-C, Wu J-C, et al. Thoracic epidural anesthesia for pain relief and post-operative recovery with modified radical mastectomy. *World J Surg*. 1999;23:256–261.

107

CONSIDER CONTINUOUS PARAVERTEBRAL BLOCK AS YOUR PRIMARY ANALGESIC TECHNIQUE

BRUCE BEN-DAVID, MD

SCENARIO

Your colleagues who are surgeons and your hospital administration are increasingly pushing the limits on what can be done as an ambulatory surgical procedure. Plans are now taking shape to perform mastectomies as same-day surgery. You are asked for your input into realizing this goal.

CONSIDERATIONS

Although the anesthetic can be done appropriately to achieve rapid recovery, the two primary problems to be expected in discharging these patients are pain and postoperative nausea and vomiting (PONV). These problems are not unrelated. Postoperative pain can itself lead to PONV, and so can its treatment with opiates. In fact, we now know that opiate side effects are linearly correlated with opiate consumption. Since this is a very painful procedure, we can anticipate significant need for opiate analgesics postoperatively.

We also know that opiates may adequately control pain at rest but, because of limited mu-agonist-receptor participation in the relevant pathways, they are less effective in controlling pain with movement. Opiates alone therefore may be insufficient to get patients mobilized and discharged home. Moreover, we cannot ignore the significant correlation between severe postoperative pain and the development of persistent or chronic postoperative pain. This is a serious concern in mastectomy surgery; a high percentage of patients having mastectomy develop chronic pain known as "postmastectomy syndrome." Trying to shuffle our patients quickly out of the hospital without aggressively addressing pain management beyond the immediate hours after surgery clearly is not only likely to fail in the short term but also in the long term.

OPTIONS

Multiple intercostal blocks or local-anesthetic wound infiltration can be expected to provide analgesia of only limited duration. A "soaker" catheter infusing local anesthetic into the wound may add modestly to the analgesia, but the technique generally has not been shown to provide the same level of analgesia as do neural-blockade techniques.

© 2006 Mayo Foundation for Medical Education and Research

The most commonly used neural-blockade technique today for procedures of the thorax and abdomen is thoracic epidural analgesia (TEA). While TEA can be expected to provide analgesia far superior to that possible with patient controlled analgesia (PCA) opiate, it is not a practicable solution here. TEA use is associated with several side effects, some of them quite common, which render the technique unacceptable for the ambulatory surgical patient. These side effects include pruritis, urinary retention, nausea and vomiting, respiratory depression, and hypotension. Though probably not relevant here, TEA use is a particular concern in the patient who will be administered anticoagulants postoperatively. In the United States, epidural hematoma has rendered dozens of patients paraplegic when, postoperatively, low-molecular-weight heparin was administered in conjunction with the use of epidural analgesia.

An alternative technique of neural blockade, continuous paravertebral block (CPVB), is at least as effective an analgesic as TEA but is nearly devoid of TEA's side effects. Originally described more than 100 years ago, paravertebral block has found renewed popularity in recent years and has proven most useful as a continuous technique. Its advantages include its ability to achieve a high degree of sensory and analgesic blockade without causing urinary retention, respiratory depression, pruritis, or hypotension. In addition, CPVB better preserves forced vital capacity (FVC) following thoracotomy. It preserves lower-limb strength, thus facilitating early mobilization of patients. It affords the possibility of unilateral or bilateral blockade, as needed. Lastly, its offset from the midline promises less risk of spinal cord injury as a result of either needle trauma or hematoma. In fact, a second and newer technique of CPVB, the lateral intercostal approach, is even feasible in situations of coagulopathy, spine abnormality, or spinal trauma.

ANATOMY OF THE PARAVERTEBRAL SPACE

The thoracic paravertebral space is a triangular space bounded anteriorly by the parietal pleura, posteriorly by the superior costotransverse ligament, and medially by the vertebral body, intervertebral disc, and intervertebral neural foramen. The apex of the triangle laterally is continuous with the intercostal space. The space is bisected by the very thin endothoracic fascia, which effectively creates two "compartments." The anterior compartment contains the sympathetic chain, and the posterior compartment contains the intercostal nerve, dorsal ramus, intercostal blood vessels, and rami communicants. Spinal nerves in the paravertebral space are relatively devoid of fascial covering, making them uniquely and exceptionally sensitive to local anesthetic blockade. The paravertebral space openly communicates cephalocaudad, thereby making it possible to effect multiple-dermatomal blockade via a single catheter positioned in the space.

TECHNIQUE OF CPBV

Placing the continuous paravertebral catheter preoperatively is recommended, because it is technically easier, it affords the chance to use the block as part of the anesthetic, and it allows recovery room nurses immediate access for postoperative pain control. The patient is positioned sitting, with feet dangling over the side of the bed. An intravenous infusion is established, standard monitors applied, and mild sedation administered. The relevant spinal process is identified (note that the steep angulation of thoracic spinous processes brings them opposite the transverse processes of the adjacent more caudad vertebra) and the needle-entry point is marked 2.5 cm lateral to the spinous process. Catheter placement should be at a dermatomal level that represents the midpoint of the surgical wound. Patients may exhibit a vagal response during performance of the block. A prepared syringe of an anticholinergic drug (e.g., glycopyrrolate) and a syringe with a pressor agent (e.g., ephedrine) therefore should be immediately at hand.

The skin is disinfected and local anesthesia is injected subcutaneously at the needle-entry point. A 9-cm 18-gauge Tuohy needle with 1-cm graduated markings is introduced and walked caudally off the transverse process to a depth 1 cm beyond the transverse process. Often one feels a confirmatory "pop" upon penetration of the costotransverse ligament. A drop of fluid is placed in the needle hub, and the patient asked to inspire deeply. Correct placement is confirmed by lack of movement of the fluid bubble. A drawing inward of the fluid indicates intrapleural needle placement, in which case the needle should be immediately withdrawn. After negative aspiration for blood, 5 ml of 0.5% ropivacaine is injected. Having an assistant inject through an extension tube is helpful, as this helps avoid significant movement of the needle. Following the injection, the extension tube is disconnected and a polyamide, 20-gauge, closed-tip, multiport catheter is inserted to a depth of 3 to 5 cm beyond the tip of the needle. The catheter is affixed in standard fashion.

Postoperatively, a pump containing 0.2% ropivacaine is attached to the CPVB catheter and is infused at a rate of between 6 and 10 mL/h. A disposable infusion pump can be used for this purpose just as for other continuous peripheral-nerve blocks in patients having ambulatory surgery. Before discharge, patients should receive a set of written instructions and a phone number to call with questions or concerns. Catheters can be easily removed by the patients themselves at home and may be discarded along with the disposable pumps.

MULTIMODAL ANALGESIA: MAKING THE MOST OF YOUR NERVE BLOCK

CPVB and all other nerve blocks, for that matter, are only a temporary and a very incomplete treatment of postoperative pain. Even complete neural blockade does not inhibit the accumulation of inflammatory mediators in the peripheral tissues and their influence on nociceptors. Nor will it block the access of inflammatory mediators to the central nervous system where nociceptive processing will be altered as well. Therefore, once the neural blockade is lifted, the patient is still left in a hyperalgesic state. In this sense, neural blockade can be viewed as simply a window of opportunity. It allows us a several-day window during which to mobilize the patient rapidly, control her pain effectively, and minimize opiate consumption. But neural blockade can provide only a partial answer to postoperative pain.

By combining the nerve block with other analgesic agents, one can achieve better short-term and long-term pain relief. These agents include nonsteroidal anti-inflammatory drugs, COX-2 antagonists, alpha-2-delta calcium-channel blockade (gabapentin or pregabalin), N-methy-l-D-aspartase (NMDA) blockade (e.g., intraoperative low-dose ketamine, dextromethorphan, magnesium), single-dose dexamethasone, alpha-2 agonists (clonidine, dexmedetomidine), and, of course, short-acting opioids for breakthrough pain. Use of multimodal analgesia not only enhances the success of early analgesia and discharge of patients but also profoundly reduces patients' chances of developing a chronic pain state.

TAKE HOME POINTS

- CPVB is a remarkably effective analgesic technique, with many advantages over TEA.
- For bilateral breast surgery, as for surgery of the abdomen or retroperitoneum, one needs to place bilateral CPVB catheters.
- Heavy reliance on opioid analgesia is contrary to many of our modern goals of postoperative care.
- Do not rely solely on neural blockade for postoperative analgesia. The best results, in the short and long terms, are achieved by using a multimodal approach.

SUGGESTED READINGS

Davies RG, Myles PS, Graham JM. A comparison of the analgesic efficacy and side-effects of paravertebral vs. epidural blockade for thoracotomy–a systematic review and meta-analysis of randomized trials. *Br J Anaesth*. 2006;96:418–426.

Ganapathy S, Nielsen KC, Steele SM. Outcomes after paravertebral blocks. *Int Anesthesiol Clin*. 2005;43:185–193.

Karmakar MK. Thoracic paravertebral block. *Anesthesiology*. 2001;95:771–780.

Lönnqvist PA. Pre-emptive analgesia with thoracic paravertebral blockade? *Br J Anaesth*. 2005;95:727–728.

Naja Z, Lonnqvist PA. Somatic paravertebral nerve blockade: incidence of failed block and complications. *Anaesthesia*. 2001;56:1184–1188.

Naja MZ, Ziade MF, Lonnqvist PA. General anaesthesia combined with bilateral paravertebral blockade (T5-6) vs. general anaesthesia for laparoscopic cholecystectomy: a prospective, randomized clinical trial. *Eur J Anaesthesiol*. 2004;20:489.

Richardson J, Lonnqvist PA. Thoracic paravertebral block. *Br J Anaesth.* 1998;81: 230–238.

Richardson J, Sabanathan S, Jones J, et al. A prospective, randomized comparison of preoperative and continuous balanced epidural or paravertebral bupivacaine on post-thoracotomy pain, pulmonary function and stress response. *Br J Anaesth.* 1999;83:387–392.

Vogt A, Stieger DS, Theurillat C, et al. Single-injection thoracic paravertebral block for postoperative pain treatment after thoracoscopic surgery. *Br J Anaesth.* 2005;95: 816–821.

108

WET TAP? WHAT NOW?

DAVID Y. KIM, MD, IHAB R. KAMEL, MD AND
RODGER BARNETTE, MD, FCCM

When a puncture occurs in the course of placing an epidural, causing the patient to have headache after the procedure, such headache is called postdural puncture headache (PDPH). The puncture may be accidental or intentional (for example, an intentional puncture is made for lumbar drains for abdominal aortic aneurysm surgery). A PDPH may also result from a spinal anesthetic; however, this is much less common due to the smaller size of the needle puncturing the dura mater of the spinal cord.

PDPH is defined by the International Headache Society as follows: "Bilateral headache that develops within 7 days after lumbar puncture and disappears within 14 days after the lumbar puncture. Headache worsens within 15 minutes of upright position and disappears or lessens within 30 minutes of supine position. Usually is frontal, occipital, or both and may involve the neck and upper shoulders."

Note that the differential diagnosis for an acute headache after dural puncture must include cortical venous thrombosis, meningitis, and intracranial hematomas (intracerebral and subdural). PDPH characteristically depends on position and is usually noted within 48 hours after dural puncture; however, PDPD may develop in approximately one third of cases more than 72 hours after dural puncture and, in rare instances, several weeks after dural puncture. Symptoms associated with this type of headache are nausea, emesis, back pain, and visual and hearing alterations.

WHY IS A "SIMPLE HEADACHE" SO IMPORTANT?

Unintentional dural puncture in the obstetric patient is a complication. In an Obstetric Anesthesiology closed-claim study published in the American Society of Anesthesiologists newsletter in 1999, PDPH was the third most common reason for claim (15% of obstetric claims). Such headaches are more common than nerve damage, pain during anesthesia, and maternal brain damage. The median duration of untreated PDPH is 5 days, with a range of 1 to 12 days.

Note that other complications may result from neuraxial anesthesia for obstetrics, and always consider the possibility of concomitant complications. Some of the other complications of epidurals include epidural catheter complications, unintentional subarachnoid injection, intravascular injection of

© 2006 Mayo Foundation for Medical Education and Research

local anesthetic, direct spinal cord injury, bloody tap, epidural abscess, local anesthetic toxicity, and epidural hematoma.

WHAT CAUSES THIS TYPE OF HEADACHE?

Two proposed pathophysiologic mechanisms for PDPH are (a) continued leak of cerebrospinal fluid (CSF) leads to loss of brain support and results in traction on the meninges of the brain, which are pain-sensitive structures; and (b) loss of CSF results in intracranial hypotension, causing compensatory cerebral vasodilatation and dilatation of intracerebral veins, which, in turn, results in a downward sagging of the brain and subsequent tension on the meninges. Activation of adenosine receptors is another, less widely accepted, postulated mechanism.

Significant risk factors include age, gender, needle diameter, needle-tip design, orientation of the tip during puncture, previous PDPH, history of migraine, and repeated attempts to achieve puncture. Younger patients are more prone to PDPH. Premenopausal women are twice as likely as men to have PDPH. The risk for PDPH relates directly to the diameter of the needle used. The smaller the gauge of the needle used, the lower the incidence of PDPH is. Needle-tip design is also important. Pencil-point needles (Sprotte, Whitacre) have a side orifice on the needle and result in a lower incidence of PDPH than do those with a cutting-point (Quincke). Needle-bevel orientation during insertion is also important. The frequency nearly doubles when the bevel of the needle is inserted perpendicularly instead of parallel to the longitudinal dura fibers. Lastly, the more attempts that are made at a neuraxial technique, the greater the risk for PDPH is, and patients with a history of migraine headaches and previous PDPH are more prone to PDPH.

SO WHAT DO I DO IF I AM PLACING AN EPIDURAL AND CAUSE AN UNINTENTIONAL DURAL PUNCTURE?

Most anesthesiologists recommend removing the needle and placing the epidural in a new interspace, either above or below the previous attempt. Some anesthesiologists recommend placing an intrathecal catheter and using this for obstetrical anesthesia.

Historically, conservative treatment modalities for PDPH were bed rest; hydration; lying in a prone position; abdominal binders; caffeine, oral, or intravenous; theophylline; serotonin agonists; and corticosteroids.

WHICH OF THESE TREATMENTS HAVE EFFICACY AND WHICH HAVE BEEN DISCOUNTED?

Continued bed rest and lying in the prone position often result in a "trend toward increased headache." Allowing early ambulation does not increase the risk for PDPH; on the contrary, early ambulation is recommended.

Additional hydration does not decrease incidence of PDPH. Anecdotal evidence for abdominal binders has been theorized to work by increasing intra-abdominal pressure, thereby equalizing CSF compartment pressures with epidural space pressures. Caffeine (500 mg, intravenously) resolved the symptoms in over two thirds of subjects tested in one trial. Oral dosing of 300 mg of caffeine resulted in only brief relief of symptoms in most patients. A single study using oral theophylline was done, but benefits have not been confirmed, and most anesthesiologists would say the risks outweigh the possible benefits. Trials of serotonin agonists have been done but have not had reproducible results. Lastly, there is only anecdotal evidence for use of corticosteroids.

More aggressive treatments for PDPH include the placement of intrathecal catheters with saline infusion; epidural saline infusions; epidural blood patch (EBP); and epidural colloid infusions.

Studies of continuous epidural infusions of saline have had inconsistent results. Some trials have shown that a saline bolus infused into the intrathecal space does not reduce the risk for PDPH but may decrease the need for an EBP. Several studies have shown that placement of an intrathecal catheter and continuous infusion of local anesthetic for labor analgesia may decrease the incidence of PDPH. Many practitioners would consider using Epidural Dextran 40 as nonstandard therapy.

An EBP should be reserved for patients for whom conservative treatment fails, and the primary indication for doing an EBP is moderate to severe PDPH. A previous EBP is not a contraindication to epidural anesthesia, and human immunodeficiency virus infections are not a contraindication to doing an EBP. In addition, as with any procedure, an EBP has its own subset of complications, the most common of which are back pain, bradycardia, cauda equina syndrome, pneumocephalus, arachnoiditis, abdominal pain and diarrhea, and cerebral ischemia.

HOW AND WHEN DO I DO AN EPIDURAL BLOOD PATCH?

An EBP is a sterile procedure in which a new or existing epidural is used to inject sterile blood into the epidural space. Using 15 to 20 cc of sterile blood, with the patient remaining recumbent for 1 to 2 hours after the EBP, is the standard of care. The most widely accepted etiology for relief of symptoms from use of an EBP is equalization of compartment pressures and normalization of physiologic compartment pressures.

Early studies noted significant benefits in prophylactic use of an EBP. Unfortunately, the majority of the studies were not prospective. More recent reports suggest that the success rate of EBP may be as low as 65%. Studies indicate that the best time to place a prophylactic EBP is 48 hours after a postdural puncture. The authors recommend using conservative treatment first and using an EBP after failure of conservative treatment for moderate to severe PDPH or for recurrent headaches after a postdural puncture.

TAKE HOME POINTS

- Note the general contraindications for epidural placement: Patient refusal, coagulopathy, local infection, systemic sepsis, and anatomic abnormalities. Avoid dealing with PDPH in someone who should not have had an epidural at all.
- PDPH is fairly rigorously defined. Remember that not all headaches occurring after dural puncture are "spinal headaches." Always evaluate the patient for other conditions.
- Closed-claim analyses show that malpractice claims relating to PDPH are quite common, especially in obstetrics cases.
- Several mechanisms are proposed for the pathophysiology of PDPH.
- Significant risk factors for PDPH include age, gender, needle diameter, needle-tip design, orientation of the tip during puncture, previous PDPH, history of migraine, and repeated attempts to achieve puncture.
- The authors recommend reserving use of an EBP, which carries its own significant risk, for patients for whom conservative treatment has failed.

SUGGESTED READINGS

Aldrete JA. Epidural dextran for PDPH. *Reg Anesth Pain Med*. 1993;18:325–326.

Ayad S, Demian Y, Narouze SN, et al. Subarachnoid catheter placement after wet tap for analgesia in labor: Influence on the risk of headache in obstetric patients. *Reg Anesth Pain Med*. 2003;28:512–515.

Berger CW, Crosby ET, Grodecki W. North American survey of the management of dural puncture occurring during labour epidural analgesia. *Can J Anaesth*. 1998; 45:110–114.

Camann WR, Murray RS, Mushlin PS, et al. Effects of oral caffeine on postdural puncture headache. A double-blind, placebo-controlled trial. *Anesth Analg*. 1990;70:181–184.

Chadwick HS. Obstetric anesthesia closed claim update II. *ASA Newsletter*. 1999;63:6.

Chestnut DH. *Obstetric Anesthesia Principles and Practice*. New York: Mosby; 1999;354–375.

Choi A, Laurito CE, Cunningham FE. Pharmacologic management of postdural puncture headache. *Ann Pharmacother*. 1996;30:831–839.

Choi PT, Galinski SE, Takeuchi L, et al. PDPH is a common complication of neuraxial blockade in parturients: A meta-analysis of obstetrical studies. *Can J Anaesth*. 2003;50:460–469.

Davies JM. Obstetric anesthesia closed claim–trends over three decades. *ASA Newsletter*. 2004;68:6.

Dieterich M, Brandt T. Incidence of post-lumbar puncture headache is independent of daily fluid intake. *EUR Arch Psychiatry Clin Neurosci*. 1988;237:194–196.

Despond O, Meuret P, Hemmings G. Postdural puncture headache after spinal anaesthesia in young orthopaedic outpatients using 27-g needles. *Can J Anaesth*. 1998;45:1106–1109.

Duffy PJ, Crosby ET. The epidural blood patch. Resolving the controversies. *Can J Anaesth*. 1999;46:878–886.

Eledjam JJ, Viel E, Aya G, et al. Postdural puncture headache. *Can Anesthesiol*. 1993;41:579–588.

Eriksson AL, Hallen B, Lagerkranser M, et al. Whitacre or Quincke needles: Does it really matter. *Acta Anaesthesiol Scand Suppl*. 1998;113:17–20.

Evans RW, Armon C, Frohman EM, et al. Assessment: Prevention of post-lumbar puncture headaches. In: *Report of the Therapeutics and Technology Assessment.*

Subcommittee of the American Academy of Neurology. *Neurology.* 2000;55:909–914.

Fleisher LA. *Evidence-Based Practice of Anesthesiology.* New York: Saunders; 2004:314–322.

Hess JH. Postdural puncture headache: A literature review. *AANA J.* 1991;59:549–555.

Lambert DH, Hurley RJ, Hertwig L, et al. Role of needle gauge and tip configuration in the production of lumbar puncture headache. *Reg Anesth Pain Med.* 1997;22:66–72.

Lybecker H, Moller JT, May O, et al. Incidence and prediction of postdural puncture headache. A prospective study of 1021 spinal anesthesias. *Anesth Analg.* 1990;70:389–394.

Norris MC, Leighton BL. Continuous spinal anesthesia after unintentional dural puncture in parturients. *Reg Anesth Pain Med.* 1990;15:285–287.

Ross BK, Chadwick HS, Mancuso JJ, et al. Sprotte needle for obstetric anesthesia: Decreased incidence of post dural puncture headache. *Reg Anesth Pain Med.* 1992;17:29–33.

Seeberger MD, Kaufmann M, Staender S, et al. Repeated dural punctures increase the incidence of postdural puncture headache. *Anesth Analg.* 1996;82:302–305.

Sha JL. Epidural pressure during infusion of saline in the parturient. *Int J Obstet Anesth.* 1993;2:190–192.

Turnbull DK, Shepherd DB. Post-dural puncture headache: Pathogenesis, prevention, and treatment. *Br J Anaesth.* 2003;91:718–729.

Vallejo MC, Mandell GL, Sabo DP, et al. Postdural puncture headache: A randomised comparison of spinal needles in obstetric patients. *Anesth Analg.* 2000;91:916–920.

Wiesel S, Tessler MJ, Easdown LJ. Postdural puncture headache: A randomised prospective comparison of the 24 gauge Sprotte and the 27 gauge Quincke needles in young patients. *Can J Anaesth.* 2002;40:607–611.

Yucel A, Ozyalcin S, Talu GK, et al. Intravenous administration of caffeine sodium benzoate for postdural puncture headache. *Reg Anesth Pain Med.* 1999;24:51–54.

109

A PATIENT UNDER REGIONAL ANESTHESIA WHO SUDDENLY CANNOT SPEAK ABOVE A WHISPER HAS A HIGH BLOCK UNTIL PROVEN OTHERWISE

RYAN J. BORTOLON, MD AND JURAJ SPRUNG, MD, PhD

Use of regional anesthesia has grown in recent years, due in large part to the benefits of improved postoperative pain management. Regional anesthesia also continues to be the preferred technique for management of pain during labor and is considered the safest approach for elective cesarean section. Despite adoption of safer regional anesthetic dosing practices, catastrophic complications from inadvertent intrathecal or intravascular injection are still reported.

INADVERTENT INTRATHECAL INJECTION

High spinal or "total" spinal block is one of the most feared complications of neuraxial anesthesia and other regional techniques. Total spinal block is typically caused by excessive cephalad spread of local anesthetic. Severity of block is variable and depends primarily on baricity and duration of local anesthetic action. Patient characteristics, such as age, height, and anatomic considerations (e.g., pregnancy) also have a role in the level of spinal block. The most common cause of excessive anesthetic spread is unintentional dural puncture and subsequent injection of a large volume of local anesthetic intrathecally. Mechanisms of total spinal block include the following:

1) Migration of the epidural catheter into the intrathecal space after proper placement;
2) Repeated spinal anesthetic administration;
3) Large volume expansion of the epidural space, leading to compression of the dura;
4) Intrathecal spread of an epidural bolus after a previous dural puncture;
5) Unrecognized subdural placement of the epidural catheter; and
6) Inadvertent injection or catheter placement into the dural sleeve surrounding the nerve root.

The onset of total spinal block may be quick or delayed, depending on the type, volume, rate of injection, and location of injection of local anesthetic. In a patient who is awake, the first signs of high spinal block may include dyspnea, loss of speech, feeling of impending doom, or restlessness. These signs may then be followed by hypotension, bradycardia, unconsciousness, and, ultimately, circulatory (cardiac) arrest.

Anesthesiologists must keep in mind that a total spinal block may occur in patients under general anesthesia who have had epidural or peripheral nerve blocks for perioperative pain management. In these patients, a total spinal block presents only as hypotension or bradycardia intraoperatively. In the postoperative setting, these patients remain unconscious with fixed, dilated pupils and require full ventilatory support until brainstem and respiratory functions return.

INTRAVASCULAR INJECTION

In general, local-anesthetic toxicity results in benign transient symptoms; however, with large doses of anesthetic, central nervous system (CNS) and cardiovascular toxicity can lead to catastrophic consequences. The most common cause of local-anesthetic toxicity is unrecognized intravascular injection of bolus doses of local anesthetics from a misplaced catheter or needle during a regional anesthetic block. The surest sign of intravascular injection is aspiration of blood, but this test is far more sensitive than specific (resulting in a higher false-negative rate). Several case reports have described intravascular injection despite negative aspiration from the catheter. Most authors of these case reports suspect migration of the needle or catheter tip intravascularly as the primary cause. Others theorize that a catheter tip flush against an intravessel wall may also give a falsely negative aspirate. Less commonly, local anesthetic uptake by highly vascular tissues can lead to toxic plasma levels. Understanding the relationship between anesthetic dose, body weight, and speed of systemic absorption is important in clinical practice to help avoid high plasma concentrations of local anesthetic.

The initial symptoms of CNS toxicity may be excitatory and include tinnitus, perioral numbness, metallic taste, visual disturbances, peripheral motor twitching, and, eventually, grand mal seizures. As plasma levels of anesthetic increase, CNS depressant effects predominate, with disorientation, drowsiness, or unconsciousness being most common.

The cardiovascular effects of local-anesthetic toxicity are seen at serum concentrations of local anesthetic higher than those necessary to elicit CNS toxicity. All local anesthetics directly depress cardiac contractility through their inhibitory action on voltage-gated sodium channels in cardiac muscle. Local anesthetics have a variable effect on the fast-conducting tissues that predispose the heart to dysrhythmias. Although all anesthetics at high plasma levels cause dose-dependent cardiac depression, bupivacaine and tetracaine are the most potent inhibitors and are associated most frequently with severe cardiac collapse. Bupivacaine-associated cardiac arrest is often refractory to normal resuscitative efforts; prolonged cardiopulmonary support is often required.

PREVENTION AND TREATMENT

Focusing on prevention is of the utmost importance for the anesthesiologist. No single test can guarantee proper needle or catheter placement. Several case reports involving total spinal anesthesia or large bolus intravascular injection have been reported despite use of proper preventive techniques. Possible causes of false-negative aspiration include obstruction of the catheter tip (by tissue or vascular wall), partial dural puncture, or subdural placement. Most false-negative test doses are the result of insufficient wait time or inadequate concentration of epinephrine in solution.

The use of dilute anesthetic solutions and the practice of slow, incremental dosing are both very effective methods of preventing serious complications of local anesthetics. The use of dilute anesthetic solutions for epidurals has been clearly supported in the obstetric literature and is most likely responsible for the sharp decrease in morbidity and mortality associated with epidurals placed on patients in labor. Similarly, the practice of fractional dosing, typically 5 mL, has very effectively avoided these complications. The ideal incremental dose is one sufficient to elicit mild toxicity symptoms while avoiding the life-threatening sequelae from a large-dose intravascular or intrathecal injection. The addition of epinephrine to local anesthetic provides a means to identify reliably an intravascular injection–namely, if the systolic blood pressure increases by more than 15 mm Hg in healthy patients, such an injection is deemed to have occurred. The efficacy of this method may be less reliable in certain subsets of patients, such as those taking β-blockers and those in active labor.

The American Society of Regional Anesthesia and Pain Medicine recommends taking the following steps to enhance safety:

1) Gentle aspiration at the needle or catheter;
2) Slow, incremental injection;
3) Dose limitation based on established per-kg guidelines (*Table 109.1*); and
4) Use of intravascular markers.

Even with strict adherence to these guidelines, the anesthesia provider should always be prepared to treat the most severe complications of regional anesthesia. The treatment for total spinal block is always supportive and often requires ventilatory assistance with 100% oxygen via mask or endotracheal intubation and circulatory support with intravenous fluids and vasopressors. In the laboring patient, reducing aortocaval compression by positioning the patient in the lateral (tilt) position is necessary.

The treatment for intravascular injection is also mainly supportive, with the use of benzodiazepines, thiopental, or propofol for cessation of seizures and prolonged cardiopulmonary resuscitation for severe cardiotoxicity. Anesthesiologists must remain vigilant for signs of toxicity and must

TABLE 109.1	DOSE LIMITATION BASED ON ESTABLISHED PER-KG GUIDELINES	
DRUG	PLAIN (MG/KG)	WITH EPI (MG/KG)
Amides		
Bupivacaine	2.5	3
Dibucaine	1	—
Etidocaine	4	5
Lidocaine	4.5	7
Mepivacaine	4.5	7
Prilocaine	6	9
Ropivacaine	2.5	2.5
Esters		
Chloroprocaine	12	15
Cocaine	3	—
Procaine	7	8
Tetracaine	1.5	2.5

rely on safe practice guidelines to avoid these untoward effects of local anesthetics.

TAKE HOME POINTS

- Know the situations in which total spinal blocks typically occur–in laboring patients, in elderly patients, etc.
- Don't do a block without having pharmacologic intervention to treat both CNS and cardiac toxicity immediately available.
- A patient who suddenly starts whispering is deemed to have a high block until proven otherwise.
- Remember that high blocks and intravascular injections can and do occur in patients under general anesthesia–consider this as a possible etiology if the patient suddenly becomes unstable or fails to emerge as expected.

SUGGESTED READINGS

American Society of Regional Anesthesia and Pain Medicine. Park Ridge, Illinois: American Society of Regional Anesthesia and Pain Medicine; 2006. Available from: http://www.asra.com.

Chadwick HS. An analysis of obstetric anesthesia cases from the American Society of Anesthesiologists closed claims project database. *Int J Obstet Anesth*. 1996;5:258–263.

Chestnut DH, ed. *Obstetric Anesthesia: Principles and Practice*. 3rd ed. Philadelphia: Mosby; 2004.

Guinard JP, Mulroy MF, Carpenter RL. Aging reduces the reliability of epidural epinephrine test doses. *Reg Anesth Pain Med*. 1995;20:193–198.

Kopp SL, Horlocker TT, Warner ME, et al. Cardiac arrest during neuraxial anesthesia: Frequency and predisposing factors associated with survival. *Anesth Analg*. 2005;100:855–865.

Korman B, Riley RH. Convulsions induced by ropivacaine during interscalene brachial plexus block. *Anesth Analg*. 1997;85:1128–1129.

Mulroy MF. Systemic toxicity and cardiotoxicity from local anesthetics: Incidence and preventive measures. *Reg Anesth Pain Med*. 2002;27:556–561.

Mulroy MF, Norris MC, Liu SS. Safety steps for epidural injection of local anesthetics: Review of the literature and recommendations. *Anesth Analg*. 1997;85:1346–1356.

Park PC, Berry PD, Larson MD. Total spinal anesthesia following epidural saline injection after prolonged epidural anesthesia. *Anesthesiology*. 1998;89:1267–1270.

Richardson MG, Lee AC, Wissler RN. High spinal anesthesia after epidural test dose administration in five obstetric patients. *Reg Anesth Pain Med*. 1996;21:119–123.

Ruetsch YA, Fattinger KE, Borgeat A. Ropivacaine-induced convulsions and severe cardiac dysrhythmia after sciatic block. *Anesthesiology*. 1999;90:1784–1786.

110

CONSIDER LIPID EMULSION RESCUE FOR LOCAL ANESTHETIC OVERDOSE

HEATH A. FALLIN, MD AND DAVID A. BURNS, MD

Regional anesthesia—the injection of local anesthetics to block or treat pain—continues to grow in popularity. Regional techniques can provide complete nerve blockade, leading to superior analgesia with relatively few side effects. In rare cases, however, use of regional techniques leads to an overdose of local anesthetic through unintentional intravascular injection of anesthetic or through systemic absorption following local anesthetic infiltration. Systemic overdose is a potentially devastating complication characterized by seizures, cardiovascular collapse, and, possibly, death. Until recently, the standard treatment available to treat local anesthetic overdose was the standard advanced cardiac life support (ACLS) protocol for cardiopulmonary resuscitation (CPR) and, especially in the case of bupivacaine toxicity, these measures were often not enough and cardiopulmonary bypass was necessary. Now, however, new evidence supports using lipid infusion to treat local anesthetic overdose.

BACKGROUND

Local anesthetics produce their effects by blocking sodium channels. The effect is desirable during regional anesthesia when local anesthetics are infiltrated around nerves to provide analgesia and, if desired, motor blockade. If a local anesthetic is absorbed intravenously, however, the same sodium-channel blockade can occur in all tissues, including the brain and the heart, producing similar dose-dependent attenuation of action potentials throughout these structures.

In the central nervous system (CNS), local anesthetics first depress the inhibitory pathways in the amygdala and hypocampus. Symptoms of such depression begin with visual, auditory, or sensory hallucinations (including circumoral numbness, metallic taste, and tinnitus); progress to irritability, lightheadedness, tremors and muscle twitching; and finally culminate in generalized tonic-clonic seizures. As blood levels increase, the excitatory pathways are also suppressed, leading to loss of consciousness, coma, and eventual respiratory arrest. In general, CNS changes are an early indicator of local anesthetic toxicity and are seen before cardiac toxicity develops.

Local anesthetics also cause direct vasodilation and cardiac depression. The cardiac tissue response to local anesthetics is similar to the nerve tissue

© 2006 Mayo Foundation for Medical Education and Research

response: Blockade of sodium channels inhibits the cardiac action potential, leading to myocardial depression. Lidocaine is frequently used to decrease myocardial irritability through this mechanism. More potent anesthetics, such as bupivacaine and etidocaine, however, can actually act as proarrhythmic agents, since these anesthetics bind to sodium channels in a state-dependent fashion, leading to bradycardia and conduction delay through the myocardium, thereby allowing re-entrant arrhythmias, ventricular fibrillation, or asystole. These cardiac complications resist normal resuscitative measures, and multiple deaths from systemic local anesthetic toxicity, especially with bupivacaine, have been reported.

PREVENTION/PREVENTION

So how do we treat local anesthetic overdose? The primary method of treatment is prevention. Use the least potent and least toxic drug available to achieve the desired affect, and alter the dose based on patient age, weight, and comorbidities to prevent systemic toxicity. Bupivacaine is very cardiotoxic, and the dextro enatiomer seems to possess the most potent effects. This is why the levobupivacaine enatiomer was developed as a separate preparation. Bupivicaine, particularly in high doses or high concentrations, should be avoided. Premedication of patients with benzodiazepines, such as midazolam or lorazepam, may facilitate patient cooperation and can raise the seizure threshold and the level of local anesthetic required to cause CNS symptoms. Remember, however, that these symptoms usually occur early with local anesthetic toxicity and benzodiazepine use may mask these early warning signs without raising the cardiac toxicity threshold.

Before administering local anesthetic, ensure adequate intravenous (IV) access is available, standard monitors are in place, and resuscitative drugs and equipment are readily available. Airway equipment must also be readily available in the event of an overdose, as rapid intubation may be required.

Consider using the following techniques while placing a block to prevent overdose. Avoid transvascular approaches, if possible, and use ultrasound imaging, if available, to confirm needle position before injection. Aspirate before injection and frequently during block placement, and remember to allow adequate time for blood to become visible in the hub of the needle or catheter. Inject a small test dose after aspiration, and evaluate the patient for symptoms before giving the full dose to the patient. Fractionation, the splitting of the total dose into smaller aliquots with aspiration between them, helps ensure that the needle or catheter has not migrated into a nearby vessel during the block placement. Finally, monitor the patient throughout the block, and maintain verbal communication, if possible, to ascertain early signs of intravascular injection (tinnitus, metallic taste in mouth, anxiety or faintness).

To prevent systemic absorption, you may mix a vasoconstrictor with the anesthetic to slow systemic absorption. Epinephrine is a popular choice, although other vasoactive medications are also used. Epinephrine has the added advantage of causing a rapid increase in heart rate during test-dose administration if it is absorbed systemically.

TREATMENT

Despite the best techniques, however, systemic injection or toxic absorption of local anesthetics still occurs, perhaps in as many as 20 of every 10,000 peripheral nerve blocks. In the case of overdose, treatment measures are largely supportive and follow established treatment protocols for the symptoms experienced. First and foremost, evaluate the airway: Apply supplemental oxygen, ventilatory support, or intubation, if necessary. Ventilate the seizing patient to limit acidosis and to ensure adequate tissue oxygenation. Treat seizures with thiopental, 50 mg IV, or midazolam, 2 mg IV, and titrate up, as necessary, until seizures cease. Succinylcholine may help relax the seizing patient, but remember that muscle blockade only stops the muscular symptoms of seizures; the CNS will have continued seizure activity along with increased metabolic and oxygen demands.

If cardiovascular symptoms occur, begin CPR and ACLS resuscitation measures immediately. Local anesthetic overdose may lead to refractory cardiovascular symptoms, and prolonged CPR may be necessary—CPR of 1 hour or more may be required until clearance of the anesthetic occurs and the heart can begin to beat again; do not give up too quickly! Use a cardioverter to treat malignant ventricular arrhythmias, as required, and provide pharmacological support as necessary: Atropine for bradycardia; ephedrine for hypotension; and epinephrine, as required, for cardiovascular collapse. Multiple doses of these drugs may be required and are indicated in local anesthetic overdose. If available, consider instituting cardiac bypass to allow the patient time to clear the drug from the circulatory system and regain normal cardiac function.

TWENTY-PERCENT LIPID EMULSION
AS A POTENTIAL TREATMENT

In many cases, however, all of these methods have failed to restore a normal cardiac rhythm, and multiple patients have died secondary to local anesthetic overdose. Recently, a new treatment has emerged, which is showing great promise. Twenty-percent lipid emulsion may provide a "magic bullet" for cardiac collapse secondary to local anesthetic overdose. This milky mix of soybean oil and water (similar to the emulsion in which propofol is mixed) has been in use for many years for total parenteral nutrition (TPN). (Note that propofol is currently supplied in a 10% soybean emulsion, equivalent to 10% lipid emulsion.) Some authors have therefore suggested propofol infusion as a lipid rescue agent. However, using a dose of 3 mL/kg of propofol (equivalent to the lipid content of 1.5 mL/kg of 20% Intralipid), a 70-kg patient would require injection of 100 cc of propofol–a dose of 1 g (1,000 mg) of propofol! Clearly, propofol is not a suitable substitute for 20% lipid emulsion for treatment of local anesthetic overdose and is contraindicated in cardiovascular collapse; see comment in Weinberg (Suggested Reading, item 16). Sold under the trade names Intralipid and Liposyn, the emulsion is used in thousands of patients daily as a lipid nutritional replacement. Its short-term side effects are minimal, and long-term effects, such as pancreatitis and hypertriglyceridemia, would be expected due to the high fat load in the bloodstream. The drug is inexpensive and readily available in most hospital pharmacies (20% Intralipid retails for approximately $20.00 for a 500 mL bag [in bulk] and bags may be stored at room temperature for approximately 2 years according to the product label). While the required dosage for local anesthetic toxicity is not fully established, a currently suggested protocol uses a loading dose of 1.5 mL/kg IV of 20% lipid emulsion followed by infusion of 0.5 mL/kg/min until cardiac recovery. The patient should be closely monitored until all symptoms resolve.

The above dosing protocol has been used successfully in case reports of adult patients and in studies of adult animals. No evidence exists to suggest a safe dosing regimen in special populations such as pediatric or pregnant patients. However, intravenous lipid emulsions are an established treatment for patients in all stages of life and, in general, the daily dose of lipid for TPN is much greater than the lipid bolus described above.

In pediatric patients, daily lipid doses of 1 to 2 g /kg have been used for decades, well in excess of the above-proposed bolus of 1.5 mL/kg of 20% Intralipid (equivalent to 300 mg/kg). Even in low-birthweight neonates, starting dosages of 1 to 1.5 g/kg/d are well tolerated and levels are often titrated to above 2 g/kg/d without side effects.

In pregnant patients, the safety of lipid infusion has recently become slightly less clear. A 2004 retrospective study suggested that pregnant patients with hyperemesis gravidarum undergoing total parenteral nutrition therapy may have much higher rates of complications directly related to TPN therapy. However, this study is limited to a retrospective analysis of a small number of patients at a single hospital. Multiple other studies and decades of clinical experience have demonstrated the safety of total parenteral nutrition in pregnant patients. Parenteral infusions, including lipid dosing of 1 to 2 g/kg/d or more, have been demonstrated as safe for both the mother and the fetus, particularly since soybean emulsions have replaced older cottonseed-oil emulsions. In light of this evidence, and the potentially catastrophic effects of local anesthetic overdose, there appears to be little to contraindicate lipid infusion as a last resort in a pregnant patient, and no adjustment in dosing is suggested by existing data.

POTENTIAL MECHANISM

The action of the lipid infusion is unknown, but at least two mechanisms are proposed. The first theory is that the lipid infusion provides a lipid phase in the plasma that absorbs the lipophilic local anesthetic and sequesters it away from body tissues. Indeed, in a study by Weinberg et al., lipid infusion sped the efflux of bupivacaine from isolated rat hearts, supporting this "lipid sink" hypothesis. Other authors have suggested that a different mechanism may be responsible: Since the heart derives most of its energy from lipids and since bupivacaine interferes with lipid metabolism, some have suggested that a massive lipid load simply overwhelms the bupivacaine interference and provides the heart with ample energy supplies to function. Of course, neither of these hypotheses is exclusionary; both could be correct or perhaps another reason lies behind the success of lipid infusion for local anesthetic overdose.

EVIDENCE

While further investigation into the exact mechanism of action proceeds, the limited evidence so far is that it does work. Besides the study mentioned above, additional studies have shown lipid infusion to be potentially lifesaving in the event of local anesthetic overdose. In a study with dogs, Weinberg et al. once again demonstrated the efficacy of lipid infusion. Twelve dogs were given toxic overdoses of bupivacaine, the local anesthetic notorious for refractory cardiac collapse. In the study, all 12 dogs experienced cardiac collapse. All dogs were aggressively resuscitated; half were given lipid infusions, and half were given saline boluses. Remarkably, all six of the lipid-infused dogs survived, whereas the non-lipid-infused animals all died. These are striking results even in a small study.

Now, too, case reports of lipid infusions reversing local anesthetic overdose in human beings are starting to appear. In July of 2006, Rosenblatt et al. reported the first use of lipid infusion to treat bupivacaine cardiac arrest successfully, and, in August of 2006, Litz et al. reported a similar success after ropivicaine-induced asystole. These case reports are promising and support the use of lipid infusion to reverse cardiovascular symptoms of local anesthetic toxicity.

Of course, the use of lipid infusion is not yet a proven, established method for treating local anesthetic overdose. Until more data becomes available, its use must still be considered experimental. The mainstay of safe local anesthetic use in regional anesthesia remains prevention of overdose, and, in the case of toxicity, to follow established ACLS protocols, as needed to resuscitate patients. However, given the promising track record of lipid infusion and the extremely limited downside of its use in the event of refractory local anesthetic-induced cardiac arrest, its use should be considered early on in the event of an overdose, and a 500-ml bag of 20% lipid emulsion should be readily available in areas in which regional blocks are performed. After all, the drug is relatively harmless, and it just might provide the "magic bullet" required to rescue a patient from a devastating complication.

TAKE HOME POINTS

- Intravascular injection or absorption of local anesthetics can be a catastrophic complication of regional anesthesia.
- Bupivacaine overdose is particularly dangerous because of its cardiac toxicity profile.
- The primary method of treatment of local anesthetic overdose is preventative.
- Supportive measures, including the possibility of cardiopulmonary bypass, are the mainstays of therapy once local anesthetic toxicity occurs.
- 20% lipid emulsion is a promising treatment for local anesthetic toxicity.

SUGGESTED READINGS

Amato P, Quercia RA. A historical perspective and review of the safety of lipid emulsion in pregnancy. *Nutr Clin Pract.* 1991;6(5):189–192.

Barash PG, Cullen BF, Stoelting RK, eds. *Clinical Anesthesia.* 5th ed. Philadelphia: Lippincott Williams & Wilkins; 2006:463–467.

Folk JJ, Leslie-Brown HF, Nosovitch JT, et al. Hyperemesis gravidarum: Outcomes and complications with and without total parenteral nutrition. *J Reprod Med.* 2004;49(7):497–502.

Graf BM. The cardiotoxicity of local anesthetics: The place of ropivacaine. *Curr Top Med Chem.* 2001;1(3):207–214.

Kerner JA Jr, Poole RL. The use of IV fat in neonates. *Nutr Clin Pract.* 2006;21(4):374–380.

Weinberg G. LipidRescue™. 27 November 2006. Copyright © 2006. http://www.lipidrescue.org.

Litz RJ, Popp M, Stehr SN, et al. Successful resuscitation of a patient with ropivacaine-induced asystole after axillary plexus block using lipid infusion. *Anaesthesia.* 2006;61:800–801.

Mulroy MF. Systemic toxicity and cardiotoxicity from local anesthetics: Incidence and preventive measures. *Reg Anesth Pain Med.* 2002;27:556–561.

Rayburn W, Wolk R, Mercer N, et al. Parenteral nutrition in obstetrics and gynecology. *Obstet Gynecol Surv.* 1986;41(4):200–214.

Tasch MD, Butterworth JF. Toxicity of local anesthetics. In: Schwartz AJ, ed. *ASA Refresher Courses in Anesthesiology.* Philadelphia: Lippincott Williams & Wilkins; 2006:167–168.

Rosenblatt MA, Abel M, Fischer GW, et al. Successful use of a 20% lipid emulsion to resuscitate a patient after a presumed bupivacaine-related cardiac arrest. *Anesthesiology.* 2006;105: 217–218.

Russo-Stieglitz KE, Levine AB, Wagner BA, et al. Pregnancy outcome in patients requiring parenteral nutrition. *J Matern Fetal Neonatal Med.* 1999;8(4):164–167.

Spencer SL, Joseph RS. Local anesthetics. In: Barash PG, Cullen BF, Stoelting RK, eds. *Clinical Anesthesia.* 5th ed. Philadelphia: Lippincott Williams & Wilkins; 2006:453–471.

Weinberg G. Lipid infusion resuscitation for local anesthetic toxicity: Proof of clinical efficacy. *Anesthesiology.* 2006;105(1):7–8.

Weinberg G, Ripper R, Feinstein DL, et al. Lipid emulsion infusion rescues dogs from bupivacaine-induced cardiac toxicity. *Reg Anesth Pain Med*. 2003;28(3):198–202.

Weinberg G, VadeBoncouer T, Ramaraju GA, et al. Pretreatment or resuscitation with a lipid infusion shifts the dose–response to bupivacaine-induced asystole in rats. *Anesthesiology*. 1998;88(4):1071–1075.

Widhalm K. Current status of parenteral feeding with fat emulsions. Clinical experience in children. *Infusionsther Klin Ernahr*. 1983;10(4):225–228.

Zibell-Frisk D, Jen KL, Rick J. Use of parenteral nutrition to maintain adequate nutritional status in hyperemesis gravidarum. *J Perinatol*. 1990;10(4):390–395.

111

REMEMBER THAT POSTOPERATIVE PAIN MANAGEMENT SHOULD BE STARTED PREOPERATIVELY

J. TODD HOBELMANN, MD

Postoperative pain is a significant issue in the anesthesia provider's management of patients. A survey mailed to 56 anesthesiologists stated that the principal endpoints they believed to be the most important to patients were postoperative incisional pain, nausea, vomiting, preoperative anxiety, and pain related to intravenous access placement. A key part of the recovery period is appropriate control of both pain during rest and pain with activity (incident pain). With the continued advances in anesthesia practice, anesthesiologists now have a growing armament to combat postoperative pain, including use of neuraxial anesthesia, nerve blocks, and perioperative analgesic medications. We will discuss some of the pharmaceutical interventions at the anesthesiologists' disposal for the time after surgery.

Planning is an integral, and arguably the most important, component of anesthesia management. As anesthesiologists, our job frequently demands preventing an undesirable situation, like a postinduction hypotension, a difficult airway, patient's movement at the time of skin incision, or postoperative nausea and vomiting. Similarly, postoperative pain management starts with pre-emptive analgesia. Pre-emptive analgesia is an antinociceptive therapy aimed at preventing both peripheral and central sensitization, thereby attenuating the postoperative amplification of pain. Regional anesthesia (both neuraxial and peripheral-nerve blockade) and even local infiltration for superficial procedures are excellent examples of pre-emptive analgesia. Preoperative use of certain nonsteroidal anti-inflammatory drugs (NSAIDs) (piroxicam, 20 mg, taken orally 2 hours before the procedure; intravenous ketorolac), antiepileptic drugs (gabapentin, 600 mg, taken orally 2 hours before the procedure) as well as intravenous opioids and receptor antagonists (ketamine) at the time of induction have all been shown to reduce postoperative analgesic requirements. The pre-emptive analgesic plan should be titrated according to the type of surgery and patients' characteristics. Whenever possible, a multimodal approach should be used.

After adequate preventative steps have been taken, the next step is often dealing with postoperative pain. Opioids are the most commonly used medications under these circumstances. Titrations of morphine, fentanyl, dilaudid, etc. are often used as a first-line agent. Ethnicity (white race),

© 2006 Mayo Foundation for Medical Education and Research

emergency surgery, major surgery, surgery lasting more than 100 minutes, and high pain score on arrival to the PACU are factors predictive of increased opioid requirements. Titration to effect is the goal; however, it is important to realize that the presence of pain does not prevent narcotic-induced respiratory depression, the most worrisome side effect of narcotics. Opioids also have other potential adverse effects, such as pruritis, nausea, vomiting, and constipation. The PACU anesthesiologist must always remain vigilant when administering any opioid dose. Patient-controlled analgesia (PCA) allows patients to determine the timing of analgesic doses and allows for improved titration of analgesia while minimizing patient anxiety. When used correctly, pain management may occur with less risk of side effects. Common intravenous (IV) PCA orders used at the Johns Hopkins Hospital are listed in *Table 111.1*.

NSAIDs can be used as part of an effective multimodal analgesia regimen. NSAIDS are beneficial postoperatively, because surgery causes both pain and inflammation. These medications can be divided into three groups: NSAIDs with predominantly analgesic effects (Naproxen, Ketorolac), NSAIDs that are mainly anti-inflammatory (oxicams), and those that confer both benefits (Diclofenac, Ketoprofen, Indomethacin). The one most often used in the PACU is Ketorolac (Toradol). It has been estimated that the use of Toradol in pain management may reduce opioid requirements by up to a third (range of 0% to 79%, depending on the type of surgery) and may improve the patient's pain relief. Nonsteroidal medications have their own set of risk factors, including bleeding from platelet dysfunction, gastrointestinal (GI) upset, and renal impairment. These risks increase with higher dosages, prolonged therapy (more than 3 to 5 days), and, in susceptible patients (i.e., those with a history of GI bleeding or renal insufficiency). The newer class of selective COX-2 inhibitor nonsteroidals (celecoxib, rofecoxib, valdecoxib) was believed to have fewer side effects; however only celecoxib is still on the

TABLE 111.1	OPIOID NAÏVE PATIENTS		
DRUG NAME	DEMAND DOSE	LOCKOUT	LOADING DOSE
Hydromorphone	0.1–0.3 mg	5–10 min	0.4 mg prn
Fentanyl	5–20 mcg	5–8 min	25 mcg prn
Morphine	0.6–2 mg	5–10 min	2–5 mg prn

Demand dose, the dose administered whenever the patient presses the dosing button; lockout, the timeframe in which no medication will be injected, regardless of how many time the patient presses the button; loading dose, the initial bolus given before beginning the PCA. Advanced pain specialists may also use a continuous infusion that runs at a set rate (low dose) throughout. With permission from Jeffrey Richman, MD.

TABLE 111.2	OPIOID CONVERSION CHART			
DRUG NAME	**IV DOSE (MG)**	**PO DOSE (MG)**	**DURATION (HRS) IV**	**DURATION (HRS) PO**
Morphine	10	30	4–5	4–7
Hydromorphone	1.5	7.5	4–5	4–6
Methadone	10	20	4–5	4–8
Meperidine	75	300	3–5	4–6
Fentanyl	0.1	–	1–2	–
Codeine	130	200	4–6	4–6
Hydrocodone	–	30	–	4–5
Oxycodone	–	20	–	4–5
Propoxyphene	–	65	–	4–6
Nalbuphine	10	–	4–6	–
Butorphanol	2	–	4–6	–

With permission from Jeffrey Richman, MD.

market as the other two have been show to cause cardiac events in susceptible patients.

After discharge, patients may take pain medications for various reasons. In addition, hospital pharmacies may stock certain medications, and not others, limiting physicians' choice of drugs. Understanding how opioids are converted thus is important in the perioperative setting, in the postoperative setting, and upon patient discharge from the hospital. The opioid conversion chart is outlined in *Table 111.2*. The steps for opioid conversion are discussed in another chapter of this book.

In addition, those patients who are seen on an outpatient basis may take drugs included in other families of pain medications, which must be considered in the perioperative setting. Whether the patient has Complex Regional Pain Syndrome (CRPS), low-back pain, or postherpetic neuralgia, many other classes of pharmaceuticals may be seen. The groups most likely to be encountered (besides narcotics and NSAIDs) include the tricyclic antidepressants (TCAs: Amitriptyline, nortripyline, desipramine); anticonvulsants and membrane stabilizers (gabapentin, pregabalin); and NMDA receptor antagonists (dextromethorphan). TCAs are used in "subclinical" doses to improve overall pain control. The older forms of the drugs, like amytriptyline, carry significant side effects, ranging from anicholinergic phenomenon (dry mouth, sedation) to orthostatic hypotension. The anticonvulsants also have untoward side effects of sedation and potential liver damage (it is essential for the primary provider to follow liver function tests on patients using this class of medication). They are believed to relieve pain by decreasing the overall electrical activity in the brain. The NMDA receptor antagonists are believed to exert their effects by decreasing the sensitization of the central nervous system to pain. The main side effect of this class of drugs is sedation.

TAKE HOME POINTS

- Postoperative pain control plays a vital role in patient satisfaction.
- Postoperative pain management is an integral part of anesthetic management and should be started pre-emptively. Whenever feasible, a multimodal approach should be chosen.
- Some of the patients are already taking pain medications preoperatively, and such medications should be taken into account when planning postoperative pain management. Administration of such medications should not be discontinued before surgery, unless side effects are unmasked during the interview or laboratory values demonstrate areas of concern.
- As our understanding of the pain pathways emerges, our tools for treating pain perioperatively will grow, and patient satisfaction may increase as well.

SUGGESTED READINGS

American Pain Society. *Principles of Analgesic Use in the Treatment of Acute Pain and Cancer Pain.* 5th ed. Glenview, Illinois: American Pain Society; 2003.

Kelly DJ, Ahmad M, Brull SJ. Preemptive analgesia II: Recent advances and current trends. *Can J Anaesth.* 2001;48(11):1091–1101.

Rowlingson JC. Postoperative pain: To diversify is to satisfy. *Anesth Analg.* 2005;101(5 Suppl): S1–4.

112

SEEK OUT HYPERCAPNEA IN THE PACU AND REMEMBER THAT AN ACCEPTABLE PULSE OXIMETER READING IS *NOT* ASSURANCE OF ADEQUATE VENTILATION

MICHAEL P. HUTCHENS, MD, MA

"Global warming is not the only downside of elevated CO_2 concentration"

Respiratory complications are common events in the postanesthesia care unit (PACU) – as many as 7% of patients require upper-airway support of some kind during their PACU course. Although pulse oximetry provides excellent monitoring of arterial oxygen saturation, it is an anesthesia truism that reduced arterial oxygen saturation due to hypoventilation in patients receiving supplemental oxygen is a late finding. The physiologic manifestations of hypercapnea are truly protean, and although central nervous system effects are noticeable in patients who are awake, these findings, and others, may be masked by the shifting perioperative milieu. Hypercapnea both results from and causes respiratory arrest and is usually easily reversible in the PACU patient if caught in time.

Carbon dioxide (CO_2) is an odorless, colorless, heavier-than-air gas, which, apart from oxygen and water, may be the most ubiquitous drug in medicine. Anesthesiologists routinely manipulate the CO_2 content of blood to achieve physiologic goals. It is endogenously produced as a byproduct of energy production by degradation of carbohydrates in the Krebs cycle. Although physiologic investigation of the effects of CO_2 began during the Enlightenment, its toxic effects were known in antiquity from the occasional (sometimes intentional) lethal encounter between living beings and caves with elevated CO_2 concentration. Indeed, CO_2 is itself a general anesthetic; it is currently used for laboratory animal euthanasia and sedation of livestock before slaughter. Experimentation in the 1960s using monkeys and cats breathing a 50:50 mix of CO_2 and oxygen demonstrated electroencephalogram (EEG) slowing to isoelectricity after initial activation. Unlike the mechanism of conventional inhalational anesthetics, the mechanism of CO_2 anesthesia is thought to be an effect of locally induced brain acidosis. In an elegant paper published in 1967, Eisele et al. measured the $PaCO_2$ at which response to surgical stimulus was abolished in 50% of experimental dogs as 222 mmHg; this is, in essence, the MAC in dogs of CO_2. Thirty-percent CO_2, in oxygen administered by mask to human beings, produces

© 2006 Mayo Foundation for Medical Education and Research

anesthesia, but produces a foul acidic taste in the mouth and feelings of anxiety and dyspnea. As $PaCO_2$ rises above 90 mmHg, human beings exhibit stupor and, ultimately, loss of consciousness.

CO_2, whether exogenously or endogenously sourced, has significant physiologic effects apart from those on consciousness. Hypercapnea increases cerebral blood flow and, thus, intracranial pressure. CO_2 is a pulmonary vasoconstrictor, however, and causes a predictable increase in pulmonary-artery pressures at elevated levels. Because of the Bohr effect, hypercapnea decreases hemoglobin affinity for oxygen. An increased CO_2 level also causes systemic hypertension, both from increased cardiac output and arteriolar vasoconstriction. An elevated $PaCO_2$ is proarrythmic, particularly in the presence of halothane. Hyperkalemia can result from release of cellular potassium stores, and at a very high $PaCO_2$, glomerular filtration rate is reduced by afferent arteriolar vasoconstriction. Interestingly, a brief review of the literature reveals multiple cases of $PaCO_2$ levels of more than 200; these patients (mostly children) were stuporous or comatose but, in the absence of hypoxemia, recovered without permanent deficit.

In the immediate perioperative period, it is not unusual to encounter a stuporous (or anxious) patient with abnormal vital signs. While these aberrations are most commonly caused by residual anesthetic, pain, or medication, they can all be caused by hypercapnea as well. Since extubated patients in the PACU do not usually have their end-tidal CO_2 displayed on the monitor, it is up to the clinician to suspect and diagnose hypercapnea from clinical data. Patients in the PACU have two excellent reasons to become hypercapneic. They almost universally receive medications that depress their respiratory drive, and they therefore frequently hypoventilate. Secondly, as patients emerge from anesthesia, their basal metabolic rate increases, and, as a result, they may have increased production of CO_2, thus increasing the relative impact of hypoventilation. Shivering increases this effect, as do agitation and fever. Malignant hyperthermia causes a sustained increase in CO_2 production, but other systemic signs are usually present.

While reduced respiratory rate is one mechanism for hypoventilation, patients who are splinting may hypoventilate while breathing rapidly and taking small breaths. Patients with obstructive sleep apnea or postanesthetic airway obstruction may have a normal respiratory rate but only transport gas during a short part of the respiratory cycle, thus reducing their alveolar ventilation. Regardless of the etiology, the clinician must have a high index of suspicion for hypercapnea in the postoperative patient. Since it often results in end-organ dysfunction, it must be treated quickly. Patients who have decreased respiratory drive from opioid administration should receive naloxone, 40 mcg every 1 to 2 minutes, intravenously, until their respiratory rate and level of consciousness increase. Patients who are apneic from opioids, or imminently apneic, should of course receive bag-mask ventilation, and the clinician should consider administering a larger dose of naloxone intravenously (the maximum single dose is 400 mcg). Patients with obstructive sleep apnea may benefit from the application of noninvasive ventilation. Patients with splinting can be the most challenging; their hypercapnea paradoxically improves with opioid administration. The clinician must be confident of this etiology before treating it, and, ultimately, these patients may benefit most from regional analgesia. As always, endotracheal intubation and mechanical ventilation are the definitive treatments and should be considered early, while they are still optional, rather than late, when control of the airway becomes emergent.

CO_2 is a powerful drug that affects the physiology and care of the postoperative patient. Regardless of the etiology, the clinician must have a high index of suspicion for hypercapnea. Since it often results in end-organ dysfunction, it must be diagnosed and treated quickly to prevent such dramatic physiologic consequences as intracranial hypertension, confusion, stupor, coma, respiratory arrest, and death.

TAKE HOME POINTS

- Respiratory events in the PACU are common.
- Patients in the PACU are at high risk of hypercapnea.
- The onset of hypercapnea may be masked by other perioperative conditions.
- CO_2 is a general anesthetic and loss of consciousness occurs above a $PaCO_2$ level of about 90.
- CO_2 is a powerful drug that affects intracranial pressure, hemodynamics, oxygen transport, renal function, and other physiologic parameters.

SUGGESTED READINGS

Eisele JH, Eger EI 2nd, Muallem M. Narcotic properties of carbon dioxide in the dog. *Anesthesiology.* 1967;28(5):856–865.

Fu ES, Downs JB, Schweiger JW, et al. Supplemental oxygen impairs detection of hypoventilation by pulse goniometry. *Chest.* 2004;126(5):1552–1558.

Goldstein B, Shannon DC, Todres ID. Supercarbia in children: clinical course and outcome. *Crit Care Med.* 1990;18(2):166–168.

Hines R, Barash PG, Watrous G, et al. Complications occurring in the postanesthesia care unit: a survey. *Anesth Analg.* 1992;74(4):503–509.

Leake CB, Waters RM. The anesthetic properties of carbon dioxide. *J Pharmacol Exp Ther.* 1928;3:280–281.

Meyer JS, Gotoh F, Tazaki Y. CO_2 narcosis. An experimental study. *Neurology.* 1961;11: 524–537.

113

CONSIDER ACUPUNCTURE AS AN ADJUNCT FOR THE PROPHYLAXIS AND TREATMENT OF POSTOPERATIVE NAUSEA AND VOMITING

LEENA MATHEW, MD

Unfortunately, postoperative nausea and vomiting (PONV) is still a common side effect of anesthesia despite the availability of newer-generation antiemetics and shorter-acting anesthetics and opioids. PONV is one of the two most significant factors leading to patient dissatisfaction (the other, of course, being pain). The incidence of PONV is approximately 70% in those patients who are at high risk for this complication and 30% in the general population. Even though postoperative vomiting is self-limited, it can cause significant morbidity, including dehydration, wound dehiscence, aspiration, and electrolyte imbalance. PONV also increases costs since each episode of emesis in the postanesthesia care unit (PACU) delays discharge by an average of 20 minutes.

The following factors place a patient at high risk for PONV:

1) Patient-related factors: Female, nonsmoking, dehydrated, and with prior episodes of PONV.

2) Procedure-related factors: Ear, nose, or throat surgery, intra-abdominal surgery, laparoscopic surgery, strabismus repair, and obstetric or gynecologic surgery. A 30-minute increase in the duration of surgery increases the baseline risk for PONV by 60%. Any surgical procedure needing large fluid administration can cause gastrointestinal edema, which can also increase the incidence of PONV.

3) *Anesthesia-related factors*: The use of volatile agents, nitrous oxide, neostigmine (more than 2.5 mg) and long-acting opioids.

At present, the most common modalities for the prophylaxis and treatment of PONV include ensuring adequate, but not excessive, hydration; avoidance of risk factors; and the use of pharmacologic agents, such as metoclopromide, dexamethasone, and 5 HT 3 antagonists. Acupuncture is an additional approach that shows great promise in prophylaxis and treatment of PONV. In 1997, a National Institutes of Health Consensus Development Panel on acupuncture reviewed the available evidence from randomized controlled trials and concluded that clear evidence indicates that needle acupuncture is efficacious for postoperative and chemotherapy-related nausea and vomiting and probably also for pregnancy-related nausea.

© 2006 Mayo Foundation for Medical Education and Research

Americans are now spending approximately $27 billion annually on complementary and alternative medical treatments. Statistical reports published as early as 1997 suggest that visits to complementary practitioners outnumber those to conventional practitioners by 12 to 1. Acupuncture is only one of many complementary and alternative modalities, but it is one that is already somewhat familiar to patients. A great degree of integration exists between "standard" medical techniques and acupuncture in the East, especially in China, and there is now a growing recognition of the need for such integration in the Western health system.

To review briefly, acupuncture is accomplished by stimulating acupoints. There are 14 major meridians corresponding to internal organs, along which there are a total of 365 acupoints. Acupuncture involves the placement of fine, disposable, stainless-steel needles (*Fig. 113.1*) at select acupuncture points. Acupuncture needles range from 1/4 inch to several inches in length and a few thousandths to several thousandths of an inch in diameter. One inch and 1.5 inch are the most commonly used lengths of needle. The vast majority of needles used in the United States are of stainless steel; however, copper, gold, and silver also are used. The placement of needles is followed by a stimulation technique done to the needle to elicit a characteristic sensation called *De Qi*. Stimulation is usually done by manual twirling or electrical stimulation but can also be done by laser or by moxibustion. Moxibustion involves the burning of fine herbs to apply gentle heat at the free end of the

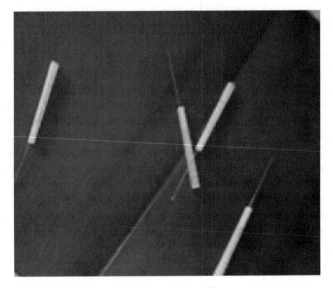

FIGURE 113.1. Stainless-steel acupuncture needles.

needle. The choice of specific needle stimulation technique depends upon the therapist's experience, preference, and patients' concerns and condition.

Manual acupuncture involves manipulating the inserted needles by lifting, thrusting, twisting, twirling, or doing other complex combinations. It is a traditional method of acupuncture and is most commonly used in clinical practice.

Electroacupuncture (EA) is achieved by attaching the acupuncture needles to an electrical-pulse generator and stimulating the acupoints with electrical pulses. EA appears to be more consistent and to generate more reproducible results, and it is more efficacious than manual acupuncture. The procedure for EA is to insert the acupuncture needle as would normally be done, attain the *De Qi* reaction by hand manipulation, and then attach an electrode to the needle to provide continued stimulation. The benefits of using electrical stimulation are absence of prolonged hand maneuvering, reduction of total treatment time by providing continued stimulus, and better control of the frequency of the stimulus. It can also produce a stronger stimulation, without causing the tissue damage associated with twirling and lifting the needle.

Transcutaneous electrical acustimulation (TEAS) or transcutaneous electrical nerve stimulation (TENS) refers to electrical stimulation performed via skin-surface electrodes placed on the acupoints or nerve dermatomes. TEAS and TENS are very similar because acupoints are very likely distributed along the nerve dermatomes.

The mechanism of action of acupuncture is still unknown. It is hypothesized that, with low-frequency stimulation at certain acupoints, there is activation of A-ß and A-alpha fibers, which may influence neurotransmission in the dorsal horn or higher centers. Increased concentrations of ß-endorphins have been reported in human cerebrospinal fluid after acupuncture in patients with chronic pain. Different frequencies of stimulation have been shown to be associated with the release of specific opioids. Stimulation at a level of 2 Hz releases enkephalin and ß-endorphin, whereas stimulation at a level of 100 Hz releases dynorphin. Acupuncture also decreases gastric-acid secretion and promotes forward peristalsis. It is well understood that the analgesic effect of acupuncture can be reversed completely by administration of naloxone.

Many studies indicate that acupuncture at the P6 acupuncture point is effective in ameliorating postoperative nausea and also nausea and vomiting associated with chemotherapy and pregnancy. Acupressure at P6 has also been shown to be antiemetic, and there is fairly extensive literature on the use of P6 acupressure for treating pregnancy-related nausea and vomiting. This point is specifically designated in traditional Chinese medicine for the treatment of vomiting.

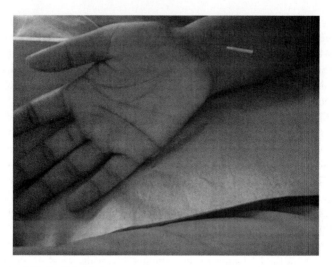

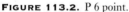

FIGURE 113.2. P 6 point.

The Neiguan or P6 acupoint is located along the pericardial meridian on the volar aspect of the forearm, 2 Cun proximal to the distal wrist crease and approximately 1 to 1.5 cm below the surface of the skin. It lies in between the tendons of the flexor carpi radialis and palmaris longus (*Fig. 113.2*). A Cun is a unit of traditional Chinese medicine measurement–1 Cun is equal to the middle finger's middle interphalangeal distance and 2 Cun is equal to three times the diameter of the patient's little finger.

Prophylaxis of PONV by acupuncture is more efficacious than treatment of PONV by acupuncture and involves the placement of bilateral P6 needles. These needles are inserted in a sterile fashion immediately after induction of anesthesia and are kept in place for 15 to 30 minutes. If patient positioning or operation timing precludes this, the acupuncture may be done in the postoperative recovery unit after surgery. The needles can then be manually or electrically stimulated.

Acupressure may also be applied by the application of "sea bands," which do not have the same degree of efficacy as acupuncture; however, placement is easily done and does not require professional training. Other techniques of stimulation include TEAS38 and even laser stimulation, although these are not yet well-described techniques.

Studies done of pediatric patients having tonsillectomy have shown that acupuncture is unsuccessful in preventing or treating postoperative nausea and vomiting. However, in these studies, only a unilateral P6 point was used without uniformity in the exact location of P6 as 2 Cun above the wrist. In adult patients, Dundee performed a series of well-designed studies, including prospective, randomized, sham-controlled trials. These studies provided reliable evidence on the efficacy of acupuncture in treating postoperative nausea and vomiting by TEAS at PC6 as an adjuvant to antiemetic use in more than 100 patients in whom chemotherapy-induced sickness was not adequately controlled by antiemetic use alone. In a randomized, controlled trial with concealed allocation, sham control, and careful blinding, EA was found to control emesis effectively in 104 patients with breast cancer receiving chemotherapy. In a recent single-blinded study involving 593 women with early pregnancy, nausea was significantly reduced with acupuncture at P6 alone. No side effects have been reported to date, other than local soreness at the site of needle placement.

The mechanism of acupressure or acupuncture at P6 to prevent PONV is not clearly understood. Because the P6 point is located near the median nerve, stimulation of this point has been postulated to release neurotransmitters that desensitize the chemo trigger receptor zone (CTZ) and thus prevent nausea and vomiting. However, once the CTZ is sensitized, it is difficult to desensitize it. Accordingly, for prophylaxis of PONV, it may be better for acupuncture to be done after induction but before emergence.

TAKE HOME POINTS

- Acupuncture is an excellent adjunct with minimal side effects in the treatment and prophylaxis of postoperative nausea and vomiting. It is more effective in the prophylaxis than in the treatment of PONV.
- The P6 point is stimulated bilaterally by acupressure or acupuncture with manual or electrical stimulation.
- Placement of the needles can be done after induction or in the PACU.
- The mechanism of action of acupressure or acupuncture at P6 is not completely understood.
- Some providers have had good results with "sea bands," which can be applied by the nursing staff.

SUGGESTED READINGS

Al-Sadi M, Newman B, Julious A. Acupuncture in the prevention of postoperative nausea and vomiting. *Anaesthesia*. 1997;52:658–661.

Anonymous. NIH consensus development panel on Acupuncture. *JAMA*. 1998;280:1518–1524.

Carlsson CP, Axemo P, Bodin A, et al. Manual acupuncture reduces hyperemesis gravidarum: A placebo-controlled, randomized, single-blind, crossover study. *J Pain Symptom Manage*. 2000;20:273–279.

Carroll NV, Miederhoff PA, Cox FM, et al. Costs incurred by outpatient surgical centers in managing postoperative nausea and vomiting. *J Clin Anesth*. 1994;6:364–369.

Clement-Jones V, McLoughlin L, Tomlin S, et al. Increased beta-endorphin but not metenkephalin levels in human cerebrospinal fluid after acupuncture stimulation for recurrent pain. *Lancet*. 1980;2:946–948.

Flake ZA, Scalley RD, Bailey AG. Practical selection of antiemetics. *Am Fam Physician.* 2004;69:1169–1174.

Gan T. Postoperative nausea and vomiting: Can it be eliminated? *JAMA.* 2002;287(10): 1233–1236.

Han JS. Acupuncture and endorphins. *Neurosci Lett.* 2004;361:258–261.

Ho RT, Jawan B, Fung ST, et al. Electro-acupuncture and postoperative emesis. *Anaesthesia.* 1990;45:327–329.

Jewell D, Young G. Interventions for nausea and vomiting in early pregnancy. *Cochrane Database Syst Rev.* 2003;4:CD000145.

Lewis IH, Pryn SJ, Reynolds PI, et al. Effect of P6 acupressure on postoperative vomiting in children undergoing outpatient strabismus correction. *Br J Anaesth.* 1991;67:73–78.

Ouyang H, Chen JDZ. Therapeutic roles of acupuncture in functional gastrointestinal disorders. *Aliment Pharmacol Ther.* 2004;20:831–841.

Roscoe JA, Matteson SE. *Am J Obstet Gynecol.* 2002;186:S244.

Shenkman Z, Holzman RS, Kim C, et al. Acupressure—acupuncture antiemetic prophylaxis in children undergoing tonsillectomy. *Anesthesiology.* 1999;90:1311–1316.

Yentis SM, Bissonnette B. P6 acupuncture and postoperative vomiting after tonsillectomy in children. *Br J Anaesth.* 1991;67:779–780.

114

NEVER DELAY IN RESPONDING TO A CALL FROM THE PACU ABOUT AN EYE COMPLAINT

ANAGH VORA, MD

INCIDENCE AND ETIOLOGY

Eye complications during the perioperative period are actually quite common. In one study, the incidence was 44% after general anesthesia when appropriate protective measures for the eye were not taken. Although ophthalmic complications after anesthesia are often less dramatic than the airway and cardiopulmonary issues that receive so much focus, the importance of promptly recognizing and appropriately managing ophthalmic complications in the perioperative period cannot be overestimated.

Remember that the American Society of Anesthesiologists (ASA) Closed Claim Study demonstrates that there is a significant cost to ignoring or trivializing the patients' risk of perioperative eye injuries. *Of the total claims against anesthesia providers for ocular injuries, an astonishing 81% of cases did not meet the standard of care and could have been prevented.*

Common anesthesia-related eye injuries include corneal abrasions, exposure keratitis, chemical keratitis, movement during ophthalmic surgery, or improper positioning with direct pressure on the eyes. Other less common, but much more serious, ocular complications include postoperative visual loss (POVL) from ischemic optic neuropathy or central retinal artery occlusion.

The underlying etiology of perioperative eye injuries, as with most complications in medicine, is often multifactorial. General anesthesia causes changes in ocular physiology that predispose the eye to injury. These changes include a decrease in both tear production and tear-film stability, suppression of the Bell's phenomenon (normal upward gaze upon closure of the eyelids), inactivation of the blink reflex, and an increase in lagophthalmos (incomplete closure of the eyes). The suppression of these reflexes abolishes the innate protective mechanism of the eye that guards against direct trauma and corneal desiccation and can lead to an increased incidence of corneal abrasions and exposure keratitis.

CORNEAL ABRASIONS AND KERATITIS

Corneal Abrasions. Corneal abrasions result from disruption of the corneal epithelium, usually as the result of direct trauma to the cornea. Common

© 2006 Mayo Foundation for Medical Education and Research

scenarios include direct injury from stethoscopes, identification badges, and watches during intubation; improper face-mask positioning or surgical draping; and even the patient himself rubbing his eyes.

Exposure Keratitis. Exposure keratitis (EK) is inflammation of the cornea from exposure and drying of the corneal epithelial surface. The most common cause of EK during anesthesia is lagophthalmos or incomplete closure of the eyelids for prolonged periods. Partial exposure of the eye, coupled with decreased tear-film production and stability, leads to breakdown of the corneal epithelium. Sequelae of EK include epithelial defects, corneal infiltrates, ulceration, perforation, and even endopthalmitis.

Chemical Keratitis. Chemical keratitis is serious eye condition, resulting from exposure of the eye socket and globe to potentially toxic substances, such as surgical preparatory solutions. A commonly used agent for surgical scrubs is Hibiclens, a preparation of 4% chlorhexidine antiseptic solution and detergent. Remember that in *very dilute* concentrations (0.005%), chlorhexidine is a valuable ophthalmologic agent and has been used as a preservative for soft and gas-permeable contact-lens solutions. Also, concentrations of 0.02% can be used with propamide to treat *Acanthamoeba* keratitis. However, the 4% solution should be considered toxic to the eye. Injuries usually involve epithelial defects associated with epithelial-cell death and desquamation, which is potentiated by the presence of the detergent. Other described injuries include conjunctival hyperemia, chemosis, hypotony, anterior-chamber flare, and corneal edema. Rarely, exposure to large amounts of chlorhexidine has necessitated corneal transplant.

SIGNS AND SYMPTOMS

Symptoms

- Foreign-body sensation (usually described as a gritty sensation);
- Pain, burning, itching;
- Decreased vision; and
- Photophobia.

Signs

- Dye uptake of the cornea on fluroscein staining;
- Specific pattern of staining related to etiology;
- Circumcorneal injection (limbal reaction); and
- Severe cases may manifest as corneal epithelial defects or ulcerations.

Management

- Prompt recognition of corneal abrasion and keratitis;
- For mild symptoms, administration of preservative-free drops during the day and ointment at night;
- Reassurance that condition is temporary and should resolve in 2 to 3 days; and

- For moderate to severe symptoms, early ophthalmic consultation (possible treatments by the ophthalmologist include addition of antibiotics to lubricating regimen, temporary tarsorrhaphy, and definitive surgical therapy).

Prevention

- Patients' eyes should be taped shut upon loss of consciousness, except in cases in which securing the airway should take precedence (e.g., patients with obstructive sleep apnea, morbidly obese patients with rapid desaturation, and patients requiring rapid-sequence intubation);
- Prevent direct pressure on the eyes in patients having surgery in the prone position (consider using molded eye shields if they are available at your hospital);
- Maintain neutral position of the head as a head in the lateral position increases intraocular pressure in the dependent eye and increases the likelihood of corneal edema and epithelial breakdown; and
- Anticipate possible eye injuries during administration of anesthesia and remain vigilant in the PACU for signs and symptoms of postoperative ocular complications.

CASE SCENARIOS

Scenario 1. Your parents are in town, and your spouse has just paged you to tell you that they will meet you at the restaurant. You are happily changing out of scrubs when you are paged by the postanesthesia care unit (PACU). The nurse tells you that your last patient of the day had been dozing but is now awake and complaining of right-eye pain and foreign-body sensation. She is a 27-year-old woman who had repair of a compound fracture of the left tibia and fibula. She has minimal pain in her leg after the excellent epidural you placed earlier. You ask the nurse how bad the eye pain is, and she says, "The patient's crying pretty hard and the light hurts her eyes."

Do:

- See the patient yourself as soon as possible–your mom and dad will have to wait! Understand that this is actually a fairly common clinical scenario, one that you will encounter intermittently in your practice. The patient is not experiencing incisional or surgical pain because of the epidural; therefore, she may have a heightened perception of the eye pain. Remember also that people in general are usually very careful and anxious about their eyes and eyesight and the fear of being blinded is a universal one—it is not unheard of for a patient to describe for you an eye injury that caused them great distress that they suffered years ago.
- Review the basic history of the patient, including the ophthalmologic history, and try to establish the temporal associations of the eye symptoms as well as descriptive characteristics and alleviating and exacerbating stimuli.

- Try assessing visual acuity (counting fingers, reading name badge, etc.). You do not need a Snellen card (the little pocket card with the black letters), unless a medical student happens to have one handy.
- Reassure the patient that, most likely, this is a benign process (probably a corneal abrasion), but you will consult ophthalmology to make sure. Inform the patient that the ophthalmology consultant is likely to repeat the exam you just did as well as to do some additional testing after adding some drops to the eye.

Don't:

- Never avoid the complaint or wait for the patient to leave the PACU.
- Don't tell the PACU nurses that a significant percent of corneal abrasions happen after the patient has left the operating room and that, therefore, this is not a true anesthetic complication. This *is* a perioperative complication, and, as the anesthesia provider, you are responsible for medical care in the PACU.
- Don't call an ophthalmology consultant before seeing the patient yourself. The ophthalmology consultant will rightfully expect you to give a brief synopsis of the current situation.

Scenario 2. You are on call, and, at about midnight, you receive a page from the intensive care unit (ICU), asking you to see the patient whose anesthesia you provided earlier that day. The patient is a 70-year-old man with a history of diabetes and hypertension who had lumbar-spine fusion and instrumentation and who is now complaining of decreased vision in his right eye. During the procedure (which lasted about 8 hours), the patient had a significant blood loss of 3200 mL and, despite transfusion during the procedure, had an initial hematocrit in the ICU of 27%. The patient was not placed in Mayfield pins; instead, the patient's head was placed in a foam headrest. In your anesthesia record, you were careful to make sure that you wrote "the face was padded without direct pressure on the eyes" (which it was). After completion of the surgery, the anesthesia team agreed that there was significant facial edema, and the patient was left intubated. After a short course of postoperative ventilation, the patient was extubated. He had no initial complaints, until the patient's daughter mentioned that the patient told her he could not see her standing by the side of the bed.

Do:

- Recognize that this is potentially a much more serious situation than a corneal abrasion.
- See this patient immediately. Document your assessment as above.
- Call the surgeons immediately to discuss the risks inherent in cases in doing a lengthy procedure on a patient in the prone position, with significant blood loss, and with a decreased mean arterial pressure (MAP) from

baseline. Recommend that the surgeons obtain an ophthalmology consultation immediately. Document your conversation.

- Openly express your concern about postoperative visual loss (POVL) with the patient and family.
- Reassure the patient that you will get all the "specialists" involved in conjunction with the surgeons.
- Explain to the patient that POVL is very unusual, with the highest complication rate reported in the literature of just 0.2% of all spinal cases.
- Review your anesthetic record for periods of hypotension, documented eye exams, and transfusions. Give your legal department an early notice of incidents and possible medical and legal issues.
- Register the case with the POVL registry (www.asa.closedclaims.org).

Don't:

- Do not accept responsibility for negligence of care.
- Do not change any anesthetic or other patient record ever.

In the future:

- Always discuss possible catastrophic complications in high-risk surgeries.
- Discuss possible eye-related complications with surgeons intraoperatively when doing a procedure on a patient in the prone position if the patient has a decreased MAP or a decreased hematocrit. Suggest that the surgeon stage the procedure and come back a second time. Document your suggestion.
- Discuss POVL complications with the surgeons prior to speaking with the patient.

TAKE HOME POINTS

- Understand the resources available in your practice location with respect to managing perioperative eye injuries. In private practices or smaller hospitals, there may not always be an ophthalmologist immediately available to see the patient in the PACU. In that case, it is usually both reasonable and feasible to apply saline eye drops and patch the eye while awaiting the consultant's input.
- Mention possible eye-related complications in your preanesthetic evaluation, especially when a procedure is to be done on a patient in the prone position or coronary bypass is to be done.
- Tape the patient's eyes shut as early in the procedure as the patient's medical condition allows.
- *Watch your watch*; better still, don't wear a watch (the anesthesia machine states the time).
- Be cognizant of your personal paraphernalia (e.g., stethoscopes, identification badges, pens, etc.).

- Tape the patient's eyes *completely* shut; incomplete closure leads to dehydration of the cornea.
- Consider not placing the syringe on the endotracheal tube (ETT) while intubating; the syringe might be scratching the cornea while you are looking for the vocal cords.
- Place the pulse oximeter on the ring finger instead of the index finger, as patients invariably rub their eyes with the index and middle finger.
- Avoid putting direct pressure on the globe.
- Avoid lubricating ointments like "Lacrilube" that have been sitting in your anesthesia machine for several years–they're great vectors for adenovirus.
- Watch the surgeons carefully; if you suspect that Hibiclens has been administered inadvertently to the patient's eyes, irrigate them immediately with a sterile wash and contact an ophthalmology consultant.
- Check the position of the patient's head and eyes after the patient is placed in the prone position; don't forget to check again after you move the patient into an airplane position.
- Specifically *ask* the patient about ocular symptoms after anesthesia.
- *Never* discount patients' complaints about foreign-body sensations or altered vision.
- When in doubt, seek ophthalmic consultation early.

SUGGESTED READINGS

Batra YK, Bali IM. Corneal Abrasions during general anesthesia. *Anesth Analg.* 1977:56(3): 363–365.

Cha SM. Do not use chlorhexidine to prep the face. In: Marcucci L, Moritz M, Chen H, eds. *Avoiding Common Surgical Errors.* Philadelphia: Lippincott Williams & Wilkins; 2006: 107–108.

Gild WM, Posner KL, Caplan RA, et al. Eye injuries associated with anesthesia. *Anesthesiology.* 1992;76:204–208.

Web Page Resource www.asaclosedclaims.org.

White E, Crosse MM. The aetiology and prevention of peri-operative corneal abrasions. *Anaesthesia.* 1998;53:157–161.

115

BE AWARE OF THE ISSUES AND CRITERIA PERTAINING TO DISCHARGE OF THE POSTSPINAL PATIENT

ERIK A. COOPER, DO AND LI MENG, MD, MPH

It is your first day on rotation in the operating room suite that covers orthopedics, urology, and gynecology cases. At 4 PM, you are paged by the agency nurse who is working in the Post-Anesthesia Care Unit (PACU) that day. She tells you that she collected 400 cc of urine about 2 hours ago via straight catheter from Mr. Johnson (who had a diagnostic knee scope in the middle of the day), but that he still has not been able "to go on his own." He is getting "antsy" and his family would like to get back to the Eastern Shore before dark. She requests that you come over to sign out the patient. What do you do?

Because regional anesthesia has grown in popularity and allows surgical facilities to discharge patients quickly, more surgical procedures are being performed using peripheral nerve blocks as well as epidural or spinal anesthesia. Spinal anesthesia is less technically difficult and has a faster onset time than epidural techniques; however, a surprising number of complications exist with spinal anesthetics. As these procedures increase in number, the astute clinician must be able to manage complications that arise and be aware of the specific PACU discharge criteria related to spinal anesthesia.

COMPLICATIONS

In general, light sedation is often administered with spinal anesthetics, and such administration decreases the incidence of postoperative respiratory complications as compared to the use of general anesthetics. In one study, nearly two thirds of complications related to general anesthetic use involved postoperative respiratory events. Conversely, the most common complications associated with spinal anesthetics are postdural puncture headache (PDPH) and backache.

POSTDURAL PUNCTURE HEADACHES

PDPH is the most common complication in patients receiving spinal anesthesia, with incidences as high as 25% reported in some studies. Small-bore, 25-gauge, pencil-point needles decrease the incidence of PDPH. The greatest incidence of PDPH occurs when large-bore epidural needles accidentally

ⓒ 2006 Mayo Foundation for Medical Education and Research

puncture the dura. PDPH is believed to result from a loss of cerebrospinal fluid, which places traction on the meninges and, thus, on the brain. Patients with a PDPH typically present with orthostatic, position-related headaches. Valsalva maneuvers, such as coughing and sneezing, exacerbate the head pain. The patients may complain of nausea, vomiting, dizziness, visual and auditory changes, paresthesias, weakness, and cranial-nerve palsies. The pain typically resolves in several days. Conservative measures, such as rest, hydration, and caffeine can alleviate symptoms. More long-standing symptoms can be managed through an autologous epidural blood patch, with success rates approaching 90% for the first blood patch and up to 98% with repeat patches.

BACKACHE

In general, the delivery of anesthesia of any kind is associated with postoperative backache, but the incidence is higher following spinal anesthesia. Epidurals have been associated with a higher incidence and a longer duration of backache than have spinal blocks. The etiology of such backache is unknown, but local anesthetic irritation, direct trauma, and ligamentous strain related to muscle relaxation have been postulated.

SYSTEMIC TOXICITY

Although systemic toxicity is continually a concern with epidural anesthesia, systemic toxicity does not occur with spinal anesthesia, because drug doses are generally considered too low to cause toxic reactions, even if injected intravenously.

TOTAL SPINAL

Total or high spinals occur when excessive amounts of medication are injected intrathecally. The anesthetic spreads to the entire spinal cord and the brain stem, resulting in total sympathetic blockade with resultant bradycardia, hypotension, and respiratory depression. Ponhold and Vicenzi found that the patient's operative position helps determine the incidence of bradycardia and, thus, of sympathetic blockade. Patients in the Trendelenburg position were more likely to develop bradycardia than were those in the supine or hammock position. Respiratory arrest can also occur as the primary and accessory respiratory muscles are paralyzed, and the lower-respiratory brain centers are affected. Adequate supportive measures with antimuscarinics, vasopressors, intravenous fluids, and ventilation can effectively treat high-spinal blocks.

NEUROLOGIC INJURY

Neurologic injury is a feared complication of both spinal and epidural anesthesia. The incidence of serious injury to the cauda equina roots and paraplegia is extremely low, but persistent paresthesias and limited motor weakness are the most common injuries among neurologic complications. Barash and Stoelting state that, "Injury may result from direct needle trauma to the spinal cord or spinal nerves, from spinal cord ischemia, from accidental injection of neurotoxic drugs or chemicals, from introduction of bacteria into the subarachnoid or epidural space, or very rarely from epidural hematoma."

Transient neurologic symptoms (TNS) can result from clinical administration of high concentrations of local anesthetics, causing pain to radiate down the back and lower extremities. The pain occurs within 24 hours after spinal anesthesia and generally lasts 48 hours. As the number of procedures done using spinal anesthetics has increased over the past decade, so has awareness and concern about TNS. Hyperbaric lidocaine is a major culprit in causing TNS, and the lithotomy position and knee arthroscopy position increase the rate of TNS. Although the dose of a solution does not appear to affect the incidence of TNS, anesthesiologists believe that hyperbaric solutions surrounding neurologic components pool in dependent locations and fail to mix adequately with cerebrospinal fluid, causing cauda equina syndrome. Anesthesiologists speculate that neural stretching compromises blood flow and can exacerbate sciatic-type symptoms. Pollack et al. compared various concentrations of lidocaine and found no difference in their associated incidences of TNS. TNS is, however, a rare complication. In a retrospective study examining the risk of neurologic symptoms in 4,767 subjects, Horlocker et al. showed the safety of spinal anesthesia.

ANTICOAGULATION

Spinal hematoma and other central nervous system (CNS) hematomas are potentially disastrous complications of spinal anesthesia in patients receiving anticoagulation therapy, which is commonly administered to various patients, including those with atrial fibrillation and hypercoagulable disorders; those with orthopedic fractures; and those who are bedridden and debilitated. Antiplatelet-drug use and traumatic or prolonged needle placement also can lead to CNS hematomas. The American Society of Regional Anesthesia and Pain Management has developed practice guidelines for treating neuroaxial anesthesia. The extremely low incidence of neuroaxial hematomas precludes prospective randomized studies. Using these guidelines and understanding the relevant pharmacology permits well-informed clinical decision-making (http://www.asra.com/publications/consensus-statements-2.html).

DISCHARGE CRITERIA

After having general or regional anesthesia, a patient can be evaluated for discharge from the Post-Anesthesia Recovery Unit (PACU), using the Aldrete score, which assigns scores of 0, 1, or 2 in five categories, including extremity movement; the ability to breathe deeply and cough; orientation and consciousness; oxygen saturation; and systemic blood pressure (*Table 115.1*).

TABLE 115.1	ALDRETE SCORE	
CATEGORY	**PARAMETERS**	**SCORE**
Activity	Moves four extremities on command	2
	Moves two extremities on command	1
	Moves no extremities on command	0
Breathing	Breathes deeply and coughs deeply	2
	Dyspnea	1
	Apnea	0
Circulation	Blood pressure within 20% of preanesthetic level	2
	Blood pressure within 20% to 49% of preanesthetic level	1
	Blood pressure within 50% of preanesthetic level	0
Consciousness	Fully awake	2
	Arousable	1
	Nonresponsive	0
Oxygen saturation	>92% on room air	2
	Supplemental oxygen to maintain saturation >90% on room air	1
	<90% with supplemental oxygen	0

Adapted from Aldrete JA. The post anaesthesia recovery score revisited. *J Clin Anesth.* 1995;7:89–91, with permission.

Typically, a score of 9 or greater is required for discharge from the PACU. Peripheral perfusion, including heart rate and blood pressure, should be stable for at least 15 minutes before discharge. Hypothermia can persist, but shivering should resolve. Patients should also understand that their activities, including driving, are restricted postoperatively for at least 24 hours.

Regional-anesthetics techniques with decreased parenteral opioid requirements minimize postoperative nausea and vomiting (PONV), pain, and somnolence, which are the most common symptoms necessitating PACU admission following general anesthesia. Numerous randomized studies have shown that general anesthesia is associated with a high incidence of PONV, sore throat, longer recovery time and higher opioid requirements; whereas spinal anesthesia is associated with a high incidence of pruritis and urinary retention. Postoperative symptoms, such as pain, nausea, and vomiting, generally resolve within 24 hours, but vomiting should resolve before discharge.

Patients receiving neuroaxial anesthesia, including spinals, must be evaluated for the regression of motor, sympathetic, and sensory blockade before ambulating. The clinician can test the sacral nerves (S4-5) for perineal sensation, first-toe proprioception, and pedal-plantar flexion. Before ambulating, residual motor, sympathetic, and sensory blockade should have resolved. Patients should ambulate without dizziness or difficulty before discharge.

Delayed voiding commonly delays discharge from the PACU. In one study, 18% of patients receiving spinal anesthesia had delayed voiding that delayed their discharge. Motor and sensory functions typically return before sympathetic nerve function, and residual sympathetic blockade to the bladder and urethra can lead to urinary retention. Once the third sacral dermatome blockade ceases, the micturition reflex generally returns. Epinephrine is not recommended for use when administering spinal anesthetics to ambulatory patients, because, although it can increase the duration of the spinal anesthetic, it further compromises the micturition reflex. Avoidance of long-acting spinal and epidural anesthetics allows bladder function to return before bladder distention begins. *A consensus does not exist on whether voiding should be a criterion for PACU discharge.* Recent trials have shown that those at low risk for urinary retention do not need to void before discharge, whereas those at high risk for urinary retention should void before discharge. Marshall et al suggested that even patients with a high risk for urinary retention could be discharged home before voiding with specific follow-up if voiding fails to occur in a given time interval.

Jin et al. showed no correlation between drinking and not drinking and its association to nausea and vomiting. In a review, Marshall et al concluded that withholding fluid intake shortens the postoperative recovery period without evidence of adverse effects. The medical staff should be educated that drinking before discharge may not be needed in ambulatory patients.

A modification of the Aldrete PACU scoring system, termed the Postanesthesia Discharge Scoring System (PADS), "establishes a pattern of routine, repetitive evaluation of patients home readiness, that is likely to contribute to improved outcome." The PADS scoring system lacks requirements for drinking and voiding. Chung recommended initially using the Aldrete score, followed by home-readiness evaluation with the PADS scoring system, which includes categories for vital signs, activity level, nausea and vomiting, pain, and surgical bleeding.

TAKE HOME POINTS

- Use of spinal anesthetics represents a safe, efficient, and inexpensive technique that offers lower postoperative morbidity when compared with general anesthetics for some of the complications of anesthesia; however, use of spinal anesthetics introduces new postoperative issues that must be confronted.
- Spinal anesthetics are ideally suited for use in ambulatory surgical cases, given their short duration and limited complications; however, they also can serve well in chronically debilitated, hospitalized patients.
- *Although all surgical facilities should have established PACU discharge requirements, no standard exists.*
- At minimum, patients should meet the Aldrete scoring system's requirements.

■ An anesthesiologist must ultimately decide a patient's postanesthetic disposition, with the ultimate goal of returning the patient to his preanesthetic state.

SUGGESTED READINGS

Acharya R, Chhabra SS, Ratra M, et al. Cranial subdural haematoma after spinal anaesthesia." *Br J Anaesth.* 2001;86(6):893–895.

Barash PG, Cullen BF, Stoelting RK, eds. *Clinical Anesthesia.* 5th ed. Philadelphia: Lippincott Williams & Wilkins; 2005.

Chakravorty NJR, Chakravorty D, Agarwal RC. Spinal anaesthesia in the ambulatory setting—a review. *Indian Journal of Anaesthesia.* 2003;47(3):167–173.

Chung F, Chung F. Are discharge criteria changing? *J Clin Anesth.* 1993;5(6 Suppl 1): 64S–68S.

Dahl JB, Schultz P, Anker-Moller E, et al. Spinal anaesthesia in young patients using a 29-gauge needle: Technical considerations and an evaluation of postoperative complaints compared with general anaesthesia. *Br J Anaesth.* 1990;64:178–182.

Freedman JM, Li DK, Drasner K, et al. Transient neurological symptoms after spinal anesthesia: An epidemiologic study of 1863 patients. *Anesthesiology.* 1998;89:633–641.

Horlocker TT, Wedel DJ, Benzon H, et al. Regional anesthesia in the anticoagulated patient: Defining the risks (the second ASRA Consensus Conference on Neuraxial Anesthesia and Anticoagulation). (See comment.) *Reg Anesth Pain Med.* 2003;28(3):172–197.

Jin F, Norris A, Chung F, et al. Should adult patients drink fluids before discharge from ambulatory surgery? *Anesth Analg.* 1998;87(2):306–311.

Korttila K. Recovery and driving after brief anaesthesia. *Anaesthesist.* 1981;30:377–382.

Liu SS, Mulroy MF. Neuraxial anesthesia and analgesia in the presence of standard heparin. *Reg Anesth Pain Med.* 1998;23(6 Suppl 2):157–163.

Marshall SI, Chung F. Discharge criteria and complications after ambulatory surgery. *Anesth Analg.* 1999;88(3):508–517.

Miller RD, ed. *Miller's Anesthesia.* Philadelphia: Churchill Livingstone; 2000.

Pavlin DJ, Pavlin EG, Fitzgibbon DR, et al. Management of bladder function after outpatient surgery. *Anesthesiology.* 1999;91(1):42–50.

Pavlin DJ, Pavlin EG, Gunn HC, et al. Voiding in patients managed with or without ultrasound monitoring of bladder volume after outpatient surgery. *Anesth Analg.* 1999;89(1): 90–97.

Pollock JE, Liu SS, Neal JM, et al. Dilution of spinal lidocaine does not alter the incidence of transient neurologic symptoms. *Anesthesiology.* 1999;90(2):445–450.

Pollock JE, Neal JM, Stephenson CA, et al. Prospective study of the incidence of transient radicular irritation in patients undergoing spinal anesthesia. *Anesthesiology.* 1996;84(6):1361–1367.

Ponhold H, Vicenzi MNl. Incidence of bradycardia during recovery from spinal anaesthesia: Influence of patient position. *Br J Anaesth.* 1998;81(5):723–726.

Vaghadia H. Spinal anesthesia for outpatients: Controversies and new techniques. *Can J Anaesth.* 1998;45:R64–R70.

Van der walt JH, Webb RK, Osborne GA, et al. The Australian incidence monitoring study: Recovery room incidents in the first 200 incident reports. *Anaesth Intensive Care.* 1993;21(5):650–652.

Acharya R, Chhabra SS, Ratra M, et al. Cranial subdural haematoma after spinal anaesthesia. [Review] [16 refs] [Case Reports. Journal Article. Review] *British Journal of Anaesthesia.* 2001;86(6):893–895.

PEDIATRIC ANESTHESIA

116

FASTING GUIDELINES FOR CHILDREN SHOULD BE SIMPLE BUT NOT TOO SIMPLE

JUSTIN B. HAUSER, MD

Among the many routine decisions that must be made concerning the preoperative care of pediatric patients, perhaps none is as consistently complicated as the preoperative fasting guidelines. The anesthesiologist must always balance the risks of a full stomach and pulmonary aspiration against the threat of prolonged fasting, dehydration, and hypoglycemia. While making the safest medical decision, the anesthesiologist must also consider the probability of irritable children, disgruntled parents, and a constantly evolving operating room schedule. Large retrospective studies have shown that, although perioperative pulmonary aspiration is more common in children than in adults, it is still rare. Significant morbidity resulting from aspiration is seen even less frequently.

Practices regarding preoperative fasting guidelines vary significantly, as reported in a recent survey of major pediatric hospitals. Most centers agreed on allowing clear fluids for as many as 2 hours and breast milk for as many as 4 hours before a planned procedure. However, there was less concurrence regarding the appropriate fasting period for infant formula and solids. Some institutions restricted intake of formula in a manner similar to solids. Others recommended a fasting period for formula the duration of which was between the durations recommended for clear liquids and solids and was similar to the duration recommended for breast milk. In addition, certain policies dictated fasting intervals based on the patient's age whereas others placed definitive limits on volumes of ingestible items. These discrepancies, along with frequently unclear policies within individual institutions, have created a great deal of confusion for both parents and health care providers.

In 1999, in an effort to establish clear recommendations regarding nothing by mouth (NPO) status, the American Society of Anesthesiologists (ASA) published Practice Guidelines for Preoperative Fasting and the Use of Pharmacologic Agents to Reduce the Risk of Pulmonary Aspiration. These guidelines provide clinical recommendations based on a review of current literature, a large survey of physicians, and a consensus among anesthesiologists within the Task Force on Preoperative Fasting. As part of their recommendations, the task force emphasizes the importance of a preoperative evaluation of each patient and recognition of comorbidities that may increase the risk of pulmonary aspiration. Gastroesophageal reflux, ileus, and bowel obstruction

© 2006 Mayo Foundation for Medical Education and Research

are prevalent among the pediatric surgical population and certainly warrant individualized preoperative fasting orders based on the severity of the patient's condition.

The task force's guidelines are intended for healthy patients who are scheduled for elective procedures and provide appropriate fasting intervals for each type of ingested material. Accordingly, clear liquids may be given as many as 2 hours before a planned procedure. Clear liquids frequently given to pediatric patients include water, ginger ale, popsicles without fruit chunks, fruit juices without pulp, and oral rehydration solutions. For breast milk, the recommended fasting interval is 4 hours. Regarding infant formula, the task force recommends a fasting interval of 6 hours. Similar to that for formula, the recommended fast for solids and milk other than breast milk is 6 hours before the procedure.

For patients requiring preoperative or daily medications, decisions must be made on an individual basis. Pediatric patients generally can safely be given their medications on the morning of surgery with a small amount of water. A prospective study in pediatric surgical patients showed no significant change in gastric pH or residual volume in those given oral midazolam mixed with 5 mL of water. Pediatric anesthesiologists generally accept the risk associated with ingestion of premedications, such as midazolam, just before induction of anesthesia due to the other desirable attributes of these drugs. Special consideration must be given to medications that involve the administration of a larger volume of liquid. The Task Force on Preoperative Fasting does not recommend the routine preoperative use of gastrointestinal stimulants, histamine-2 receptor antagonists, antacids, or antiemetics due to insufficient evidence suggesting a role of these agents in reducing the risk of pulmonary aspiration. The guidelines instead emphasize the importance of the fasting intervals for the specific types of ingested liquids and solids.

These NPO recommendations are most easily remembered as the "2, 4, 6" rule (*Table 116.1*): 2 hours for clear liquids, 4 hours for breast milk, and

TABLE 116.1	NPO INTERVALS RECOMMENDED BY TASK FORCE ON PREOPERATIVE FASTING	
TWO HOURS BEFORE PROCEDURE	**FOUR HOURS BEFORE PROCEDURE**	**EIGHT HOURS BEFORE PROCEDURE**
Water, ginger ale	Breast milk	Formula
Fruit juices (no pulp)	–	Milk other than breast milk
Oral rehdyration solutions	–	Solids
Popsicles	–	–

TABLE 116.2	PROPOSED NPO TIMES FOR PREPRINTED NPO ORDERS
AM PROCEDURE	**PM PROCEDURE**
Midnight—solids, formula, milk other than breast milk	Midnight—solids, formula, milk other than breast milk
3 AM—breast milk	8 AM—breast milk
5 AM—clear liquids	10 AM—clear liquids

6 hours for formula, milk other than breast milk, and solids. Another way to simplify these guidelines is to provide two sets of standardized NPO orders, one for all pediatric patients with procedures scheduled to occur before noon and another for those with procedures scheduled to occur after noon (*Table 116.2*). For patients having procedures in the morning, no solids, milk other than breast milk, or formula are permitted after midnight. Breast milk is permitted until 3 AM, and clear liquids are permitted until 5 AM. For children scheduled for procedures after noon, no solids, milk other than breast milk, or formula are permitted after midnight. However, breast milk may be given until 8 AM, and these children may have clear liquids until 10 AM. Undoubtedly, conflicts with operating-rooms schedules due to a child's NPO status will forever persist. Nonetheless, these standardized orders are aimed at ensuring that pediatric patients may be safely anesthetized at the time of their procedure while minimizing the number of irritable children and frustrated parents in the surgical waiting room. As with every clinical decision, deciding on the appropriate fasting interval must include consideration of each patient's medical condition and the urgency of the planned procedure. Any significant divergence from these guidelines requires that the anesthesiologist consider the probability of a full stomach and the need for techniques to prevent pulmonary aspiration.

TAKE HOME POINTS

- Implementing reasonable NPO guidelines for children involves considering many factors, including the fact that aspiration of gastric contents is rare but, potentially, very serious.
- Most centers are agreed on guidelines for clear liquids and breast milk.
- The ASA published Practice Guidelines in 1999 to provide clinical guidelines for anesthesia providers. This document stresses awareness of factors that can increase risk of aspiration of gastric contents. These factors, gastroesophageal reflux, ileus, and bowel obstruction, are prevalent among the pediatric surgical population.

- The Task Force on Preoperative Fasting does not recommend the routine preoperative use of gastrointestinal stimulants, histamine-2 receptor antagonists, antacids, or antiemetics.
- NPO guidelines for children are most easily remembered as the "2,4,6" rule.
- One way to simplify the NPO guidelines is to provide two sets of standardized NPO orders, one for all pediatric patients with procedures scheduled to occur before noon and another for those with procedures scheduled to occur after noon.

SUGGESTED READINGS

Ferrari LR, Rooney FM, Rockoff MA. Preoperative fasting practices in pediatrics. *Anesthesiology*. 1999;90(4):978–980.

Riva J, Lejbusiewicz G, Papa M, et al. Oral premedication with midazolam in paediatric anaesthesia. Effects on sedation and gastric contents. *Paediatr Anaesth*. 1997;7:191–196.

Warner MA, Caplan RA, Epstein BS, et al. Practice guidelines for preoperative fasting and the use of pharmacologic agents to reduce the risk of pulmonary aspiration: Application to healthy patients undergoing elective procedures-a report by the American Society of Anesthesiologists Task Force on Preoperative Fasting. *Anesthesiology*. 1999;90:896–905.

Warner MA, Warner ME, Warner DO, et al. Perioperative pulmonary aspiration in infants and children. *Anesthesiology*. 1999;90(1):66–71.

117

DO NOT AUTOMATICALLY CANCEL THE PROCEDURE IF THE CHILD HAS A RUNNY NOSE

ANN G. BAILEY, MD

One of the most common dilemmas for the pediatric anesthesiologist is deciding whether to anesthetize a child who has just recovered from or currently has an upper-respiratory-tract infection (URI). This situation is challenging even for experienced providers who have lots of judgment and experience in this area—junior anesthesiologists should not be at all hesitant about seeking help and advice.

The first problem is to determine if the child has an URI at all. When is a runny nose secondary to an URI, and when is it due to allergic rhinitis? Remember that the symptoms that the parents are most likely to tell you about ("he's had a runny nose" or "a little bit of a cold") can be very similar to those of other illnesses or allergies. The most reliable way to tell the difference between an URI and allergic rhinitis or other benign entities is to get further history from the parents. If they relate that the child developed symptoms while in daycare or that he has sick siblings, it is probably an URI. Also, you should suspect that the child has an URI if the parents tell you that their child's symptoms are new and not a routine occurrence. There are, however, some children who "keep a cold." In one study, the probability of having an URI in a child younger than 3 years, in daycare, with parents who smoke in crowded house was 0.61 in any given 2-week period! Signs that are associated with an URI include purulent rhinorrhea, fever, sore throat, productive cough, and other lower-tract signs, such as wheezing or rhonchi. Allergic rhinitis is not associated with fever or productive cough, rhinorrhea is usually clear, and it is often associated with a history of atopy.

The second problem is determining whether the URI will affect the child's anesthetic course. Early studies demonstrated that what is thought to be purely an URI might also involve the lower airways and be associated with decreased pulmonary function, and increased reactivity for up to 6 weeks after the infection. In viral airway infections, much of the bronchial hyper-reactivity is vagally mediated. Some viruses are thought to produce a viral neuraminidase that decreases the function of M_2 muscarinic receptors. As a result, there is increased release of acetylcholine in virus-infected airways. There may also be a decrease in the activity of airway neutral endopeptidase, an enzyme responsible for inactivating tachykinins. These effects render the

© 2006 Mayo Foundation for Medical Education and Research

lower airways more susceptible to smooth-muscle contraction, thus increasing airway reactivity.

The typical URI also is associated with more airway secretions. The combination of increased secretions with increased reactivity leads to the adverse events often described in clinical studies of anesthetized children with URIs: coughing, breath-holding, laryngospasm, bronchospasm, and episodes of desaturation.

The next question is which procedures should be cancelled to avoid serious complications in the child with a URI? Children who present for an elective procedure with moderate-to-severe signs and symptoms of fever, myalgias, lassitude, wheezing, or rhonchi are easily discerned as being at high risk, and their procedures should be delayed. However, those who present with mild or recent symptoms are also at risk for adverse events. One study evaluated more than 1,000 children scheduled for elective surgery who were either well, had a recent URI (within 4 weeks), or had an active URI. The incidence of adverse respiratory events was greater in the children with recent or active URIs than in the children who were well. Independent risk factors for respiratory complications in children with an URI were copious secretions, presence of an endotracheal tube (ETT) in children less than 5 years of age, history of premature birth, nasal congestion, paternal smoking, history of reactive airway disease, and airway surgery. The more serious complications of laryngospasm and bronchospasm were not different among the groups. A second study compared the cases of 1,280 children with preoperative URIs with those of 20,876 children without preoperative URIs and demonstrated that there was an 11-fold increase in the risk of a respiratory complication if the child with an URI required intubation. The first study also confirmed that an ETT in the presence of an URI contributed to more adverse respiratory events, although these events were primarily breathholding.

Does the increased risk of adverse respiratory events mean that, in every case in which a child has a recent or current URI, the procedure should be delayed for at least 4 weeks (6 weeks for lower-tract symptoms)? Absolutely not, since the vast majority of children with an URI do well upon having an anesthetic. Identifying children who are at higher risk for adverse outcomes and delaying those surgeries is reasonable. The child who has a runny nose for 3 days, who is otherwise well, and who is scheduled for an adenoidectomy will probably do fine. One can improve the likelihood of an uneventful anesthetic by tailoring it to minimize reactivity (See Take Home Points). Sevoflurane, with its mild airway pungency, causes fewer respiratory events when used as a maintenance agent in children with an URI. Additionally, the use of a laryngeal mask airway (LMA) or facemask, when feasible, decreases complications. Administering a dose of atropine (10 mcg/kg intravenously

[IV]) or glycopyrrolate (5 to 10 mcg/kg IV), to serve both as an antisialogue and as a vagolytic agent, may decrease risk. Giving a bronchodilator prophylactically to prevent wheezing has not been shown to be effective. In a younger child who will require intubation, one should anticipate a higher incidence of postoperative croup and should consider giving dexamethasone (0.3 to 0.5 mg/kg IV; maximum dose, 10 mg) intraoperatively.

With such a small amount of scientific evidence regarding the risks of anesthesia for the child with an URI, clinical experience and common sense must help to determine our course of action. Charles Cote, MD, summarized it best in an editorial about this dilemma: "We are left to our best clinical judgment about an individual patient undergoing a specific procedure for a specific duration of time by a specific surgeon that requires intubation that may or may not involve admission to the hospital who also has or has had a recent URI."

TAKE HOME POINTS

Strategies for minimizing risks when the patient has an URI include the following:

- Use a LMA or mask instead of ETT, if possible;
- Administer atropine or glycopyrrolate, preoperatively or intraoperatively;
- Use sevoflurane rather than desflurane or isoflurane;
- Use propofol rather than thiopental for an IV induction;
- Have albuterol available, but do not use it prophylactically; and
- Consider dexamethasone in small children who require intubation.

SUGGESTED READINGS

Cohen M, Cameron C. Should you cancel the operation when a child has an upper respiratory tract infection? *Anesth Analg*. 1991;72:282–288.

Cote C. The upper respiratory tract infection (URI) dilemma: Fear of a complication or litigation? *Anesthesiology*. 2001;95:283–285.

Empey DW, Laitinem LA, Jacobs L, et al. Mechanisms of bronchial hyperreactivity in normal subjects after upper respiratory tract infection. *Am Rev Respir Dis*. 1976;113:131–139.

Fleming D, Cochi S, Hightower A, et al. Childhood upper respiratory tract infections: To what degree is incidence affected by day-care attendance? *Pediatrics*. 1987;79:55–60.

Tait AR, Malviya S, Voepel-Lewis T, et al. Risk factors for perioperative adverse respiratory events in children with upper respiratory tract infections. *Anesthesiology*. 2001;95:299–306.

Tait AR, Randit UA, Voepel-Lewis T, et al. Use of the laryngeal mask airway in children with upper respiratory tract infections: A comparison with endotracheal intubation. *Anesth Analg*. 1998;86:706–711.

118

PUT SOME THOUGHT INTO WHICH CHILD, AND WITH WHICH DRUG, YOU PREMEDICATE

M. CONCETTA DeCARIA, MD

The amount of literature on the subject of preoperative medication can be overwhelming. This may be because there is no "ideal" medication available that is free from unwanted side effects. When deciding whether to administer medication to a child before surgery, one should consider, first, whether that child is a candidate for such medication, and, secondly, which medication would be most appropriate for that child. There is no perfect formula for this, but one general rule is to consider both the comfort and the safety of the child when making these choices. This is yet another situation where much can be learned from observing the senior pediatric anesthesia providers. Experienced pediatric anesthesiologists start like the rest of us—with the general rule that both the safety and the comfort of the child must be considered. But they then know how to use the available agents to take an anxious, upset child and transition smoothly to an anesthetized patient.

When choosing whether to give medications preoperatively to a child, it is imperative to consider the consequences of doing so. The advantages of administering medication before surgery are well described and include the dissipation of preoperative anxiety, for both the child and the parent. Preoperative medication can facilitate separation from the parents and can smooth induction in the operating room. Of course, there are also disadvantages to giving medication to children preoperatively, which can include anything from inconvenient side effects, such as prolonged recovery, to dangerous side effects, like oxygen desaturation and loss of airway control.

The perfect preoperative medication would have the following characteristics:

- It would have a relatively rapid and reliable onset;
- It would be free of side effects, such as nausea, the risk for excessive sedation, increased oral secretions, and discomfort from administration;
- It would readily be accepted by the child and would have a route of administration that is not traumatic;
- It would last long enough to accommodate operating-room delays but not prolong recovery or delay discharge; and
- It would not require constant nursing supervision due to side effects.

For outpatient pediatric patients about to have anesthesia, a medication that does not require intravenous (IV) administration would be most useful.

ⓒ 2006 Mayo Foundation for Medical Education and Research

One of a child's worst fears associated with coming to the hospital is being stuck by needles. It logically follows that it would be best to avoid administering drugs via the intramuscular route. Other options then include giving a medication by the oral, rectal, or transmucosal route. The most commonly sited classes of medications used for preoperative purposes are hypnotics, opiods, N-methyl-D-aspartate (NMDA) receptor antagonists, and alpha-2 agonists. As a general rule, most children under approximately 10 months of age do not require sedation preoperatively because they have yet to develop separation anxiety.

HYPNOTICS

The medication used most frequently preoperatively in pediatrics is midazolam, largely due to its safety profile, reliability, anxiolytic effect, ability to be given orally, and its effect on antegrade recall. While it is possible to administer midazolam by virtually any route, in the pediatric population, the oral route is most commonly used.

A common and effective dose for oral administration is 0.5 mg/kg. When given intranasally, it has been shown that a dose of 0.2 to 0.3 mg/kg has been helpful in reducing preoperative anxiety. Another efficient method of administration is sublingual (0.2 mg/kg), which works better for older children who can comply with this technique. Rectal midazolam (0.5 mg/kg to 1 mg/kg) is anxiolytic, but approximately 20% of patients who receive midazolam rectally develop hiccups.

Compared to other benzodiazepines, midazolam has a more rapid onset and shorter duration of action. While relatively free of unwanted side effects, oral midazolam does have one problem. It has a very bitter aftertaste, and many children will refuse to finish their doses if they have gotten a little taste of it. Many flavored syrups, the most common of which is cherry, have been used to mask the taste. Encourage your patients to take it all down at once and not to "sip" it. The period between oral administration and onset is 10 to 15 minutes.

For patients who refuse to take the medication orally, it can be given intranasally. Intranasal midazolam causes a burning sensation, and, when oral and intranasal routes of administration were compared in one study, patients preferred oral administration. For short procedures, orally administered midazolam can prolong recovery and delay discharge.

Barbituates have also been historically used for preoperative medication in the pediatric population. The most common of these is the shorter-acting pentobarbital, which can be given safely by both the oral and rectal routes. It can also be given intramuscularly, but this has been associated with prolonged pain at the injection site. The dose of pentobarbital is 2 to 4 mg/kg. It is best given rectally in children younger than 3 years of age. Given orally, it can take from 1 to 1.5 hours to become effective, which can be an obvious drawback to its use. We do not use barbituates as preoperative medication in our practice.

OPIOIDS

Narcotics, such as sufentanil and fentanyl, have been studied for the purposes of preoperative medication. Problems with the routine usage of opioids include respiratory depression, decreased oxygen saturation, delay in the tolerance of oral intake postoperatively, dysphoria, nausea, and vomiting. Routes of administration are broad and include oral, nasal, rectal, intravenous, and intramuscular administration. In some cases, the transmucosal route (fentanyl oralet) has been used.

When given intranasally, sufentanil can be given in increments of 2 mcg/kg. Compared with the intranasal administration of midazolam, intranasal administration of sufentanil appears to be less unpleasant. However, its administration has been shown to result in an increased difficulty in ventilation in approximately one third of patients, due to chest-wall rigidity.

KETAMINE

An NMDA-receptor antagonist, ketamine, can be used for the induction and maintenance of anesthesia. As a preoperative medication, it can be given intramuscularly, orally, rectally, nasally, and intravenously. Advantages of ketamine are good anxiolysis, facilitation of mask induction, and sedation. Potential disadvantages are emergence delirium, increased salivation, and, in some studies, delayed discharge from the postanesthesia care units.

An effective intranasal dose of ketamine for preoperative sedation is 6 mg/kg, with an onset time of approximately 20 to 40 minutes. A rectal dose of ketamine (5 to 10 mg/kg) has been shown to provide adequate sedation within 7 to 30 minutes after administration. Ketamine is given orally in doses from 3 to 6 mg/kg with good effect within 20 to 25 minutes. Notably, there seems to be an absence of emergence delirium associated with the oral administration of ketamine. The ketamine "dart" is still used in some special circumstances. Usually 1 to 2 mg/kg is sufficient, although some use a true induction dose of 4 mg/kg. The addition of glycopyrolate or atropine is recommended.

CLONIDINE

Clonidine, an alpha-2 receptor agonist, has been shown to have many desirable effects, including perioperative sedation, hemodynamic stability, reduced anesthetic requirements, and even postoperative analgesia. The use of clonidine in adult patients is well described. Interest in pediatric use is growing. At doses of 4 mcg/kg, oral clonidine has been shown to provide sedation and analgesia and to facilitate separation from parents. It requires administration 60 minutes before induction when given orally. Determining an optimum dose and providing other safe routes of administration, such as intranasal administration, may increase preoperative use of clonidine.

CHILDREN WITH AN IV LINE

If a child has an IV line, by all means use it for preoperative medication. Remember, with IV administration, doses required will be much smaller and the period between administration and onset will be much shorter.

TAKE HOME POINTS

- Choose which patients need preoperative medication: Determine whether the patient has had surgery before; whether the patient appear to be anxious; and whether the patient will return for repeated procedures.
- Consider which medication would best suit the needs of and be least dangerous to the patient: Determine whether the patient has a history of a difficult airway, breathing problems, or paradoxical reactions to certain sedative medications.
- Consider using methods other than preoperative medication to relieve a child's anxiety. Such methods may include familiarizing the child with the operating room before the date of surgery, when possible, and demonstrating the mask induction on a stuffed animal. Consider allowing a parent to accompany the child to the operating room, realizing that sometimes this creates more anxiety, depending on the child and the parent.
- Keep the safety and personal needs of the child at the forefront of your mind when considering preoperative medication.

SUGGESTED READINGS

Gregory G. *Pediatric Anesthesia.* 3rd ed. New York: Churchill Livingstone; 1983:188–193.

Karl H, Keifer A, et al. Comparison of the safety and efficacy of intranasal midazolam or sufentanil for the preinduction of anesthesia in pediatric patients. *Anesthesiology.* 1992;76: 209–215.

Karl H, Rosenberger J, Larach MG, et al. Transmucousal administration of midazolam for premedication of pediatric patients. *Anesthesiology.* 1993;78:885–891.

Krane EJ, Davis PJ. Preoperative preparation for infants and children. In: *Smith's Anesthesia for Infants and Children.* Philadelphia: Mosby Elsevier; 2006:266–268.

McMillan CO, Spahr-Schopfer, Sikich N, et al. Premedication of children with oral midazolam. *Can J Anaesth.* 1992;39(6):545–550.

119

PARENTS ARE PRESENT IN THE OPERATING ROOM BY INVITATION OF THE ANESTHESIOLOGIST ONLY

JUANITA P. EDWARDS, MD, MS AND ROBERT D. VALLEY, MD

Surgery can be a time of *intense* psychological stress, for both the child and the parents, and the stress comes from several sources. First, there is often a lot of anticipatory anxiety leading up to arrival at the operating room (OR). Second, a significant percentage of children may experience anxiety when separated from their parents. Finally, induction can be one of the most challenging times of the perioperative period for the child. The anesthesia provider's job is to minimize all of these stresses for both the parent and the child and still accomplish a safe and expeditious induction.

A number of different interventions, which are discussed elsewhere (see Chapter 118), are useful to reduce preoperative anxiety. These interventions include play therapy with distraction techniques and pharmacologic interventions. For relieving separation anxiety for both the patient and the parent as well as for increasing the patient's compliance in the OR, it has become common practice in many centers to allow one parent to accompany the child to the operating suite. The decision to allow parents into the operating room is still controversial—there are advantages and disadvantages. The obvious benefit of parental presence during induction is that it eliminates the need to separate the child from the parent while the child is still awake. In some cases, parental presence in the OR may eliminate the need for preoperative medication of the child, which can be particularly useful when the risks of using such medication may outweigh the benefits. A parent's presence in the OR decreases the child's fears relating to the unfamiliar OR environment. In both pre-school and school-age children, watching the parent dress up in the gown, mask, and cap can be a humorous distraction. It can be comforting for the child to have his parent with him while being introduced to the unfamiliar OR environment and to sit in the parent's lap until induction is complete.

There are also several potential drawbacks to parental presence at induction of anesthesia. The presence of an anxious parent can actually increase the anxiety of the child, even at very young ages. During the preoperative interview, the anxiety level of the parents must be assessed and taken into account when deciding whether a parent should be invited to accompany

© 2006 Mayo Foundation for Medical Education and Research

the child. A parent should not be allowed into the operating suite solely to calm his or her own fears. It is better to calm the parent's fears by engaging them in an open and relaxed discussion about the procedure and the risks and benefits of anesthesia.

The presence of parents in the OR depends, to a certain extent, on the institution's culture. At some hospitals, a parent almost always comes into the OR, with very few exceptions, whereas, at other hospitals, parents quite rarely enter the OR. Regardless of what the local culture is, the final decision of whether to invite the parent into the OR for induction is the anesthesiologist's decision. In making this decision, the anesthesiologist must balance the needs of the parents, patient, OR staff, and anesthesia staff. Most experienced anesthesiologists evaluate each family on a case-by-case basis in the preoperative area, taking into account the child's age, activity level, and overall temperament as well as the baseline anxiety level of the parent. You should consider your options carefully before inviting a parent to enter the OR. Parents that are very upset or hostile are best not brought back to the OR. Non-English speaking parents are generally not good candidates to be present at induction. Generally, only one parent is invited to enter the OR; virtually all experienced anesthesiologists feel that having more than one family member present is a mistake. Finally, in certain emergent or trauma cases, having a parent present might not be appropriate. Once a decision is made, it should be clearly and openly communicated to the parent, with a focus on the child's safety as the ultimate goal.

The anesthesiologist is responsible for informing the parent who is coming into the OR about what to expect. Anesthesia residents and nurse-anesthetist students should expect that the majority of the parent-doctor interaction in the OR will probably be done by the senior anesthesia provider. The parent should be told that the mask may upset the child, the child may thrash briefly and appear to be disoriented, the child's eyes may roll back as the child goes to sleep, and the child's breathing may become noisy. There are different styles of doing this—the authors prefer to "brief" the parents as the induction proceeds. The important thing is that the parent needs to be assured that these events are normal. The parent also needs to know that he will be escorted out of the OR as soon as the child is asleep. Occasionally, during a completely routine induction, the child's response to induction may cause a very emotional response in the parent, which can occasionally lead to a vasovagal reaction. For this reason, the parent should *always* be seated during the induction of the child.

There should be a designated OR staff member (not the anesthesiologist!) to escort the parent out of the OR immediately after induction and to be available to comfort and reassure the parent if needed. Parents are sometimes uncertain when to leave the OR, particularly in cases in which the child's eyes remain open after induction. The parent may wish to confirm that the child is "asleep" or to ask questions. A simple signal that cues both the parent as well as the designated OR staff is extremely helpful in keeping everyone informed in the steps of the process. An example would be "Okay, Mom, she is asleep now. You can give her a kiss. The nurse will show you back to the waiting area."

For hospitals that offer parental presence at induction, an educated surgical staff is vital. It is very important that the OR staff be clear that the anesthesiologist makes the decision on whether the parent may enter the OR. Staff should avoid inadvertently misleading parents by suggesting that they are welcome to be present for induction before the anesthesiologist has made that determination. It is important to establish a consistent, hospital-wide policy that is well known by surgeons and their staff and that can be communicated early to parents during their child's preoperative workup in the surgery clinic. In this way, there are no unrealistic expectations on the day of surgery. At some institutions, no parent is allowed to accompany a child younger than 10 to 12 months of age. The rationale is that children younger than 10 to 12 months of age have not developed stranger anxiety and can separate from their parents relatively easily.

There are several nonpharmacologic interventions that can be adjuncts or alternatives to parental presence at induction. The effectiveness of these options is determined primarily by the child's age. For some children, particularly those under 4 years of age, bringing both the child's mother and the child's teddy into the OR may provide extra comfort, so the rule about no siblings is suspended if the additional "family member" is a small stuffed animal (the mother takes the sleep buddy with her when she goes out of the room). For school-age children, allowing the child to choose among various scents for their face mask or printing out an electrocardiogram strip once monitors are placed makes the experience more intriguing. Offering a child the opportunity to be the line leader walking into the operating suite may allow them to display independence and is also a good way to assess the child's ability to separate successfully from parents. Providing adolescents with options regarding the procedure gives them some control and reduces anxiety. One example would be to give them the option of an IV or an inhalational induction when either method would be appropriate.

An interesting question is whether the parent should enter the OR when pharmacologic agents have been successfully administered to the child preoperatively. Studies have not shown any clear benefit to the child in combining parental presence in the OR with administration of oral midazolam. Oral midazolam, at a dose of 0.25 to 0.5 mg/kg (maximum dose, 20 mg), results in less patient anxiety than does parental presence in the OR without any preoperative medication.

To summarize, parental presence at induction of anesthesia reduces the child's anxiety level at induction and avoids having to separate the parent and child in the preoperative area. Although being in the OR reduces anxiety and increases satisfaction in parents, these are not the primary reasons to have them in the OR. For a successful experience, the anesthesiologist should make plans clear to the parents as soon as possible and the OR staff should be organized and skilled in having a parent present at a child's induction. Ultimately, the anesthesiologist's goal is to ensure a perioperative experience for the pediatric patient that is safe and not psychologically traumatic.

TAKE HOME POINTS

- The anesthesiologist makes the final decision on whether to have a parent present at induction—don't do it if you are inexperienced or uncomfortable dealing with parents or if the case has high clinical acuity.
- Watch the senior pediatric anesthesiologists—they all have certain tricks and techniques. Borrow freely the techniques you think will work for you.
- The needs of the child are more important than the needs of the parent.
- Be *very* calm when you have a parent in the OR!

SUGGESTED READINGS

Brosius KK, Bannister CF. Oral midazolam and premedication in preadolescents and adolescents. *Anesth Analg.* 2002;94:31–36.

Cote CJ, Cohen IT, Suresh S, et al. A comparison of three doses of a commercially prepared oral midazolam syrup in children. *Anesth Analg.* 2002;94:37–43.

Kain ZN, Caldwell-Andrews AA, Krivutz DM, et al. Trends in the practice of parental presence during induction of anesthesia and the use of preoperative sedative premedication in the United States, 1995-2002: Results of a follow-up national survey. *Anesth Analg.* 2004;98:1252–1259.

Kain ZN, Caldwell-Andrews AA, Maranets I, et al. Postoperative anxiety and emergence delirium and postoperative maladaptive behaviors. *Anesth Analg.* 2004;99:1648–1654.

Kain ZN, Mayes LC, Bell C, et al. Premedication in the United States: A status report. *Anesth Analg.* 1997;84:427–432.

Kain ZN, Mayes LC, Caramico LA, et al. Parental presence during induction of anesthesia: A randomized control trial. *Anesthesiology.* 1996;84(5):1060–1067.

Kain ZN, Mayes LC, Wang S, et al. Parental presence during induction of anesthesia versus sedative premedication: Which intervention is more effective? *Anesthesiology.* 1998;89(5): 1147–1156.

Kain ZN, Mayes LC, Wang S, et al. Parental presence and a sedative premedicant for children undergoing surgery: A hierarchical study. *Anesthesiology.* 2000;92(4):939–946.

McCann ME, Kain ZN. The management of preoperative anxiety in children: An update. *Anesth Analg.* 2001;93:98–105.

Cullen BF, Stoelting RK, Barash PG, eds. *Clinical Anesthesia.* 3rd ed. Philadelphia: Lippincott-Raven Publishers; 1996:1115–1124.

120

PAY SCRUPULOUS ATTENTION TO ELIMINATING AIR BUBBLES IN PEDIATRIC INTRAVENOUS TUBING

ERICA P. LIN, MD

Fetal intracardiac and extracardiac shunts that persist after birth provide a natural setup for paradoxic emboli. Right-to-left shunting allows blood to bypass the inherent filtering action of the lungs, and emboli arising from the venous system can pass directly into the systemic arterial circulation. *Remember always that even a small air embolus can have devastating results.*

ANATOMY AND PHYSIOLOGY

In utero, blood flows in a parallel circuit with respect to the right and left ventricles. The highest oxygen content is in blood returning from the placenta via the umbilical vein. The ductus venosus is the first shunt encountered and connects the umbilical vein with the inferior vena cava, allowing roughly half of this oxygen-rich blood to be diverted away from the liver. Within the right atrium, a pressure gradient enables a significant portion of this oxygenated blood to be preferentially streamed across the foramen ovale to the left atrium. This allows the blood with the most oxygen content to be efficiently delivered, via the left ventricle and aorta, to the coronary and cerebral circulations. Right-ventricular outflow consists of a mixture of oxygenated blood from umbilical veins and desaturated blood from the superior and inferior vena cavi. Only 10% of right-ventricular blood actually passes into the pulmonary circuit because of high vascular resistance (the combined result of fluid-filled fetal lungs and medial-muscle hypertrophy in the small pulmonary arterioles). The remaining 90% of right-ventricular output is shunted away from the lungs through the ductus arteriosus and into the descending aorta, where it supplies the lower body or returns to the placenta.

The transition between fetal and neonatal circulation occurs primarily in response to changes in resistance throughout the circulatory system. The parallel circulation of the fetus is converted to a series system. Clamping of the umbilical cord eliminates the low-resistance placenta, and systemic vascular resistance increases. Without venous return from the placenta, right-atrial pressure decreases. As breathing is initiated, pulmonary vascular resistance falls dramatically, resulting in an increase in blood flow to the pulmonary circulation. In addition, higher pulmonary arterial oxygen tension (compared to the relatively hypoxemic fetal environment) contributes to lower pulmonary

© 2006 Mayo Foundation for Medical Education and Research

vascular resistance. Due to remodeling of the pulmonary vasculature, a continued gradual reduction in pulmonary vascular resistance occurs during the first months of life. More blood flow to the lungs translates to greater pulmonary venous return to the left atrium. Elevated left pressure relative to the right atrium facilitates closure of the flap-like foramen ovale. Higher arterial oxygen concentration stimulates closure of the ductus arteriosus. Removal of the placenta also lowers circulating prostaglandin levels, which further facilitates ductal closure. The ductus arteriosus is functionally closed within the first 24 hours after birth; however, permanent closure requires thrombosis and fibrosis, which can take several months.

Anatomic closure of these alternate pathways does not occur immediately after birth, meaning that the shunts reopen in response to physiologic stimulation. For example, premature infants demonstrate less sensitivity to the effects of oxygen on ductus-arteriosus closure. Similarly, the existence and, often, the pharmacologic maintenance of these shunts are necessary for the survival of infants with congenital heart disease until surgical correction is possible. The drawback, however, is that these shunts provide a route for paradoxic emboli. Multiple case reports have described the source of emboli as varying from air bubbles entrained in intravenous lines to thrombus dislodgement from the ductus venosus, umbilical vessels, or renal veins. Such emboli can be catastrophic, resulting in permanent neurologic damage, myocardial infarction, and even death.

PREVENTION

Simple measures can be taken by health care providers to minimize the risk of iatrogenic emboli. While these maneuvers are second nature for practicing pediatric anesthesia providers, the beginning or occasional pediatric provider should allow for extra time for "de-airing the lines" when setting up the room. These preparations should not be rushed.

Intravenous catheters are an especially frequent culprit. Disconnection of the line, fracture of the hub, or a break in the tubing can allow air entry. Medication administration through peripheral veins can also introduce air. Wald et al. demonstrated in their experimental model that an average volume of 0.02 mL of air is delivered per injection, even when careful attention is paid to remove all air before mounting syringes onto connecting lines. Special care should always be taken when preparing infusions. Ideally, fluids should not be prepared in a cold room and then brought into a warm environment. As the temperature is raised, gas bubbles may form because of reduced solubility and the size of existing bubbles will increase. This same principle applies to the infusion of fluids through a warming system. As the solution passes through the warmer, microbubbles can form and tend to coalesce into larger bubbles that can be passed to the patient. Studies have shown that higher rates of infusion through warmers correspond with decreased amounts of gas escaping from solution. This is presumably due to the shorter amount of time the solution spends in the warming tubing, which, in turn, limits the time for gas to diffuse out of solution. Using distally placed bubble traps or a stopcock for aspiration of any collected air has been suggested. Efforts should also be made to remove air from intravenous fluid bags prior to infusion, as there have been case reports of massive air embolism, especially when such bags are used with pressurized infusion devices.

The risk of paradoxic air embolism is greater in newborns with transitional circulation and patients of any age with cardiac lesions that allow right-to-left shunting to occur. However, as many as 25% of adults have a patent foramen ovale, which can allow paradoxic emboli. For that reason, it is imperative that caretakers always be meticulous in preparing all intravenous infusion systems.

TAKE HOME POINTS

- Newborns are at high risk for right to left shunting.
- Up to 25% of adults have a patent foramen ovale.
- IV setups are a significant source of air.

SUGGESTED READINGS

Adhikary GS, Massey SR. Massive air embolism: A case report. *J Clin Anesth.* 1998;10:70–72.

Stevenson GW, Tobin M, Hall SC. Fluid warmer as a potential source of air bubble emboli (letter). *Anesth Analg.* 1995;80(5):1061.

Wald M, Kirchner L, Lawrenz K, et al. Fatal air embolism in an extremely low birth weight infant: Can it be caused by intravenous injections during resuscitation? *Intensive Care Med.* 2003;29:630–633.

Woon S, Talke P. Amount of air infused to patient increases as fluid flow rates decrease when using the Hotline HL-90 fluid warmer. *J Clin Monit Comput.* 1999;15:149–152.

Wolin J, Vasdev GM. Potential for air embolism using Hotline Model HL-90 fluid warmer (letter). *J Clin Anesth.* 1996;8:81–82.

121

IN CHILDREN, IMPROPER PLACEMENT, USE, AND MAINTENANCE OF VASCULAR ACCESS CAN RESULT IN SERIOUS MORBIDITY AND EVEN MORTALITY

ANGELA KENDRICK, MD

Anesthesia providers must always be diligent in limiting vascular cannulation errors in kids. Serious morbidity or even mortality can result from the placement, the use, or the improper maintenance of vascular access lines. An important resource for tracking information about anesthesia complications is the American Society of Anesthesiologists (ASA) Closed Claim Project (the editors feel it's in the required reading category). The Closed Claims Project allows a retrospective comparison of past legal claims for different categories of injury. This data base includes data on vascular cannulation complications.

COMPLICATIONS ASSOCIATED WITH PERIPHERAL CATHETERS

The most common intravenous (IV) complications reported in the Closed Claim Project include skin sloughing or necrosis, as well as swelling, inflammation, infection, nerve damage, and fasciotomy scars resulting from the treatment of compartment syndromes. Frequently, in cases of compartment syndromes, an extremity was tucked or covered and the peripheral IV was not visually or tactilely monitored. The infiltration therefore was not noted in a timely manner. Peripheral IVs can also be a source of other complications, such as air embolism, fluid overload, and infection.

PERIPHERAL SITE SELECTION

In addition to the usual extremity sites, scalp veins may be selected for use in infants. Often, a branch of the superficial temporal vein is selected. This vein may have many branches helping to form the superficial venous network seen on the infant scalp. Most centers no longer shave the scalp prior to IV insertion. Stroking the vein with one end of the vein occluded by finger pressure may help you establish the direction of flow in the vein; drainage usually is toward the neck. Smaller tourniquets (even rubber bands) may be appropriately used on infants, and angiocath sizes used in infants are typically 22 or 24-gauge.

© 2006 Mayo Foundation for Medical Education and Research

The saphenous vein deserves special mention as a site "of choice" for IV placement. The vein has a reliable anatomic location, lying just in front of the medial malleolus, and is often palpable, even in pudgy toddlers.

Before line placement, you should wash your own hands with an alcohol based solution prior to donning your gloves. Nonsterile gloves may be used for peripheral IVs, but maximum sterile barrier precautions (caps, masks, gowns, gloves, and drapes for the field) are required for central venous lines.

MAINTENANCE OF LINE

Proper securing of the line with clear, occlusive dressing, tape, a padded arm (or leg) board; and, then, an over wrap of gauze dressing prevents a carefully won site from being dislodged by vigorous thrashing. Be sure to leave the insertion site exposed so that it can be monitored for signs of leaking or infection. Infectious complications occur in as many as 25% of patients with indwelling intravenous catheters and can result in serious morbidity and mortality. If an infant or child arrives in the operating room with a covered IV site and a flush fluid needle is not easily injected into the infant or child, the IV site should be uncovered and inspected for skin infiltration. Heated compresses should not be used to treat an infiltration; serious burns have occurred with their use.

To prevent excessive fluid administration, microdrip delivery devices should be used. For patients weighing less than 10 kg, it is best to use a device with a calibrated delivery chamber (e.g., Buretrol). These devices should have a valve or seal that prevents air from entering the IV tubing once the chamber is empty. Careful flushing of all lines, including stopcocks, also is important to help to prevent air embolus. For very small patients (e.g., premature infants), placing all fluids on a regulated pump and avoiding gravity drips altogether is best.

CENTRAL LINES

Mechanical Complications. Arterial puncture, hematoma and pneumothorax are the most common complications of central venous catheters. Serious morbidity, such as perforation of the heart with subsequent pericardial tamponade and catheter or wire embolization, have declined in the most recent closed-claims analysis. Hemothorax, hydrothorax, and injury to the carotid or subclavian artery continue to be significant problems following central line insertion. Ultrasound guidance (see Chapter 21) has been shown to reduce the number of mechanical complications, the number of catheter placement failures, and the time required for placement.

Thrombotic Complications. Catheter related thrombosis occurs at a relatively high rate (around 15%), depending on insertion site, with femoral venous catheters having the highest rate. The risk of blood clot embolism from catheter-related venous thrombosis in this group is still undefined.

Infectious Complications. Maximal sterile-barrier precautions have been shown to reduce the rate of catheter related blood-stream infections. Use of chlorhexidine gluconate (2%) for preparation of the skin prior to insertion of central lines in children older than 2 months of age has been shown to reduce line-related infections. There is a theoretic concern about using this preparatory solution in children younger than 2 months of age because of their higher skin permeability.

Site Selection. Data are available to suggest optimal sites for CVC in adults (subclavian). The jugular, subclavian, or femoral veins may all be used for central access in children. Preference is really dependent on what sites are available and who is placing the line. Cuffed and tunneled central-venous catheters or peripherally inserted central catheters (PICCS) are preferred for patients requiring prolonged venous access.

Size and Depth. Central lines are sized in "French units." The size in French units is roughly equal to the circumference in millimeters of the external surface of the catheter. A size 1 F catheter is 1 mm in circumference and 0.33 mm in diameter. One should select the smallest diameter catheter that will provide the flow rate needed. Infants and small children often take a 3 F or a 5 F catheter. The depth to which the catheter is to be inserted is determined by calculating the length needed so that the tip of the catheter lies at the superior vena cava (SVC) and the right atrial junction (RA). Formulas exist to calculate this depth based on the infant's height or weight. For example, for either the right internal jugular (IJ) or the subclavian approach, for example, length of insertion in cm = height in cm/10 − 1 for children <100 cm in height.

PICC LINES

You may be asked to insert a PICC line or you may want to use one as access during a procedure. PICC lines are designed for long-term access and may have a single or a double lumen. As with other central lines, maximal sterile-barrier precautions apply for the insertion of these lines. PICCs are usually placed via the arm using the Seldinger approach, feeding a stylet-type catheter a measured distance measured in advance to the SCV-RA junction through an angiocatheter guide. The placement is confirmed by a chest x-ray prior to final securing of the catheter to the skin. Ultrasound guidance may facilitate identification of an appropriate peripheral vein, or it may be used to identify a catheter that has angled up in the neck rather than flowing centrally.

MAINTENANCE OF CENTRAL LINES

Flush solution and dressing change protocols vary from center to center and are device dependent. Some use 10 units of heparin per mL of flush, whereas others up to 1000 units per mL of flush. Percutaneously inserted central line catheters used for dialysis require special caution. Dialysis catheters may have 1000 to 5000 units of heparin in the line. You must draw off the heparin solution prior to using the line; do not flush it to the patient. The incidence of central line infections may be reduced by using antimicrobial impregnated catheters, selecting the site properly, taking maximal sterile barrier precautions during insertion, not using topical ointment at the insertion site, disinfecting catheter hubs carefully before use, and removing catheters promptly when they are no longer needed.

Arterial Access. This type of access is indicated for measuring beat-to-beat blood pressure and sampling arterial blood gas. Mechanical complications include injury to the vessel, thrombosis of the vessel, and embolization. Nerve injury can also result from puncture of a nerve or as a result of hematoma formation near the nerve.

Site Selection. The radial artery is usually the preferred site in children, as in adults; however, other sites may be used. The radial artery is not an "end artery" to the hand because of the collateral circulation offered by the ulnar artery. It is estimated that 10% of patients do not have good collateral flow to the hand. Use a modified Allen test (occlude both the radial and ulnar arteries, then release the ulnar artery and observe whether the hand's color returns to normal within 6 seconds) to identify those without significant collateral flow to the hand. Other vessels used include the dorsalis pedis, the posterior tibialis, the ulnar, and the femoral. Catheters (22- or 24-gauge) are appropriately sized to reflect the smaller size of the target vessel. Thrombosis is estimated to occur in 1% to 4% of cannulations. Complications increase with the use of larger catheters and prolonged use. Distal perfusion, including capillary refill, skin temperature, and skin color, needs to be checked every 8 hours. If poor perfusion is detected, the catheter should be removed immediately and the extremity should be monitored closely for the return of adequate perfusion.

UMBILICAL CATHETERS

Using the umbilical artery results in mechanical complications similar to those of using other arterial sites; such complications include thrombosis, (which can involve the aorta), infection, and hemorrhage. It also carries a risk of organ infarction. The infectious risks for umbilical artery catheters and umbilical vein catheters (despite a high colonization rate) are about the same, around 5%.

Using umbilical artery catheters placed in a high position (above the diaphragm at a T5 level) results in a lower incidence of vascular sequelae than does using those placed in a low position (below the diaphragm and above the aortic bifurcation).

The single umbilical vein extends from the umbilicus to the ductus venosus and through the liver to the inferior vena cava (IVC). The preferred location of the tip of the umbilical venous catheter is usually in the cephalad portion of the IVC or at the IVC –RA junction. Air may be introduced into the intrahepatic circulation with insertion of an umbilical venous line; however, this is usually a transient finding and should not be confused with the portal venous air associated with necrotizing enterocolitis.

In general, umbilical or arterial catheters may be left in place for as long as 5 days. Umbilical venous catheters may remain for as long as 14 days. If there is a suspicion of a catheter-related infection, vascular insufficiency, or thrombosis, the catheter should be removed.

TAKE HOME POINTS

- Use of vascular-access devices poses the same or an even greater risk for children as it poses for adults.
- Remember the saphenous and scalp veins when searching for a peripheral IV site.
- Peripheral IV catheters are not changed routinely in children.
- Children can be burned from hot compresses applied to infiltrated IV sites.
- Central-line placement in children requires maximum sterile barrier techniques and can be facilitated by ultrasound guidance.
- Flushing and dressing-change protocols for pediatric central lines are institution and device specific.
- Perfusion distal to an arterial line must be checked every 8 hours.
- The umbilical artery is a unique cannulation site and involves special and potentially serious risks.

SUGGESTED READINGS

Andropoulos DB, Bent ST, Skjonsky B, et al. The optimal length of insertion of central venous catheters for pediatric patients. *Anesth Analg.* 2001;93:883–886.

Bowdle TA. Central line complications from the ASA closed claims project: An update. *ASA Newsletter.* 2002;66(6):11–12, 25.

Garland J, Hendrickson K, Maki D. The 2002 Hospital Infection Control Practices Advisory Committee Centers for Disease Control and Prevention guideline for prevention of intravascular device—related infection. *Pediatrics.* 2002;110:1009–1013.

Liau DW. Injuries and liability related to peripheral catheters: A closed claims analysis. *ASA Newsletter.* 2006;70(6):11–13, 16. Also on www.asaclosedclaims.org.

McGee D, Gould M. Preventing complications of central venous catheterization. *N Engl J Med.* 2003;348:1123–1133.

Rothschild JM. Ultrasound guidance of central vein catheterization. *Evidence Report/ Technology Assessment, no 43. Making Health Care Safer. A Critical Analysis of Patient Safety Practices.* Agency for Healthcare and Quality Publication No.01–E058; 2001; Ch21:245–253. Also available on the web through the Agency for Healthcare and Quality (part of the US Health and Human Services Department at www.ahrq.gov/clinic/ptsafety/chap21).

122

Always make sure you see the intubation and airway equipment you plan to use and the equipment you think you might use

Eugene E. Lee, MD

Because pediatric patients come in a variety of sizes (from a 500-gm neonate to a 100-kg teenager), the pediatric anesthesia provider is confronted with a variety of airway issues and must work with a variety of sizes of airway equipment. Preparedness is very important when securing a child's airway; because babies and children desaturate so quickly, there is not much time to look through the anesthesia cart for airway equipment. Having a little foresight and preparing your anesthesia cart with the equipment you *plan* to use and equipment you think you *might* use will increase patient safety and save a lot of stress.

Understanding the anatomic differences between the pediatric and adult airway is the first step in pediatric airway management. Children have a proportionally larger head and tongue, narrow nasal passages, an anterior and cephalad larynx (at a vertebral level of C4, compared with C6 in adults), a long epiglottis, slanted vocal cords, and a cone-shaped larynx, with the narrowest point being at the cricoid cartilage. Remember also that infants are obligate nose breathers and the upper airway is relatively more prone to collapse. The relatively larger head and prominent occiput of children places the head in a naturally flexed position when the patient is placed supine. It is helpful to elevate the shoulders with a roll–this lets the head extend back slightly on the shoulders and optimizes the airway for mask ventilation and laryngoscopy. It also allows easier access to the neck if external laryngeal or cricoid pressure is required.

Remember always that children as well as adults can have difficult airways and that problems can occur both with establishing a mask airway and intubating. Oral and nasal airways are quite useful in children and should always be readily available in a variety of sizes. The appropriately sized oral airway should reach from the angle of the mandible to the corner of the mouth. Nasal airways should not be so long that they enter the esophagus. Laryngeal mask airways (LMAs) have become a mainstay in managing difficult airways in children, much as in adults.

Both curved and straight laryngoscope blades should be available prior to induction—each has its advantages. A curved blade can sweep the tongue

© 2006 Mayo Foundation for Medical Education and Research

out of the way to improve the view when there is an obscured view of the larynx due to prominent adenoidal and tonsillar tissue. Straight blades are useful when the larynx is particularly anterior and cephalad; for example, a small Miller blade can be helpful in infants in picking up the epiglottis if it obscures the view of the larynx.

There are several issues to consider when selecting endotracheal tubes (ETT) for pediatric patients. The ETT must be large enough to permit spontaneous or controlled ventilation but not so large as to damage the trachea. Selecting the largest tube that will enter the patient's trachea will decrease resistance, lessen the likelihood of plugging, allow the passage of suction catheters, and lessen the chance of airway aspiration. However, an ETT that is too large can cause tracheal damage when the pressure of the ETT against the wall of the trachea exceeds the capillary pressure of the mucosa. This pressure is believed to be 25 to 35 mmHg in adults; however, no values are available for children. Since the cricoid cartilage is the narrowest point of the airway in children and the only complete tracheal ring, mucosal trauma from placing too large an ETT usually occurs here. This can result in postoperative mucosal edema and swelling, which presents clinically as stridor, croup, airway obstruction, and increased work of breathing. According to Poiseuillle's law:

$$R = \frac{8lv}{\prod r^4}$$

where R is resistance, l is length (of the airway), v is gas viscosity, and r is the radius (of the airway). Therefore, small changes in airway radius lead to large changes in airway resistance. The appropriate size of ETT can be estimated by a formula based on age: $4 + \text{age}/4 = \text{ETT}$ size (internal diameter [ID] in mm). One should always have at least three different-sized endotracheal tubes available: The tube you think is the correct size and a tube 0.5 mm ID larger and one 0.5 mm ID smaller. Correct size is confirmed by easy passage of the ETT and gas leakage of 15 to 25 cm H_2O. No leakage indicates an oversized tube that should be replaced, while excessive leakage may make ventilation difficult, require excessive fresh-gas flows, and pollute the operating room. Traditionally, uncuffed ETTs have been the tubes of choice for children younger than 8 years of age. This was because the funnel-shaped larynx resulted in a natural seal at the level of the cricoid ring and the concern that a cuffed tube would require a small ID ETT, hence more resistance. Practitioners are also concerned that excessive cuff pressures can cause mucosal damage. Cuffed ETTs are available in pediatric sizes and have a number of advantages. They allow for an "adjustable fit," permitting fewer tube changes to get the right size. A better seal allows higher inspiratory pressure in children with reduced lung compliance. The better seal also results in less leakage, reduced fresh-gas flows, less operating room contamination, and a reduced risk of aspiration. To avoid tracheal damage, a number of precautions should be taken. The initial choice of tube size should be at least one-half size smaller than that for an uncuffed tube. The tube should be placed so that the cuff is distal to the cricoid ring. The cuff pressure should be monitored to make sure it is *less than* 25 to 30 cm water pressure, and the cuff should be inflated no more than is necessary to prevent a leak at the patient's peak inspiratory pressure.

Use the following formula to estimate the correct depth of ETT placement: 12 + age (years)/2 = depth of tube (cm) at the lip. Another easy rule of thumb follows: Depth at the lip is equal to three times the size of the tube. One can also intentionally place the ETT into the right main-stem bronchus and slowly withdraw it until breath sounds are equal. One final note: A stylet is usually not needed for routine intubations in older children but may be useful with a smaller (flimsier) ETT or if there is anterior or other abnormal airway anatomy. If used, stylets should be malleable and soft, with a flexible tip in order to avoid airway trauma.

TABLE 122.1	ESTIMATES FOR USE IN PLACING PEDIATRIC AIRWAY DEVICES
AIRWAY DEVICE	**SIZE AND DEPTH ESTIMATE**
Nasal airways	Best estimate is a tube that extends from the ala nasi to the tragus of the ear
Oral airways	Best estimate is a tube that extends from the lips to the angle of the mandible
Endotracheal tube size	Uncuffed: 4 + age (years)/4
	Cuffed: 3.5 + age (years)/4
	Premature infant: 2.5 to 3.0
	Term infant: 3.0 to 3.5
	Depth at lip: 6 plus the weight (kg) for infants weighing from 1 to 4 kg = depth in cm at the lip (e.g., for a 2-kg infant, 2 + 6 = 8 cm at the lip); for older infants and children, roughly three times the size of endotracheal tube placed = the depth in cm at thelip
Laryngoscope blades	Premature infant: "0" Straight Blade (Miller)
	Term infant: "1" Straight Blade
	Toddler: "0" to "1" Robert Shaw or "2" Curved (Macintosh) Blade
	Older children: 2 to 3 curved or straight blade, depending on user preference and patient size
Laryngeal mask airways	Up to 5 kg: 1
	>5 to 10 kg: 1.5
	>10 to 20 kg: 2
	>20 to 30 kg: 2.5

TAKE HOME POINTS

- Understanding the anatomic differences between the pediatric and adult airway is the first step in pediatric airway management.
- Remember always that children as well as adults can have difficult airways and that problems can occur with both establishing a mask airway and intubating.
- Be familiar with the size and depth estimates associated with the use of the most common pediatric airway devices (*Table 122.1*).
- Be prepared with the appropriate airway devices and always have a backup readily available!

SUGGESTED READINGS

Gregory GA, ed. *Pediatric Anesthesia*. 4th ed. Philadelphia: Churchill Livingstone; 2002.

Morgan GE, Mikhail MS, Murray MJ. *Clinical Anesthesiology*. 4th ed. New York: McGraw-Hill; 2006:850–861.

Motoyama EK, Davis PJ, eds. *Smith's Anesthesia for Infants and Children*. 7th ed. Philadelphia: Mosby; 2006.

123

ALWAYS EXPECT AND BE PREPARED TO TREAT HYPOXEMIA DURING THE INDUCTION AND EMERGENCE OF A PEDIATRIC PATIENT

MICHAEL J. STELLA, MD

The "blue baby" is one of the most urgent and potentially disastrous complications an anesthesiologist may face. The term describes the rapid oxygen desaturation of a child, usually occurring at induction or upon emergence. What is especially difficult about this clinical situation is how *quickly* a pediatric patient can turn blue—it is common to hear the pulse oximeter reading described as "dropping like a stone." Recognition and preparation can save lives. Never be reluctant to call for help when dealing with a baby who has turned blue—these are challenging situations for even the most experienced pediatric anesthesiologists.

PHYSIOLOGY AND ANATOMY

Toddlers, infants, and neonates are all at significant risk for intraoperative hypoxemic events. Remember that babies are not just small adults; they have important differences in both anatomy and physiology, particularly in the circulatory and respiratory systems. Compared with adults, babies have higher rates of oxygen consumption (6 mL/kg/min in babies, 3 mL/kg/min in adults), as well as lower oxygen reserves or functional residual capacity (FRC). This higher ratio of oxygen consumption to FRC is one of the primary factors affecting the increased rate of desaturation when a baby is apneic or has upper-airway obstruction. Neonates and infants also have fewer alveoli and reduced elastic recoil and compliance of the lung. Coupled with greater chest-wall compliance, these factors create an increased risk of atelectasis and intrapulmonary shunt. A patent foramen ovale (PFO) or a patent ductus arteriosus (PDA) in a newborn creates anatomic shunt, which may cause more rapid desaturation. Also, a newborn can revert to a transitional circulation during the first day or so of life. Therefore, anything that causes an increase in pulmonary vascular resistance (PVR) can result in right-to-left shunting via a PDA or PFO.

Anatomic differences, including a relatively larger tongue, pharyngeal hypotonia, and less rigid supraglottic structures, are present in the airway as well. These contribute to a greater chance of airway obstruction. Negative airway pressure results in pharyngeal obstruction from the tongue sticking to the palate and pharyngeal soft-tissue collapse.

© 2006 Mayo Foundation for Medical Education and Research

WHAT CAN GO WRONG

A number of events can lead to hypoxic episodes in babies. For some infants and in some situations, even a slight prolongation in the time to intubate the trachea can result in significant desaturation episodes. This may be especially common with rapid-sequence inductions when mask ventilation is avoided. A relatively common cause of airway obstruction, especially during the cold-and-flu season is laryngospasm. Laryngospasm is frequently the result of extubation during the "excitement" or stage II depth of anesthesia. Pediatric patients also commonly hold their breath during emergence, which can lead to rapid and deep desaturation. This breath holding, or Valsalva-like phenomenon, results in increased intra-abdominal and intrathoracic pressure with glottic closure. Ventilation is difficult, and the resulting increase in PVR causes right-to-left intracardiac shunting via a PFO. Finally, another common cause of airway obstruction during both induction and emergence is relaxation of the genioglossus muscle, which allows the tongue to fall back and occlude the oropharynx.

HOW TO AVOID THESE PROBLEMS

Avoiding these problems is clearly preferable to managing them. Always have appropriately sized oral and nasal airways and a tongue depressor immediately available. Use the proper size and type of laryngoscope blade and proper head and neck positioning to facilitate visualization of the vocal cords. Consider using glycopyrrolate (10 mcg/kg, intravenously [IV]) or atropine (10 mcg/kg IV) as a premedicant to dry oropharyngeal secretions. Administering oxygen in advance is an important adjunct to "buy" time for your intubation attempts. To avoid obstruction due to relaxation of the genioglossus muscle, open the mouth and "unstick" the tongue from the roof of the mouth. Upon emergence, clear the airway and be certain the patient meets extubation criteria and is fully awake. Be certain that the patient remains deeply anesthetized if you are doing a deep extubation. If the patient is emerging from airway surgery, be sure there is adequate hemostasis. Be prepared to provide positive airway pressure if initial respiratory efforts are ineffective due to upper-airway obstruction. Have succinylcholine (1 to 2 mg/kg IV or 3 to 4 mg/kg, intramuscularly [IM]) and atropine (10 mcg/kg IV or 20 mcg/kg IM) readily available.

WHAT TO DO WHEN HYPOXEMIA OCCURS

Even with proper planning, babies may become hypoxemic secondary to difficulty with ventilation. Upper-airway obstruction is treated with an oral or nasal (or both) airway and jaw thrust with continuous positive airway pressure (CPAP) or positive-pressure ventilation. Breath holding is best treated with 100% oxygen and CPAP. This allows the child to receive an assisted breath upon spontaneous inhalation. Laryngospasm is initially treated with positive-pressure ventilation and 100% oxygen, with jaw thrust and temporomandibular joint pressure sometimes being needed. If this fails to break the laryngospasm, succinylcholine and atropine should be readily available and administered. If none of the above maneuvers works, remember the difficult airway algorithm and proceed accordingly. With proper preparation and vigilance, a "blue baby" scenario can be managed safely.

TAKE HOME POINTS

Always expect and be prepared to treat hypoxemia during the induction and emergence of a pediatric patient:

- Pediatric patients can desaturate *fast* due an increased ratio of oxygen consumption to FRC, which leads to rapid desaturation.
- Never be reluctant to call for help with a hypoxic patient.
- Neonates can be very susceptible to shunting (due to PDA, PFO, and increased PVR).
- Laryngospasm is relatively more common in pediatric than in adult patients, especially during stage II.
- With genioglossus laxity, a larger tongue can obstruct the oropharynx.
- Be prepared:
  - Have the proper equipment ready.
  - Have the proper medications drawn up beforehand.
  - Administer oxygen in advance appropriately.
- Use CPAP, a jaw thrust, and 100% O_2 for obstructions and laryngospasm.

SUGGESTED READINGS

Barash PG, Cullen BF, Stoelting RK, eds. *Clinical Anesthesia*. 4th ed. Philadelphia: Lippincott Williams & Wilkins; 2001.

Cote CJ, Todres ID, Ryan JF, Goudsouzian NG, eds. *A Practice of Anesthesia for Infants and Children*. 3rd ed. Philadelphia: Saunders; 2001.

124

THE PEDIATRIC AIRWAY IS A SCARY REPOSITORY FOR ALL KINDS OF FOREIGN BODIES

JANEY P. MCGEE, MD AND ROBERT D. VALLEY, MD

So... you are on call with that new ear, nose, and throat surgeon—the one who is new to your hospital and maybe new to the profession (just out of residency!). He wants you in to anesthetize a 10-month-old little girl who choked on "something she picked up off the rug" about 12 hours ago. Her chest X-ray is clear. She has had an intermittent cough and sounds wheezy in Mom's arms. You don't do a lot of little children and wonder if this is the right thing to do. You try talking to the surgeon, but he is distracted as he tries to piece together the seldom-used pediatric rigid bronchoscope. The surgeon assures you he did a "bunch of these" as a resident. Do you proceed or call the hospital administrator on call?

The potential for total airway obstruction, as well as the need to share the airway with the surgeon, makes anesthesia for foreign-body removal challenging. Commonly aspirated foods include peanuts, beans, hotdogs, watermelon seeds, and popcorn. Peanuts are the most common and can be difficult to remove because of the tendency to break into pieces upon attempted retrieval. Aspirated beans are challenging because they often swell once inside the airway and lead to further obstruction and edema. Nonfood items are more commonly aspirated by older children and include small plastic toys, balloon pieces, balls, and marbles.

Foreign-body aspiration should be considered in any child presenting with respiratory distress or with a pulmonary infection that is not responding to standard interventions. A history of a choking episode is found in 80% to 90% of confirmed cases. Chest radiographs are often normal during the first 24 hours. In one large retrospective series of 1,068 cases of foreign-body aspiration in children, radiographs were normal in nearly two thirds of cases. If an inspiratory film is normal, an expiratory film or fluoroscopy may be helpful. These views may demonstrate expiratory mediastinal shift away from the lung field containing the foreign body or postobstructive hyperinflation secondary to air trapping distal to the foreign body.

When foreign-body aspiration is suspected, rigid bronchoscopy is the gold standard. Rigid bronchoscopy permits control of the airway, good visualization, and manipulation of the object with a wide variety of forceps.

© 2006 Mayo Foundation for Medical Education and Research

Removal of a foreign body from the airway is considered an urgent to emergent procedure, depending on the degree of respiratory distress. A fasting patient is optimal, but the procedure should not be delayed if the airway is compromised or if the foreign body is of organic origin because of its potential to swell and produce asphyxia. The anesthesiologist should decide between using mask induction and intravenous (IV) induction on an individual basis. Most experts recommend mask induction followed by IV placement; however, rapid-sequence induction should be considered if the child has a full stomach. The use of nitrous oxide is a relative contraindication in the presence of air trapping, although most authors conclude that its use during a mask induction poses little risk. Using atropine or glycopyrrolate is recommended to reduce secretions before bronchoscopy, and a dose of a glucocorticoid can be given to reduce inflammation. After a deep plane of anesthesia is obtained, the airway should be examined with a laryngoscope to exclude any posterior pharyngeal foreign bodies and to spray the vocal cords and trachea with lidocaine in order to reduce irritation once the rigid bronchoscope is introduced.

Clinicians are divided over their approach to ventilating these patients. Some prefer spontaneous ventilation, others are equally adamamt that controlled ventilation, with or without muscle relevants, is the safest approach. There is a theoretical risk that a foreign body can be pushed more distally with positive-pressure ventilation. In a prospective randomized clinical trial to compare spontaneous and controlled ventilation during removal of airway foreign bodies in 36 children, it was concluded that routine use of controlled ventilation with muscle relaxants is the better technique. Ventilating a patient through the side port of a rigid bronchoscopy can be difficult, and the amount of inhaled anesthetic administered is unpredictable. Many clinicians would argue that having the patient breath spontaneously is safer. Airway leaks and resistance are highly variable depending on the bronchoscopic instrumentation, patient size, level of the foreign body, depth of anesthesia and relaxation of the patient. Communication between the anesthesiologists and surgeon is essential during the procedure because the distal end of the bronchoscope may need to be occluded. Adequate oxygenation frequently requires the administration of 100% oxygen.

Sixty percent of airway foreign bodies are located in the right lung. Of the remainder, 23% are in the left lung, 3% are in the larynx, 13% are in the trachea or carina, and 2% are in both lungs. During removal of a foreign body, total-airway obstruction may occur. If a single object breaks into multiple pieces, the uninvolved lung may become obstructed. An object, such as a bean, that has swollen can become lodged in the trachea upon attempted removal. The complication of total-airway obstruction is a possibility whenever a foreign body is being removed. Immediate recognition and treatment is essential. If the surgeon can remove the foreign body, it must be done in a timely fashion. If that is not possible, the foreign body can be pushed distally until ventilation is reestablished. If a foreign body is pushed distally to obtain adequate ventilation and can no longer be retrieved bronchoscopically, a thoracotomy may be required.

Maintenance of deep anesthesia, with or without muscle relaxants, is essential for successful removal of an airway foreign body. Complications during bronchoscopy include laryngospasm, bronchospasm, laryngeal edema, arterial desaturations, and upper-airway damage. A retrospective review was done to quantify adverse events in 287 cases in which children had rigid bronchoscopy after mask induction and muscle paralysis for foreign-body aspiration. Anesthesia-related adverse events were seen in 0.7% of cases, whereas complications from rigid bronchoscopy were observed in 7.6% of cases. In this study, the most common anesthesia-related adverse event was laryngospasm upon extubation.

TAKE HOME POINTS

Anesthesia for airway foreign-body removal is challenging, and keys to success include the following:

- Open communication with the surgeon;
- A deep level of anesthesia, with or without paralysis;
- Quick recognition and treatment of total airway obstruction;
- Full emergence in the operating room with the otolaryngologists present; and
- Recognition and treatment of laryngospasm and postextubation stridor.

SUGGESTED READINGS

Eren S, Balci AE, Dikici B, et al. Foreign body aspiration in children: Experience of 1160 cases. *Ann Trop Paediatr*. 2003;23:31.

Soodan, A, Pawar D, Subramanium R. Anesthesia for removal of inhaled foreign bodies in children. *Pediatric Anesthesia*. 2004;14:947–952.

Tomaske M, Gerber A, Weiss M. Anesthesia and periinterventional morbidity of rigid bronchoscopy for trachebronchial foreign body diagnosis and removal. *Pediatric Anesthesia*. 2006;16:123–129.

125

EFFECTIVE EPIDURAL ANESTHESIA FOR CHILDREN DOES NOT ALWAYS REQUIRE A CATHETER

DENNIS YUN, MD AND ROBERT D. VALLEY, MD

Pediatric anesthesiologists at major centers often place epidural catheters for complex ureteral implant surgeries and many major lower-abdominal procedures. These catheters are used for both adjunctive anesthesia and postoperative pain control and are best managed by the experienced pediatric anesthesiologist. However, a one-time caudal epidural injection with local anesthetic (the "single-shot caudal") is a reliable and generally safe technique for patients undergoing smaller abdominal and lower-limb surgeries, such as inguinal hernia repair, hypospadias repair, circumcision, orchiopexy, and club foot repair. The authors feel that the single-shot caudal block is an underused technique, but that it should not be—its technical ease puts it well within the practice parameters of pediatric anesthesiologists who have less experience and anesthesiologists who provide care to pediatric patients only occasionally.

INDICATIONS

The single-shot caudal block is indicated for treating children ranging in age from infancy to approximately 8 years. Single-shot caudal blocks are usually placed at the end of the procedure to maximize the duration of postoperative analgesia; however, practice varies. If this block is placed at the beginning of the procedure, be aware that total anesthetic requirements will be decreased. *Always* discuss the planned block with the pediatric patient's parents. The older child should also be made aware that his or her legs may be difficult to feel after the surgery or that he or she may have trouble walking for a few hours.

CONTRAINDICATIONS

The single-shot caudal block is contraindicated for treating children with infection around the sacral hiatus, coagulopathy, increased intracranial pressure (ICP), uncorrected hypotension, or known anatomic abnormality and children whose parents refuse to consent.

ANATOMY

In patients younger than 1 year of age, the caudal extent of the dura and spinal cord ends at S3-4. The caudal space can be accessed through the

© 2006 Mayo Foundation for Medical Education and Research

sacral hiatus, which is flanked laterally by the prominent sacral cornu and covered by the sacral-coccygeal ligament.

TECHNIQUE

The patient should be placed in lateral decubitus position (left lateral for the right-handed anesthesiologist and right lateral for the left-handed anesthesiologist), with hips and knees flexed to help spread the gluteal muscles away from the sacral hiatus. Using aseptic technique, a 22-gauge needle (or 22-gauge Teflon intravenous catheter) is placed approximately 45 degrees to the skin until a "pop" is felt, which indicates penetration of the sacrococcygeal ligament. The needle should be slightly withdrawn and the angle lowered before advancing a few more millimeters into the canal. Aspiration is necessary to check for blood or cerebrospinal fluid. An initial test dose of 0.1 mL/kg of local anesthetic with 1:200,000 epinephrine can be used to exclude intravascular placement (see below). Resistance to injection should be minimal. Any resistance strongly suggests that the needle tip is not in the epidural space.

DOSING

For single-shot caudal epidural injection, long-acting local anesthetics, such as bupivacaine (0.125% to 0.25%) and ropivacaine (0.2%), are typically used. The volume of local anesthetic depends on the desired blockade level. 0.5 mL/kg can be adequate for sacral blockade, whereas 1.0 mL/kg is needed for upper-abdominal blockade. The maximum volume is 1.25 mL/kg, which will give you a low thoracic level in an infant. The maximum recommended dose for bupivacaine or ropivacaine is 3.0 mg/kg. For older children, the maximum volume of anesthetic injected into the epidural space (regardless of concentration) is usually about 20 mL. To prolong the block's duration, clonidine (1 to 2 mcg/kg) can be added to the local-anesthetic solution.

COMPLICATIONS

Dural Puncture Unintentional dural puncture can lead to total spinal. Symptoms include apnea, blown pupil, hypotension, and unresponsiveness. Younger children (less than 6 years of age) usually do not exhibit unstable hemodynamics due to an immature sympathetic system and greater centralization of their intravascular space. Treatment is supportive: Airway management, ventilation or oxygenation (or both), and circulatory support (fluids and vasopressors, as indicated).

Intravascular Injection. Intravascular injection is the most common serious complication of caudal anesthesia. Using a test dose and looking only for heart-rate changes is not a sensitive indicator of intravascular injection in anesthetized children. Changes in electrocardiogram (EKG) morphology, especially peaked T-waves and broadening of the QRS complex, are more sensitive indicators of intravascular (or intraosseous) injection. A caudal block should *never* be placed without continuous EKG monitoring. Even after a negative response to an initial test dose, the anesthesiologist must give the remaining local anesthetic incrementally, looking for EKG changes after administration of each dose. Local-anesthetic toxicity manifests as seizures, hypotension, arrhythmia, and cardiovascular collapse. Support includes airway management, ventilation or oxygenation (or both), circulatory support, and antiseizure medication. The importance of chest compressions cannot be over emphasized, since the primary offset to toxicity is redistribution, which cannot occur if circulatory support is not provided. Also, 20% lipid emulsion has recently been identified as a useful treatment for bupivacaine toxicity (see Chapter 128).

Intraosseous Injection. Intraosseous injection can lead to systemic toxicity similar to that caused by intravascular injections. The thin cortical bone of the sacrum is easily penetrated in pediatric patients. Treatment is the same as for intravascular injection.

TAKE HOME POINTS

Consider incorporating the single-shot caudal injection into your practice even if you are a pediatric anesthesiologist who has less experience or are an anesthesiologist who provides care to pediatric patients only occasionally.

- The typical age range of patients who are good candidates for single-shot caudal blocks is from infancy to approximately 8 years of age.
- Caudal blocks can be performed at the beginning or end of a procedure.
- Always discuss the block with the pediatric patient's parents and tell older children they may have "wobbly legs" when they wake up.
- Dosing varies according to agent, weight, and level of block desired. Maximum doses are given above.
- Maintain high vigilance for dural puncture (total spinal). Children become unresponsive and apneic but may not manifest overt hemodynamic signs.
- Avoidance of intravascular injection depends on close observation of the continuous EKG trace.
- Peaked T-waves and widening of the QRS complex are both sensitive indicators of intravascular or intraosseous injection.

SUGGESTED READINGS

Ansermino M, Basu R, Vandebeek C, et al. Nonopioid additives to local anaesthetics for caudal blockade in children: A systematic review. *Paediatr Anaesth.* 2003;13(7):561–573.

Markakis DA. Regional anesthesia for pediatrics. *Anesthesiol Clin North America.* 2000;18(2):355–381.

Mulroy MF. *Caudal Anesthesia in Regional Anesthesia: An Illustrated Procedural Guide.* 3rd ed. Philadelphia: Lippincott Williams & Wilkins; 2002:119–125.

Rosenblatt MA, Abel M, Fischer GW, et al. Successful use of a 20% Lipid Emulsion to Resuscitate a Patient after Presumed Bupivacaine-related Cardiac Arrest. *Anesthesiology.* 2006;105(1):217–218.

126

KEEPING BABIES WARM IN THE PERIOPERATIVE PERIOD IS IMPORTANT, CHALLENGING, AND, AT TIMES, DANGEROUS!

KATHLEEN A. SMITH, MD

Virtually all pediatric patients become hypothermic in the perioperative period, unless measures are taken to maintain normothermia. Hypothermia leads to a variety of complications, including delayed emergence, prolonged neuromuscular blockade, platelet dysfunction, increased oxygen consumption upon emergence, and poor wound healing. Thus, the anesthesiologist must continuously monitor core temperature and actively prevent heat loss in the operating room (OR), as well as in the postanesthesia care unit (PACU). Keep in mind that there are actually a number of reasons for heat loss. Also, cooling begins with exposure of the patient upon removal of his clothing; accordingly, do not have the baby undressed until it is necessary.

The most important type of heat loss is via radiation, but convection, conduction, and evaporation also play a role. Most ORs are kept extremely cold, which allows for tremendous radiant heat loss to the OR environment. Next, the surgical site is prepped with cold solution, which partially evaporates from the skin, decreasing the body's temperature further. Other evaporative losses occur from surgical incisions as well as from the airway. Volatile anesthetics cause vasodilation, which brings heat to the cutaneous surface where it can participate in heat exchange with the environment. During the first half hour of anesthesia, it is this redistribution of heat from the core to the periphery that causes the patient's temperature to drop 0.5° to 1.5° C. General anesthesia also impairs normal function of the body's thermoregulatory center, the hypothalamus. Under normal circumstances, the vessels of the body constrict to conserve heat, while metabolic heat production is increased. Peripheral vasodilation is combined with a 20% decease in heat production, thus altering the thermal steady state.

Heat loss is directly proportional to surface area. Because infants and neonates have a very large surface-area-to-volume ratio, they are particularly prone to becoming hypothermic. In addition, metabolic heat production is a function of mass. Therefore, not only do they lose heat faster, but they are less capable of producing heat. Infants and neonates do not shiver. Instead, they produce heat via nonshivering thermogenesis, which takes place primarily in brown fat. This mechanism of heat production, which continues until 2 years of age, is inhibited by anesthesia and sympathetic blockade.

© 2006 Mayo Foundation for Medical Education and Research

For the many aforementioned reasons, anesthesiologists often battle intraoperative hypothermia on a regular basis. This has led to the development of various mechanisms that can be used to maintain normothermia during anesthesia. Some of the methods are simple and can be of tremendous benefit. Warming the operating room by 1° C will decrease the patient's heat loss by 7%. This is an easy and effective means of preventing heat loss form the start of the procedure. Passive insulators, such as blankets or plastic bags wrapped around the exposed surfaces of the body, may reduce heat losses up to 30%. An infant's head is a major source of heat loss, given its large surface area, and should be wrapped to decrease radiant heat losses. Warming intravenous fluids helps prevent hypothermia during longer procedures with greater fluid requirements. It has been shown that 1 L of room-temperature fluid given to an adult reduces core temperature between 0.25° and 1.0° C. A similar result is seen in children receiving a comparable volume of unwarmed fluid. Circulating water mattresses are used less often to reduce conductive heat losses. Their effectiveness is limited, given that they only reduce the already minimal heat loss from a patient's back. Warming lights, infrared heaters, and warm preparatory and irrigation solutions may also be of benefit.

Perhaps the most popular means of preventing hypothermia intraoperatively is the forced-air warmer. These devices work via convective heat transfer and depend on a device-skin temperature gradient. As helpful as this device can be, improper use may have an effect opposite of that intended and may even be dangerous. The Food and Drug Administration notes several reports of patient injury resulting from the use of warming hoses that are not attached to a warming blanket. This so-called "free-hosing" has led to third-degree burns in several patients. A second pitfall with forced-air warming devices is unintentional patient cooling when either the skin beneath the blanket or the blanket itself becomes wet as a result of messy surgical preparation or leakage of irrigation fluid or body fluids. Little information has been published regarding this phenomenon. To quantify the degree of patient cooling that can result when this occurs, we performed our own miniature experiment. Skin-temperature probes were placed on two warm saline bottles, before covering each of them with a forced-air warming blanket. Both forced-air warming blankets were turned on, set to 43° C, and allowed to equilibrate for 10 minutes. Following this, 125 mL of warm irrigation fluid was poured over the blanket covering bottle A. Bottle B remained dry. The starting temperatures for bottles A and B were 37.8° and 37.3° Celsius, respectively. Ten minutes later, bottle A had cooled from 37.8° to 35.5° C, whereas bottle B remained at 37.3° C. After 15 minutes, bottles A and B were at 34.9° and 37.2° C, respectively.

Clearly, the soiled blanket was not only ineffective at heating but actually might have cooled a patient significantly in a short period of time.

Steps must be taken to prevent forced-air warming blankets from becoming soiled. This starts with awareness of all personnel, especially surgeons. A preparatory job that is sloppy and uses an excessive amount of solution is the anesthesiologist's enemy. In addition, a plastic sheet is included with each forced-air warming blanket. This sheet may be used to make a barrier between the operative field and the blanket itself. This step may reduce the incidence of saturating the blanket, both during the surgical preparation and throughout the surgery. If a warming blanket does become wet, it should be removed and, if possible, replaced with a new blanket. If a warmer must be removed, the OR temperature should be increased. This may be an incentive for all OR personnel to be cautious not to allow the blanket to become wet.

Finally, be aware of iatrogenic hyperthermia. Many practitioners, in an effort to prevent hypothermia, overuse warming techniques, resulting in hyperthermia. This is not uncommon in dental surgery, for example, where virtually the entire body is covered and no body cavities are exposed. This results in very minimal, if any, heat loss. These procedures tend to be long, and the child's basal metabolic rate naturally generates heat. If atropine has been given, sweating is reduced, preventing dissipation of this heat and increasing body temperature. In this situation, a forced-air warming blanket may actually be used to help cool a febrile patient, using the warming blanket's ambient setting.

TAKE HOME POINTS

- We want our pediatric patients to be warm, but not too warm, and we need to keep them warm effectively and safely.
- Don't let the warming blankets get wet!

SUGGESTED READINGS

Badgwell JM, ed. *Clinical Pediatric Anesthesia*. Philadelphia: Lippincott-Raven; 415, 472–473.
Davis P, Motoyama EK, Davis PJ, eds. *Anesthesia for Infants and Children*. 7th ed. Philadelphia: Mosby; 2006:158–163, 166–173.
Food and Drug Administration. http://www.fda.gov. Medical devices database.
Gregory GA. *Pediatric Anesthesia*. 4th ed. Philadelphia: Churchill Livingstone; 2002:63 –77.

127

FOCUS ON PREVENTION AND TREATMENT OF EMERGENCE DELIRIUM

WARREN K. ENG, MD AND ROBERT D. VALLEY, MD

Emergence delirium can be a frustrating and stressful situation for everybody involved, including the patients' families and the nurses. A scenario might unfold as follows: A 5-year-old patient with a history of mild attention deficit and hyperactivity disorder has come to your operating room for an emergency esophago gastroduodenoscopy (EGD) to rule out ingestion of a foreign body. The patient is given a midazolam premedication which helps some with the induction. The endoscopist finds nothing in the esophagus or stomach. You wake the child up from the sevoflurane anesthetic and, on the way to the postanesthesia care unit (PACU), he begins crying and thrashing. He catches the PACU nurse on the lip with the back of his head. There is blood. This doesn't look good for you. He is crying and moaning. You can't seem to get his attention even though his eyes are open. Mom comes in and says she has never seen him like this. She starts to cry because her child doesn't recognize her. The nurse looks at you and whispers, "You better do something to make this better!"

Emergence Delirium (ED), also frequently called emergence agitation, is a *diagnosis of exclusion*. A disoriented patient who is incognizant of his or her surroundings and of previously familiar individuals and objects and who is generally inconsolable and uncooperative is diagnosed as having ED, absent another diagnosis. Behavior ranges from incoherence and moaning, to thrashing, agitation, and paranoia or hallucinations. While usually self-limited (<1 hour in duration), ED can lead to many undesirable consequences, such as an inability to monitor the patient, disconnected intravenous (IV) lines, and significant physical trauma to the patient or caregivers (or both).

Hypoxia, inadequate analgesia, hypoglycemia, severe hypercarbia, increased intracranial pressure, nausea, and bladder distention are all factors to consider prior to settling on ED as the diagnosis for a pediatric patient's disorientation and agitation.

The incidence of ED is estimated to range from 5% to 55% and is higher in children who are 2 to 5 years of age than in younger and older children. One of the problems in recognizing and treating the disease has been the lack of a reliable and valid instrument for measuring ED in children. Previously, this precluded comparisons between trials and raised serious questions about the reliability and validity of research results. The development and evaluation

© 2006 Mayo Foundation for Medical Education and Research

of the Pediatric Anesthesia Emergence Delirium (PAED) Scale in 2004 will enable researchers to characterize ED in children accurately and to compare treatment options in future studies.

Various mechanisms have been postulated to cause ED; a definitive causality has yet to be identified. Volatile anesthetics (halothane, isoflurane, sevoflurane, and desflurane) are associated with an incidence of ED as high as 50%. Sevoflurane and desflurane have been extensively studied. Their low blood-gas-solubility quotient with rapid emergence has been theorized to lead to a higher incidence of ED. Numerous studies have yielded conflicting data but suggest that sevoflurane may be associated with a higher incidence of ED than desflurane. Ketamine, droperidol, atropine, and scopolamine also are associated with ED. Propofol, when used for maintenance of anesthesia, is associated with a very low incidence of ED.

Administering pain medication (fentanyl, 1 to 1.5 mcg/kg IV; or clonidine, 2 mcg/kg IV) may reduce the incidence of ED. Administering midazolam in advance does not consistently reduce the incidence of ED. In pediatric patients, ranging in age from 18 months to 10 years, having outpatient magnetic resonance imaging (a painless procedure) with use of sevoflurane, administering fentanyl (1 mcg/kg IV) 10 minutes before anesthetic discontinuation reduced the incidence of ED by 56%, whereas administering a placebo reduced the incidence of ED by 12%. Similar results were found in a group of 110 developmentally delayed American Society of Anesthesiologists (ASA) Physical Status 1-2 patients having dental restoration (with sevoflurane general anesthesia administered using laryngeal mask array [LMA]). These patients were randomly assigned to receive either fentanyl, 1 to 1.5 mcg/kg, or saline at induction of anesthesia. Notably, administering this dose of narcotic did not increase nausea and vomiting or delay discharge.

Intraoperative use of the alpha-2 adrenergic agonist clonidine, which has sedative and analgesic properties, can also provide ED prophylaxis. A prospective double-blind study examined the cases of 40 2- to 7-year-old boys having circumcision with penile block and sevoflurane general anesthesia. The boys were randomly assigned to receive clonidine, 2 mcg/kg IV, or placebo. Sixteen patients in the placebo group and two in the clonidine group developed agitation. Another prospective study examined the cases of 169 ASA Physical Status 1-2 patients having day surgery (with midazolam, 0.5 mg/kg, administered orally before the procedure and with sevoflurane general anesthesia administered using LMA). These patients were randomly assigned to receive clonidine, 2 mcg/kg IV, or saline prior to induction. The clonidine group had a lower incidence of ED (14.2%) than did the placebo group (33.3%), with no increase in the clonidine group's time to emergence.

The treatment options for ED in the PACU (i.e., rescue therapy) are controversial, even among clinicians with a special interest in this area. There is a lack of published data comparing fentanyl, clonidine, and propofol in formal clinical trials for rescue therapy; however, prospective observational studies are forthcoming. At present, fentanyl is the drug most frequently reported to be used for rescue therapy. Clonidine, besides being reported to be efficacious for prevention, has also been used anecdotally for treatment. Whatever the true efficacy of clonidine for rescue therapy, its use is not widely reported. Other pediatric anesthesiologists feel they have ample anecdotal evidence that small doses of propofol (1 mg/kg) are successful in treating ED in the PACU and prefer it to clonidine since it is generally a more readily available and familiar drug. Midazolam is thought to simply delay emergence and is not considered very useful for treating ED. Remember that, with time, ED usually resolves; therefore, a commonly employed strategy is gentle restraint of the patient until the ED passes. The decision to wait rather than treat depends on the severity of the ED, the availability of extra PACU staff to restrain the child, and the risk of injury or morbidity secondary to loss of invasive catheters or surgical drains.

TAKE HOME POINTS

- All that is agitation is not pain.
- The price of a rapid emergence may be delirium.
- A little narcotic can make for a smooth landing.

SUGGESTED READINGS

Cohen IT, Hannallah RS, Hummer KA. The incidence of emergence agitation associated with desflurane anesthesia in children is reduced by fentanyl. *Anesth Analg.* 2001;93:88–91.

Cravero JP, Beach M, Thyr B, et al. The effect of small dose fentanyl on the emergence characteristics of pediatric patients after sevoflurane anesthesia without surgery. *Anesth Analg.* 2003;97:364–367.

Hung WT, Chen CC, Liou CM, et al. The effects of low-dose fentanyl on emergence agitation and quality of life in patients with moderate developmental disabilities. *J Clin Anesth.* 2005;17:494–498.

Kulka PJ, Bressem M, Tryba M. Clonidine prevents sevoflurane-induced agitation in children. *Anesth Analg.* 2001;93:335–338.

Sikich N, Lerman J. Development and psychometric evaluation of the pediatric anesthesia emergence delirium scale. *Anesthesiology.* 2004;100(5):1138–1145.

Tesoro S, Mezzetti D, Marchesini L, et al. Clonidine treatment for agitation in children after sevoflurane anesthesia. *Anesth Analg.* 2005;101:1619–1622.

Uezono S, Goto T, Terui K, et al. Emergence agitation after sevoflurane versus propofol in pediatric patients. *Anesth Analg.* 2000;91:563–566.

Valley RD, Ramza JT, Calhoun P, et al. Tracheal extubation of deeply anesthetized pediatric patients: A comparison of isoflurane and sevoflurane. *Anesth Analg.* 1999;99:742–745.

Viitanen H, Annila P, Viitanen M, et al. Midazolam premedication delays recovery from propofol-induced sevoflurane anesthesia in children 1–3 years. *Can J Anaesth.* 1999;46:766–771.

128

REMEMBER THAT BABIES REALLY DO FEEL PAIN

ANGELA KENDRICK, MD

Pediatric pain management may be as "simple" as providing a single-shot caudal with local anesthetic for postoperative pain relief or as "complex" as providing consultative and management services for children with sickle cell disease, cancer pain, or complex regional pain syndromes.

This chapter is intended to provide you with some strategies for evaluating pediatric pain, to remind you of important pharmacokinetic and anatomic differences between infants and children, on the one hand, and adults, on the other, and to provide you with some tips on avoiding common mishaps associated with the treatment of acute pain in children.

EVALUATION OF PAIN

You must choose the appropriate pain scale. Pain scales are the tools you use to document the presence and severity of pain and the effectiveness of your treatment.

There are a number of behavior-based pain scales. The Children's Hospital of Eastern Ontario Pain Scale (CHEOPS) (*Table 128.1*) was developed by McGrath et al. to assess pain in the postanesthesia care unit (PACU). Six categories of behavior (crying, facial expression, verbal expression, movement of torso, touching of wound, and movement of legs) are observed and scored, and an appropriate number is charted to indicate the presence or intensity of a response.

The Face, Legs, Activity, Cry and Consolability (FLACC) scale (*Table 128.2*) is simpler than CHEOPS and is popular for the assessment of both infants and older, nonverbal patients. Parents or chronic caregivers of children with cognitive impairment have been shown to be sensitive to their child's method of expressing pain. This input can be invaluable for interpreting the developmentally disabled child's responses.

Observing physiologic parameters (heart rate, respirations, blood pressure, body temperature) is standard practice in evaluating a patient's overall condition. Physiologic variables are also incorporated into pain assessment, with rapid shallow breathing, elevated heart rate, and increased blood pressure possibly indicating the presence of pain.

Other methods of pain assessment, such as verbal self report, use of numeric scales, and use of the faces scale, are appropriate for use in older

© 2006 Mayo Foundation for Medical Education and Research

TABLE 128.1

CHILDREN'S HOSPITAL EASTERN ONTARIO PAIN SCALE (CHEOPS). RECOMMENDED FOR CHILDREN 1 TO 7 YEARS OF AGE; A SCORE GREATER THAN 4 INDICATES PAIN.

ITEM	BEHAVIORAL	POINTS	DEFINITION	SCORE
Crying	No crying	1	Child is not crying.	
	Moaning	2	Child is moaning or quietly vocalizing; silent cry.	
	Crying	2	Child is crying, but the cry is gentle or whimpering.	
	Scream	3	Child in a full-lunged cry; sobbing; may be scored with complaint or without complaint.	
Facial	Composed	1	Neutral facial expression.	
	Grimace	2	Score only if definite negative facial expression.	
	Smiling	0	Score only if definite positive facial expression.	
Verbal	None	1	Child not talking.	
	Other complaints	1	Child complains, but not about pain, e.g., "I want to see mommy" or "I am thirsty."	
	Pain complaints	2	Child complains about pain.	
	Both complaints	2	Child complains about pain and about other things, e.g., "It hurts; I want my mommy."	
	Positive	0	Child makes any positive statement or talks about others things without complaint.	
Torso	Neutral	1	Body (not limbs) is at rest; torso is inactive.	
	Shifting	2	Body is in motion in a shifting or serpentine fashion.	
	Tense	2	Body is arched or rigid.	
	Shivering	2	Body is shuddering or shaking involuntarily.	
	Upright	2	Child is in a vertical or upright position.	
	Restrained	2	Body is restrained.	
Touch	Not touching	1	Child is not touching or grabbing at wound.	
	Reach	2	Child is reaching for but not touching wound.	
	Touch	2	Child is gently touching wound or wound area.	
	Grab	2	Child is grabbing vigorously at wound.	
	Restrained	2	Child's arms are restrained.	
Legs	Neutral	1	Legs may be in any position but are relaxed; includes gentle swimming or serpentine-like movements.	
	Squirming or kicking	2	Definitive uneasy or restless movements in the legs or striking out with foot or feet (or both).	
	Drawn up or tensed	2	Legs tensed or pulled up tightly to body and kept there.	
	Standing	2	Standing, crouching, or kneeling.	
	Restrained	2	Child's legs are being held down.	

From McGrath PJ. *Medical Algorithms*. www.medal.org, with permission.

TABLE 128.2	FACE, LEGS, ACTIVITY, CRY AND CONSOLABILITY (FLACC) BEHAVIORAL PAIN ASSESSMENT TOOL	
CATEGORY	DESCRIPTION	SCORE
Face	0 = No particular expression or smile	0
	1 = Occasional grimace/frown, withdrawn or disinterested	1
	2 = Frequent/constant quivering chin, clenched jaw	2
Legs	0 = Normal position or relaxed	0
	1 = Uneasy, restless, tense	1
	2 = Kicking or legs drawn up	2
Activity	0 = Lying quietly, normal position, moves easily	0
	1 = Squirming, shifting back and forth, tense	1
	2 = Arched, rigid, or jerking	2
Cry	0 = No cry	0
	1 = Moans or whimpers, occasional complaint	1
	2 = Crying steadily, screams or sobs, frequent complaints	2
Consolability	0 = Content and relaxed	0
	1 = Reassured by occasional touching, hugging or being talked to, distractable	1
	2 = Difficult to console or comfort	2

From Voepel-Lewis T, Merkel S, et al. The reliability and validity of the FLACC Observational Tool as a measurement of pain in children with cognitive impairment. *Anesth Analg.* 2002;95:1224–1229, with permission.

children but have their disadvantages. For example, the child may want to avoid a potential painful encounter (fear of needles), so the child denies any pain. A child may fail to understand ordinal numbers and pick a higher "better" number, or the child may pick the smiley face on the faces scale because it is the face he or she likes the best.

KNOW YOUR HIGH-RISK POPULATIONS

Infants younger than 3 months of age, infants born prematurely that are less than 60 weeks postmenstrual age (formerly called postconceptual age), and any child with a history of apnea or airway compromise, cardiac compromise, or neuromuscular disease are at risk for cardiorespiratory complications following opioid or sedative administration. You need to carefully titrate your dose and monitor these children after administration of opioids or sedatives. *Premature Infants and Neonates Require Special Consideration.* We now know that the preterm infant has the neurophysiologic pathways to experience pain and the inhibitory pathways for modulating the pain response are less developed. Inadequate relief of pain in the neonatal intensive care unit may lead to an accelerated catabolic response, with increased secretion of stress hormones and altered sleep-wake cycles. Inadequate pain relief in the very young may lead to a long-term altered response (increased sensitivity) to pain.

Drug Metabolism in the Neonate. Newborns have lower levels of plasma proteins, including albumin and alpha (1) acid glycoprotein, than do adults. When protein-bound drugs are administered, newborns have a higher free fraction of drug, which is the pharmacologically active form, than do adults.

Infants may have physiologic processes that impair renal or portal blood flow (necrotizing enterocolitis, abdominal compartment syndrome, reduced systemic cardiac output), so metabolism and elimination of drugs may become unpredictable.

Newborns are slow metabolizers due to liver immaturity. This ability rapidly increases during the first 3 months of life. Hepatic metabolism occurs in two phases:

a) Phase 1 (oxidation, hydroxylation, and hydrolysis or reduction) involves the cytochrome P-450 enzyme system.

b) Phase II enzymes conjugate the metabolites of the phase 1 reactions. Phase II conjugation with glucuronyl transferases may be also be impaired in the newborn.

Since the kidney clears both parent drug and metabolites produced by the liver, renal failure causes accumulation and potential toxicity.

DRUG THERAPY FOR ACUTE PAIN

Opioid Infusions in the Neonate. Pain from a variety of causes can be managed via a continuous IV infusion with bolus supplementation. The two opioids most frequently used in the neonate are morphine and fentanyl. Neonates who are not intubated need particularly careful monitoring

a) Morphine does not require Phase I metabolism but undergoes Phase II glucuronidation, producing morphine 3 glucuronide (nonactive) and morphine 3,6 diglucuronide (active). Morphine has a prolonged half-life in neonates (6.8 hours and up to 10 hours in the preterm infant). The loading dose range for IV administration is 50 to 100 mcg/kg. The amount of drug used in constant-infusion doses depends on the patient's rate of metabolism, degree of pain, and other individual characteristics.

b) Fentanyl is highly bound to alpha (1)-acid glycoprotein. Its elimination half-life is prolonged in premature infants and newborns and is even more prolonged after a continuous infusion. The "context-sensitive half time" refers to the time for drug concentration at the sites of action to decrease by half. Newborns receiving fentanyl infusions for longer than 36 hours have a context sensitive half time of greater than 9 hours. Initial IV dosing for acute pain is 0.5 to 1 mcg/kg. Continuous-infusion rates are highly variable and depend on the degree of pain, the duration of administration, and the development of tolerance (see below).

PCA for Children

a) Use of standard preprinted Patient-Controlled Analgesia (PCA) order sheets, with suggested dose ranges, monitoring standards, and discontinuation of other sedative medications, is important in the care of any infant or child receiving continuous opioid therapy. The orders, the infusions, and their pumps must be reviewed on a daily basis.

b) If true PCA is to be used (rather than a continuous nonadjustable infusion), the child must understand how to push the button .The lockouts must be preset so that only a safe hourly maximum dose is delivered. "PCA by proxy," with the parents or nurse pressing the "pain button," is also used in a number of hospitals. This form of "PCA" is very controversial.

c) Infants and children receiving continuous infusions of opioids develop tolerance and require increasing doses to maintain the same effect. Data from studies done on animals show that young animals develop tolerance at a quicker rate than do adult animals. If continuous opioid infusion therapy has been used for longer than 5 to 7 days, abrupt discontinuation may result in withdrawal symptoms. The duration of drug exposure and the accumulated amount of drug administered are factors to consider when planning your weaning protocol. Weaning protocols usually reduce opioids by 10% to 20% per day, with careful observation for tachycardia, diarrhea, irritability, or other signs of opioid withdrawal. Long-acting opioids, such as methadone and the alpha agonist clonidine, are sometimes useful to assist with the weaning process.

Adjuncts Other than Opioids. Multimodal therapy is important in treating postoperative pain. Acetaminophen (orally or rectally) given as a scheduled medication (not on an as-needed basis) has a significant opioid-sparing effect. Other nonsteroidal analgesics (Ketorolac) should also be considered for use. Ketamine (small dose, <0.5 mg /kg IV) has also been used in the PACU and in low-dose infusions postoperatively. It is a noncompetitive antagonist of the N-methyl-D-asparate (NMDA) receptor and produces a synergistic effect to opioid analgesia.

REGIONAL ANESTHESIA FOR POSTOPERATIVE PAIN

In contrast to blocks for adults, the majority of blocks for children are placed after the induction of general anesthesia. Detecting an intravascular injection with a test dose of local anesthetic (5 mcg/mL of epinephrine) is less reliable in the presence of inhalational anesthetics. You must watch carefully for an increase in heart rate, a decrease in heart rate, or a change in T-wave morphology (peaked T waves); blood pressure may not increase with intravascular injection. Because the child is anesthetized, central nervous system symptoms may be masked and cardiovascular collapse may seem to occur without warning.

There are important anatomic differences to remember when placing caudal blocks or lumbar epidurals in pediatric patients. The subarachnoid space extends to S3-4 in the newborn before rising to the adult level of S1 at about the age of 1 year. This means the cerebrospinal fluid space is easy to enter when placing a caudal block in an infant. The neonatal spinal chord also extends to a lower lumbar level as low as L3 before receding to the adult level of L1.

Single shot caudal blocks are widely used to provide postoperative pain relief for operations done below the level of the patient's umbilicus. Intravascular injection, intrathecal injection, and intraosseous injection are all complications associated with this block. Careful advancement of the needle, with gentle aspiration after advancement, test dosing, continuous electrocardiogram monitoring, and incremental dosing will help you avoid catastrophic events.

As noted above, local anesthetic toxicity may develop acutely if the local anesthetic is inadvertently given intravenously or intraosseously. Toxicity may also be the result of accumulation of the local anesthetic with continuous, repeated, or inappropriately large dosing.

As with opioids, the pharmacokinetics of local anesthetic metabolism are different in infants. The amide anesthetics are metabolized through the immature cytochrome p 450 system. Infants have a higher steady-state volume of distribution for local anesthetics than do adults, which leads to a prolonged half-life in infants. Local anesthetics are bound by alpha (1) acid glycoproteins; accordingly, a higher fraction of free drug exists in infants.

Infants younger than 4 months of age who receive continuous infusions of local anesthetics (e.g., caudal epidural infusions of bupivacaine) develop increasing plasma levels of bupivacaine. The toxic plasma level of bupivacaine is in the range of 4 mcg/mL. The increasing plasma levels over time, as well as case reports of infants having toxic reactions (seizures, cardiac toxicity) while receiving higher dose infusions, have led to recommendations that infants younger than 4 months of age receive no more than 0.2 to 0.25 mg/kg/hr of bupivacaine. The duration of the infusion should be 48 hours or less. Older infants and children may receive bupivacaine infusions of 0.4 to 0.5 mg/kg/hr.

Ropivacaine has been studied in infants and similar pharmacokinetics apply. An initial epidural dose of 1 to 2 mg/kg, followed by an infusion of 0.2 mg/kg/hr for infants younger than 180 days of age and 0.4 mg/kg for infants older than 180 days of age, is considered safe.

Cardiac toxicity with bupivacaine can be very difficult to treat. Recent reports of adult cases and results from studies done in dogs have suggested that a 20% intralipid infusion may be the first-line therapy. The recommended dose for treatment of local anesthetic toxicity is 1 mL/kg over

1 minute, and it may be repeated twice every 3 to 5 minutes, followed by an infusion at 0.25 mL/kg/min until the patient is hemodynamically stable.

TAKE HOME POINTS

- Select an appropriate pain scale for evaluating the child's pain.
- Family or care giver feedback is necessary in evaluating the child who has cognitive impairment.
- Premature infants, infants younger than 3 months of age, and children with cardiopulmonary compromise, sleep apnea, or neuromuscular disease have a higher risk of adverse events from opioid administration.
- Withdrawal symptoms may occur if administration of opioids is abruptly discontinued after 5 to 7 days of continuous infusion.
- The potential for local-anesthetic toxicity with use of bupivacaine limits the infusion dose for infants to 0.2 to 0.25 mg/kg/hr.

SUGGESTED READINGS

Bosenburg AT, Thomas J, Cronje L, et al. Pharmacokinetics and efficacy of ropivacaine for continuous epidural infusion in neonates and infants. *Paediatr Anaesth.* 2005;15(9): 739–749.

Freid EB, Bailey AG, Valley RD. Electrocardiographic and hemodynamic changes associated with unintentional intravascular injection of bupivacaine with epinephrine in infants. *Anesthesiology.* 1993;79:394–398.

McCloskey JJ, Haun SE, Deshpande JK. Bupivacaine toxicity secondary to continuous caudal bupivacaine infusion in children. *Anesth Analg.* 1992;75(2):287–290.

McGrath PJ, Johnson G, Goodman JY, et al. CHEOPS: A behavioral scale for rating postoperative pain in children. In: Fields HW, Dubner R, Cervero F, eds. *Advances in Pain Research and Therapy.* New York: Raven Press; 1985:395–402.

Merkel SI, Voepel-Lewis T, Shayevitz JR, et al. The FLACC: A behavioral scale for scoring postoperative pain in young children. *Pediatr Nurs.* 1997;23(3):293–297.

Yaster M, Krane EJ, Kaplan RF, et al, eds. *Pediatric Pain Management and Sedation Handbook.* St. Louis, Missouri: Mosby Year Book; 1997.

129

DON'T LET THE SURGEONS DISCHARGE EVERY PEDIATRIC PATIENT!

PEGGY P. DIETRICH, MD AND ROBERT D. VALLEY, MD

You are at your outpatient surgery center. You run in to see your last patient of the day. It's a 3.5-month-old baby who is scheduled to have an inguinal hernia repair; this case should be a piece of cake! You are confused though when you see the baby. He is awfully little, weighing only 2.1 kg. Speaking with the mother, you find out that she has only had little Tommy at home for the last 2 weeks and that this hernia popped up 2 days ago. Tommy is so tiny because he arrived 14 weeks early. While talking to both the mother and the surgeons, you quickly calculate that he was born at 26 weeks gestation and that he is now just 40 weeks postconceptual age (26 weeks of gestational age plus 14 weeks of chronologic age). Except for the hernia, the mother says all is well. Use of the apnea monitor was discontinued just before Tommy went home. The surgeon says that the hernia needs to be fixed because it is hard to reduce. He asks you, "Can't you just watch him for a couple of hours here then let them go home?" What should you do?

Idiopathic apnea occurs in up to 55% of infants born prior to 37 weeks of gestation and in up to 2% to 3% of full-term infants. All infants, especially those born prematurely, are at risk for postoperative apnea. It is crucial to identify those infants at increased risk for postoperative apnea in order to provide extended monitoring and intervention when necessary.

Apnea is defined as an unexplained pause in breathing lasting 15 to 20 seconds or one lasting less than 15 seconds when associated with bradycardia (heart rate <80), cyanosis, pallor, or marked hypotonia. There are three identifiable types of apnea. Central apnea is characterized by a lack of respiratory effort. Obstructive apnea exists when respiratory effort is present without airflow. Mixed apnea is a combination of both central and obstructive mechanisms.

The most common pattern of apnea in infants has a mixed etiology, withcentral apnea playing the predominant role. Infants, particularly those born prematurely, have an immature central nervous system that manifests as a decreased response to carbon dioxide and a paradoxic response to hypoxia, leading to apnea rather than hyperventilation. Other contributing factors to neonatal apnea include immature intercostal and diaphragmatic musculature, an unstable pliable rib cage, an easily obstructed upper airway, and a lower airway prone to collapse. The long-term consequences of apnea

© 2006 Mayo Foundation for Medical Education and Research

are largely undefined. However, it is reasonable to conclude that hypoxemia associated with repeated apnea increases the likelihood of central nervous system damage.

Anesthesia accentuates a neonate's propensity for apneic events. The first apneic spell can occur up to 12 hours postoperatively. Both inhalational and intravenous anesthetics alter respiratory function. Inhaled anesthetics compromise the infant's immature central nervous system. They have been shown to reduce the central response to respiratory stimulants, including hypercarbia and hypoxia, and to enhance the response to inhibitory afferents. Furthermore, inhaled anesthetics relax pharyngeal musculature, promoting upper-airway obstruction in the neonate who is already prone to obstructive apnea. Intravenous anesthetics, including opioids, also depress the central-nervous-system respiratory centers.

One option for preventing or reducing postoperative apnea in preterm infants is perioperative administration of caffeine citrate (10–20 mg/kg). Caffeine, a methylxanthine, is thought to stimulate breathing by promoting central nervous system excitation, increasing intercostal and diaphragmatic muscle performance, and augmenting chemoreceptor responsiveness to hypercarbia and hypoxemia. Two small studies have demonstrated the usefulness of caffeine to prevent postoperative apnea in infants. Nonetheless, absolute indications for perioperative administration of caffeine remain to be determined by larger studies intended to identify those infants who would most benefit from the drug.

Investigators have attempted to determine whether using regional anesthesia rather than general anesthesia reduces the incidence of postoperative apnea in infants. A recent meta-analysis included four small studies comparing spinal anesthesia and general anesthesia with respect to the incidence of postoperative apnea following inguinal hernia repair. This meta-analysis failed to demonstrate a statistically significant difference in the percentage of infants with postoperative apnea or postoperative oxygen desaturation based upon anesthetic technique. However, when the patients given preoperative sedatives were excluded, the meta-analysis suggested a lower incidence of postoperative apnea in the spinal anesthetic group. It was concluded that larger studies are needed to clarify the risks and benefits of regional versus general anesthesia in the prevention of postoperative apnea.

Postoperative apnea is reported to have occurred in infants as old as 55 weeks of postconceptual age (postconceptual age = gestational age + age after birth) following extensive surgical procedures. Identifying at-risk infants and determining their need for postoperative monitoring following anesthesia is a great challenge. Many investigators have attempted to identify those infants at greatest risk. In a meta-analysis of eight published reports involving 255 prematurely born infants following inguinal hernia repair, the data revealed that there is a strong inverse relationship between apnea and gestational age and also between apnea and postconceptual age. The authors estimate that the risk of apnea is not less than 1% until postconceptual age is 54 weeks and gestational age is 35 weeks. The meta-analysis found that apnea continuing after hospital discharge and anemia (hematocrit <30), especially for infants older than 43 weeks of postconceptual age, are additional risk factors for postoperative apnea. Finally, the authors determined that the majority of apneic spells resolve without intervention; however, they were unable to identify predictors of the likelihood of self-recovery from an apnea spell.

Based upon reported investigations, general recommendations and guidelines employed at our institution include the following:

1) An infant's need for extended postoperative monitoring is evaluated on a case-by-case basis, considering the patient's gestational and postconceptual age, ongoing apneic events, hematocrit, other comorbidities, and type of surgery.

2) Elective surgery for term infants is delayed until infants are older than 44 weeks of postconceptual age.

3) Premature infants younger than 50 weeks of postconceptual age are admitted and monitored or for at least 18 hours postoperatively. Infants whose postconceptual age is between 50 and 60 weeks are monitored in our postanesthesia care unit for a minimum of 2 hours prior to discharge.

TAKE HOME POINTS

- Postoperative apnea in infants is real.
- The risk increases with decreasing gestational age at birth and chronologic age at the time of surgery.
- Your facility should have a policy to deal with these high-risk patients in a consistent manner.

SUGGESTED READINGS

Berman RE, Kliegman RM, Jenson HB, eds. *Nelson Textbook of Pediatrics*. 17th ed. Philadelphia: Saunders; 2004.

Craven PD, Badawi N, Henderson-Smart DJ, et al. Regional (spinal, epidural, caudal) versus general anesthesia in preterm infants undergoing inguinal herniorrhaphy in early infancy. In: *The Cochrane Database of Systematic Reviews*. 2003;3:.

Cote CJ, Zaslavsky A, Downes JJ, et al. Postoperative apnea in former preterm infants after inguinal herniorrhaphy: A combined analysis. *Anesthesiology*. 1995;82(4):809–822.

Gregory GA, ed. *Pediatric Anesthesia*. 4th ed. Philadelphia, PA: Churchill Livingstone; 2002.

Henderson-Smart DJ, Steer P. Prophylactic caffeine to prevent postoperative apnea following general anesthesia in preterm infants. *The Cochrane Database of Systematic Reviews*. 2001; 4:CD000048. Review.

Motoyama EK, Davis PJ, eds. *Smith's Anesthesia for Infants and Children*. 7th ed. Philadelphia: Mosby Elsevier; 2006.

130

RECOGNIZE PREDICTORS AND PATTERNS OF CARDIAC ARREST IN THE ANESTHETIZED CHILD

KIRK LALWANI, MD, FRCA

A simple Child,
That lightly draws its breath,
And feels its life in every limb,
What should it know of death?
('We are Seven' – William Wordsworth, 1770–1850)

The death of a child is a tragedy for everyone involved. Unexpected cardiac arrest may occur in anesthetized children despite optimal care. Several factors are known to be associated with an increased risk of anesthesia-related cardiac arrest in children, and the pediatric care provider should be familiar with them in order to minimize the potential risk.

Following the dramatic decline in anesthesia-related mortality rates over the last 50 years, there has recently been a change in the profile of anesthesia-related cardiac arrest in children. Many studies have identified predictors of increased risk for anesthesia-related cardiac arrest in children, but detailed analysis of the root cause of the arrests is based on data collected in the Pediatric Perioperative Cardiac Arrest Registry (POCA). POCA was initiated in 1994 as an offshoot of the American Society of Anesthesiologists (ASA) Closed-Claims Project to identify the most common causes of anesthesia-related cardiac arrest in children and to outline strategies for prevention. The initial POCA findings reported details of 150 cases of anesthesia-related cardiac arrest, which occurred between 1994 and 1997 in 63 North American institutions. The latest report summarizes approximately 300 additional cases submitted from 1998 to 2003.

PREDICTORS OF ANESTHESIA-RELATED CARDIAC ARREST IN CHILDREN

American Society of Anesthesiologists Physical Status. The strongest predictor of anesthesia-related cardiac arrest in the POCA study was ASA physical status of 3 to 5; such status was associated with a 12-fold increase in the odds of cardiac arrest. ASA physical status as a predictor of increased risk is also supported by data from other studies.

Emergency Surgery. Emergency surgery was associated with a three-fold increase in risk for cardiac arrest in the POCA study, as well as with

© 2006 Mayo Foundation for Medical Education and Research

an increased risk of other anesthetic complications in a landmark French study.

Age. The risk of anesthetic complications and cardiac arrest in children varies inversely with age. Neonates and infants are particularly at risk. Approximately 50% of all arrests in the POCA registry occurred in infants (<1 year of age), and 15% occurred in neonates (<1 month of age). Of note, however, is that when underlying disease severity was accounted for (i.e., ASA status), age alone was not a predictor of death in the POCA study.

CHANGING PROFILE OF ANESTHESIA-RELATED CARDIAC ARREST IN CHILDREN

Causes of Cardiac Arrest. Of the 150 cases of cardiac arrest submitted to POCA, 37% were related to medication. Two thirds were likely due to halothane, alone or in combination with other drugs. Medications were also deemed responsible for 64% of arrests in patients whose ASA physical status was 1 or 2. Based on the analysis of an additional 163 anesthesia-related cases added to the registry, medication-related causes declined from 37% to 20%, primarily due to a decline in cardiac depression induced by volatile agents. Cardiovascular causes of arrest are now the most common, increasing from 32% to 36%. In this category, hypovolemia (frequently due to hemorrhage) and hyperkalemia (secondary to massive transfusion) were the most frequent causes of arrest. Respiratory causes increased from 20% to 27%, with laryngospasm, airway obstruction, inadvertent extubation, difficult intubation, and bronchospasm being the most frequent events. Equipment-related arrests (4%) were commonly due to complications of central-venous-pressure (CVP) catheter placement. Assorted other causes included complex cyanotic congenital heart disease, pulmonary hypertension, myocarditis, prolonged QT syndrome, coronary artery disease, hypertrophic cardiomyopathy, topical vasoconstrictor use, and anaphylactic reactions.

Demographics of Cardiac Arrest. The percentage of patients whose ASA physical status was 1 or 2 decreased from 33% in 1998 to 27% in 2003, along with the percentage of infants younger than 1 year of age (55% to 36%, $p<0.05$). The POCA investigators attribute the decline in medication-related arrests to these changes; halothane was often responsible for cardiac arrest in infants whose ASA physical status was 1 or 2. The mortality rate did not change significantly from 1998 to 2003 (26% in 1998, 28% in 2003), despite the altered profile of reported cases.

STRATEGIES TO PREVENT CARDIAC ARREST IN ANESTHETIZED CHILDREN

Specific Measures

Sevoflurane. Halothane has potent negative inotropic and chronotropic effects that can easily produce profound myocardial depression and a precipitous fall in cardiac output in infants and neonates, particularly when the ability of the halothane vaporizer to deliver concentrations in excess of six MAC-multiples is taken into account. The dramatic decline in medication-related deaths in the POCA study has been attributed to the widespread replacement of halothane with sevoflurane for pediatric anesthesia; sevoflurane has minimal effects on heart rate and myocardial contractility.

Local Anesthetics. Local anesthetics were used in 3.3% of cases of cardiac arrest reported in the initial POCA series. Meticulous technique is essential to prevent inadvertent intravascular injection of local anesthetics, which may result in cardiac arrest. Accurately placing the needle, carefully aspirating before injecting, using epinephrine-containing test doses, continuously monitoring electrocardiograms during dosing, and incrementally injecting the local anesthetic solution are some of the precautions used to reduce the incidence of this complication. In the future, widespread adoption of ultrasound-guided regional nerve blocks may significantly decrease the incidence of local anesthetic–related cardiac arrest. Should intravascular injection occur, studies done in animals and anecdotal case reports suggest that recovery from cardiac arrest may be more likely after ropivacaine use than after bupivacaine use. In addition, the use of 20% injectable fat emulsion such as Intralipid® (Fresenius Kahi) reduces the mortality of local anesthetic–induced arrest in animals. Anecdotal reports of human cases suggest Intralipid may be clinically useful and, given its innocuous nature, should be available in locations where regional-anesthetic blocks are placed.

Hypovolemia. In the POCA study, cardiac arrest due to hypovolemia occurred as a result of failure to manage hemorrhage adequately or as a result of hyperkalemia precipitated by massive transfusion. Inadequate intravenous access and failure of the anesthesiologist to keep up with blood loss were implicated in the hypovolemic arrests that occurred secondary to hemorrhage. Hyperkalemia related to massive transfusion occurs as a result of potassium leakage from stored red cells into the plasma. It can be minimized by using packed red blood cells instead of whole blood, requesting the freshest cells available, and avoiding irradiated blood unless indicated. In high-risk situations, such as cases involving infants and children requiring more than one blood volume of replacement and cases in which irradiated blood is necessary (e.g., an immunocompromised child), packed red cells should be washed by the blood bank, and intraoperative serum potassium levels should be carefully monitored.

Central venous pressure Catheter Placement. Cardiac arrest secondary to CVP catheter placement occurred as a result of cardiac tamponade, pneumothorax, or hemothorax in the POCA study. The closed-claims study reported that either ultrasound guidance or pressure waveform analysis would have prevented almost 50% of CVP catheter-placement–related complications. Routine use of an ultrasound device for placement is strongly recommended to increase success rates and decrease complications.

Succinylcholine. Use of succinylcholine is indicated in pediatric anesthesia cases with difficult or emergency airway management, and rapid-sequence induction is indicated for pediatric patients with a full stomach. However, routine use of succinylcholine has caused several deaths from hyperkalemia in children with undiagnosed muscular dystrophies, such as Duchenne's muscle dystrophy (DMD), prompting the manufacturer to change the recommended indications for succinylcholine use in children. Succinylcholine should not be used in children except as described above. Rocuronium provides adequate intubating conditions for rapid-sequence induction, and can be used in most instances.

Muscular Dystrophy. Children with progressive muscular dystrophy (Duchenne's and Becker's) are prone to rhabdomyolysis following the use of succinylcholine or volatile anesthetic agents. A recent editorial has questioned the use of volatile anesthesia (without muscle relaxants) for these patients following the report of yet another death in a child with undiagnosed DMD. Since we are unable to predict which children with DMD will develop clinical rhabdomyolysis following volatile anesthesia, avoiding use of volatile agents in these children and using an intravenous technique instead would be prudent. Since 90% of children with DMD have a family history of DMD, careful questioning about family members and eliciting the child's developmental milestones may trigger suspicion in asymptomatic children that merits preoperative creatine phosphokinase measurement.

General Measures

Perioperative Environment. The American Academy of Pediatrics has issued guidelines for the creation of a specialized environment for the provision of care for children. These guidelines encompass provider training, experience, and credentialing and the availability of appropriate equipment, drugs, and necessary support services, such as radiology and intensive care.

The Scope of Practice. Anesthetic outcomes for children are improved when anesthesiologists who are trained or experienced in the care of children are involved. Similarly, for specialized areas, such as congenital heart surgery, high-volume centers have lower mortality rates. Therefore, it is appropriate to transfer such patients to referral centers. The United Kingdom recognized this issue many years ago and has formulated criteria for specialist pediatric centers and providers in the National Health Service.

Continuous Quality Improvement. Continuous Quality Improvement (CQI) programs include morbidity and mortality conferences and critical incident registries to monitor key quality indicators, identify systematic problems, and implement strategies for the prevention of bad outcomes. Institutional and departmental compliance with professional society guidelines establishes a standard to use in comparing the quality of care among institutions.

CONCLUSION

Rita Mae Brown, the social activist and author, once said that "good judgment comes from experience, and often experience comes from bad judgment." Pediatric care providers would be wise to study the collective experience of others afforded by elegant database tools such as POCA to heighten their awareness of the risk factors for cardiac arrest, so as to make good judgments without the burden of personal experience.

TAKE HOME POINTS

- Beware of high-risk situations such as cases involving children whose ASA physical status is 3 to 5, cases involving neonates and infants, and cases involving emergency surgery.
- Use sevoflurane instead of halothane.
- Take care to avoid laryngospasm, and treat it promptly; be vigilant for respiratory obstruction or inadequate ventilation.
- Pay meticulous attention to needle placement and technique for regional anesthesia; use ropivacaine instead of bupivacaine, and become proficient with ultrasound-guided blocks.
- Ensure adequate intravenous access, and assess blood loss relative to blood volume frequently.
- Order fresh or washed packed red cells for infants, and monitor serum potassium levels.
- Place all CVP lines with ultrasound guidance, and don't forget to order a postoperative chest X-ray.
- Use succinylcholine only when absolutely necessary.
- Avoid succinylcholine and volatile agents with suspected or known muscular dystrophy.

SUGGESTED READINGS

Arul GS, Spicer RD. Where should paediatric surgery be performed? *Arch Dis Child.* 1998;79(1):65–70, discussion 70–72.

Braz, LG, Modolo NS, do Nascimento P Jr, et al. Perioperative cardiac arrest: A study of 53,718 anaesthetics over 9 yr from a Brazilian teaching hospital. *Br J Anaesth.* 2006;96(5):569–575.

Chazalon P, Tourtier JP, Villevielle T, et al. Ropivacaine-induced cardiac arrest after peripheral nerve block: Successful resuscitation. *Anesthesiology.* 2003;99(6):1449–1451.

Cohen MM, Cameron CB, Duncan PG. Pediatric anesthesia morbidity and mortality in the perioperative period. *Anesth Analg.* 1990;70(2):160–167.

Crone RK. Frequency of anesthetic cardiac arrest in infants: Effect of pediatric anesthesiologists. *J Clin Anesth.* 1991;3(6):431–432.

Domino KB, Bowdle TA, Posner KL, et al. Injuries and liability related to central vascular catheters: A closed claims analysis. *Anesthesiology.* 2004;100(6):1411–1418.

Feldman HS, Arthur GR, Pitkanen M, et al. Treatment of acute systemic toxicity after the rapid intravenous injection of ropivacaine and bupivacaine in the conscious dog. *Anesth Analg.* 1991;73(4):373–384.

Keenan RL, Boyan CP. Cardiac arrest due to anesthesia. A study of incidence and causes. *JAMA.* 1985;253(16):2373–2377.

Keenan RL, Shapiro JH, Dawson K. Frequency of anesthetic cardiac arrests in infants: Effect of pediatric anesthesiologists. *J Clin Anesth.* 1991;3(6):433–437.

Keenan RL, Shapiro JH, Kane FR, et al. Bradycardia during anesthesia in infants. An epidemiologic study. *Anesthesiology.* 1994;80(5):976–982.

Klein SM, Pierce T, Rubin Y, et al. Successful resuscitation after ropivacaine-induced ventricular fibrillation. *Anesth Analg.* 2003;97(3):901–903. Erratum in: *Anesth Analg.* 2004;98:200.

Kong AS, Brennan L, Bingham R, et al. An audit of induction of anaesthesia in neonates and small infants using pulse oximetry. *Anaesthesia.* 1992;47(10):896–899.

Litz RJ, Popp M, Stehr SN, et al. Successful resuscitation of a patient with ropivacaine-induced asystole after axillary plexus block using lipid infusion. *Anaesthesia.* 2006;61(8):800–801.

Mason LJ. An update on the etiology and prevention of anesthesia-related cardiac arrest in children. *Paediatr Anaesth.* 2004;14(5):412–416.

Morray JP, Geiduschek JM, Ramamoorthy C, et al. Anesthesia-related cardiac arrest in children: Initial findings of the Pediatric Perioperative Cardiac Arrest (POCA) Registry. *Anesthesiology.* 2000;93(1):6–14.

Morray JP, Bhanaker SM. Recent Findings from the Pediatric Perioperative Cardiac Arrest (POCA) Registry. *ASA Newsletter.* 2005;69(6):10–12.

Murat I, Constant I, Maud'huy H. Perioperative anaesthetic morbidity in children: A database of 24,165 anaesthetics over a 30-month period. *Paediatr Anaesth.* 2004;14(2):158–166.

Ohmura S, Kawada M, Ohta T, et al. Systemic toxicity and resuscitation in bupivacaine-, levobupivacaine-, or ropivacaine-infused rats. *Anesth Analg.* 2001;93(3):743–748.

Rosenblatt MA, Abel M, Fischer GW, et al. Successful use of a 20% lipid emulsion to resuscitate a patient after a presumed bupivacaine-related cardiac arrest. *Anesthesiology.* 2006;105(1):217–218.

Schulte-Sasse U, Eberlein HJ, Schmucker I, et al., [Should the use of succinylcholine in pediatric anesthesia be re-evaluated?]. *Anaesthesiologie und Reanimation.* 1993;18(1):13–19. German.

Tiret L, Nivoche Y, Hatton F, et al. Complications related to anaesthesia in infants and children. A prospective survey of 40240 anaesthetics. *Br J Anaesth.* 1988;61(3):263–269.

Weinberg G, Ripper R, Feinstein DL, et al. Lipid emulsion infusion rescues dogs from bupivacaine-induced cardiac toxicity. *Reg Anesth Pain Med.* 2003;28(3):198–202.

Weinberg GL, Ripper R, Murphy P, et al. Lipid infusion accelerates removal of bupivacaine and recovery from bupivacaine toxicity in the isolated rat heart. *Reg Anesth Pain Med.* 2006;31(4):296–303.

Weinberg GL, VadeBoncour T, Ramaraju GA, et al, Pretreatment or resuscitation with a lipid infusion shifts the dose-response to bupivacaine-induced asystole in rats. *Anesthesiology.* 1998;88(4):1071–1075.

Yemen TA, McClain C. Muscular dystrophy, anesthesia and the safety of inhalational agents revisited; again. *Paediatr Anaesth.* 2006;16(2):105–108.

131

CLINICIANS CANNOT RELY SOLELY ON THE LEGAL DOCTRINE OF *PARENS PATRIAE* WHEN PROVIDING CARE FOR MINORS WHO ARE JEHOVAH'S WITNESSES

ANNE T. LUNNEY, MD

Caring for minors who are members of the Jehovah's Witness (JW) faith requires understanding the basic premises of the JW faith; thoroughly reviewing the patient's baseline medical condition in view of the proposed surgery; honestly and respectfully communicating with the family to formulate a collaborative plan; and using (when necessary) the legal doctrine of *parens patriae*.

It is sometimes difficult for anesthesia providers to understand that refusing to consent to the administration of blood products for their minor children is an entirely logical extension of the faith of JW parents. JW members believe that, when the end of life on earth has come, a chosen few will be resurrected for a life on earth that will be both physical and eternal. When JW members refuse blood products, they are living according to their faith, choosing eternal life over earthly life. Therefore, they regard refusal of blood products for their children as a positive act, not as neglect or martyrdom.

Preoperative optimization of the patient's medical status is of paramount importance when caring for minor patients who are JW members, especially when the patient has a baseline anemia. The source of the anemia, whether from a medical condition or from a previous surgery, should be elucidated. The patient may require a course of erythropoietin and iron supplementation. It is also important that conditions such as asthma and seizure disorders be under good surveillance and appropriately managed. The anesthesia provider should be willing to request delay of the case (if not emergent) and to seek the advice of consultants, if necessary.

The nature of the surgical case and the modalities available to minimize blood loss should be firmly established. Is the surgery urgent or emergent? Is the procedure one that typically has considerable blood loss? How well will the child tolerate anemia? What is the best estimate of the lowest "permissible" hemoglobin level in the intraoperative and perioperative period? Answering these questions generally requires collaborative discussion with the surgeon. Similarly, several blood loss-sparing modalities can be used in minor and adult patients who are JW members, and there should

© 2006 Mayo Foundation for Medical Education and Research

be a consensus between the surgical and anesthesia staff about their use as well. These modalities include controlled hypotension, tourniquet use, acute normovolemic hemodilution, and cell-salvage techniques.

The specific beliefs of the patient's parents must be established to develop a collaborative plan of care. To review, some JW members refuse primary blood components, including red blood cells, white blood cells, plasma and platelets, but will accept albumin, fibrin, clotting factors, acute normovolemic hemodilution, and cell salvage. All pertinent members of the perioperative care team should meet with the patient and the patient's parents. It is important that the anesthesiologists clearly communicate the plan to minimize the possibility of transfusion to the parents and to assure them that their beliefs are understood and respected. The anesthesiologist should ask for help from the ethics committee, hospital administrative staff, or JW liaison office if he or she feels uncomfortable in this or if there is significant disagreement or discord between the parents. Many pediatric centers also have an informational form that the parents must read and sign, acknowledging the parents' religious beliefs and respectfully promising to do everything medically possible to avoid blood-product administration. The form usually states the legal obligation of the health-care providers to avoid jeopardizing the life of the child by not giving blood products when they are deemed absolutely necessary and reiterates that, regardless of the parental consent status, moral responsibility and legal precedence requires transfusion if it is necessary to prevent harm or death.

Normally, the ethical standards of beneficence and nonmalfeasance are preserved when parents maintain decision-making authority for their children. It is well established that these standards are not preserved when parental decisions will result in harm or death. The doctrine of *parens patriae* allows the state to assume decision-making authority for individuals and is based on the state's obligation to protect those who are not competent to make their own decisions.

To implement the doctrine of *parens patriae*, the following requirements, all based on the ethical framework of "do no harm," must be met:
a) there is significant risk for serious harm;
b) harm is imminent and requires immediate action;
c) an intervention is required to prevent harm;
d) the refused intervention has proven efficacy;
e) the projected outcome outweighs harm;
f) there is not a more acceptable option;
g) the intervention is generalizable to similar situations; and
h) most parents would agree that the intervention is reasonable.

The legal precedent setting limits on parental authority and religious rights was established in 1944, in Prince v Massachusetts. The decision, made with regard to a 9-year-old child selling JW magazines on the street, stated that "neither the rights of religion nor the rights of parenthood are beyond limitation" and that "parents may be free to make martyrs of themselves, but they are not free to make martyrs of their children before they have reached the age when they can make that choice for themselves." As early as 1951, the Illinois Supreme Court upheld a decision to transfuse an infant with erythroblastosis fetalis after the parent's refusal of blood products. In the United States and abroad, the doctrine of *parens patriae* has consistently been upheld in the courts.

SUGGESTED READINGS

Bible. Revised standard version.

Busuttil D, Copplestone A. Management of blood loss in Jehovah's Witnesses. *BMJ*. 1995;311:1115–1116.

Diekema DS. Parental refusals of medical treatment: The harm principle as the threshold for state intervention. *Theor Med Bioeth*. 2004;25:243–264.

Elder L. Why some Jehovah's Witnesses accept blood and conscientiously reject official Watchtower Society blood policy. *J Med Ethics*. 2000;26:375–380.

Oates L. The court's role in decisions about medical treatment. *BMJ*. 2000;321(7271): 1282–1284.

Penson RT, Amrein PC. Faith and freedom: Leukemia in Jehovah Witness minors. *Onkologie*. 2004;27(2):126–128.

Sheldon M. Ethical issues in the forced transfusion of Jehovah's Witness children. *J Emerg Med*. 1996;14(2):251–257.

Tovarelli T, Valenti J. The pregnant Jehovah's Witness: How nurse executives can assist in providing culturally competent care. *JONAS Healthc Law Ethics Regul*. 2005;7(4):105–109.

Wooley S. Children of Jehovah's Witnesses and adolescent Jehovah's Witnesses: What are their rights? *Arch Dis Child*. 2005;90(7):715–719.

NEUROANESTHESIA

132

THE NEUROPHYSIOLOGY YOU LEARNED IN MEDICAL SCHOOL REALLY DOES MATTER DURING CRANIOTOMIES

JENNIFER J. ADAMS, MD AND LAUREL E. MOORE, MD

You're a new CA-2 carrying the code pager for the *first* time. You are called to the neurosurgical intensive care unit (ICU) for an emergent intubation. On arrival, you find serious badness. Seems a middle-age man scheduled to undergo craniotomy for tumor the next day has become progressively more unresponsive, and in the last 5 minutes, his right pupil has dilated and become unresponsive to light. The ICU team wants to transport him for an emergent head CT but wisely called you first. What is your management plan?

In caring for the patient with intracranial hypertension, the role of the anesthesiologist is ultimately to maintain a favorable balance between the delivery of oxygen (and glucose) and the brain's metabolic requirements. Under normal circumstances, flow and metabolism are elegantly controlled to maintain a physiological balance. Under pathological conditions, however, anesthesiologists have a unique role in affecting oxygen delivery and metabolism in order to try to improve oxygen delivery to potentially ischemic brain. For key terms and definitions, see *Table 132.1.*

When considering oxygen delivery to the brain, it is important to remember that the brain is contained within the indistensible skull. Under normal circumstances, the contents of the skull can be divided into three categories: Brain (80% of intracranial volume), cerebrospinal fluid (CSF) (15%), and blood (5%). Under pathological conditions, tumor or hematoma may gradually or acutely increase intracranial volume. Under chronic conditions, compensatory mechanisms to offset this increasing intracranial volume include increased reabsorption of CSF or diversion of CSF to the spinal canal. Once these compensatory mechanisms are exhausted, however, intracranial pressure (ICP) rapidly increases within the intracranial vault (*Fig. 132.1*) and cerebral perfusion pressure (CPP) is compromised:

$$CPP = MAP - ICP$$

where MAP is mean arterial pressure. Acute increases in intracranial volume, such as seen with head trauma or intracranial hemorrhage, are much more poorly tolerated, and ICP may rise precipitously.

© 2006 Mayo Foundation for Medical Education and Research

TABLE 132.1 KEY TERMS AND DEFINITIONS

TERM	ABBREVIATION	DEFINITION	UNITS	NORMAL RANGE
Cerebral blood flow	CBF		mL/min/100 g	45–65 mL/min/100 g globally
Mean arterial pressure	MAP	MAP = [SBP + 2(DBP)]/3	mm Hg	Adults: 60–90 mm Hg
Intracranial pressure	ICP		mm Hg	8–12 mm Hg
Cerebral perfusion pressure	CPP	CPP = MAP − ICP	mm Hg	50–70 mm Hg
Cerebral metabolic rate of oxygen	CMRO$_2$	CBF X (CaO$_2$ − C$_{jv}$O$_2$)	mL/min/100 g	3.0–3.8 mL/min/100 g
Cerebral vascular resistance	CVR	CPP/CBF	mm Hg/mL/min/ 100 g	1.5–2 mm Hg/mL/min/100 g

CaO$_2$, oxygen content arterial blood; C$_{jv}$O$_2$, oxygen content jugular venous blood.

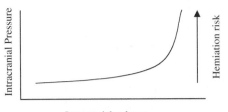

FIGURE 132.1. The intracranial compliance curve demonstrating a stable intracranial pressure (ICP) until some critical intracranial volume is reached, at which time ICP increases exponentially.

Increasing ICP not only places the brain at risk for inadequate oxygen delivery, but there is also the danger of herniation of cerebral tissue, which can rapidly produce death. Cerebral herniation may be associated clinically with Cushing's triad, which includes (a) hypertension, (b) bradycardia, and (c) breathing irregularities.

Under normal circumstances, there are four major determinants of cerebral blood flow (CBF):

1) $PaCO_2$: Carbon dioxide is the major determinant of CBF, and CBF varies directly with $PaCO_2$ between the range of approximately 20 and 80 mm Hg. Below a $PaCO_2$ of 20 mm Hg or above 80 mm Hg, vasoconstriction or vasodilation, respectively, is near maximal, and no further effect of $PaCO_2$ is seen on CBF beyond these limits (*Fig. 132.2*). It is important to remember that this effect is *temporary*, lasting only 6 to 8 hours. The result of this is that increased hyperventilation can afford additional benefit in patients with intracranial hypertension 6 to 8 hours after initiating hyperventilation. Conversely, rapidly normalizing CO_2 can markedly increase CBF in patients with abnormal intracranial compliance who have been treated with hyperventilation for hours to days.

2) PaO_2: Under normal circumstances, arterial oxygenation has little to no effect on CBF. However, under hypoxic conditions (PaO_2 <50 mm Hg), CBF rapidly increases to maintain oxygen delivery to the brain (*Fig. 132.2*).

3) $CMRO_2$: As described previously, CBF and $CMRO_2$ are closely aligned in normal brain. Drugs that reduce $CMRO_2$ and thus may benefit patients with intracranial hypertension include barbiturates, etomidate, propofol, benzodiazepines, opioids, and lidocaine. The potent inhaled vapors (excluding nitrous oxide) not only reduce $CMRO_2$ but also act as cerebral vasodilators. Thus, they are not generally considered beneficial in patients with abnormal compliance. Hypothermia is also highly effective at reducing $CMRO_2$. Its clinical relevance, however, is unproven.

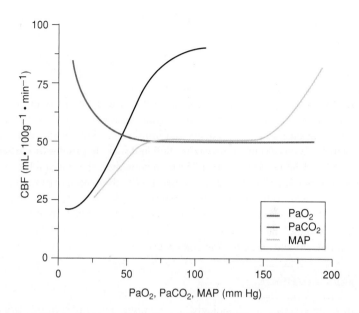

FIGURE 132.2. Cerebral blood flow (CBF) regulation. MAP, mean arterial pressure.

4) CPP: Normal brain is capable of autoregulation, which means that it maintains a constant CBF over a wide range of CPPs (*Fig. 132.3*, uninterrupted line). Under pathological conditions, however, autoregulation may be impaired or absent (*Fig. 132.3*, interrupted line). Some of these conditions include severe brain trauma or subarachnoid hemorrhage. It is critical to maintain a normal or even elevated CPP in these patients so

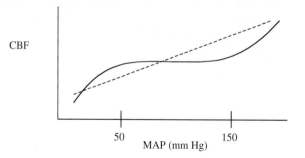

FIGURE 132.3. Diagram depicts cerebral autoregulation (solid line) defined as capacity to maintain a constant cerebral blood flow (CBF) over a wide range of mean arterial blood pressures (MAP). Interrupted line demonstrates pathologic loss of autoregulation in which CBF becomes dependent upon adequate MAP.

as to maintain adequate oxygen delivery to ischemic regions as perfusion becomes "pressure passive."

These factors, generally controlled by anesthesiologists, have addressed the control of arterial blood flow that, as stated previously, represents a small percentage of total intracranial volume. It is important to remember other modes of reducing ICP, thus optimizing CPP. Reduction of the brain/tissue component contributing to intracranial hypertension falls into the realm of the neurosurgical team. Maneuvers that improve cerebral venous drainage are extremely important to managing ICP and include placing the patient head up and minimizing obstruction to venous drainage (i.e., minimizing airway pressures and intrathoracic pressure). Cerebral interstitial fluid may be rapidly reduced by agents such as mannitol or furosemide. Mannitol, an osmotic diuretic, draws fluid from the interstitial space into the intravascular space. Steroids, when appropriate (e.g., brain tumors), may be administered to minimize tissue inflammation and edema.

TAKE HOME POINTS

- In summary, the anesthesiologist has a unique role to play in the care of patients with intracranial hypertension.
- In the patient example at the beginning of this chapter, it is appropriate to emergently intubate the patient to initiate hyperventilation.
- Drugs to reduce $CMRO_2$ will also be helpful in the acute control of CBF and ICP.
- At this point in time, our understanding of cerebral physiology remains trivial at best. What is occurring in this patient at the level of the microcirculation remains a mystery, essentially a "black box." Until we have ways to evaluate and quantify the balance of oxygen delivery and demand at the cellular level, however, these principles apply to the care of our patients. It is the challenge presented by this "black box" that makes our role as anesthesiologists so exciting and challenging.

SUGGESTED READING

Miller RD, ed., *Miller's Anesthesia* 6th edition, Chapter 21. Churchill Livingstone, Philadelphia PA; 2005.

133

ANESTHETIC GOALS FOR CEREBRAL ANEURYSM ARE NOT THE SAME AS FOR ROUTINE CRANIOTOMY

JAMES S. DEMEESTER, MD

Cerebral aneurysms typically arise in the circle of Willis at vascular bifurcation points where hemodynamic stress is maximal. Ninety percent of aneurysms occur in the anterior circulation, and only 10% occur in the basilar system. Although cerebral aneurysms, if large enough, can manifest with symptoms of neural compression, the greatest concern is the occurrence of rupture and subarachnoid hemorrhage.

Intracranial aneurysms (ICAs) are responsible for 75% to 80% of episodes of subarachnoid hemorrhage (SAH), which has an incidence of 10–20/100,000, and is associated with high morbidity and mortality. One-third of patients will die from their initial bleed, with another third having severe disability or delayed death. Only the remaining third will have minimal morbidity and an acceptable outcome.

The prevalence of undiagnosed, asymptomatic aneurysms is estimated at 4%; however, surgical clipping only confers significant outcomes benefit when aneurysm size exceeds 10 mm. Timing of surgical intervention becomes more critical after a hemorrhage because the initial 72 hours presents a window for operative management, after which surgery is delayed 10 to 14 days until the risk of vasospasm has decreased. When surgery is indicated, the anesthesiologist must realize that anesthetic considerations for SAH and ICA are unique from those of routine craniotomy.

The primary concern of an anesthesiologist during surgery for aneurysm clipping is the prevention of rupture. ICA rupture at the time of induction has a mortality exceeding 75%. The likelihood of rupture is based on aneurysm size, wall strength, history of prior rupture, and transmural pressure. Transmural pressure is

$$CPP = MAP - ICP$$

where CPP is cerebral perfusion pressure and MAP is mean arterial pressure. Although mathematically equal to CPP, the concept of transmural pressure and its concern with aneurysmal wall stress is unique to aneurysms. The periods commonly associated with intraoperative rupture are at induction, dura and arachnoid exposure, hematoma evacuation, and during dissection to the aneurysm. Rupture during dissection, or at the time of aneurysm clipping,

© 2006 Mayo Foundation for Medical Education and Research

carries with it much lower morbidity because it is usually rapidly controlled. Anesthetic priorities after a rupture are to maintain cerebral perfusion. Controlled hypotension in an attempt to reduce bleeding is detrimental *but may be necessary under emergent conditions (e.g., aneurysmal rupture) to enable the neurosurgeon to clip the feeding vessel or aneurysm itself.*

Anesthetic induction should be free from acute increases in blood pressure while preserving CPP. An awake arterial line and an induction with adjunct agents, such as lidocaine, beta blockade, and narcotic, facilitate a smooth induction. A modification from our management of routine craniotomy is the avoidance of aggressive hyperventilation and hypocapnia at induction. This prevents precipitous decreases in ICP, further increasing the transmural pressure gradient and the risk for rupture. Likewise, aggressive cerebrospinal fluid drainage at this stage can also have similar consequences.

Patients who have experienced a subarachnoid hemorrhage may have regional ischemia and dysfunctional cerebral blood flow (CBF) autoregulation. Accumulation of extravascular blood increases ICP close to MAP, diminishing the perfusion gradient. Extravasated blood also contributes to localized vasospasm and furthers the risk for ischemia. Vasospasm is rare in the first 3 days following a bleed. Risk peaks around day 7 and generally resolves around days 10 to 14. Clues to the presence of vasospasm, especially preoperatively, might include changes in mentation or new neurologic deficits. Newly evolving hemiplegia may indicate involvement of the middle cerebral artery because hemodynamic and respiratory changes may suggest involvement of the posterior circulation. The diagnosis is also made, more accurately, with angiography and transcranial Doppler. Vasospasm has been seen angiographically in 70% to 90% of patients with SAH; however, most symptoms are absent under anesthesia, making its diagnosis challenging.

Preventative and therapeutic interventions for vasospasm include hemodilution, hypertension, and hypervolemia, referred to as "triple H" therapy or HHH. HHH therapy is a strategy to augment CBF past strictures by increasing CPP and intravascular volume. Although acute hypertension should be avoided, maintenance of MAP and volume should be kept high-normal. Pressors are indicated if hypervolemia alone is insufficient. A rule of thumb should be to keep the MAP at normal prior to aneurysm clipping, and high-normal after both temporary and definitive clipping. Remember that HHH therapy is not indicated for elective aneurysm clipping because vasospasm only occurs after the accumulation of *subarachnoid blood.*

Once induction is complete, further positioning, head pinning, and additional neuromonitoring is placed (somatosensory-evoked potential, electroencephalogram). These carry the risk of acute hypertension, and require aggressive blood pressure control and a stable plane of anesthesia. The anesthetic goals during the maintenance period of anesthesia are similar to that of routine craniotomy in that cerebral relaxation is desired. Gentle hyperventilation with the addition of osmotic diuresis facilitates a slack brain, facilitating surgical dissection. The technique of controlled hypotension during dissection of the aneurysm has been largely supplanted by the use of temporary clips. This lessens the risk of aneurysm rupture or rebleeding during the dissection phase. MAP should be increased after the clip is deployed to enhance collateral perfusion. An isoelectric EEG may be requested during this time, and is achieved by bolus and infusion of propofol. Vasopressors are commonly needed to prevent hypotension.

The goals for anesthesia wake up are to have a comfortable patient free from straining, coughing, and hemodynamic lability. *Patients who are status post subarachnoid hemorrhage and at risk for vasospasm should be intravascularly replete with a normal-to-high normal mean arterial blood pressure.* If surgery was indicated for SAH, then patients who are Hunt-Hess grades I and II should be able to be extubated, facilitating a prompt neurologic examination. Patients who are Hunt-Hess grades III and IV are usually left intubated.

TAKE HOME POINTS

- Anesthetic considerations for surgery for SAH and ICA are unique from those of routine craniotomy.
- The overriding concern is to avoid rupture of the aneurysm and/or subarachnoid hemorrhage.
- ICA rupture at induction carries a mortality rate exceeding 70%!
- Avoid aggressive hyperventilation and hypocapnia at induction.
- Controlled hypotension during routine dissection of the aneurysm has been largely replaced by the use of temporary clips, but be prepared for controlled hypotension in the case of emergent clipping of an acutely ruptured aneurysm.
- Extubation after aneurysm surgery generally depends on the preoperative Hunt-Hess grade—patients who are grades I or II are generally extubated, whereas patients who are grades III or IV usually have a course of postoperative intubation.

SUGGESTED READING

McGrath BJ, Guy J, Borel CO, et al. Perioperative management of aneurismal subarachnoid hemorrhage. Part 1. Operative management. *Anesth Analg* 1995;81(5):1060-1072.

134

EVOKED POTENTIALS: DON'T APPROACH THE SURGEON AND NEUROPHYSIOLOGIST UNTIL YOU KNOW THESE PRINCIPLES

ALAN C. FINLEY, MD, ANTHONY PASSANNANTE, MD, AND LAUREL E. MOORE, MD

Intraoperative neurophysiological monitoring is used to decrease neuro-surgical morbidity and detect neurologic compromise before the damage becomes irreversible. There are numerous modalities for intraoperative monitoring, including somatosensory-evoked potentials (SSEPs), motor-evoked potentials (MEPs), brainstem auditory-evoked potentials (BAEPs), and visual-evoked potentials (VEPs). Their selection is based on the area at risk for injury. Monitoring evoked potentials (EPs) can be challenging for the anesthesia provider because many of the anesthetic agents currently used affect signal quality. The anesthesiologist or anesthetist must communicate with the surgeon and neurophysiologist prior to surgery regarding what EPs will be monitored in order to decide on an anesthetic plan that will optimize this monitoring.

EPs are measurements of the electrical potentials produced when the nervous system is stimulated in contrast to the electroencephalogram [EEG], which records spontaneous electrical activity generated by the central nervous system. EPs may be generated by sensory, magnetic, electrical, or cognitive stimulation. They are characterized by both latency and amplitude. The latency of an EP is measured in milliseconds and is the time between a stimulus and the occurrence of the EP. The amplitude is measured in millivolts and is the magnitude of the EP. EPs can be monitored noninvasively from electrodes on the skin or invasively by monitors placed within the surgery field.

SSEPs are in the form of intraoperative neurophysiological monitoring with the widest clinical application. This technique includes stimulating a peripheral sensory nerve repetitively (e.g., median nerve or posterior tibial nerve) and recording the response with electrodes placed over the primary sensory cortex. SSEPs use signal averaging (e.g., repetitive stimulation and response recording) to cancel out background noise (e.g., EEG). In certain surgeries, the recording electrodes can be placed directly in the epidural space immediately proximal to the site of interest. SSEPs monitor the well-being of the dorsal column functions (position, vibratory sense, and light touch) as well as portions of the brainstem and cerebral cortex. Specifically, the

© 2006 Mayo Foundation for Medical Education and Research

pathway includes the peripheral sensory nerves (cell bodies in the dorsal root ganglia) → which ascend via the ipsilateral dorsal column to synapse in the medulla → secondary fibers decussate and ascend to the contralateral thalamus → tertiary fibers ascend from the thalamus to the primary sensory cortex (postcentral gyrus). Note that SSEPs provide little to no information on the anterior columns (read: Motor function), and there are reports of patients with normal intraoperative SSEPs who awaken with new motor deficits. Fortunately, this is rare despite the dorsal columns having a different blood supply (posterior spinal arteries) than the anterior columns (anterior spinal artery). However, it is theoretically possible to have hypoperfusion to the anterior columns (e.g, during a thoracic aortic aneurysm repair) that SSEPs may fail to recognize. SSEPs are monitored during aneurysm surgery (median nerve during middle cerebral artery aneurysms, posterior tibial nerve during anterior circulation aneurysms—remember your homunculus!), brain tumors including the posterior fossa, and some spine surgeries.

As spine surgery becomes more complex, the need to monitor the anterior columns is becoming increasingly important. Fortunately, our technical ability to monitor MEPs has improved rapidly since the 1990s. MEPs entail applying a current directly or transcranially to the primary motor cortex (precentral gyrus) or spinal cord to initiate an action potential. The action potential then descends from the motor cortex through the pyramidal decussation to the contralateral lateral corticospinal tract. These neurons then synapse on the ventral horn with an alpha motor neuron that travels to the muscle. MEPs can be measured at numerous points along this pathway. Neurogenic MEPs are responses recorded in the periphery following stimulation of the spinal cord. Myogenic MEPs are EPs recorded over the muscle belly as compound muscle action potentials (CMAPs).

BAEPs and VEPs are two additional forms of EPs that may be monitored intraoperatively. BAEPs record subcortical responses from auditory stimuli and monitor the entire auditory pathway, including brainstem nuclei. These prove useful in surgeries near the cerebellopontine angle and particularly help with auditory preservation during resection of acoustic neuromas. VEPs record cortical responses from visual stimuli and monitor the visual pathway. This form of EPs is useful in surgeries near this pathway (i.e., parasellar region). Unlike BAEPs, VEPs are exquisitely sensitive to anesthetic agents.

Because all anesthetic agents have effects on the central nervous system, the anesthetic management of patients undergoing neurophysiological monitoring is vital. Synaptic transmission is more sensitive to anesthetic agents than mere axonal conduction. Therefore, those pathways with multiple synapses (e.g., MEPs, VEPs) are more sensitive to anesthetic agents than those pathways with few (e.g., subcortical SSEPs or BAEPs). The typical effect of most anesthetic agents is to decrease the amplitude and increase the latency of EPs. Anesthetic agents with these effects include the halogenated inhalational agents, propofol, benzodiazepines, and barbiturates. Nitrous oxide has depressant effects on amplitude and minimal effects on latency. Conversely, ketamine and etomidate have minimal effects on EPs and may enhance SSEP amplitude. Opioids also have minimal effects on SSEPs and MEPs, making them a popular choice in EP monitoring.

Neuromuscular blockade must also be carefully considered when planning anesthetic management. By decreasing neuromuscular transmission, neuromuscular blockers produce a dose-dependent decrease in CMAP amplitude, thus affecting the MEP. Similarly, if electromyography (EMG) is being done (e.g., facial nerve monitoring), profound relaxation will limit signal strength. As one might expect, neuromuscular blockers have no effect on sensation, and therefore, do not interfere with the transmission of an electric potential from the periphery to the central nervous system. Paralysis, in fact, aids in SSEP monitoring because it decreases electromyographic interference. Although neuromuscular blockade decreases the ability to monitor MEPs and EMGs, some degree of relaxation may be needed to help with surgical exposure and to prevent patient movement. Working with the neurophysiologist, a balance can be found to satisfy both the needs of the surgeon and the neurophysiologist. Care should be taken to pad extremities and pressure points, as well as to protect the tongue and oropharynx, to prevent injury during MEP stimulation in patients who are not fully relaxed.

Once the surgical procedure and type of neurologic monitoring is known, anesthetic management can be planned. The anesthetic should provide for hemodynamic stability and patient comfort, while permitting optimal conditions for neuromonitoring. This entails the use of a stable anesthetic and avoidance of medication boluses. If a change is noted in amplitude or latency, it is vital that there be no confusion as to whether the change is due to surgical manipulation or a change in anesthetic management. Furthermore, in the event of a significant change in signals, the possibility of an intraoperative wake-up test should be considered when planning the anesthetic. Medications that are rapidly titrated, such as desflurane, nitrous oxide, short-acting opioids, and low-dose propofol, generally provide for good signals and a rapid wake up should this become necessary. For MEPs, particularly in myelopathic patients who have abnormal signals, consideration should be given to using propofol in combination with ketamine, although whether this is better than low-dose volatile agent is unclear. If there is a need to determine whether a loss of signals is real or artifact (e.g., needle displacement), a bolus of etomidate may accentuate poor signals provided that the hardware is in place.

A variety of nonsurgical factors such as temperature, hypotension, anemia, and even brain shrinkage (from cerebral spinal fluid drainage) can affect signals over time. When do these changes become significant? In general, a decrease in amplitude of $\geq 50\%$, or a $\geq 10\%$ increase in latency, deserves investigation. Sudden or unilateral changes certainly suggest surgical trespass. More gradual or bilateral changes are suggestive of anesthetic or physiological change. Regardless of the circumstances, when there is a significant change in signals, the anesthesia team should evaluate (a) whether MAP is adequate and consider increasing MAP 20% above baseline, (b) check hemoglobin and oxygen saturation to ensure adequate oxygen delivery, and (c) ensure that the anesthetic technique has remained stable.

Last, communication is a vital portion of successful EP monitoring. The anesthesiologist must communicate with the neurophysiologist and surgeon about changes in anesthetic management or physiological parameters that may result in changes in signals. Likewise, the neurophysiologist must communicate with the anesthetic and surgical teams of any significant change in signals so they may respond appropriately.

TAKE HOME POINTS

- EP monitoring is actually a "family" of intraoperative monitoring modalities used to decrease neurosurgical morbidity and detect neurologic compromise before the damage becomes irreversible.
- The anesthesia provider should expect to interface with the surgeon, the neurologist, and the EP technician concerning the specific technique to be used for a given case.
- Noninvasive monitoring on the extremities is usually done by placing pad electrodes on the skin, but **beware,** often needle electrodes are used on the scalp.
- SSEPs are the form of intraoperative neurophysiological monitoring with the *widest* clinical application.
- The use of MEPs has increased as spine surgery has become more complex.
- The typical effect of most anesthetic agents is to decrease the amplitude and increase the latency of EPs. Anesthetic agents with the most pronounced effects include the halogenated inhalational agents, propofol, benzodiazepines, and barbiturates. Opioids have minimal effects on SSEPs and MEPs, making them a popular choice in EP monitoring cases.
- Always be ready to re-evaluate your anesthetic if a significant change occurs in the EPs, and always be ready for a wake-up test.

SUGGESTED READINGS

Kumar A, Bhattacharya A, Makhija N. Evoked potential monitoring in anaesthesia and analgesia. *Anesthesia* 2000;55:225–241.

Lotto ML, Banoub M, Schubert A. Effects of anesthetic agents and physiologic changes on intraoperative motor evoked potentials. *J Neurosurg Anesthesiol* 2004;16(1):32–42.

Sloan TB. Anesthetic effects on electrophysiologic recordings. *J Clin Neurophysiol* 1998;15(3):217–226.

Sloan TB, Heyer EJ. Anesthesia for intraoperative neurophysiologic monitoring of the spinal cord. *J Clin Neurophysiol* 2002;19(5):430–443.

135

DON'T TREAT HYPERTENSION IN NEUROSURGERY CASES BEFORE CONSIDERING THE CAUSE(S) AND RISKS, AND ALWAYS RECOGNIZE THAT AN ABRUPT CHANGE IN THE PATIENT'S BLOOD PRESSURE NEEDS TO BE INVESTIGATED

JOHN S. MARVEL, DO

The appropriate management of hypertension during neurosurgical cases requires knowledge of normal and pathological cerebrovascular physiology and consideration of the multiple causes of increased blood pressure. Like all things in anesthesia, simply "treating a number" without considering a cause risks worsening the patient's condition.

Cerebral blood flow (CBF) depends on an adequate cerebral perfusion pressure (CPP) and is well maintained via autoregulation over a wide range of mean arterial pressures (MAPs) in the normally functioning brain. CPP is determined by the difference between MAP and intracranial pressure (ICP):

$$CPP = MAP - ICP$$

Simply put, the body's blood pressure, minus the pressure inside a nonexpanding calvaria, gives the perfusion pressure, which drives blood into the cerebral vasculature. Classically, CBF is maintained at a relatively constant level between MAPs of 50 to 150 mm Hg. Because the "average" ICP rests around 10 mm Hg and MAP for healthy adults is generally around 80 mm Hg, a goal CPP of 70 mm Hg should keep normotensive patients safely within the range of autoregulation. Some investigators have therefore adopted this CPP goal; however, there is no "standard" CPP target due to individual variability and disease state.

Chronic hypertension shifts the autoregulatory curve to the right (*Fig. 135.1*). This means that even "normal" MAPs may be relatively too low to maintain adequate CBF. This stresses the importance of knowing the patient's baseline blood pressure values and taking them into consideration before treating hypertension. Also, autoregulation may be obliterated by certain conditions, such as ischemia (either by stroke or manual surgical retraction), and trauma. Without this ability to constrict blood vessels to maintain adequate CPP, MAPs that are adequate to perfuse a normal brain may be insufficient in the injured one.

© 2006 Mayo Foundation for Medical Education and Research

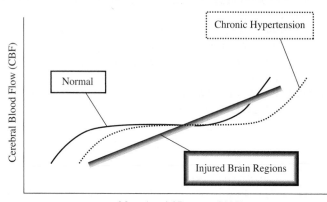

FIGURE 135.1. Autoregulatory curves in three different scenarios: Normal brain function, chronic systemic hypertension resulting in a right-shift of MAPs to maintain cerebral blood flow, and injured brain, resulting in a loss of cerebral vascular autoregulation. (Adapted from Miller RD. *Miller's Anesthesia*. 6th ed. Philadelphia, Pa.: Elsevier/Churchill Livingstone; 2005.)

From the previous formula, one can easily see how intracranial mass, hydrocephalus, or edema, each causing an increase in ICP, will lower CPP, possibly compromising CBF if the MAP is not adequately maintained. The body accommodates for elevated ICP by elevating blood pressure. The Cushing reflex, a triad of hypertension, bradycardia, and respiratory changes, demonstrates the body's attempt to maintain an adequate CPP when ICP increases. Because higher MAPs are necessary to maintain CPP, one can see how treating mild to moderate hypertension in this instance could be detrimental.

For prophylaxis and treatment of subarachnoid hemorrhage (SAH), "triple H" therapy, or hypertension, hypervolemia, and hemodilution (HHH), has traditionally been used to prevent cerebral vasospasm. In theory, increasing CBF by elevating the CPP would improve ischemia caused by cerebral vasospasm, a common complication following SAH. Although no "hard" evidence exists to support routine use of HHH, there is likely benefit in maintaining moderate hypertension in certain patients, and more important, in avoiding hypotension in this patient population.

Of course, like all things in medicine, context is everything. There are certainly times in neurosurgical cases when you want to reach for your labetalol. Keeping CPP adequately elevated is a good thing, but there are limits. Although no standard CPP goal has been established, many neuroanesthesiologists try to keep the CPP between 70 and 100 mm Hg, and usually closer to 70 mm Hg in certain brain injuries. Higher CPP (beyond the bounds of autoregulation) leads to an increase in CBF, causing a possible increase in ICP in a poorly compliant cranium.

So how do you decide which numbers to treat and which to watch? The best answer is to gather all the information you can about a patient. Ideally, one should consult with the surgery team to discuss CPP goals, the potential for increased ICP, and the surgery plan. Also, preoperative blood pressures and nature of the patient's neurologic diseases and comorbidities are necessary to make an informed decision on when to treat.

For certain neurosurgical procedures, hypertension can be almost expected. For example, percutaneous treatments for trigeminal neuralgia have traditionally been performed with an awake or partially awake patient to facilitate placement. This often painful procedure, combined with a patient population that has a higher proportion of chronic hypertensives, leads to increased intraoperative blood pressures. Knowing this, one can see how preoperative antihypertensives combined with vigilant pain control may be more effective than treating hypertension acutely intraoperatively.

TAKE HOME POINTS

- Don't just treat the numbers—think through the physiology and investigate the cause.
- Start your management decisions with firm knowledge of the patient's baseline blood pressure and remember that chronic hypertension shifts the curve to the right.
- There is likely some benefit to at least the hypertension component of "triple H" therapy in subarachnoid hemorrhage, although there are no concrete data.
- Expect a significant degree of acute hypertension with surgery for trigeminal neuralgia. In some institutions, it has been the practice to employ powerful, very short-acting vasodilating or venodilating agents to lower the blood pressure.

SUGGESTED READINGS

Chan KH, Dearden NM, Miller JD, et al. Monitoring as a guide to treatment of intracranial hypertension after severe brain injury. *Neurosurgery* 1993;32(4):547–552; discussion 552–553.

Chang HS, Hongo K, Nakagawa H. Adverse effects of limited hypotensive anesthesia on the outcome of patients with subarachnoid hemorrhage. *J Neurosurg* 2002;97(1):241.

Raabe A, Beck J, Keller M, et al. Relative importance of hypertension compared with hypervolemia for increasing cerebral oxygenation in patients with cerebral vasospasm after subarachnoid hemorrhage. *J Neurosurg* 2005;103(6):974–981.

Rose JC, Mayer SA. Optimizing blood pressure in neurological emergencies. *Neurocrit Care* 2004;1:287–300.

Schmidt EA, Czosnyka M, Steiner LA, et al. Asymmetry of pressure autoregulation after traumatic brain injury. *J Neurosurg* 2003;99(6):991-998.

Tietjen CS, Hurn PD, Ulatowski JA, et al. Treatment modalities for hypertensive patients with intracranial pathology: Options and risks. *Crit Care Med* 1996;24(2):311–322.

Torbey MT, Bhardwaj A. How to manage blood pressure in critically ill neurologic patients. *J Crit Illness* 2001;16(4):179–191.

136

AWAKE CRANIOTOMY CAN BE DONE HUMANELY

ALEXIS BILBO, MD AND LAUREL E. MOORE, MD

It's 7:00 AM when you learn that your supposedly routine craniotomy for tumor resection is actually an awake craniotomy because of the proximity of the tumor to Broca's area. The patient has been coached by the surgeon, but the family is agitated and fails to understand why anyone would need to have their head opened while awake. What do you need to prepare the room for anesthesia, and what do you say to the family to reassure them?

Awake craniotomies are relatively uncommon procedures that are generally performed in large-volume neurosurgical centers. The usual indication is to facilitate intraoperative electrocorticography to map eloquent brain regions involved in speech, motor, and sensory function in order to minimize neurologic injury to these critical regions during tumor resection. The main objectives of the anesthetic employed for awake craniotomies are to (a) minimize patient discomfort associated with painful portions of the procedure and prolonged restriction of movement, (b) ensure patient responsiveness and compliance during phases of the procedure that require assessment of speech or motor function, and (c) produce minimal inhibition of spontaneous seizure activity. These objectives are achieved by using a variety of techniques that range from minimal sedation to asleep-awake-asleep techniques using a laryngeal mask airway (LMA). There are many important considerations when performing anesthesia for an awake craniotomy. These include pain control, airway management, the possibility of hypoventilation in the setting of increased intracranial pressure, the onset of seizures, the possible complication of venous air embolism (VAE), and patient selection.

Pain control is critical to the care of patients undergoing awake craniotomies. Certain parts of the procedure, such as pin fixation of the head, temporalis muscle dissection, and traction on the dura close to the middle meningeal artery territory can be especially painful. In most institutions, pain control is accomplished with a combination of narcotics and regional anesthesia. Narcotics can be administered as a bolus or as an infusion. The narcotics used should be short acting with minimal effects on electroencephalogram (EEG) monitoring. Fentanyl and remifentanil are appropriate choices. Also, a scalp block is necessary to control pain. Scalp blocks are performed using a 22-gauge intradermal needle with circumferential injection, following a line from the glabella to the occiput and dividing it into four parts

© 2006 Mayo Foundation for Medical Education and Research

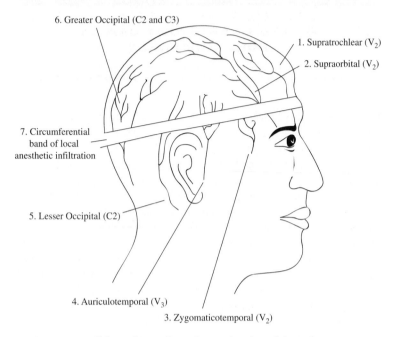

6. Greater Occipital (C2 and C3)

1. Supratrochlear (V₂)

2. Supraorbital (V₂)

7. Circumferential band of local anesthetic infiltration

5. Lesser Occipital (C2)

4. Auriculotemporal (V₃)

3. Zygomaticotemporal (V₂)

FIGURE 136.1. Schematic anterior and posterior view of the scalp.

at the intersection of the sagittal and frontal planes (*Fig. 136.1*). Mayfield pin sites generally require supplementation and should be done in conjunction with the neurosurgeon placing the head holder. The local anesthetic used for injection should have a prompt onset of action, provide analgesia for a significant period of time, and not interfere with electrocorticography. Lidocaine and bupivacaine may be used in combination to achieve rapid onset, long duration and minimal toxicity. Because the scalp block requires a large volume of local anesthetic (as much as 60 cc), it is important for the anesthesiologist to be vigilant in calculating dosages of local anesthetics and monitoring for toxicity. The addition of a third drug such as chloroprocaine or ropivacaine may be necessary to safely achieve the necessary volume of local anesthetic. Avoidance of local anesthetic toxicity is obviously critical in patients immobilized in a Mayfield head holder. It is also important to realize that even with a perfect scalp block and in the absence of somatic pain, many patients will still have a vague (or even severe) headache that will require opioid supplementation.

In addition to analgesia, most patients require sedation in order to tolerate the emotional stress of awake craniotomy and simply lying still with an immobilized head for several hours. Many anesthesiologists use an asleep-awake-asleep technique, inserting an LMA for the most stimulating portions of the procedure (line insertion, Mayfield head holder application, and craniotomy) and removing it when patient cooperation becomes necessary. Alternatively, a continuous infusion of propofol or dexmedetomidine with spontaneous ventilation is generally adequate (in conjunction with scalp block and opioids) for even the most stimulating portions of the procedure and does not involve removing the LMA (and thus the potential for coughing) in the immobilized patient. Regardless of whether an LMA is planned, final head position needs to be determined jointly between neurosurgery and anesthesiology so the airway is accessible and so an LMA could be inserted emergently if needed.

Patients undergoing awake craniotomy are at increased risk of VAE because they are breathing spontaneously. VAE can occur whenever a noncollapsable vein is opened and a pressure gradient exists favoring air entrapment rather than bleeding. This can occur whenever the operative site is above the level of the heart (atmospheric pressure > cerebral venous pressure) or in spontaneously breathing patients where negative intrathoracic pressure is transferred to the cerebral venous system. VAE involves entrainment of air into the venous system, right heart, and pulmonary vasculature. This causes sympathetic reflex vasoconstriction leading to ventilation-perfusion abnormalities. The increased pulmonary vasculature resistance can lead to increased right ventricular afterload, increased pulmonary artery pressure, and increased central venous pressure as the right ventricle begins to fail. Hypotension develops as cardiac output falls. Adult respiratory distress syndrome can be a late sequela. Signs and symptoms in the awake patient include tachypnea, cough, chest pain, hypoxemia, decreased end tidal CO_2, and the classic mill wheel murmur, which can be detected by a precordial stethoscope. Patients may express anxiety or a sense of impending doom. Precordial Doppler is the most commonly used VAE monitoring technique, although it is not quantitative. Once a VAE is suspected, the field should be flooded with saline, the patient placed in the Durant position (Trendelenburg with right side up), nitrous oxide discontinued, the central venous catheter aspirated in an attempt to retrieve entrained air, vasopressors and volume given to treat hypotension, and bilateral jugular vein compression applied to increase cerebral venous pressure and minimize air entry into the heart. Fortunately, this complication remains rare during awake craniotomy.

Another potential consideration during awake craniotomy is the onset of seizures. They can result from cortical stimulation or from local anesthetic toxicity. Treatment includes protection of the airway to maintain respiration and administration of drugs to stop the seizure. Thiopental is an appropriate drug to treat seizures, but it should be held until it is clear that the seizure is not self-limited because the drug may interfere with subsequent EEG localization of the seizure focus. Benzodiazepines may also be used to treat seizures. Generalized tonic-clonic seizures should be managed aggressively in patients immobilized in a Mayfield head holder.

The final and possibly most important consideration is patient selection. Children and extremely anxious adults are not good candidates for awake craniotomy, although this prohibition is not absolute. It is important that the patient and family understand exactly why the procedure is best performed while the patient is awake. All aspects of the procedure, including the potential for discomfort, must be explained in detail to the patient and his or her family prior to entering the operating room. To maintain credibility, an absolutely honest discussion must be held between the patient and the anesthesiologist, with the assurance that the anesthesiologist will be there to work to keep the patient comfortable throughout. Recognition of the patient's fears and concerns is essential. A comfortable professional relationship with the patient and ongoing conversation and reassurance are the keys to successful completion of the awake craniotomy.

In summary, awake craniotomies are uncommon procedures performed when neurosurgical resection may place eloquent areas of brain at risk for injury. For an awake craniotomy procedure to be a success, the anesthesiologist must take into account many considerations, including pain control, airway management, the onset of seizures, the possible complication of a VAE, and patient selection.

TAKE HOME POINTS

- A scalp block involving circumferential administration of large volumes and adequate concentrations of local anesthesia is required for successful completion of an awake craniotomy. Even when performed by an experienced clinician, patients may experience headache during the awake portions of the procedure and should be prepared in advance for this. Opioid administration is helpful to manage headache.

- Plans for sedation versus general anesthesia by LMA are determined in advance. In both scenarios, the patient is breathing spontaneously with an open calvaria and dura, placing the patient at risk for both hypoventilation and increased intracranial pressure and VAE.

- Head position, determined in conjunction with neurosurgery, should always allow for emergent access to the airway and LMA placement, if necessary.

- An honest and thorough discussion of plans, expectations, and risks needs to be had with the patient and his or her family before entering the operating room. An open relationship between clinician and patient with discussion and reassurance intraoperatively is paramount to patient comfort and safety.

SUGGESTED READINGS

Balki M, Manninen PH, McGuire GP, et al. Venous air embolism during awake craniotomy in a supine patient. *Can J Anesth* 2003;50:835–838.

Costello TG, Cormack JR. Anaesthesia for awake craniotomy: A modern approach. *J Clin Neurosci* 2004;11(1):16–19.

Deogaonkar A, Avitsian R, Henderson J, et al. Venous air embolism during deep brain stimulation surgery in an awake supine patient. *Stereotact Funct Neurosurg* 2005;83:32–35.

Faust RJ. *Anesthesiology Review.* 3rd ed. Philadelphia, Pa.: Mayo Foundation; 2002:389–391.

Manninen PH, Balki M, Lukito K, et al. Patient satisfaction with awake craniotomy for tumor surgery: A comparison of remifentanil and fentanyl in conjunction with propofol. *Anesth Analg* 2006;102:237–242.

Manninen PH, Contrearas J. Anesthetic considerations for craniotomy in awake patients. *Int Anesthesiol Clin* 1986;24(3):157–174.

Miller RD, ed. *Miller's Anesthesia.* 6th ed. Philadelphia, PA: Churchill Livingstone; 2005.

Tangier WK, Joshi GP, Landers DF, et al. Use of the laryngeal mask airway during awake craniotomy for tumor resection. *J Clin Anesth* 2000;12(8):592–594.

137

DON'T BE CAUGHT UNPREPARED FOR A WAKE-UP TEST

SARAH MERRITT, MD, PETER ROCK, MD, MBA, AND
LAUREL E. MOORE, MD

You are about to induce anesthesia on a 15-year-old girl for a thoracolumbar fusion when the surgeon casually mentions that, given the degree of kyphoscoliosis, a wake-up test might be required intraoperatively. Yikes! How does this affect your preoperative discussion with the child (and her parents) and your intraoperative management?

A wake-up test is one of several monitoring methods used to evaluate brain and spinal cord function during general anesthesia. The wake-up test allows an intraoperative neurologic examination, which is useful during surgery that may cause reversible central nervous system (CNS) injury. Wake-up tests are traditionally associated with scoliosis procedures during which significant spinal cord distraction may occur. Evoked potential monitoring is commonly performed during these procedures; however, the possibility of false-positive and false-negative results remains. A satisfactory motor response (achieved by asking the patient to *"wiggle your toes"* or *"squeeze my fingers"*) during a wake-up test reassures that both afferent and efferent spinal cord pathways are intact. Furthermore, a wake-up test is indicated in patients with persistent suppression of their evoked potentials despite correction of any identifiable cause and in cases of technical failure. Wake-up tests are rarely done during craniotomy when eloquent regions of brain are at risk (e.g., speech or motor regions). This subtopic is discussed more fully in Chapter 136.

The anesthesia provider must recognize that the potential complications of intraoperative wake-up testing are generally related to overzealous patient movement. These include injury to the patient, injury to operating room personnel, and dislodgement of monitors, intravenous lines, or airway equipment. Patient awareness of the wake-up test postoperatively is *not* necessarily an adverse event unless it is accompanied by awareness of discomfort. It is imperative that the anesthesiologist and patient discuss the wake-up test during the preoperative evaluation, both to acquire informed consent and to decrease potential for undesired patient movement. Patients should be reassured that the wake up will be brief, with maximum attention to their comfort level, and that recall of the wake-up test is possible but not likely.

© 2006 Mayo Foundation for Medical Education and Research

In addition to discussing the plan with the patient, the anesthetic regimen should be chosen to facilitate a rapid and smooth emergence for the wake-up test. The earliest anesthetic techniques combined nitrous oxide, opioid, and a volatile anesthetic, allowing for rapid awakening. Since then, there has been some evolution in what is considered the optimum anesthetic technique for major neurosurgical procedures, driven by the use of more sophisticated intraoperative monitoring techniques. For example, motor-evoked potentials (MEPs) are rapidly becoming the standard of care for major spine surgery. Unfortunately, transcranial MEPs are exquisitely sensitive to volatile anesthetics; thus, total intravenous anesthesia (TIVA), with some combination of propofol, ketamine, and opioid, is generally believed to provide the best MEP recordings under general anesthesia. Unfortunately, wake up from such an anesthetic may be prolonged. One recent trial compared two anesthetic techniques for wake-up testing and showed volatile anesthetic plus opioid (desflurane and remifentanil) allowed patient reawakening more rapidly than TIVA (propofol infusion with remifentanil or sufentanil).

At the authors' institution, the most common practice during spinal surgery involves volatile anesthetic, low-dose propofol infusion, and remifentanil infusion. The propofol decreases volatile anesthetic requirements, thus improving evoked potential recordings. When it is time for the wake-up test, the propofol and desflurane are discontinued. Remifentanil continues to infuse, providing a baseline level of analgesia throughout the wake-up test. Wake-up tests are done so rarely that surgeons may need to be reminded that it may take up to 30 minutes for a patient to awaken from TIVA.

Neuromuscular blockers must be titrated carefully during cases in which a wake-up test is performed. During the wake-up test, two to three twitches on a train of four nerve stimulators are optimal. This can be accomplished most predictably with a continuous infusion of muscle relaxant throughout surgery. This level of blockade should be sufficient to allow neurologic examination yet produce a weakened patient with less risk of injury or equipment dislodgement. Once the patient's function has been examined, a rapid induction of general anesthesia is desirable. A bolus dose of propofol is our preferred agent, and then the maintenance anesthetic regimen is resumed.

Finally, although the wake-up test is an accepted method to verify motor function in spinal surgery, a normal wake-up test does not guarantee an optimal neurologic outcome. Several cases exist in the literature of patients with normal intraoperative wake-up tests having postoperative complications, including vertebral artery dissection and delayed anterior spinal artery syndrome. Continued vigilance in maintaining stable hemodynamics and neuromonitoring are imperative until the end of the case.

- It is imperative that the wake-up test be discussed preoperatively with the patient if planned or considered likely during surgery.
- TIVA, a commonly employed anesthetic regiment used to facilitate MEP monitoring, is not ideal for a rapid wake up.
- A basal level of analgesia and incomplete reversal of neuromuscular blockade minimize the risk of vigorous patient movement and subsequent injury during wake-up testing.

SUGGESTED READINGS

Cucciara RF, Black S, Michenfelder, JD. *Clinical Neuroanesthesia.* 2nd ed. New York, NY: Churchill Livingstone; 1998.

Dickerman RD, Zigler JE. Atraumatic vertebral artery dissection after cervical corpectomy: A traction injury? *Spine* 2005;30:E658–E661.

Eroglu A, Solak M, Ozen I, et al. Stress hormones during the wake up test in scoliosis surgery. *J Clin Anesth* 2003;15:15–18.

Grottke O, Dietrich PJ, Wiegels S, et al. Intraoperative wake up test and postoperative emergence in patients undergoing spinal surgery: A comparison of intravenous and inhaled anesthetic techniques using short-acting anesthetics. *Anesth Analg* 2004;99:1521–1527.

Jaffe RA, Samuels SI, eds. *Anesthesiologist's Manual of Surgical Procedures.* 3rd ed. Philadelphia, Pa.: Lippincott Williams & Wilkins; 2004.

Miller RD, Fleisher LA, Johns RA, et al, eds. *Miller's Anesthesia.* 6th ed. Philadelphia, Pa.: Elsevier/Churchill Livingstone; 2005.

Noonan KJ, Walker T, Feinberg JR, et al. Factors related to false- versus true-positive neuromonitoring changes in adolescent idiopathic scoliosis surgery. *Spine* 2002;27:825–830.

Stockl B, Wimmer C, Innerhofer P, et al. Delayed anterior spinal artery syndrome following posterior scoliosis correction. *Eur Spine J* 2005;24:906–909.

138

REMEMBER THAT LOSS OF VISION IS ONE OF THE MOST FEARED AND DEVASTATING COMPLICATIONS OF SPINE SURGERY

LAUREL E. MOORE, MD

It is the first day of your first neuroanesthesia rotation and you're all set to start a major spinal reconstruction. You're about to wheel your patient back to the operating room when the patient's spouse (an attorney) tells you that she's recently read about blindness after spine surgery and wants to know what you think and, *specifically*, what you are going to do to prevent blindness?

Postoperative visual loss (POVL) is a devastating injury that fortunately remains rare, with an occurrence rate of between 1/1,000 to 3/10,000 spine surgeries. The time of presentation is variable—patients may present with painless loss of vision immediately post surgery or up to 3 to 4 days postoperatively. The deficit can vary from a mild field cut to complete loss of light perception. Historically, POVL was most closely associated with cardiac surgery and cardiopulmonary bypass. However, with the advent of increasingly complex spine surgeries, the incidence of POVL may also be increasing. This is somewhat surprising because the eye has a dual blood supply: (a) the central retinal artery (CRA), and (b) a series of posterior ciliary arteries. The anterior optic nerve (*Fig. 138.1*) (anterior to the lamina cribrosa) is supplied by branches of posterior ciliary arteries. These are end arteries and therefore may produce watershed regions, placing the retina at risk for ischemia. The posterior optic nerve is supplied by pial vessels and, occasionally, branches of the CRA. Notably, up to 20% of normal individuals have minimal or absent autoregulation of the optic nerve blood supply.

Unfortunately, the mechanisms of POVL are poorly understood, but they may be categorized into at least two general subgroups. The first of these is central retinal artery occlusion (CRAO). CRAO is the predominant mechanism of POVL following cardiac surgery and is almost certainly embolic following cardiopulmonary bypass. CRAO following spine surgery may not only be embolic, but it may also result from reduced perfusion pressure to the retina by other mechanisms, such as direct pressure on the orbit while in the prone position ("head rest syndrome"). CRAO is generally unilateral and may present with periorbital edema suggesting decreased venous outflow from the orbit, thus reducing retinal perfusion

ⓒ 2006 Mayo Foundation for Medical Education and Research

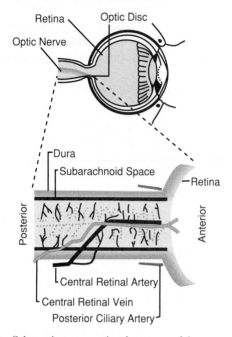

FIGURE 138.1. Schematic cross-sectional anatomy of the eye.

pressure. Funduscopic exam classically reveals a cherry red spot. The prognosis with CRAO is poor, and there is rarely significant improvement in vision.

More common than CRAO after spine surgery is ischemic optic neuropathy (ION). ION is subdivided into anterior ischemic optic neuropathy (AION) and posterior ischemic neuropathy (PION), depending on whether the ischemic optic nerve is anterior or posterior to the lamina cribrosa (e.g., intraorbital or retro-orbital). These may be distinguished on funduscopic exam. With AION, the funduscopic exam is generally abnormal at presentation, whereas the funduscopic exam with PION is normal at presentation and then becomes abnormal over several weeks as the optic nerve dies. Also, PION is generally more common in spine surgery. The mechanism of ION is poorly understood, but known patient risk factors include (a) history of diabetes and/or atherosclerotic disease, (b) preoperative anemia, (c) *intraoperative hypotension and anemia*, (d) prolonged surgical procedures with large blood loss, and (e) possibly the intraoperative use of vasoconstrictors. ION is more likely to be bilateral than CRAO. In one review of cases, approximately 40% of patients with ION had some return of vision, unlike

CRAO patients. AION has a better prognosis than PION in terms of vision recovery.

Because of the devastating nature of POVL, the American Society of Anesthesiologists recently convened a subcommittee on POVL with the goal of formulating a practice advisory for spine patients. This practice advisory was recently completed and includes the following recommendations[1]:

1) Systemic blood pressure should be continuously monitored in high-risk patients (read: Arterial monitoring). Although all committee members believed that deliberate hypotension was contraindicated in patients with chronic hypertension, there was disagreement as to whether deliberate hypotension was safe in patients without chronic hypertension.

2) A combination of crystalloids and colloids should be used to maintain euvolemia. Central venous pressure monitoring should be considered in high-risk patients.

3) Hemoglobin should be monitored intermittently. The subcommittee could not determine a lower limit below which the risk of POVL could be eliminated. It is the author's belief that hemoglobin should be maintained above 9.0 g/dL at all times for major spine surgery in adults.

4) Although subspecialty neuroanesthesiologists believed that the prolonged use of alpha-agonists could contribute to POVL, the subcommittee believed that there was insufficient evidence to make a statement regarding the use of alpha-agonists.

5) Avoid direct pressure on eye to prevent CRAO. The high-risk patient's head should be maintained in a neutral position with the head higher than the heart whenever possible.

6) For complex spine surgery, consideration should be given to the use of staged procedures in high-risk patients.

7) When POVL is suspected, immediate ophthalmologic consultation should be obtained.

Unfortunately, once POVL is recognized postoperatively, there are few treatment options. For suspected CRAO, some have suggested eye massage or intravenous acetazolamide to reduce intraocular pressure and local thrombolytic therapy, although these maneuvers are of questionable benefit. In general, optimization of hemoglobin and mean arterial pressure are probably of greater benefit. Magnetic resonance imaging (MRI) should be considered to rule out other possible causes of postoperative blindness, including pituitary apoplexy or cortical blindness. Edema of the optic nerve may be visualized on MRI with PION.

---

[1] High-risk patients are specifically defined as those patients undergoing spine procedures with predicted long duration, large blood loss, or both.

- Optimization of mean arterial pressure and hemoglobin with careful presurgical patient positioning are probably the best ways to minimize the risk of POVL.
- Surgeons should consider staged procedures in high-risk patients.
- Because the mechanisms are not fully elucidated, it is probably impossible to completely eliminate the risk of POVL.
- Two clinical practices are recommended: (a) discussion of POVL preoperatively with patients at high risk, and (b) confirmation (and documentation) that the eyes are free of pressure every 15 minutes during prolonged procedures in the prone or lateral position.

SUGGESTED READINGS

American Society of Anesthesiologists Task Force on Perioperative Blindness. Practice advisory for perioperative visual loss associated with spine surgery: A report by the American Society of Anesthesiologists Task Force on Perioperative Blindness. *Anesthesiology* 2006;104: 1319–1328.

Lee LA, Roth S, Posner KL, et al. The American Society of Anesthesiologists Postoperative Visual Loss Registry: Analysis of 93 spine surgery cases with postoperative visual loss. *Anesthesiology* 2006;105:652–759.

139

CANNULATION FOR CARDIOPULMONARY BYPASS—BE CAREFUL WHERE YOU POINT THAT THING!

JASON Z. QU, MD AND EDWIN G. AVERY, IV, MD

A 64-year-old female insulin-dependent diabetic with severe aortic atheromatous disease and peripheral vascular disease presents for coronary revascularization. Surgery is planned to include the use of cardiopulmonary bypass (CPB). Intraoperative pre-CPB transesophageal echocardiography exam reveals a "mine field" of an ascending aorta with multiple mobile elements and protruding atheromatous plaques. The surgeon requests your help to find an appropriate site for insertion of the arterial perfusion cannula. What is your move in this situation? An epiaortic scan will help better define the extent of atheromatous disease in the ascending aorta. The epiaortic scan did not suggest that it would be safe to place the cannula in the ascending aorta because the stroke risk would be as big as the state of Texas! The surgeon begins to prepare for cannulation of the left femoral artery. Is your left radial arterial line appropriate for systemic pressure monitoring? Yes, but given that the surgical plan involves femoral cannulation in a severely diseased aorta, the patient still has a high risk of stroke from retrograde emboli (e.g., like kicking your foot upstream in a brook where the bottom is covered with moss and loose sand, the upstream current stirs up a load of dirt and debris). The key to placing the cannula in this patient is to recognize that it is going to be difficult to minimize the stroke risk, *and* iatrogenic aortic dissection will also be of major concern.

Cannulation for more complex cardiac surgical operations is not quite as "cookbook" as it may be for coronary surgery. Although the ascending aorta is the most common site of arterial cannulation for CPB, the presence of ascending aortic aneurysms, dissections, severe atherosclerosis, or previous ascending aortic surgery may preclude safe cannulation in this region. *In cannulating an ascending aorta that has severe atheromatous disease, one must ensure that the major force of the arterial cannula flow stream is not directed at a focus of aortic atheromatous disease (i.e., creating "the sand blasting effect") in order to minimize the risk of stroke.* Optimal selection of the aortic cannulation site is facilitated with epiaortic ultrasound assessment. Alternative sites for arterial cannulation include the femoral artery, axillary artery, innominate artery, common carotid artery, and cardiac apex. The different

© 2006 Mayo Foundation for Medical Education and Research

cannulation sites will have unique implications for perfusion techniques and hemodynamic monitoring.

FEMORAL ARTERY CANNULATION

The femoral artery is the most common alternative site for CPB cannulation. This vessel is readily accessible and is therefore often used for cannulation to emergently initiate CPB, or when the ascending aorta is not suitable for cannulation such as in an acute ascending aortic dissection. CPB can be initiated with cannulation of the femoral artery and femoral vein or vena cava. On initiation of CPB, the arterial blood flows retrograde through the aorta. *In select emergent cases (e.g., massive pulmonary embolism), femoral cannulation can be accomplished under local anesthesia to avoid the potential hemodynamic collapse that may accompany induction of general anesthesia (related to the blunting of sympathetic outflow) and the initiation of positive-pressure ventilation.*

In the case of aortic dissection or severe aortic atherosclerosis, the descending aorta and femoral artery are often involved. Retrograde perfusion via femoral cannulation may elevate the dissected intima, causing malperfusion with consequent neurologic injury or visceral organ ischemia, or it may cause retrograde embolization from the atherosclerotic aortic wall. *Commonly, the right femoral artery is cannulated in preparation for CPB in patients with an aortic dissection that involves the descending thoracic aorta because it is more common for the dissection to extend into the left femoral artery.*

AXILLARY ARTERY CANNULATION

In comparison to the femoral artery, the axillary artery is usually less affected by atherosclerosis or dissection. Axillary artery cannulation minimizes the need to manipulate an atherosclerotic ascending aorta, which may help reduce the potential for atheroembolic sequelae.

For an operation that requires deep hypothermic circulatory arrest (DHCA), it is also necessary to have a cannulation strategy that promotes cerebral protection. Retrograde cerebral perfusion is accomplished by cannulating the superior vena cava (SVC) and providing retrograde venous blood flow to the brain while concurrently monitoring SVC pressure with an internal jugular central venous line. *Be sure to keep the SVC pressure <25 mm Hg during retrograde cerebral perfusion to protect the cerebral capillary beds.* A designated central venous catheter (e.g., the side arm of the pulmonary artery introducer is often used for this purpose) should be used for monitoring the retrograde cerebral perfusion pressure. The tip of the catheter has to be cephalad to the end of the SVC cannula to guide the retrograde perfusion pressure because inaccurate pressures put the cerebral capillary beds at risk for pressure-related trauma.

However, it may be difficult to control the SVC in surgical procedures that involve a redo sternotomy. Axillary artery cannulation provides

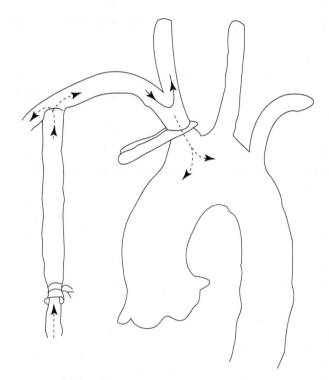

FIGURE 139.1. Right axillary artery cannulation with interpositional graft and antegrade selective cerebral perfusion. Through the right axillary artery, the cardiopulmonary bypass (CPB) pump provides systemic blood flow via an interpositional graft (with clamp off the innominate artery). The arterial pressure recorded from right radial artery will be significantly higher than that of the left radial or femoral arteries. The CPB pump provides antegrade cerebral perfusion via right common carotid artery when the innominate artery is clamped.

anterograde right carotid artery perfusion in conjunction with innominate artery occlusion during DHCA (*Fig. 139.1*). Axillary artery cannulation for CPB can be either direct or via an end-to-side interposition graft.

INNOMINATE ARTERY CANNULATION

This technique provides the previously mentioned advantages of right axillary artery cannulation, but with a greater simplicity, because there is no need to make an adjunctive incision. It is especially useful in emergency cases (e.g., acute type A dissection).

Line Placement and Pressure Monitoring. The radial artery is the most common peripheral artery used to monitor systemic blood pressure during CPB. In most situations, radial artery cannulation laterality does not produce a clinically significant issue. *However, when axillary or innominate arterial cannulation for CPB is planned, bilateral radial cannulation is recommended so systemic arterial pressure can be more accurately assessed.* Depending on the cannulation technique used when CPB is initiated with right axillary arterial cannulation, the right radial artery may transduce a pressure close to that of the CPB circuit. Therefore, the right radial artery pressure is much higher than the left radial artery or femoral artery pressure, which could lead to hypoperfusion of the brain and other organs. In procedures with right axillary arterial CPB cannulation that plan to employ DHCA, selective anterograde cerebral perfusion via the right common carotid artery can be used if the innominate artery is temporarily clamped. Bilateral radial artery cannulation is recommended in these cases to accurately assess cerebral and systemic blood pressures. In patients who do not need DHCA but receive axillary arterial CPB cannulation for other reasons, arterial pressure monitoring should be accomplished using the contralateral upper extremity.

Special attention should be paid to central venous pressure (CVP) monitoring while patients are on CPB with SVC cannulation. To accurately monitor the SVC pressure, be sure that the tip of the central venous line or CVP port of the pulmonary artery catheter is cephalad to the end of the SVC cannula.

TAKE HOME POINTS

- In cannulating an ascending aorta that has severe atheromatous disease, one must ensure that the major force of the arterial cannula flow stream is not directed at a focus of aortic atheromatous disease (i.e., creating "the sand blasting effect") in order to minimize the risk of stroke.

- The femoral artery is the most common alternative site for CPB cannulation. Retrograde perfusion via femoral cannulation may elevate the dissected intima in patients with aortic dissection, causing malperfusion with consequent neurologic injury, visceral organ ischemia, or retrograde embolization from the atherosclerotic aortic wall.

- In select emergent cases (e.g., massive pulmonary embolism), femoral cannulation for CPB can be accomplished under local anesthesia to avoid the potential hemodynamic collapse that may accompany the induction of general anesthesia and the initiation of positive-pressure ventilation.

- Commonly, the right femoral artery is cannulated in preparation for CPB in patients with an aortic dissection that involves the descending thoracic aorta because it is more common for the dissection to extend into the left femoral artery.

- For an operation that requires DHCA, it is necessary to have a cannulation strategy that promotes cerebral protection.

- When axillary or innominate arterial CPB cannulation is planned, bilateral radial cannulation is recommended so systemic arterial pressure can be more accurately assessed.
- The tip of a cannula used to monitor CVP should be optimally positioned relative to the CPB venous cannula to ensure accurate determination of pressure.
- For DHCA, be sure to keep the SVC pressure <25 mm Hg during selective retrograde cerebral perfusion in order to protect the cerebral capillary beds.

SUGGESTED READINGS

Eusanio MD, Quarti A, Pierri MD, et al. Cannulation of the brachiocephalic trunk during surgery of the thoracic aorta: A simplified technique for antegrade cerebral perfusion. *Eur J Cardiothorac Surg* 2004;26:831–833.

Orihashi K, Sueda T, Okada K, et al. Detection and monitoring of complications associated with femoral or axillary arterial cannulation for surgical repair of aortic dissection. *J Cardiothorac Vasc Anesth* 2006;20:20–25.

Watanabea K, Fukudab I, Osakaa M, et al. Axillary artery and transapical aortic cannulation as an alternative to femoral artery cannulation. *Eur J Cardiothorac Surg* 2003;23:842–843.

140

REMEMBER TO ASK ABOUT A HISTORY OF ESOPHAGEAL DISEASE IF TRANSESOPHAGEAL ECHOCARDIOGRAPHY IS PLANNED (OR POSSIBLE)

THOMAS R. ELSASS, MD AND ROBERT W. KYLE, DO

Fortunately, there are relatively few complications of transesophageal echocardiography (TEE). When they do occur, however, the complications can be quite serious. Untoward events include severe odynophagia, esophageal rupture, bleeding varices, bleeding ulcers, endotracheal tube dislodgement, and dental and oral trauma. The overall incidence of complications in the immediate postoperative period is ~0.2%. In 7,200 cardiothoracic (CT) surgery patients, severe odynophagia occurred in 0.1% of all patients, and upper gastrointestinal bleed (UGIB) occurred in 0.03%. It has been reported that the incidence of UGIB is even higher. They found that 1.2% of CT surgery patients who underwent TEE had a UGIB within 30 days of the surgery, compared to 0.29% of patients who underwent CT surgery only. It is important to note that bleeding complications often go unrecognized in the immediate perioperative period.

The key, as always, is to avoid complications in the first place. TEE probes should *not* be placed in patients who have an absolute contraindication. These include known or recent (<6 months) esophageal trauma, active variceal bleeding, and tracheoesophageal fistula. Placement of a probe should be considered *carefully* if the patient has any relative contraindications, including esophageal varices, history of UGIB, esophageal strictures, and Barrett esophagus (*Table 140.1*). To determine whether a patient has a contraindication to TEE, **you must ask the patient about history and look for signs and symptoms** of these disorders. Pertinent signs and symptoms include dysphagia, odynophagia, coffee-ground emesis or hematochezia, liver disease, history of banding, significant longstanding (especially untreated) gastroesophageal reflux disease, and hiatal hernia.

TEE probes are typically placed for certain cardiac surgery procedures (especially valve replacement and repair) but may also be used to evaluate the heart during emergent intraoperative events. The ultimate decision to place a TEE probe depends on the clinical indications and the risk-benefit profile that is determined by the managing anesthesia team.

© 2006 Mayo Foundation for Medical Education and Research

TABLE 140.1	RELATIVE CONTRAINDICATIONS TO TRANSESOPHAGEAL ECHOCARDIOGRAPHY
History	
Dysphagia	
Odynophagia	
Mediastinal radiation	
Recent upper gastrointestinal (GI) surgery	
Recent upper GI bleeding	
Esophageal pathology	
Stricture	
Tumor	
Diverticulum	
Varices	
Esophagitis	
Recent chest trauma	

From Hensley FA, Martin PF, Gravlee GP. *A Practical Approach to Cardiac Anesthesia.* 3rd ed. Philadelphia, Pa.: Lippincott Williams & Wilkins; 2003.

Here are the three basic guiding principles to follow when placing a TEE probe:

1) Never force the probe. If there is resistance, try something else.
2) Use a lot of lubrication.
3) Use a jaw thrust, and consider asking for help. An extra pair of hands can prove invaluable in difficult situations.

One specific technique for placing a TEE probe is to start by anteflexing the tip to help make the anatomical angle of the pharynx. Simultaneously, perform a jaw thrust and gently twist the probe side to side with careful pressure. Use of a laryngoscope is routine and will assist in displacing the tongue and mandible anteriorly. If you encounter difficulty, you may try retroflexing the probe or approaching from a different angle in the mouth. Again, use lots of lubrication and **never force the probe**. If placing the probe is difficult using standard maneuvers, creating more space for the TEE to pass may be necessary. This can be accomplished with the help of a second operator or different laryngoscope blade to assist in displacing airway structures anteriorly. Also, in smaller patients, it is advisable to empty the stomach and then discontinue the gastric tube. If this is unsuccessful, some institutions will get a STAT intraoperative esophagogastroduodenoscopy (EGD) from the thoracic or gastrointestinal services to evaluate for intrathoracic stomach, tumor, or stricture.

If you are still unable to pass the probe but believe that the surgery necessitates TEE, consider a pediatric probe. Pediatric probes come in biplane and omniplane, are often of sufficient length (especially in women), and are likelier to cause less injury due to their small diameter. Another alternative to inserting a TEE probe may be to switch strategies and perform epicardial echocardiography (for cardiac cases) or TTE for cases not involving the thorax.

The TEE probe should be considered an invasive monitoring device and care must be taken not to cause additional morbidity once the probe has been placed. One practice is to withdraw the probe to the upper esophagus for cases involving cryoablation (maze) of the posterior left atrium in order to reduce the probability of atrial rupture. Also, during the cardiopulmonary bypass and especially during circulatory arrest, the editor advises that the power to the TEE be discontinued to avoid burn injury to the esophageal tissues (rare) and to avoid unnecessarily warming the heart with the ultrasound signal (especially for cold cardioplegia protection cases).

TAKE HOME POINTS

- TEE is a valuable intraoperative monitor. Complications are rare but serious.
- There are both absolute and relative contraindications to placement of the probe.
- Insertion is facilitated by flexing the probe tip, doing a jaw thrust, removing the gastric tube, performing laryngoscopy, and switching to a smaller probe.
- *Never* force the probe.
- An intraoperative EGD may be warranted to check for significant pathology.
- Know when to withdraw the probe and/or discontinue power.

SUGGESTED READINGS

Hensley FA, Martin PF, Gravlee GP. *A Practical Approach to Cardiac Anesthesia.* 3rd ed. Philadelphia, Pa.: Lippincott Williams & Wilkins; 2003.
Kallmeyer IJ, Collard CD. *Anesth Analg* 2001;92(5):1126–1130.
Lennon MJ, Gibbs NM. *J Cardiothor Vasc Anesthesiol* 2005;19(2):141–145.

141

REMEMBER THAT IT IS NOT POSSIBLE TO COMPLETELY AVOID MYOCARDIAL ISCHEMIA ASSOCIATED WITH CARDIOPULMONARY BYPASS AND THE DELIVERY OF CARDIOPLEGIA—THE GOAL IS TO MINIMIZE IT

AMY C. LU, MD, MPH AND
GIORA LANDESBERG, MD, DSC, MBA

Myocardial protection techniques are critical in obtaining optimal results in cardiac surgery with the aim to decrease myocardial ischemia during cardiopulmonary bypass (CPB). Although some degree of myocardial damage and disturbance of cellular integrity is almost inevitable, in the majority of cases it is reversible when appropriate protection methods are performed. The normal working myocardium consumes 8 mL of O_2/100 g/minute. Oxygen (O_2) consumption decreases to 5.6 mL O_2/100 g/minute in the empty beating heart, to approximately 4 mL/100 g/minute in the fibrillating heart (at a temperature of $32°C$), and to 1.1 mL O_2/100 g/minute during CPB with potassium cardioplegia. Cooling the heart to $22°C$ may further decrease O_2 consumption to 0.3 mL O_2/100 g/minute. Typically, myocardial damage is attributed to a combination of myocardial ischemia due to oxygen supply-demand imbalance and reperfusion injury. Both mechanisms may result in intracellular acidosis, calcium overload, the formation of free radicals, initiation of inflammation, complement activation, and myocardial cellular edema. During CPB, myocardial injury can also occur due to ventricular fibrillation with concurrent ventricular distention, excessive use of inotropes and/or calcium, surgical manipulation, and coronary embolism. Normothermic ventricular fibrillation should be avoided in patients with myocardial hypertrophy because the increased wall tension compromises subendocardial perfusion. Likewise, ventricular distension is a special threat in patients with severe aortic insufficiency. Proper deairing of grafts, cardiac chambers, and venting before and during initial cardiac ejection can prevent formation of air bubbles that may lead to coronary embolism and both ventricular arrhythmias and dysfunction. Not surprisingly, those patients with more severe cardiac risk factors (e.g., severe coronary artery disease (CAD), valvular disease, ventricular hypertrophy, New York Heart Association functional class IV) are at greatest risk of sustaining myocardial injury from inadequate myocardial protection. The area of myocardial protection

© 2006 Mayo Foundation for Medical Education and Research

strategies is continually growing, and this chapter summarizes the current trends in this evolving field.

CARDIOPLEGIA

Always consider that following the initiation of CPB, it is important to discontinue the administration of all exogenous inotropes so they are not mixed into the cardioplegia because these drugs can potentially increase myocardial energy consumption. Potassium cardioplegia is the most common method of myocardial protection during CPB. Traditionally, cardioplegia is delivered in an anterograde intermittent fashion through the cross-clamped aortic root with a cold, high-potassium, crystalloid solution. The increase in extracellular potassium concentration eventually inactivates the sodium channels, abolishing action potentials and arresting the heart in diastole, thus stopping the energy expenditure associated with electrical and mechanical activity. The composition of cardioplegia varies on an institutional basis; however, all solutions contain 10 to 40 mEq/L. In addition, small amounts of calcium and magnesium and a buffer (usually bicarbonate) are needed in the cardioplegia. Alkaline buffers improve myocardial protection by preventing acid metabolite buildup. With cold cardioplegia, multiple doses are given for the effects of washout, rewarming, and prevention of metabolite buildup. Washout of high-potassium cardioplegia occurs due to the presence of noncoronary collaterals. Standard practice has been to employ systemic and topical cardiac hypothermia to reduce basal metabolic oxygen consumption. O_2 consumption decreases by 50% for every $10°C$ decrease in myocardial temperature, and myocardial cooling to $25°C$ allows the interruption of coronary blood supply (aortic cross-clamping) for longer periods of time. However, hypothermia itself may elicit myocardial injury by affecting cellular fluidity, transmembrane gradients, and these changes may result in cellular edema. Recently, it has been suggested that continuous and/or warm cardioplegia provides better protection, although severe, diffuse CAD may preclude even distribution of the cardioplegia and lead to poor protection. So far, studies have not consistently demonstrated the superiority of one method over the other. Although only anterograde cardioplegia was initially used, retrograde perfusion via the coronary sinus while carefully monitoring coronary sinus perfusion pressure (at <40 mm Hg) has become popular, with many centers using a combination of both methods and showing superior protection. Retrograde cardioplegia is particularly advantageous in valve surgery and in patients with critical CAD or total coronary occlusions. This technique is contraindicated in patients with a persistent left superior vena cava draining into the coronary sinus because of the risk of retrograde cardioplegia perfusion to the brain. Most centers currently use blood cardioplegia, a mixture of blood in crystalloids with a final hematocrit of 16% to 20%. In addition to the O_2-carrying capacity of hemoglobin, blood contains buffers, free radical scavengers, colloids, and other components that protect the myocardium.

MYOCARDIAL PRECONDITIONING WITH ANESTHETIC AGENTS

Ischemic preconditioning describes the heart's ability to be protected during periods of ischemia through an endogenously mediated mechanism. Extensive investigation in this area has demonstrated that volatile anesthetics can confer similar cardioprotective benefits through conformational changes in myocardial protein structure. Clinical research in this area has shown encouraging results for isoflurane, sevoflurane, and desflurane when compared to a primarily propofol-based anesthetic. The majority of these studies demonstrate decreased postoperative troponin elevation, reduced inotropic support, and greater preserved cardiac function. A similar incidence of postoperative complications has been observed between both groups in these trials. Current research in this area is focused on the timing of volatile anesthetic administration during cardiac surgery for maximal preconditioning benefits.

ANTI-INFLAMMATORY THERAPEUTIC STRATEGIES

CPB activates multiple contact, coagulation, fibrinolytic, and cytokine cascades, which result in a systemic inflammatory response. In recent years, this concept of myocardial injury leading to inflammatory mediated responses has prompted research to prevent CPB-induced inflammation. Numerous studies have investigated potential pharmacologic agents, such as corticosteroids, adenosine, phosphodiesterase inhibitors, antioxidants, nitric oxide donors, and complement inhibitors. Mechanical strategies that have been studied include hemofiltration, leukocyte filters, hypothermic CPB, pulsatile CBP flow, and uniquely coated circuits (e.g., heparin bonded [Carmeda Bonded Maxima; Medtronic, Inc, Minneapolis, MN] or circuits SMART; Cobe Cardiovascular, Arvarda, CO). The beneficial effects of both pharmaceutical and mechanical strategies have yet to be definitively demonstrated in large clinical studies.

In summary, myocardial protection remains one of the most critical determinants in the success of cardiac surgery. Cold intermittent potassium cardioplegia remains the mainstay of myocardial protection. New techniques include focusing on preventing systemic inflammatory responses and on myocardial preconditioning are not conclusive, and further work remains to be done in these areas. Because cardiac surgery currently carries excellent results in low-risk patients, future innovations in myocardial protection will ultimately benefit those patients with high risk, including those with poor ventricular function, severe valvular disease, and high-grade CAD.

- Myocardial protection remains one of the most critical determinants of the success of cardiac surgery.

- CPB-associated myocardial damage is attributable to O_2 supply–demand imbalance, reperfusion injury, ventricular fibrillation with ventricular distension, use of inotropes and calcium, surgical manipulation, and coronary artery embolism.

- Always consider that following the initiation of CPB, it is important to discontinue the administration of all exogenous inotropes so they are not mixed into the cardioplegia because these drugs can potentially increase myocardial energy consumption.

- Studies to date do not consistently demonstrate that "traditional" cardioplegia with a cold, high-potassium, crystalloid solution is superior to continuous and/or warm cardioplegia.

- Retrograde cardioplegia is advantageous in valve surgery or with critical CAD. Careful attention to avoiding coronary sinus perfusion pressures of >40 mm Hg is of paramount importance.

- An anesthetic based on volatile anesthetics (isoflurane, sevoflurane, and desflurane) can protectively precondition the heart against ischemia damage.

- The relationship between myocardial injury and CPB and a systemic inflammatory response is a subject of ongoing investigation.

SELECTED READINGS

Cohen G, Borger M, Weisel R, et al. Intraoperative myocardial protection: Current trends and future perspectives. *Ann Thorac Surg* 1999;68:1995–2001.

Collard CD. Modulating the inflammatory response to optimize contractility. Society of Cardiac Anesthesiology Annual Meeting & Workshop; 2006. San Diego, CA, April 2006;315–316.

De Hert SG, Van der Linden PJ, Cromheecke S, et al. Choice of primary anesthetic regimen can influence intensive care unit length of stay after coronary surgery with cardiopulmonary bypass. *Anesthesiology* 2004;101(1):9–20.

Kaplan JA, Reich DL, Lake, et al., eds. *Kaplan's Cardiac Anesthesia*. 5th ed. Philadelphia, PA: Elsevier/Saunders; 2006:901–904.

142

ON THE CUSP OF DISASTER: DISTINGUISH BETWEEN THE ANESTHETIC MANAGEMENT OF STENOTIC AND REGURGITANT CARDIAC VALVES

GEORGE A. MASHOUR, MD, PhD AND
THEODORE A. ALSTON, MD, PhD

The initial approach to the patient with cardiac valve disease involves three basic questions:

1) Which valve is affected?
2) Is the lesion stenotic or regurgitant?
3) What is the severity of stenosis or insufficiency?

This chapter reviews disease of the aortic and mitral valve and provides recommendations for anesthetic management during cardiac surgical repair.

AORTIC VALVE DISEASE

Aortic Stenosis. Stenosis is defined as a fixed obstruction preventing outflow through a valve. Stenotic lesions of the aortic valve may be either congenital or acquired. Bicuspid valve is associated with a prevalence of approximately 2% and is therefore one of the most common congenital cardiac lesions. Aortic stenosis may also be acquired due to degenerative calcification. The severity of aortic stenosis is characterized by the valve area and mean pressure gradient (*Table 142.1*).

A low cardiac index can cause underestimation of the severity of aortic stenosis; selected patients benefit from valve replacement for low-output, low-gradient aortic stenosis.

Compensatory changes in response to aortic stenosis include left ventricular hypertrophy. The associated increase in wall thickness and decrease in compliance renders the ventricle preload dependent. Adequate preload is achieved by normovolemia, maintenance of venous return, adequate diastolic filling time, and preservation of sinus rhythm and the associated "atrial kick." Anesthetic goals for the patient with aortic stenosis therefore include the following:

- Avoidance of hypovolemia
- Avoidance of precipitous decrease in systemic vascular resistance, as may happen during induction of anesthesia
- Avoidance of tachycardia, which will decrease diastolic filling time
- Maintenance of sinus rhythm and preservation of atrial kick

© 2006 Mayo Foundation for Medical Education and Research

TABLE 142.1	SEVERITY OF AORTIC STENOSIS CHARACTERIZED BY AREA AND MEAN PRESSURE GRADIENT	
SEVERITY	VALVE AREA (CM^2)	MEAN PRESSURE GRADIENT (MM HG)
Mild	1.5–2.0	<25
Moderate	1.0–1.5	25–50
Severe	0.5–1.0	>50
Critical	<0.5	

The classic technique of high-dose fentanyl induction was initially developed as a management technique for patients with aortic stenosis.

Aortic Regurgitation. Regurgitation or insufficiency is defined as the failure of a valve to prevent backflow of blood. Such lesions of the aorta are due to dilation of the aortic root or leaflet abnormalities and, like stenosis, may be congenital or acquired. Congenital root dilation is associated with Marfan disease and other connective tissue disorders, while acquired insufficiency can result from aortic dissection, chronic hypertension, atherosclerosis, and aortitis. Leaflet abnormalities include bicuspid valves (which can become regurgitant), as well as rheumatic heart disease, endocarditis, and connective tissue disease. The determinants of insufficiency include the valvular orifice area and the diastolic pressure gradient. Like stenosis, adequate preload and sinus rhythm should be maintained. Unlike stenosis, high-normal heart rate and lower systemic vascular resistance improve cardiac performance in the patient with aortic insufficiency. Faster heart rate decreases diastolic time during which insufficiency is manifested, and lower systemic vascular resistance favors forward flow rather than regurgitation.

Intra-aortic balloon counterpulsation is contraindicated in the setting of significant aortic regurgitation. The balloon increases the regurgitation.

MITRAL VALVE DISEASE

During diastole, the mitral valve allows blood to flow from the left atrium to the left ventricle, and during systole, it protects the left atrium and pulmonary circulation from high pressures. Like the aortic valve, mitral valve lesions can be stenotic or regurgitant.

Mitral Stenosis. The normal area of the mitral valve is 4 to 6 cm^2. Mitral stenosis is defined as an area of <2 cm^2 and is critical at <1 cm^2. Mitral stenosis is typically caused by rheumatic fever and may lead to elevated left atrial pressures, consequent atrial fibrillation, and pulmonary hypertension. Left atrial filling pressures are critical for patients with mitral stenosis. Thus, like aortic stenosis, anesthetic goals include the following:

- Maintenance of preload
- Avoidance of tachycardia

- Maintenance of systemic vascular resistance
- Maintenance of sinus rhythm

Mitral Regurgitation. Mitral insufficiency can be either acute or chronic. Acute regurgitation often results from the rupture of chordae tendineae, ischemic papillary muscle, or ruptured papillary rupture. Myxomatous degeneration, rheumatic heart disease, and endocarditis are other causes of mitral regurgitation. As with aortic regurgitation, high normal heart rate and decreased afterload are beneficial intraoperatively. Although preferable, sinus rhythm is not as crucial in mitral regurgitation as other valvular lesions. In fact, patients with chronic mitral regurgitation often present with atrial fibrillation due to left atrial distension.

Intra-aortic balloon counterpulsation is hemodynamically beneficial in the setting of mitral regurgitation, although atrial fibrillation can decrease the efficiency of the device. The balloon can be lifesaving in cases of acute, severe regurgitation.

INTRAOPERATIVE TRANSESOPHAGEAL ECHOCARDIOGRAPHY

Use of intraoperative echocardiography is essential to cardiac valve surgery. The initial exam should evaluate the following:

- Valve area
- Peak and mean gradients
- Color Doppler mapping of regurgitant jets
- Valve leaflet structure, movement, coaptation, and apposition
- Annular dilation

Accurate echocardiographic evaluation can help guide surgical planning, especially in the decision between mitral valve replacement and repair. After surgery is performed, echocardiographic evaluation should focus on the following:

- Degree of valvular regurgitation or stenosis
- Paravalvular leak
- Systolic anterior motion of mitral leaflet leading to obstruction of left ventricular outflow tract

---

TAKE HOME POINTS

- Stenotic lesions of the aortic and mitral valves are best managed by maintaining higher preload, higher systemic vascular resistance, sinus rhythm, and lower heart rate.
- Regurgitant lesions of the aortic and mitral valves are best managed by maintaining normal preload, lower systemic vascular resistance, and higher heart rate.

■ Accurate transesophageal echocardiographic evaluation is essential for cardiac valve surgery.

SUGGESTED READINGS

Istaphanous G. The patient with aortic stenosis. *Int Anesthesiol Clin* 2005;43(4):21–31.

Mackay JH, Arrowsmith JE. Aortic valve disease. In: Mackay JH and Arrowsmith JE, eds. *Core Topics in Cardiac Anaesthesia*. Cambridge, UK: Greenwich Medical Media Limited; 2004:169–174.

Mackay JH, Wells FC. Mitral valve disease. In: Mackay JH and Arrowsmith JE, eds. *Core Topics in Cardiac Anaesthesia*. Cambridge, UK: Greenwich Medical Media Limited; 2004:175–182.

Nishimura RA, Grantham JA, Connolly HM, et al. Low-output, low-gradient aortic stenosis in patients with depressed left ventricular systolic function: The clinical utility of the dobutamine challenge in the catheterization laboratory. *Circulation* 2002;106(7):809–813.

143

ANTIFIBRINOLYTIC AGENTS: SPARE THE CLOT BUT SPOIL THE THROMBUS

ALA NOZARI, MD, PhD AND THEODORE A. ALSTON, MD, PhD

PHYSIOLOGY OF FIBRINOLYSIS

The fibrinolytic system has evolved to dissolve intravascular thrombus and vessel-sealing clot after control of the vascular breach. The system prevents inappropriate accumulation and extension of fibrin. It is important in the repair and remodeling process following injury.

The major fibrinolytic enzyme is plasmin, which circulates as its inert proenzyme plasminogen. The conversion of plasminogen to plasmin is facilitated by the plasminogen activators, thrombin, fibrin, and factor XII (Hageman factor). Tissue-type plasminogen activator (tPA) is produced predominantly in the vascular endothelium in the presence of fibrin, while the urokinaselike plasminogen is found in urine and other secretions. The proteolytic function of tPA is inhibited by plasminogen activator inhibitor (PAI), which is produced by the vascular endothelium (PAI-1) or the placenta (PAI-2).

Plasmin can be inactivated by the serine protease inhibitor alpha 2-antiplasmin and by alpha 2-macroglobulin, a large plasma protein produced by the liver that is found in increased concentration in nephrotic syndrome. Alpha 2-antiplasmin deficiency can lead to a bleeding tendency.

Plasmin functions as a serine protease, cutting specifically C-terminal to the lysine and arginine residues on fibrin. Fibrin monomers, when polymerized, form protofibrils. These protofibrils contain two strands, antiparallel, associated noncovalently. Within a single strand, the fibrin monomers are covalently linked through the actions of coagulation factor XIII. Thus, plasmin action on a clot initially creates nicks in the fibrin, and further digestion leads to solubilization. These soluble parts, called fibrin degradation products, compete with thrombin and slow down the conversion of fibrinogen to fibrin. This effect can be seen in the thrombin clotting time test, which is prolonged in a person who has active fibrinolysis. Soluble fibrin degradation products are cleared by the reticuloendothelial system.

ANTIFIBRINOLYTIC AGENTS

Antifibrinolytic agents (aprotinin, epsilon-aminocaproic acid [EACA], and tranexamic acid) can reduce the amount of blood loss and the need for blood transfusions.

ⓒ 2006 Mayo Foundation for Medical Education and Research

Tranexamic acid (Cyklokapron) and EACA (Amicar) are antifibrinolytic amino acids with the ability to bind to plasminogen by its lysine-binding site, preventing its association with fibrin. They also inhibit the proteolytic activity of plasmin. Tranexamic acid is more potent but less well absorbed orally than EACA. Both drugs are minimally metabolized and are mainly excreted unchanged in the urine, with plasma half-time of 2 to 10 hours. Dosage reduction is indicated in renal impairment.

Besides their role in cardiac surgery, these agents are useful in conditions with bleeding tendency such as patients with von Willebrand disease, patients following prostatic or uterine surgery, and patients with gastrointestinal (GI) bleeding, and as adjunctive therapy in patients with hemophilia.

Side effects are more frequently seen with EACA and include GI symptoms and dizziness. Prolonged use of EACA can rarely cause acute necrotizing polymyositis with myoglobinuria. Antifibrinolytics should not be used in patients with gross hematuria because of the risk for clot formation in the urinary tract with subsequent obstruction and hydronephrosis.

Aprotinin (Trasylol) is a serine protease inhibitor (serpin) isolated from bovine lung tissue. It forms a reversible enzyme inhibition complex with serine proteases by binding to the proteases in a dose-dependent manner. These proteases include plasmin, trypsin, kallikrein, and activated protein C. It inhibits platelet activation by thrombin and is suggested to modulate the systemic inflammation associated with cardiopulmonary bypass (CPB). The antifibrinolytic properties of aprotinin are of particular interest in cardiac surgery because it is suggested to decrease contact activation of the intrinsic coagulation pathway during CPB.

Anaphylactic and anaphylactoid reactions are rare in patients without prior exposure to aprotinin (<0.1%), but patients who are re-exposed have an increased risk of allergic reactions (0.9%–5%). Clinically relevant creatinine elevation (0.7–2 mg/dL over baseline) has been reported in up to 7.7% of cardiac surgery patients treated with aprotinin, but in the majority (80%), renal impairment was associated with perioperative hemodynamic instability and hemorrhage. The proposed mechanism involves the effects of aprotinin on afferent arteriolar tone through inhibition of renin and kallikrein activity. Risk factors for postoperative renal failure include advanced age, duration of CPB >3 hours, preoperative ventricular dysfunction, diabetes mellitus, and pre-existing renal disease. The beneficial effect of aprotinin in achieving hemostasis must also be weighed against risk of pathological thrombosis, even though studies have not confirmed an increased risk of deep venous thrombosis or pulmonary embolism in these patients.

KEY POINTS

1) Aprotinin significantly reduces transfusion requirements compared to placebo (relative risk, 0.38–0.61) and total blood loss (35%–53%, depending on dose).

2) EACA and tranexamic acid also reduce bleeding. All three drugs significantly reduce the rate of surgical re-exploration. All three drugs refers to Aprotinin, EACA, and tranexamic acid.

3) Antifibrinolytic therapy is not associated with an increased incidence of early SVG occlusion or myocardial infarction.

4) EACA is given as a loading dose of 100 to 150 mg/kg (10 g over 30 minutes) to the patient and into the pump prime solution, followed by a 20 to 30 mg/kg/hour infusion. Aprotinin is administered as a 280-mg bolus (2 million kallikrein inhibitory units) to the patient and into pump prime, followed by 70 mg/hour during surgery.

POTENTIAL MISTAKES IN THE USE OF ANTIFIBRINOLYTICS

1) Prior to administration of full-dose aprotinin, all patients should undergo an evaluation of risk factors followed by a test dose of aprotinin 5 minutes prior to the loading dose.

2) Consider the risk of anaphylactic reaction, particularly in patients who are being re-exposed to aprotinin. For patients who have received aprotinin within the previous 12 months (the manufacturer changed this recommendation in Dec. 2006 from 6 in 12 months), do not administer the drug until the surgical ability to rapidly achieve CPB is achieved (after aortic cannulation). Do not prime the pump with aprotinin until the risk of anaphylaxis is deemed remote.

3) Postoperative renal failure may be a problem in patients with pre-existing renal disease, advanced age, preoperative ventricular dysfunction, diabetes mellitus, and expected prolonged CPB.

4) Avoid antifibrinolytic treatment in patients with disseminated intravascular coagulation.

5) Remember to correct underlying coagulopathy, factor deficiency, thrombocytopenia, or platelet dysfunction. Note that aprotinin prolongs the celite-activated clotting time and the partial thromboplastin time, and those test results do not indicate anticoagulation. The kaolin-activated clotting time and the prothrombin time are relatively insensitive to the presence of aprotinin in the blood.

SUGGESTED READINGS

Alston TA. Procoagulant action of aprotinin. *Anesth Analg* 1996;82(6):1305–1306.

Fitzsimons MG, Peterfreund RA, Raines DE. Aprotinin administration and pulmonary thromboembolism during orthotopic liver transplantation: Report of two cases. *Anesth Analg* 2001;92(6):1418–1421.

Mangano DT, Tudor IC, Dietzel C, et al. The risk associated with aprotinin in cardiac surgery. *N Engl J Med* 2006;354(4):353–365.

Royston D. High-dose aprotinin therapy: A review of the first five years' experience. *J Cardiothorac Vasc Anesth* 1992;6(1):76–100.

144

THE DOWNSIDE OF ANESTHESIA FOR THE DESCENDING THORACIC AORTA: JUST ABOUT ALL ANESTHETIC ISSUES ARE OF PARAMOUNT IMPORTANCE!

EDWIN G. AVERY, IV, MD AND DAVID A. SHAFF, MD

Patients undergoing surgery on the descending thoracic aorta (DTA) present a *great* anesthetic challenge. The general categories of aortic pathology affecting the DTA include aneurysm, pseudoaneurysm, coarctation, aortic rupture, dissection, intramural hematoma, infection, and atherosclerotic disease (with or without penetrating ulcers). Constructing a safe anesthetic plan for patients requiring DTA surgery mandates an intimate knowledge of aortic pathology, the planned procedure, and strategies to minimize the deleterious effects of surgical manipulation of the aorta. These patients often present in an urgent or emergent fashion with little time to evaluate serious comorbidities that frequently accompany aortic disease. *Emergent procedures require recruiting additional anesthesia personnel so preoperative preparation is carried out with optimal efficiency.* The anesthesiologist must review the details of all available imaging studies and create an anesthetic plan that focuses on providing protection and support for all bodily systems affected by the planned procedure.

A successful anesthetic monitoring plan for DTA surgery considers that the nature of these procedures creates hemodynamic instability and hypoperfusion of multiple organ systems. To partially circumvent the effects of interrupting blood flow with aortic cross-clamping, the distal aorta is often perfused using a Gott shunt or partial left-heart bypass (left atrium to distal aorta, iliac or femoral artery bypass with centrifugal pump assist). *Femoral arterial blood pressure monitoring is therefore necessary to assess distal arterial perfusion pressure.* Distal aortic mean arterial pressure (MAP) is commonly maintained between 60 and 70 mm Hg during the partial bypass period, while proximal MAP is maintained at approximately 90 mm Hg. The use of partial left-heart bypass does not routinely incorporate a heater/cooler exchange unit into the extracorporeal circuit and thus puts the patient at risk for developing profound hypothermia as heat is lost through the extracorporeal circuit. *Hypothermia increases the risk of coagulopathic hemorrhage and hyperglycemia (which may exacerbate ischemic injury to the cord and/or heart) in these patients, and thus patient warming systems (e.g., forced convective*

© 2006 Mayo Foundation for Medical Education and Research

air blankets or hydrogel energy conduction pads) should routinely be used in these anesthetics.

Invasive monitoring is essential for DTA surgery. Caution is warranted in choosing a site for radial arterial cannulation because atherosclerotic disease is highly prevalent in patients requiring DTA surgery. *Severe subclavian or axillary artery plaquing can result in inaccurate hemodynamic data.* Checking bilateral noninvasive cuff pressures can identify significant gradients between the upper extremities. *Central venous access is mandated for these procedures* so cardiac function and filling pressures can be monitored (e.g., by insertion of a pulmonary artery catheter). Intraoperative transesophageal echocardiography (TEE) monitoring can also be useful in this regard. A dedicated central infusion port for the rapid administration of potent inotropes, vasoconstrictors, and vasodilators is also necessary. Aortic cross-clamping places an acutely increased afterload on the left heart that can result in myocardial ischemia and/or acute left ventricular failure in susceptible patients. Careful monitoring for ischemic electrocardiogram changes and/or signs of acute left ventricular failure (e.g., an acute increase in the pulmonary capillary wedge pressure or new wall motion abnormalities observed with TEE) during aortic cross-clamping is mandatory. *Pharmacologic-based afterload reduction (e.g., administration of sodium nitroprusside, nitroglycerin, or fenoldopam) is often indicated during aortic cross-clamping.* Aortic cross-clamp removal can also be accompanied by hemodynamic instability (e.g., hypotension) related to an acute reduction in left ventricular afterload and to the release of lactic acid from ischemic tissue beds distal to the clamp if partial left-heart bypass is not employed. *The transient increase in circulating lactic acid and potassium associated with cross-clamp removal can also instigate ventricular irritability or arrhythmias. Fluid loading and pharmacotherapy (e.g., administration of α_1-agonists and sodium bicarbonate) just prior to and after unclamping can be useful to quell the hemodynamic deterioration.* Large-bore peripheral intravenous access is standard for these procedures to allow for the rapid administration of fluid and/or blood products throughout perioperative period.

The temporary interruption of aortic blood flow associated with DTA surgery to allow for aortic interposition grafting places all distal organs at risk for ischemic injury and infarction. *Potential ischemic injury to the spinal cord is of paramount concern; thus, the anesthetic plan is tailored to both monitor for and prevent such damage.* Protection of the spinal cord during DTA surgery is accomplished with maneuvers that promote blood flow to the cord. Suggested interventions include the preoperative insertion of a lumbar spinal drain, arterial pressure augmentation, neurophysiological monitoring techniques, and pharmacologic support measures. Lumbar cerebrospinal fluid (CSF) drainage is employed to both prevent cord ischemia and treat postoperative paraplegia resulting from DTA surgery. These catheters are managed *without the use of a heparinized or pressurized transducer flush apparatus*. CSF is permitted to drain if the lumbar CSF pressure exceeds 10 mm Hg. Care is taken to ensure a normal coagulation profile prior to catheter insertion and removal. *Arterial pressure augmentation is achieved by maintaining a spinal cord perfusion pressure (MAP – intrathecal pressure) of at least 70 mm Hg, which is accomplished by achieving an MAP of 80 to 100 mm Hg.* Intraoperative neurophysiological monitoring can reveal the acute development of spinal cord ischemia and is accomplished through the use of somatosensory-evoked potentials or motor-evoked potentials. Pharmacologic support measures include the intrathecal administration of preservativefree papaverine (in conjunction with lumbar CSF drainage) and the systemic administration of glucocorticoids, thiopental, mannitol, magnesium, calcium channel blockers, and naloxone. Supportive studies of these drugs in this clinical setting are difficult to interpret, and no widely used standard pharmacologic regimen has been established to date. Intravenous naloxone given at 1 μg/kg/hour has been demonstrated to be associated with improved neurologic outcomes (including reversal of paraplegic symptoms) in this clinical setting.

Left thoracotomy, or a thoracoabdominal incision, is the most common surgical incision used for exposure of the DTA. This surgical approach often necessitates selective lung ventilation, most often of the right lung. Options for selective lung ventilation include lung retraction, insertion of a left bronchial blocker, or the use of a double-lumen endobronchial tube (DLT) (i.e., commonly, a left DLT is employed). The DLT permits pulmonary maneuvers such as the ability to suction the airways and apply continuous positive airway pressure. However, its use may require transition to a single-lumen endotracheal tube at the end of the procedure with the inherent risks after a major surgery.

Consideration of postoperative analgesia is of major concern in this clinical setting because of the painful nature of a thoracotomy. The intra- and postoperative use of thoracic epidural analgesia can provide excellent pain control and permit early extubation to allow for the prompt assessment of neurologic function (e.g., rule out paraplegia related to spinal cord ischemia); care must be taken to ensure normal function of the coagulation cascade for both insertion and removal of the catheter to prevent bleeding-related neurologic complications.

TAKE HOME POINTS

- Emergent procedures on the DTA require recruiting additional anesthesia personnel so preoperative preparation is carried out with optimal efficiency.

- Potential ischemic injury to the spinal cord is of paramount concern and thus the anesthetic plan is tailored to both prevent and monitor for such damage.
- When DTA surgery involves the use of a Gott shunt, or partial left-heart bypass, femoral arterial blood pressure monitoring is necessary to assess distal arterial perfusion pressure.
- Hypothermia increases the risk of coagulopathic hemorrhage and hyperglycemia (which may exacerbate ischemic injury to the cord and/or heart) in these patients, and thus patient warming systems (e.g., forced convective air blankets or hydrogel energy conduction pads) are routinely used.
- Invasive monitoring is essential for DTA surgery. Be aware that severe subclavian or axillary artery plaquing can result in inaccurate hemodynamic data. Checking bilateral noninvasive cuff pressures can identify significant gradients in the upper extremities.
- Central venous access is mandated for these procedures so cardiac function and filling pressures can be monitored. Central access also provides a route for administration of important drugs.
- Pharmacologic-based afterload reduction (e.g., administration of sodium nitroprusside, nitroglycerin, or fenoldopam) is often indicated during aortic cross-clamping.
- The transient increase in circulating lactic acid and potassium associated with aortic cross-clamp removal can instigate ventricular irritability or arrhythmias.
- Fluid loading and pharmacotherapy (e.g., administration of α_1-agonists and sodium bicarbonate) just prior to and after aortic unclamping can be useful to quell the associated hemodynamic deterioration.
- Lumbar CSF drainage is employed to prevent and/or treat spinal cord ischemia. These catheters are managed without the use of a heparinized or pressurized transducer flush apparatus.
- Consideration of postoperative analgesia is of major concern in this clinical setting because of the painful nature of a thoracotomy.

SUGGESTED READINGS

Bittner E, Dunn PF. Anesthesia for vascular surgery. In: Hurford WE, Bailin MT, Davison JK, et al., eds. *Clinical Anesthesia Procedures of the Massachusetts General Hospital*. 6th ed. Philadelphia, PA.: Lippincott Williams & Wilkins; 2002:350–365.

Moskowitz DM, Kahn RA, Reich DL. Anesthesia for the surgical treatment of thoracic aortic disease. In: Thys DM, Hillel Z, Schwartz AJ, eds. *Textbook of Cardiothoracic Anesthesiology*. New York, NY: McGraw-Hill; 2001:680–710.

Pantin EJ, Cheung AT. Thoracic aorta. In: Kaplan JA, Reich DL, Lake CL, et al., eds. *Kaplan's Cardiac Anesthesia*. 5th ed. Philadelphia, PA.: Saunders-Elsevier; 2006:723–764.

145

ANESTHESIA FOR ASCENDING AORTIC DISSECTION: IT'S LIKE WALKING ON EGGSHELLS FOR THE ANESTHESIOLOGIST

JAMES F. DANA, MD AND EDWIN G. AVERY, IV, MD

A 74-year-old man arrives at the emergency ward (EW) at 2:31 AM. Gripping his chest, he complains of an intense tearing pain. Medical history is significant for poorly controlled hypertension, hyperlipidemia, and gout. Surgical history is significant for a right hip replacement and cholecystectomy. Vital signs are blood pressure—left: 188/124 mm Hg, right: 125/110 mm Hg; pulse 124/minute; and respirations 24/minute. Physical exam is remarkable for slight confusion, no jugular venous elevation, bilateral basilar rales, holodiastolic diastolic murmur, unremarkable abdomen, and no pedal edema. Pulses are unequal with the right radial pulse obviously weaker than the left radial pulse. Left pedal pulse is weaker than right pedal pulse. The patient has a 14-gauge intravenous catheter in the left forearm. Electrocardiogram shows ST-segment elevation in the inferior leads with a baseline sinus tachycardia. Chest film demonstrates widening of the mediastinum, and a computed tomography (CT) scan confirms a type A dissection extending to the iliac bifurcation. Now, you get paged to the EW to assist with management! Strap in and hold on because you're in for a ride! Forget about getting any sleep for the rest of the night because this patient needs to go to the operating room pronto! Establish arterial monitoring in the left radial artery, reduce the systolic blood pressure to 110 mm Hg, order some blood, and get a quick transthoracic or transesophageal echocardiogram to assess for cardiac tamponade and to determine the mechanism of his aortic insufficiency, which the holodiastolic murmur tipped you off to. Get a lot of help because time is of the essence in these cases, and even when you do your job just right, the patient can still have a bad outcome.

Dissections of the ascending aorta, representing 60% to 70% of all aortic dissections, are true life-threatening emergencies. They involve a tear of the intimal wall of the aorta, creating a false channel. *Due to the high aortic pressures and shear stress created by pulsatile perfusion, the dissection flap can continue to dissect in its proximal or distal extent (often in a spiral manner) and potentially compromise blood flow to multiple vital organs.*

Risk factors for aortic dissection include congenital unicuspid or bicuspid aortic valve, aortic aneurysm, collagen vascular disorders (e.g., Marfan

© 2006 Mayo Foundation for Medical Education and Research

syndrome), cocaine use, chest trauma, and chronic, uncontrolled hypertension. Aortic dissection usually occurs in patients of ages 30 to 80 years, with the peak occurrence in the sixth and seventh decades of life. It affects men more frequently than women. *The Stanford classification of aortic dissection designates type A as involving the ascending aorta, while type B refers to dissections that do not involve the ascending aorta.* Furthermore, using the DeBakey classification of aortic dissection, a type I (involves the entire aorta), type II (involves only the ascending aorta), or type III (involves only the descending aorta) designation can better clarify which aortic segments are involved.

The most common presentation (80% of patients) is chest pain described as "ripping," "tearing," "sharp," "stabbing," or "pressurelike." There may be pulse deficits in the extremities, suggesting limb ischemia or systemic hypoperfusion. Aortic dissection resulting in cardiac tamponade (i.e., commonly from aortic root rupture into the transverse pericardial sinus) may produce jugular venous elevation and systemic hypotension; complete cardiovascular collapse is also possible. If the dissection causes severe aortic insufficiency, signs of congestive heart failure (e.g., pulmonary edema) may be present.

Diagnosis of ascending aortic dissection is commonly made by CT, magnetic resonance imaging with angiography (sensitivity 94%–100% and specificity of 95%–100% for all dissections), aortic angiography, or transesophageal echocardiography (TEE) (sensitivity 78%–100% for type A). TEE is a particularly useful diagnostic modality to rule out cardiac tamponade, both for a more detailed analysis of the extent of the dissection and for determining the mechanism/severity of aortic insufficiency (if present). Intraoperatively, TEE can help identify both the true and false aortic lumens, which will facilitate the arterial cannulation required for the initiation of cardiopulmonary bypass (CPB). *Any attempt to perform a preoperative diagnostic TEE must be made in conjunction with an experienced cardiac anesthesiologist because inadequate sedation and blunting of sympathetic autonomic outflow could result in immediate aortic rupture with unrecoverable hemodynamic collapse.*

The mortality rates associated with Stanford type A dissections are approximately 1% to 2% per hour, in the first 48 hours, following initial onset of symptoms. This increases to 60% in the first 6 days and 74% by 2 weeks, and by 6 months, the trend levels off near 91%. The complications associated with type A dissection are listed in *Table 145.1*. The high degree of morbidity and mortality is usually related to involvement of the coronary ostia, dissection into the aortic root causing severe aortic insufficiency, and proximal dissection causing cardiac tamponade. The dissection can also cause rupture into either atria or the right ventricle.

Acute medical management is directed at control of systemic blood pressure to reduce the shear stress or change in pressure over time $(\Delta P/\Delta t)$ transmitted

TABLE 145.1	COMPLICATIONS OF ACUTE STANFORD TYPE A AORTIC DISSECTION (N = 513)
COMPLICATION	PERCENTAGE OF OCCURRENCE
All neurologic defects	18%
Coma/altered consciousness	14%
Myocardial ischemia/infarct	4%
Acute renal failure	6.2%
Hypotension	26%
Cardiac tamponade	17%
Mortality	30%

Adapted from Bossone E, Rampoldi V, Nienaber CA, et al. Usefulness of pulse deficit to predict in-hospital complications and mortality in patients with acute type A aortic dissection. *Am J Cardiol* 2002;89:851.

to the aortic wall. *Although there has not been any pressure range proven to be best, a pressure of 100 to 110 mm Hg systolic is the generally accepted goal.* This pressure will likely maintain adequate organ perfusion while minimizing the risk of aortic rupture.

Anesthetic management should be directed at establishing access and includes multiple large-bore intravenous catheters with blood warming devices, as well as a rapid infusion device (if available), central venous access (i.e., to permit monitoring of central filling pressures, assess cardiac output, and deliver both potent α-agonists and inotropes), and at least one arterial line, depending on the surgical plan for the arterial cannulation that is needed for CPB (see Chapter 139 because arterial monitoring can be complicated in these patients, depending on the extent of the dissection). Ultrasonic exam of the common carotid arteries prior to central line placement can reveal both the location of the vessel and whether the dissection has extended into the neck. Such involvement is common with type A dissections, but flow obstruction–related common carotid dissection is not common and portends increased mortality. It may be prudent to avoid cannulating the central venous system on the side of compromised arterial flow, although some experienced anesthesiologists make a sound argument for avoiding central venous cannulation on the side with normal arterial flow.

Have **at least** *4 U of appropriately typed and cross-matched packed red blood cells available in the operating room before the procedure begins.* Necessary monitoring includes standard American Society of Anesthesia monitors with the addition of a Foley catheter (for urine drainage/monitoring), orogastric tube, and temperature monitoring of both the shell and the core. High-dose narcotic induction is a preferred method due to hemodynamic instability frequently observed in these patients. *Induction of general anesthesia for patients with aortic dissection must always proceed with prevention of hypertension as a*

TABLE 145.2	MEDICATIONS FOR CONTROL OF BLOOD PRESSURE
MEDICATION	DOSAGE
Esmolol	25–300 mcg/kg/min
Sodium nitroprusside	0.5–2 mcg/kg/min
Nicardipine	1–15 mg/h

priority. If the airway necessitates a rapid sequence intubation, then esmolol can be used as an adjunct to treat the hypertensive response to laryngoscopy (these patients are often managed preoperatively with a combination of esmolol and nitroprusside infusions, as indicated in *Table 145.2*). Intravenous lidocaine (1.5 mg/kg) at the time of induction can also blunt the response to laryngoscopy. The short half-lives of esmolol and nitroprusside make them ideal for blood pressure control in these patients. A TEE probe should be placed after induction, and a complete TEE exam performed with special attention to the extent of the dissection (e.g., involves the aortic arch, coronary ostia, and aortic valve). *Depending on the distal extent of the dissection, circulatory arrest may be required to perform an adequate surgical repair.* Neuroprotection is of paramount concern in cases requiring deep hypothermic circulatory arrest (see Chapter 146).

If the dissection has caused cardiac tamponade, the transition to positive-pressure ventilation during the induction of general anesthesia can be deleterious for right heart filling and result in cardiovascular collapse. Maintain cardiac filling pressures with intravenous volume administration and a short inspiratory-to-expiratory ratio to maximize right heart filling. If pericardial tamponade is diagnosed or suspected, femoral cannulation for CPB under local anesthesia should be considered, followed by induction and immediate sternotomy. *Decompression of cardiac tamponade prior to bypass may cause rebound hypertension, resulting in aortic rupture and a tremendous increase in mortality risk.* If femoral cannulation for CPB cannot be instituted under local anesthesia prior to inducing general anesthesia, then a careful induction with the gradual transition to assisted and, finally, positive-pressure ventilation should be performed to minimize the risk of cardiovascular collapse. In such cases, prior to induction, a surgeon must be present, the patient fully prepped and draped, and the operating room team ready to establish emergent femoral bypass.

TEE is a useful post-CPB monitor to assess the adequacy of repair. Important post-CPB TEE findings include restoration of flow to the true aortic lumen, assessment of aortic valve repair/replacement, and evaluation of cardiac function. Finally, use of a cerebral oximeter (Somanetics Corporation, Troy, MI) can alert one to the presence of compromised cerebral blood flow post-CPB. Alternatively, the common carotid arteries can be directly assessed with a surface ultrasound probe via color Doppler interrogation to confirm that bilateral blood flow is present to the cerebral circulation. *Following confirmation of a successful surgical repair, the anesthesia team should be prepared to both evaluate (e.g., via thromboelastography) and aggressively treat coagulopathic hemorrhage* (see Chapter 149).

TAKE HOME POINTS

- Due to the high aortic pressures and shear stress created by pulsatile perfusion, the dissection flap can continue to dissect in its proximal or distal extent (often in a spiral manner) and potentially compromise blood flow to multiple vital organs.
- The Stanford classification of aortic dissection designates type A as involving the ascending aorta, while type B refers to dissections that do not involve the ascending aorta.
- Any attempt to perform a preoperative diagnostic TEE must be made in conjunction with an experienced cardiac anesthesiologist because inadequate sedation and blunting of sympathetic autonomic outflow could result in immediate aortic rupture with unrecoverable hemodynamic collapse.
- Acute medical management is directed at control of systemic blood pressure to reduce the shear stress, or change in pressure over time ($\Delta P/\Delta t$), transmitted to the aortic wall. Although there has not been any pressure range proven to be best, a pressure of 100 to 110 mm Hg systolic is the generally accepted goal.
- Make at least 4 U of appropriately typed and cross-matched packed red blood cells available in the operating room before the procedure begins.
- Induction of general anesthesia for patients with aortic dissection must always proceed with prevention of hypertension as a priority. The short half-lives of esmolol and nitroprusside make them ideal for blood pressure control in these patients.
- Depending on the distal extent of the dissection, circulatory arrest may be required to perform an adequate surgical repair. Neuroprotection is of paramount concern in cases requiring deep hypothermic circulatory arrest (see Chapter 146).
- If the dissection has caused cardiac tamponade, the transition to positive-pressure ventilation during the induction of general anesthesia can be deleterious for right heart filling and result in cardiovascular collapse.
- Decompression of cardiac tamponade prior to the bypass may cause rebound hypertension, resulting in aortic rupture and a tremendous increase in mortality risk.

- Following confirmation of a successful surgical repair, the anesthesia team should be prepared to both evaluate (e.g., via thromboelastography) and aggressively treat coagulopathic hemorrhage.

SUGGESTED READINGS

Moskowitz DM, Kahn RA, Reich DL. Anesthesia for the surgical treatment of thoracic aortic disease. In: Thys DM, Hillel Z, Schwartz AJ, eds. *Textbook of Cardiothoracic Anesthesiology.* New York, NY: McGraw-Hill; 2001:680–710.

Otto CM. Diseases of the great vessels. In: Otto. CM, ed. *Textbook of Clinical Echocardiography.* 3rd ed. Philadelphia, PA.: Saunders/Elsevier; 2004:431–454.

Pantin EJ, Cheung AT. Thoracic aorta. In: Kaplan JA, Reich DL, Lake CL, et al., eds. *Kaplan's Cardiac Anesthesia.* 5th ed. Philadelphia, PA.: Saunders/Elsevier; 2006:723–764.

146

FREEZE—YOU'RE UNDER DEEP HYPOTHERMIC CIRCULATORY ARREST!

STEPHEN R. BARONE, MD AND MICHAEL G. FITZSIMONS, MD

A 50-year-old male who works as an aeronautical engineer presents sporting a bicuspid aortic valve and a "grande burrito" size (63 mm) ascending aorta. He is scheduled for both aortic valve replacement and ascending aortic replacement requiring deep hypothermic circulatory arrest (DHCA). Following initiation of cardiopulmonary bypass (CPB), the heater/cooler exchange jacket is dropped to 15°C, and after the patient reaches a nasopharyngeal temperature of 18°C, the rest of the operating room team is ready for DHCA. Are you? Hopefully, he'll return to work for another 15 years after this operation, and his space shuttle will have a successful mission. To allow that, you'll have to protect that great brain of his! Cover his head with ice bags, and prepare a brain cocktail with steroids, magnesium, and mannitol. Once circulation is arrested, ensure that the selective anterograde cerebral perfusion circuit flow is appropriate for his body size. Watch the clock; time is the enemy now, and the surgeon needs to be informed of the circulatory arrest time at regular intervals. Following complete rewarming of both core and shell temperatures, make sure that platelets, plasma, and red blood cells are available for transfusion if needed. With these maneuvers and a technically successful surgery, the patient has a great chance of going right back to being a rocket scientist!

Certain adult cardiac surgical procedures, primarily involving the ascending and descending aorta, aortic arch, and pulmonary vasculature require temporary interruption of cerebral blood flow to improve visualization and technical repair. This technique is referred to as DHCA (aka "circ arrest") and is associated with high rates of neurologic compromise. Advanced age (older than 80 years) and DHCA times of >30 minutes are associated with higher rates of neurologic injury. The immediate energy-supply imbalance that occurs with "circ arrest" requires that the anesthesiologist consider the direct application of ice to the head (i.e., inducing an ice cream headache) and administration of a fancy drug cocktail in an attempt to preserve neurologic function. In addition, selective cerebral perfusion during DHCA has been observed to be of clinical benefit.

MECHANISM OF BENEFITS

The brain is exquisitely vulnerable to ischemic episodes due to its high cerebral metabolic rate of oxygen consumption ($CMRO_2$) and yet relatively

© 2006 Mayo Foundation for Medical Education and Research

limited reserve of high-energy phosphates. Hypothermia decreases the metabolic rate of neural tissue and increases the safe time that the brain can survive without oxygen and metabolic substrate. Silence of the electroencephalogram is only achieved in 50% of patients at 18°C but up to 99% at 12.5°C. Other suggested mechanisms of protection include inhibition of capsases, maintenance of microvascular integrity, prevention of glutamate-associated transient spikes in activity, suppression of inflammation, and decrease in edema formation. Most clinicians will cool systemically to between 15°C and 20°C and then maintain circulation at this temperature for approximately 5 minutes before bypass flow is ceased.

The acceptable duration of circulatory arrest depends on the degree of hypothermia. According to the Kirkland normogram, at 15°C, 30 minutes is possible, and at 10°C, up to 40 minutes is possible. There is no consensus opinion about the acceptable duration, and the limit likely varies between individuals.

Known risks of hypothermia include injury to blood elements associated with cooling and warming, platelet dysfunction, and coagulopathy.

DIRECT APPLICATION OF ICE—THE ICE CREAM HEADACHE

Direct application of ice-filled bags to the head has been advocated to facilitate cooling and to reduce passive rewarming during the period of arrest. Placement of ice-filled bags around the entire head with careful attention to protect the eyes, nose, and ears from direct contact should be done as soon as cooling is initiated. Ice should also be applied to the occiput. The ice bags should be removed on rewarming if you want to keep the respect of your surgical colleagues!

BLOOD GAS MANAGEMENT

Pediatric literature and animal experimentation supports "**pH stat**" blood gas management (temperature corrected values), in which CO_2 is added to the blood to facilitate cerebral vasodilation and more uniform distribution of cooling. The results in adult patients are not as clear. Blood gas management using "**alpha stat**" techniques (temperature uncorrected values) without additional CO_2 may be beneficial during rewarming to avoid excessive cerebral perfusion and embolic injury commonly seen due to the blood vessel–rich nature of the brain.

BRAIN COCKTAIL ANYONE? (PHARMACOLOGIC ADJUNCTS)

There is no universally accepted medical protocol for DHCA that has been validated in randomized controlled clinical trials. **Barbiturates** (Phenobarbital) may be administered in an attempt to decrease $CMRO_2$ by burst suppression.

Large doses are required and result in hemodynamic compromise and longer periods of intubation. **Volatile anesthetic agents** may provide protection by ischemic preconditioning. **Glucocorticoids** are often administered due to several potentially beneficial mechanisms, including decreased lipid, eicosanoid, free radical, and edema formation. In addition, normal cerebral blood flow may return earlier after DHCA. *The obvious risks of uncontrolled hyperglycemia must be recognized and treated.* **Magnesium** has several potential beneficial mechanisms, including inhibition of NMDA receptors, which limits the excitotoxic cascade that commonly leads to central nervous system damage. **Ketamine** also inhibits NMDA receptors, and several in vitro studies show benefit. The benefits of **mannitol** may be due to limitation of free radical formation, improved blood viscosity, and a decrease in edema formation. Volatile anesthetic agents may confer cerebral protection through inhibition of excitotoxicity, improvement in brain oxygenation, and decreasing the metabolic rate.

SELECTIVE CEREBRAL PERFUSION

Selective cerebral perfusion is proposed as a mechanism to provide the brain with substrate while the rest of the body is subject to circulatory arrest.

Retrograde cerebral perfusion is the practice of providing oxygenated blood flow and nutrients from the bypass circuit into the superior vena cava. Other benefits may include a decreased risk of air or atheromatous emboli and maintenance of cerebral hypothermia. *Care is taken to maintain a pressure <25 mm Hg (measured via an internal jugular catheter). Generally, flows of 200 to 600 mL/minute are achieved.* Risks include ineffective perfusion due to valves, edema formation, injury to the venous system, and cerebral hemorrhage.

Selective anterograde cerebral perfusion is the practice of intermittent or continuous perfusion of the brain via cannulation of the brachiocephalic vessels, axillary artery, or aortic arch vessels. This is from last page usually initiated once full cooling has occurred and the arch vessels are exposed. Flow rate is approximately 15 cc/kg/minute when perfusion is via the axillary artery. Cerebral perfusion depends on an intact circle of Willis and may prolong the period of arrest. *Potential risks include crowding of the surgical field, injury to arch vessels, embolization, and malperfusion.*

REWARMING

Rewarming starts as soon as surgical conditions warrant. Usually, the body is warmed 1°C every 3 minutes of bypass time. The bypass temperature should never be more that 10°C higher than body temperature. Warming should be terminated when the body is between 35°C and 36°C.

- Directly apply **ice** bags to head, including occiput, with protection of eyes, ears, and nose. Ice should be placed as soon as cooling is initiated
- Consider use of **corticosteroids** (methylprednisolone 30 mg/kg, generally 1,000 mg) administered at start of the case
- Provide maintenance anesthetic maintained **a volatile anesthetic agent** at 1 MAC prior to DHCA
- Empty "**pH stat**" blood gas management during cooling
- Administer intravenous **mannitol** (0.25 g/kg, usually 25 g) 5 minutes before initiation of circulatory arrest
- Administer **magnesium sulfate** (100 mg/kg) just prior to DHCA
- Carefully manage **hyperglycemia** before and after DHCA
- Consider the use of either selective anterograde or retrograde cerebral perfusion during the period of DHCA with the knowledge that the weight of existing evidence is supportive of the use of the selective anterograde technique
- Employ "**alpha stat**" management during rewarming
- Provide controlled **rewarming** no faster than 1°C every 3 minutes, with a gradient no more than 10°C between body and perfusate

SUGGESTED READINGS

Hagl C, Ergin MA, Galla JD, et al. Neurologic outcome after ascending aorta-aortic arch operations: Effect of brain protection technique in high-risk patients. *Thorac Cardiovasc Surg* 2001;121:1107–1121.

Kurth CD, Pristley M, Watzman HM, et al. Desflurane confers neurologic protection for deep hypothermic circulatory arrest in newborn pigs. *Anesthesiology* 2001;95:959–964.

Pokela M, Dahlbacka S, Biancari F, et al. pH-stat versus alpha-stat perfusion strategy during experimental hypothermic circulatory arrest: A microdialysis study. *Ann Thorac Surg* 2003;76:1215–1226.

147

REMEMBER THAT ANESTHESIA FOR LEFT VENTRICULAR ASSIST DEVICE SURGERY IS ESPECIALLY CHALLENGING: DO NOT NEGLECT THESE ESSENTIAL PRINCIPLES

MARK CHROSTOWSKI, MD AND
GIORA LANDESBERG, MD, DSC, MBA

The chronic shortage of donor hearts for transplantation has created the need for ventricular assist devices (VADs) in patients with end-stage heart failure, for either temporary (bridge to transplantation) or permanent implantation (destination therapy). Left ventricular assist devices (LVADs) support the left ventricle (LV) by diverting either the entire or partial LV blood flow via a cannula in the apex of the LV to the aorta using an external mechanical force. Anesthesia for these cases can be challenging. Consider the options for a patient on a transplant list with end-stage heart failure (ejection fraction [EF] 21%), worsening symptoms, and new signs of renal failure. An intra-aortic balloon pump is placed. What is involved in the perioperative assessment and management of this patient?

CLASSIFICATION OF LEFT VENTRICULAR ASSIST DEVICES

There are two main types of VADs: Pulsatile and nonpulsatile. The pulsatile or displacement VADs use valves and a pusher plate, displacing blood drained from the LV through a reservoir into the aorta. Pulsatile devices are further divided into extracorporeal or paracorporeal (Abiomed BVS 5000, Abiomed, Inc., Danvers, MA and the Thoratec, Thoratec Corp., Pleasanton, CA), in which the pump is external to the body. These LVADs are in use only for temporary assist (up to 30 days). The other type is intracorporeal (HeartMate I Thoratec IVAD, Thoratec Corp., Pleasanton, CA and Novacor World Heart Inc., Oakland, CA), in which the pump is implanted inside the peritoneum or the thorax, and only the power supply is external. The nonpulsatile or rotary VADs are also divided into two types: The centrifugal (either extracorporeal or intracorporeal), which are rarely used anymore, and the more modern axial flow pumps (Jarvik 2000, Jarvik Heart, Inc., New York, NY and the HeartMate II, Thoratec Corp., Pleasanton, CA), in which a small electromagnetically actuated impeller drive shaft rotates and propels blood at a flow that can be controlled according to the needs of the individual patient. The axial flow pumps are smaller, less than one-fifth the size of the

© 2006 Mayo Foundation for Medical Education and Research

pulsatile pumps, allowing their implantation in children and small adults. Axial rotary pumps can also be easily adjusted to operate in parallel to the pulsating LV, thus allowing the heart to gradually recover and wean from the LVAD.

Indications. Candidates for heart transplant are those with a cardiac index <2 L/minute/m^2 and a pulmonary capillary wedge pressure (PCWP) >20 mm Hg.

Contraindications. Contradictions include infection (blood cultures are negative, especially for fungus, at least 1 week before device placement), renal failure (creatinine >5.0 mg/dL), severe liver impairment, stroke, severe pulmonary dysfunction, and severe pulmonary dysfunction.

Anesthetic Considerations. These patients are critically ill, are often dependent on inotropes and/or intra-aortic balloon pump counterpulsation therapy, and have often had previous cardiac operations and other end-organ dysfunctions. Their fixed low stroke volume strongly depends on preload and heart rate to maintain marginal performance, which is already on the flat or even descending limb of the Starling curve. Excessive increase in afterload may decrease stroke volume and output dramatically. They are often maintained on angiotensin-converting enzyme (ACE) inhibitors and β-blockers to decrease afterload and diuretics to minimize volume overload. Amiodarone is also commonly used; this blocks the sympathetic system by noncompetitive α- and β-blockade. Its combination with ACE inhibitors that block the renin-angiotensin system and decrease cardiovascular responsiveness to catecholamines may lead to increased vasoconstrictor requirements during cardiopulmonary bypass (CPB). Circulating endogenous catecholamines are high in patients with heart failure, which makes them prone to cardiovascular decompensation during induction or maintenance of anesthesia. Changes in volume of distribution and the decreased clearance of drugs are likely due to altered metabolism by the liver and elimination by the kidney.

Monitoring. Monitoring should include standard cardiac hemodynamic monitoring, arterial line, pulmonary artery catheter (inserted either before or after induction) and transesophageal echocardiography (TEE). Large-bore intravenous lines are prudent for rapid administration of fluid and blood products. Pulmonary vascular resistance (PVR) provides an indication of the need for pulmonary vasodilators on weaning from bypass:

$$PVR = 80(MPAP - PCWP)/CO$$

where MPAP is mean pulmonary artery pressure and CO is cardiac output. Continuous CO catheters may be useful after LVAD placement for continuous assessment of right-sided CO, while the LVAD monitor continuously displays left-sided flow. Discrepant values may indicate aortic regurgitation or intracardiac shunting.

TEE has a major role in managing LVAD surgery. Before bypass, TEE helps optimize left ventricular filling; **exclude patent foramen ovale** (PFO), artial septal defects (ASD), and aortic insufficiency; evaluate right ventricular function; assess degree of tricuspid regurgitation; assess the aorta for calcification, plaque, or dilation; and examine all chambers for thrombus, particularly at the apex of the LV, where the LVAD inflow cannula is inserted. Exclusion of even the smallest PFO, ASD, or ventricular septal defect (VSD) is of paramount importance due to the risk of hypoxia secondary to the right-to-left shunt after bypass and LV decompression if the PFO/ASD/VSD is not surgically sutured. Efforts to detect a PFO should include intravenous bubble contrast injection during and following the release of a Valsalva maneuver and with increased preload (Trendelenburg position). *Caution should be exercised when executing a Valsalva maneuver in these patients because it may precipitate a malignant arrhythmia and subsequent cardiovascular collapse.* During bypass, TEE is used to assess appropriate placement of the inlet cannula and its orientation (toward the mitral valve), **device** activation, and deairing. After bypass, TEE is used to monitor right ventricular function and tricuspid regurgitation, decompression of the LV and left atrium, air entrainment if the LV collapses, and **Doppler assessment of LVAD flows** to rule out partial cannula obstruction.

Anesthetic Induction. Maximal preoxygenation is extremely important and may take time due to the low functional residual capacity. Hemodynamic stability is usually achieved with low-dose fentanyl (5–10 mcg/kg), midazolam, and etomidate. The stress of intubation, hypoxia, or hypercarbia should be avoided because they may lead to rapid decompensation, and low-dose norepinephrine or phenylephrine is often administered to augment blood pressure.

Maintenance of Anesthesia. Low-dose isoflurane (0.4%–1.0%) is often used to avoid awareness to the extent that the hemodynamic state allows. Mean blood pressure of 70 mm Hg is acceptable and is often supported by low-dose norepinephrine. Aprotinin or ε-aminocaproic acid is administered to reduce bleeding and blood product consumption.

Weaning from Bypass. The major concerns on weaning from CPB are right ventricular failure (in 25% of the patients), control of pulmonary and peripheral resistances, and bleeding. Of note, axial flow devices function best in the presence of lower systemic and PVR; therefore, drugs such as milrinone, dobutamine, or isoproterenol are preferentially used to lower resistance and support the RV. Inhaled nitric oxide or PGE_1 have been used successfully to reduce pulmonary hypertension. Conversely, some patients may require an increase in systemic vascular resistance with the use of norepinephrine

(1–20 μg/minute) or vasopressin (0.03–0.07 U/minute). RV failure may become evident only after LVAD operation due to the improved cardiac output and venous return, combined with the loss of developed LV systolic pressure related to ventricular unloading by the LVAD. Excessive decompression of the LV may cause LV collapse and LVAD inlet occlusion, which may lead to air entry through suture lines or interstices of the graft, with potential catastrophic air embolism, particularly in pulsatile LVADs. TEE is used to measure LVAD flow by continuous-wave Doppler through the inflow cannula and comparing that to the flow set on the device.

TAKE HOME POINTS

- LVAD patients are extremely sick and are often dependent on both intrinsic and extrinsic adrenergic support. Anesthesia and hemodynamic support should be carefully planned to avoid catastrophic hemodynamic collapse during induction and before going on bypass.
- TEE plays a major role during all stages of LVAD surgery and anesthesia.
- After bypass, the major issues are tuning RV function and pulmonary resistance as well as assuring proper LVAD function and hemostasis.

SUGGESTED READINGS

Hensley FA, Martin DE, Gravlee GP. *A Practical Approach to Cardiac Anesthesia.* 3rd ed. Philadelphia, PA.: Lippincott Williams & Wilkins; 2003.

Lietz K, Miller LW. Left ventricular assist devices: Evolving devices and indications for use in ischemic heart disease. *Curr Opin Cardiol* 2004;19:613–618.

Mets B. Anesthesia for left ventricular assist device placement. *J Cardiothorac Vasc Anesth* 2000;14:316–321.

Nussmeier NA, Probert CB, Hirsch D, et al. Anesthetic management for implantation of the Jarvik 2000[TM] left ventricular assist system. *Anesth Analg* 2003;97:964–971.

148

OFF-PUMP CARDIAC SURGERY: WHAT DO YOU MEAN NO PUMP BREAK FOR THE ANESTHESIOLOGIST?

BISWAJIT GHOSH, MD AND
VIPIN MEHTA, MBBS, MD, DARCS, FFARCSI

A 68-year-old male is admitted for elective coronary revascularization. Coronary angiography reveals severe three-vessel coronary artery disease. Left ventricular ejection fraction (LVEF) is 45% by echocardiogram. Preoperative chest film reveals a heavily calcified ascending aorta. Past medical history is notable for hypertension (HTN), diabetes mellitus type 2 (DM-2), stroke 3 years prior (no residuum), and a 45 pack-year smoking history prior to quitting 3 years earlier. In addition, he underwent right carotid endarterectomy (CEA) 2 years ago, and his most recent blood tests reveal chronic, moderate renal insufficiency. During your preoperative anesthesia evaluation, he informs you that the surgeon has told him that he plans an off-pump coronary artery bypass (OPCAB) surgery for him. The patient recently read an article about "beating heart surgery" and is terrified about the prospect of undergoing this procedure! He wants to know what benefits he can expect from OPCAB versus standard coronary artery bypass grafting (CABG). He asks, "Doc, am I going to have another stroke while I am asleep?" What do you tell him?

OPCAB is a good option for this patient, especially because his surgeon performs this procedure frequently. The patient's age, history of a stroke, prior CEA, DM-2, calcified ascending aorta, and history of both HTN and tobacco abuse suggest he is at great risk for perioperative stroke, especially if the diseased aorta is heavily manipulated. Avoiding aortic manipulation and cardiopulmonary bypass (CPB) may minimize the propensity for stroke in this case. The patient should be informed that OPCAB surgery could be associated with less neurologic complications than standard CABG in his case.

OPCAB surgery does not offer any additional protection to the kidneys over conventional bypass. The possibility of blood product transfusion may be less in OPCAB surgery. Time to extubation, intensive care unit (ICU) length of stay, and hospital length of stay may be reduced in OPCAB surgery.

BACKGROUND

The first CABG performed without CPB was reported by Kolessov in 1967. The advancement and standardization of CPB and myocardial

© 2006 Mayo Foundation for Medical Education and Research

perfusion techniques resulted in a waning interest for this technique during the 1970s. Since the 1990s, there has been a notable resurgence of interest in the OPCAB technique at select centers. Of note, approximately 25% of all CABG in the United States in 2003 was done without CPB.

WHO QUALIFIES FOR OPCAB?
Selection of OPCAB patients depends on multiple factors: Institutional practice, expertise of the surgeon, number of vessels to be revascularized, site and degree of stenosis, and location of the vessel (i.e., *intramyocardial vessels are technically more difficult to graft during OPCAB surgery*). Patients who may not be good candidates for OPCAB include those with a cardiothoracic ratio >0.7, vessel diameter <1.5 mm, left main disease, LVEF <35%, acute myocardial infarction with hemodynamic instability, morbid obesity, and severe pulmonary disease. Although these are all relative contraindications, experienced OPCAB surgeons are often not deterred by such risk factor profiles from attempting OPCAB.

SURGICAL TECHNIQUE
The position of the patient varies from supine (standard midline sternotomy and reverse J inferior sternotomy) to supine with right lateral tilt for the left anterior minithoracotomy in the fourth or fifth intercostal space.

The sequence of graft placement is determined in order of increased cardiac displacement, and accordingly, the anterior wall vessels are grafted initially, followed by inferior wall vessels and then lateral wall vessels. The concept behind this is that the increasingly revascularized heart tolerates a greater degree of displacement and the hemodynamic insults associated with this repositioning. Exceptions to this approach exist according to individual anatomy.

Adequate exposure and stabilization of the operative vessel is critical for the success of anastomosis completion. This goal is achieved using retractors, stabilizing devices, stabilizing sutures, and possibly intracoronary shunts. OPCAB equipment varies and may function by compression and/or suction to achieve stabilization. Development of these devices has played a significant role in the progress and safety of OPCAB surgery.

Proximal and distal occlusion of the coronary artery is accomplished by encircling suture or soft, flexible, Silastic string around the vessel. Distal occlusion is not always necessary. Intracoronary shunts are often used to reduce ischemia during this time, and along with a carbon dioxide–containing saline mister-blower, provide better visualization of the anastomosis.

ANESTHETIC MANAGEMENT
Patients should be evaluated thoroughly regarding cardiac status (e.g., number of vessels to be revascularized, site and type of lesion, LVEF, presence

of any significant valvular abnormality). A careful history, physical examination, and review of the diagnostic studies, focusing on the pulmonary, renal, hepatic, and neurologic status, are of paramount importance.

Premedication should be customized according to the patient's condition. Scopolamine should be avoided to prevent delayed anesthesia recovery.

Anesthetic management goals of OPCAB include maintenance of hemodynamic stability (especially during frequent repositioning of the heart and intermittent coronary occlusion), *maintenance of normothermia, early detection and prompt management of myocardial ischemia, provision of adequate postoperative analgesia, rapid emergence, early extubation, and early patient mobilization.*

Patient warming systems (e.g., forced convective air warming blanket [Bair Hugger, Arizant, Inc., Eden Prairie, MN] or hydrogel energy conduction pads [Kimberly-Clark Patient Warming System, Kimberly-Clark Health Care, Roswell, GA]) *and warmed intravenous (IV) fluids should be routinely used.* Room temperature may need to be adjusted to prevent passive loss of heat to the environment and the potential development of a hypothermia-related coagulopathy.

Arterial catheterization, large-bore peripheral IV access (14- or 16-gauge), and central venous access (e.g., a triple-lumen catheter or pulmonary artery catheter) are standard for OPCAB. Pacing and defibrillator capabilities should be immediately available if they are required; the pacing pulmonary artery catheter can be a useful adjunct in this regard.

Monitoring of electrocardiogram (ECG) leads II and V5 is important for detection of ischemia. Transesophageal echocardiography (TEE) is also helpful for early detection of ischemia (e.g., segmental wall motion abnormality or development of ischemic mitral regurgitation) and the development of ventricular systolic or diastolic dysfunction, and for monitoring the volume status. The cardiac displacement required for this procedure can make obtaining diagnostic TEE images challenging. The ECG diagnosis of myocardial ischemia is also challenging as a result of the frequent axis shifts of the heart that accompany repositioning.

Any of the available IV induction agents can be titrated, depending on the patient's hemodynamic status. Fentanyl 7.5 to 10 mcg/kg or sufentanil 0.5 to 1 mcg/kg is usually adequate to blunt the hemodynamic response to airway manipulation. *Always remember that high-dose, narcotic-based anesthetics are not advisable when early extubation is the goal.* Intermediate-acting muscle relaxants (e.g., vecuronium, rocuronium, cisatracurium) are preferable over the longer-acting agents.

Any of the inhalational agents (isoflurane, sevoflurane, or desflurane) can be used for maintenance. Nitrous oxide can also be used but should be turned off promptly if conversion to CPB is anticipated.

Hypotension associated with retraction and compression of the heart is primarily managed by preloading with crystalloid and/or colloid solution. In general, IV fluid is used more liberally as compared to standard CABG. Overall, fluid management should be guided by the cardiac filling pressures and echocardiographic appearance of the volume status of the heart. Hypotension can also be managed by the Trendelenburg position, lightening of anesthesia, and use of vasopressors such as Neo-Synephrine, norepinephrine, and ephedrine. Underlying arrhythmias should be corrected pharmacologically or electrically (e.g., with cardioversion or pacing). Inotropes such as milrinone, dobutamine, or epinephrine may be used in patients with a low cardiac output state. *Always consider that the hemodynamic instability associated with OPCAB positioning may be related to compromised right heart filling; therefore, it is frequently helpful for the surgeon to open the right pleural space to allow for more efficient right heart filling during maximal cardiac displacement.*

Management of intraoperative ischemia includes the IV administration of nitroglycerin and the use of beta-blockers (to reduce myocardial oxygen consumption) and alpha-adrenergic agonists to maintain coronary perfusion pressure. Endocardial or epicardial pacing may be required in the event of severe bradycardia or heart block. Coronary perfusion and cardiac output should be optimized instead of merely treating the systemic blood pressure. Use of intracoronary shunting during the distal anastomosis can be helpful. Initiation of intra-aortic balloon pump counter pulsation therapy may be needed in select cases. The surgeon can also release the coronary occlusion or pericardial compression temporarily, if feasible. Ischemic preconditioning (transient occlusion of the coronary artery) before initiating completion of the distal anastomosis has been observed to reduce myocardial damage in some studies. *In resistant cases, CPB may have to be initiated following appropriate systemic heparinization.*

Anticoagulation varies among different institutions from a full dose of heparin (3–4 mg/kg or 300–400 IU/kg) in multivessel anastomoses to often much lower doses when one or two vessel anastomoses are planned. *Heparin reversal strategies are also variable in that it is not routinely or completely reversed.* Some literature suggests that OPCAB patients are hypercoagulable, presumably due to the lack of hemodilution and platelet dysfunction associated with CPB.

Extubation in the operating suite can be contemplated with hemodynamically stable patients that demonstrate acceptable postoperative thermal and metabolic profiles. The majority of patients are extubated in the ICU within 1 to 2 hours, although this varies on case-by-case and institutional basis.

- In OPCAB, the anesthesiologist plays a more active role as compared to on-pump CABG, where the perfusionist maintains the patient's circulation during revascularization. Continuously communicating with the surgeon; observing the operative field to follow/anticipate the steps of surgery; frequently changing the position of the operating table/heart; and closely monitoring the patient's ventilation, hemodynamics, and hematologic parameters, coupled with delivery of prompt and appropriate corrective measures, requires vigilance from the anesthesia provider.

- Hemodynamic instability associated with OPCAB is common. Allowing time for the heart to adjust to the position while providing appropriate supportive measures is often all that is needed to achieve acceptable hemodynamics.

- Always consider that the hemodynamic instability associated with OPCAB positioning may be related to compromised right heart filling; therefore, it is frequently helpful for the surgeon to open the right pleural space to allow for more efficient right heart filling during maximal cardiac displacement.

- The principal advantages of OPCAB as compared to on-pump CABG are directly associated with avoiding CPB and the complications related to it, which include platelet dysfunction, coagulation abnormalities, increased blood loss, increased transfusion of blood products, metabolic/stress response related to extracorporeal circulation, and CPB-associated systemic inflammatory response.

- Avoiding aortic manipulation minimizes the complications related to it (e.g., aortic dissection, dislodgement of the atheromatous plaques and embolization).

- OPCAB may facilitate early extubation, early ICU discharge, and shorter hospital lengths of stay. OPCAB may reduce the overall cost associated with coronary surgery by as much as 15% as compared to standard CABG.

- The incidence of type I neurologic complications such as stroke, transient ischemic attack (as diagnosed on anesthesia emergence), or cerebrovascular accident occurring later in the postoperative course is significantly lower in some OPCAB cohorts as compared to standard CABG patients.

- The incidence of postoperative atrial fibrillation is lower in OPCAB patients as compared to standard CABG for patients older than 70 years. The evidence is less clear in younger patients.

- Studies have failed to show any evidence that OPCAB provides protection against postoperative pulmonary dysfunction as evidenced by observed alveolar-arterial oxygen gradients.

- The incidence of postoperative renal dysfunction is not reduced in OPCAB patients.
- Early patency of the grafts is comparable in OPCAB and standard CABG. The success of long-term OPCAB graft patency is not clear at present.

SUGGESTED READINGS

Chukwuemeka A, Weisel A, Maganti M, et al. Renal dysfunction in high-risk patients after on-pump and off-pump coronary artery bypass surgery: A propensity score analysis. *Ann Thorac Surg* 2005;80:2148–2153.

Livesay JJ. Reflections on the history of coronary surgery. *Tex Heart Inst J* 2004;31(3):208–209.

Mack MJ. Beating heart surgery: Does it make a difference? *Am Heart Hosp J* 2003;1(2):149–157.

Magee MJ, Coombs LP, Peterson ED, et al. Patient selection and current practice strategy for off-pump coronary artery bypass surgery. *Circulation* 2003;108(suppl):II9–14.

Montes FR, Maldonado JD, Paez S, et al. Off-pump versus on-pump coronary artery bypass surgery and postoperative pulmonary dysfunction. *J Cardiothorac Vasc Anesth* 2004;18(6):698–703.

Puskas JD, Williams WH, Mahoney EM, et al. Off-pump vs. conventional coronary artery bypass grafting: Early and 1-year graft patency, cost, and quality-of-life outcomes: A randomized trial. *JAMA* 2004;292(2):169–170 (author reply).

Reston JT, Tregear SJ, Turkelson CM. Meta-analysis of short-term and mid-term outcomes following off-pump coronary artery bypass grafting. *Ann Thorac Surg* 2003;76:1510–1515.

Zangrillo A, Crescenzi G, Landoni G, et al. Off-pump coronary artery bypass grafting reduces postoperative neurologic complications. *J Cardiothorac Vasc Anesth* 2005;19(2):193–196.

149

Coagulopathy in the Cardiac Surgical Patient—It's Not Just About the Numbers

Joby Chandy, MD and Edwin G. Avery, IV, MD

You are the anesthesia provider for a 71-year-old man with multivessel coronary artery disease and normal preoperative labs who is undergoing a whopper of a coronary artery bypass graft (six vessels!) on cardiopulmonary bypass (CPB). Anticoagulation was managed with appropriate heparinization and protamine reversal as dictated by the HEPCON Heparin Management System. Amicar (Medtronic, Inc., Minneapolis, MN) was given pre-CPB in anticipation of a long CPB run (187 minutes). Following heparin neutralization, the floodgates appear to burst open and profuse bleeding from the surgical field is apparent; the hemoglobin measured just before CPB separation is 10 mg/dL. The surgeon notes that there is no apparent "surgical bleeding," only diffuse oozing from all tissues and anastomoses. He requests immediate administration of fresh frozen plasma (FFP), cryoprecipitate, banked red blood cells (RBCs), and "rescue aprotinin therapy." Central laboratory coagulation studies are sent off STAT. FFP, platelets, and banked RBCs are immediately available in the operating room. What is the best course of treatment for the patient at this time?

Start a thromboelastograph (TEG) right away if available; it will help diagnose the nature of the coagulopathy within 15 minutes. Do not administer "rescue aprotinin" to patients already treated with an antifibrinolytic. In the absence of preoperative antiplatelet or antithrombotic therapy, the bleeding is most likely due to the platelets getting knocked around in the CPB circuit (mechanical shear stress activation) during the prolonged pump run. Administer 6 U of platelets pronto! Platelets should not be given too quickly to avoid hypotension associated with bradykinin release. Give crystalloid to maintain intravascular volume. Do not inject concentrated calcium solutions in the same intravenous line as the platelets because it will activate them in the tubing! Following administration of the platelets, the field becomes considerably less oozy, and the central laboratory reports a platelet count (drawn pretransfusion) of 140 th/mm^3; the activated partial thromboplastin time (aPTT) is normal, and the prothrombin time (PT) is prolonged. No additional blood products are given. The platelet count was not helpful in diagnosing the nature of this coagulopathy because many of the counted platelets were dysfunctional or "spent platelets." The PT was

© 2006 Mayo Foundation for Medical Education and Research

also misleading. Pretransfusion TEG confirms poor platelet function and normal coagulation protein function.

If anyone is going to experience a clinically significant perioperative coagulopathy, it will probably be a cardiac surgical patient. The complexity of cardiac surgical procedures distinguishes the coagulopathy seen in these patients. Remember that cardiac surgery patients are routinely exposed to variable time periods of CPB. Whether the Silastic CPB circuit is uncoated, bonded with heparin, or bonded with a uniquely charged coating (Smart tubing, SMART; Cobe Cardiovascular, Arvarda, CO), the coagulopathy observed has been shown to correlate with the length of time spent on CPB (i.e., there is an increasing incidence of coagulopathy as CPB time increases). *In general, CPB times exceeding 3 hours should alert the clinician to the potential for development of a clinically significant coagulopathy.* Blood–synthetic tubing/filter interfaces and blood–air interfaces within the CPB circuitry initiate activation of systemic inflammatory pathways. Systemic inflammation is tied to the coagulation system and can provoke imbalance toward hypocoagulability. CPB-associated mechanical trauma to the blood elements (e.g., CPB induces shear stress injury, which activates platelets) causes anemia, thrombocytopenia, and a functional platelet defect that contributes to the development of coagulopathy. In addition, the same processes associated with the conduct of cardiac surgery reproducibly manifest an antifibrinolytic state that is only partially overcome through the pre-CPB initiation of antifibrinolytic agents. Furthermore, because many cardiac surgery patients have undergone previous percutaneous coronary interventions (e.g., coronary stenting and/or angioplasty) or present with a low cardiac output syndrome, they are routinely treated with antiplatelet and/or antithrombotic agents. The cardiologists love to give these drugs that cause cardiac surgery patients to bleed! These treatments are associated with increased postoperative hemorrhage and the increased need for transfusion of allogeneic blood products. Several antithrombotic (e.g., low-molecular-weight heparin) and antiplatelet (e.g., clopidogrel) agents cannot be neutralized pharmacologically and will require the administration of allogeneic blood products to overcome their effects.

The potentially costly and morbid consequences of mistreating the coagulopathy observed in cardiac surgery patients calls for the use of point-of-care testing as well as standard central laboratory coagulation tests. The PT measures the integrity of the extrinsic and common coagulation pathways. It can be prolonged in the setting of factor VII deficiency, Coumadin therapy, or vitamin K deficiency. Unfractionated heparin can also prolong the PT due to inactivation of factor II. *The PT is a poor predictor of postoperative hemorrhage in cardiac surgery patients and is therefore not appropriate to use as an independent test of coagulation.* The aPTT tests the integrity of the intrinsic and final coagulation pathways. The aPTT is prolonged in patients being treated with unfractionated heparin as well as in patients with deficiencies of factors XII, XI, IX, and VIII; high-molecular-weight kininogen; and kallikrein. The activated clotting time (ACT) is the point-of-care test that is used in cardiac surgery to monitor the effect of blood heparin levels, and it correlates with the bleeding related to dysfunction within the intrinsic and final coagulation pathways. Of note, the ACT does not correlate well with plasma heparin levels in hypothermic, hemodiluted patients on CPB and thus may potentially mislead clinicians to underdose heparin. Patients with marked thrombocytopenia ($<50,000/\mu$L) and those treated with platelet inhibitors may exhibit an abnormally prolonged ACT. Platelet lysis, anesthesia, and surgery can decrease the measured ACT value. *The platelet count will not always predict whether a bleeding cardiac surgery patient requires a platelet transfusion because CPB frequently induces a functional platelet defect.*

Increasingly, TEG is being employed as a point-of-care test to rapidly evaluate the integrity of the coagulation cascade, platelet function, platelet–fibrin interactions, and fibrinolysis in cardiac surgery patients. TEG involves testing the viscoelasticity of a clot and the temporal nature of clot formation. TEG values include the reaction time (R), the coagulation time (K), or angle ($\propto$), the maximal amplitude (MA), and the percent lysis at 30 minutes (LY30). R represents the time for initial fibrin formation, which is a measure of the intrinsic, extrinsic, and common pathways. K or $\propto$ are measures of the speed of clot formation; they reveal the level of functional fibrinogen. MA is an index of the tensile clot strength and is predominantly determined by platelet function and platelet–fibrin interaction. LY30 indicates the percentage of clot lysis that has occurred after 30 minutes, and it can reveal abnormal fibrinolytic states. Particular coagulation defects have characteristic TEG tracings that the clinician is aided in interpreting by the software that drives the TEG device. A number of trials have confirmed that the use of TEG in cardiac surgery is more predictive of bleeding than routine coagulation studies. The concurrent use of TEG with a transfusion algorithm has been demonstrated to result in significant reductions of re-exploration for hemorrhage and in the need for transfusion of blood products.

TAKE HOME POINTS

- The complexity of the cardiac surgery–associated coagulopathy calls on the clinician to employ the results of both central laboratory coagulation tests (e.g., activated partial thromboplastin time [aPTT], prothrombin time [PT], and platelet count) and point-of-care tests (e.g., activated clotting time [ACT], thromboelastography [TEG]) to guide the administration of allogeneic blood products and ultimately restore normal coagulation function.

- The ACT does not correlate well with plasma heparin levels in hypothermic, hemodiluted patients on cardiopulmonary bypass (CPB) and is generally a poor test for use in revealing trace amounts of unfractionated heparin when compared to the aPTT.

- The platelet count will not always predict whether a bleeding cardiac surgery patient requires a platelet transfusion because CPB frequently induces a functional platelet defect.

- The post-CPB initiation of antifibrinolytic therapy (e.g., ε-aminocaproic acid, tranexamic acid, or aprotinin) has not been prospectively evaluated in cardiac surgery patients and therefore is not recommended as a primary treatment for this coagulopathy. The safety of this practice has not been determined, and administration of these agents should begin prior to CPB.

- The combined use of aprotinin with either ε-aminocaproic acid or tranexamic acid has not been prospectively studied as a treatment option for this coagulopathy and therefore should not be considered.

- Cardiac surgery–associated coagulopathy should be anticipated in patients that have experienced CPB times in excess of 3 hours.

- Several antithrombotic and antiplatelet agents cannot be neutralized pharmacologically and require the administration of allogeneic blood products to overcome their effects. Select patients treated with these agents will benefit from the delay of elective cardiac surgery.

- Rebound heparinization should be considered as a contributing cause of cardiac surgery–associated coagulopathy, and can be effectively diagnosed (e.g., through the use of the heparinase TEG or the HEPCON Heparin Management System) and treated (e.g., administration of additional protamine sulfate).

SUGGESTED READINGS

Kaplan JA, Reich DL, Lake CL, et al., eds. *Kaplan's Cardiac Anesthesia.* 5th ed. Philadelphia, PA: Saunders/Elsevier; 2006.

Shore-Lesserson L. Evidence based coagulation monitors: Heparin monitoring, thromboelastography, and platelet function. *Semin Cardiothorac Vasc Anesth* 2005;19(4):453–458.

Spiess BD, Spence RK, Shander A, eds. *Perioperative Transfusion Medicine.* 2nd ed. Philadelphia, PA: Lippincott Williams & Wilkins; 2005.

150

REMEMBER THERE ARE SPECIFIC DO'S AND DON'TS OF ANESTHESIA CARE FOR HYPERTROPHIC OBSTRUCTIVE CARDIOMYOPATHY

COSMIN GAURAN, MD AND EDWARD GEORGE, MD, PHD

A 27-year-old professional snowboarder experienced a syncopal episode while training on a closed ski slope at Snowbird. The "Dude" (as he likes to call himself) was found at the scene in ventricular tachycardia and was successfully cardioverted by the emergency medical response team. On questioning, he admitted to experiencing some vague chest discomfort and shortness of breath over the past several months that he attributed to the altitude (>8,000 ft) and some "vigorous aprés ski celebrating." Following some strong encouragement from his adoring entourage, he agreed to forego the rest of the day's snowboarding to visit the local hospital. Medical evaluation demonstrated the presence of hypertrophic obstructive cardiomyopathy (HCM).

Now, adorned with his orange lens shades, he presents to your preoperative clinic for anesthesia consult prior to surgical septal myomectomy. Review of his past medical and surgical history is unremarkable. Family history is significant for a paternal uncle and grandfather with sudden death in their twenties. He takes atenolol 100 mg each morning and has no allergies. Vital signs are blood pressure 110/62 mm Hg, heart rate regular at 64/minute, and 100% oxygen saturation on room air. Physical exam revealed a noticeable double apical impulse and III/VI systolic ejection murmur at the left sternal border with radiation to the sternal notch, but not to the common carotid arteries. The murmur intensifies with upright posture, Valsalva maneuver, and squatting. The electrocardiogram showed normal sinus rhythm with electrical criteria for ventricular hypertrophy and diffuse depression of the ST segments. Chest film revealed a minimally increased cardiac silhouette. Echocardiography revealed ventricular hypertrophy with a marked asymmetrically enlarged upper interventricular septum. The mean gradient across the left ventricular outflow tract (LVOT) was calculated to be 55 mm Hg. The mitral valve showed signs of systolic anterior motion (SAM) and mild to moderate mitral insufficiency. Cardiac catheterization revealed normal coronary anatomy and confirmed the LVOT gradient. He wants to know how soon he could be back on the slopes.

HCM (formerly known as HOCM or idiopathic hypertrophic subaortic stenosis [IHSS]) is increasingly recognized as a relatively common (i.e.,

© 2006 Mayo Foundation for Medical Education and Research

estimated incidence of approximately 1/500) and underdiagnosed congenital cardiac abnormality. Although the disease is known to be a frequent cause of sudden cardiac death in young people, the majority of affected patients is minimally symptomatic and has a normal lifespan.

HCM is an autosomal disease with variable penetrance associated with mutations in the sarcomeric proteins. The main pathological mechanisms include hypertrophy, obstruction, diastolic dysfunction, and arrhythmias. Asymmetric hypertrophy is the trademark of the disease, with the interventricular septum being the most common area of involvement. Upper septal hypertrophy creates an area of narrowing and increases the velocity of the blood in the LVOT, which in turn leads to a Venturi effect and SAM of the mitral valve. The end result of this physiological pattern is a characteristic dynamic obstruction in mid to late systole. SAM resulting in significant mitral regurgitation will decrease forward cardiac flow. Increased inotropism, chronotropism, and hypovolemia can accentuate the dynamic obstruction in HCM patients. The diastolic dysfunction associated with HCM translates into decreased ventricular compliance and leads to requirements for higher cardiac filling pressures and a dependence on the atrial contribution for adequate cardiac output. Any type of arrhythmia can be associated with HCM, particularly atrial fibrillation (i.e., there is an incidence of up to 25%) and malignant ventricular arrhythmias; thus, the risk of sudden cardiac death becomes apparent.

Medical management of HCM involves aggressive treatment with beta-blockers to reduce the inotropic state of the heart, to decrease heart rate to allow adequate filling time, and to promote maintenance of normal sinus rhythm. Therapeutic approaches available for symptomatic patients not responding to medical management are septal ablation with alcohol injection using percutaneous techniques (increasingly popular, although not an option for all HCM patients) and the Moro surgical septal myomectomy. The Moro procedure involves a transaortic approach to the LVOT and uses cardiopulmonary bypass with cardiac arrest. Complete heart block and creation of a ventricular septal defect (VSD) are associated complications of this procedure. HCM patients with a history of a malignant ventricular arrhythmia should have an implantable cardioverter-defibrillator (ICD) placed.

TAKE HOME POINTS

- In providing anesthesia care for an HCM patient, DO be certain that the patient has undergone a recent echocardiographic assessment of their cardiac anatomy to gauge progression of their risk for dynamic obstruction. A complete history (i.e., take care to inquire about shortness of breath, syncope, anginal symptoms, palpitations, and history of arrhythmias) and physical exam may provide clues to pathology progression but should not replace echocardiographic examination in elective surgeries.

- In providing anesthesia care for an HCM patient, DO be certain that if the patient has a strong family history of sudden death, a personal history of syncope, or a malignant arrhythmia that they have a functional ICD, or are cared for perioperatively in a monitored bed with the means to immediately provide electrical therapy for a perioperative malignant arrhythmia. A negative electrophysiology study is not a sensitive predictor as to whether an HCM patient will suffer a malignant arrhythmia.

- Although the preferred anesthetic approach for HCM patients requiring both cardiac and noncardiac surgery is the use of general anesthesia, DO consider that regional anesthesia can be safely used (for noncardiac surgical procedures only) as long as the patient is given adequate anxiolytics and volume loaded prior to central neuraxial blockade. Vigilant maintenance of systemic vascular resistance with alpha-agonists (e.g., phenylephrine infusion) is required with both general and regional anesthetic techniques. Arterial catheterization and monitoring promotes the success of these techniques.

- In providing anesthesia care for any procedure (cardiac surgery or noncardiac surgery) for an HCM patient, DO consider the use of central pressure monitoring (i.e., following hemodynamic trends can be useful in these patients that may have elevated cardiac filling pressures related to chamber noncompliance) or preferably transesophageal echocardiography (TEE) to assess the adequacy of ventricular filling and the degree of dynamic LVOT obstruction.

- In providing anesthesia care for an HCM patient undergoing septal myomectomy, DO consider that complete heart block and creation of a VSD are complications of this procedure. Preoperative placement of an AV Paceport pulmonary artery catheter will provide the ability to deliver cardiac pacing in the event of perioperative complete heart block. Performing a complete post cardiopulmonary bypass TEE exam is essential and will rule out the presence of an iatrogenic VSD. In addition, it is important to document the resolution of the LVOT gradient following septal myomectomy.

- In providing anesthesia care for a patient without a history of HCM who has undergone a mitral valve repair (MVR), DO consider that SAM is a potential complication in this circumstance, although the genetic sarcomeric abnormality does not exist in these patients. Medical treatment may be all that is needed, and the return to cardiopulmonary bypass for MVR revision following MVR is not always necessary. Experienced anesthesia and surgical clinicians should be involved in such a decision and base their therapy on the postcardiopulmonary bypass TEE exam results.

- In treating hypotension in HCM patients, DO NOT employ agents (e.g., dopamine, milrinone, norepinephrine, ephedrine) with mixed inotropic, chronotropic, and peripheral vascular effects. Consider that the increase in heart rate and the inotropic state of the heart can acutely worsen hypotension related to dynamic LVOT obstruction. Phenylephrine infusion, beta-blockers, and maintenance of adequate intravascular volume are the treatments of choice in HCM patients.
- In planning the anesthesia induction of an HCM patient, DO NOT rely heavily on agents (e.g., propofol or thiopental) that acutely sympathectomize the patient and abruptly reduce both venous and arterial tone. Narcotic and benzodiazepine combinations can have more subtle sympathetic depressive effects when used judiciously. Most contemporary volatile anesthetics (e.g., isoflurane, sevoflurane, desflurane) act as systemic vasodilators and myocardial depressants, and thus they should be used cautiously if at all.

SUGGESTED READINGS

Cook DJ, Housmans PR, Rehfeldt KH. Valvular heart disease: Replacement and repair. In: Kaplan JA, Reich DL, Lake CL, et al., eds. *Kaplan's Cardiac Anesthesia*. 5th ed. Philadelphia, PA: Saunders/Elsevier; 2006:660–666.

Nishimura RA, Holmes DR, Jr. Clinical practice: Hypertrophic obstructive cardiomyopathy. *N Engl J Med* 2004;350(13):1320–1327.

151

MANAGING GUESTS ON THE LABOR DECK REQUIRES CLEAR COMMUNICATION CONSISTENTLY, FIRMNESS WHEN NECESSARY, AND CALMNESS ALWAYS

CHRISTOPHER E. SWIDE, MD

The labor and delivery suite is one of the few places in the hospital where family and friends are almost universally present during procedures that are fraught with risk (the other being the induction of pediatric patients with the parent present). The obstetric anesthesiologist must have not only the clinical skills to deal with the medical management of parturients but also the social and communication skills to manage guests. In the obstetrics environment, the patient's family and friends are often in the immediate vicinity. They can be distracting to care providers and may become stressed themselves by witnessing emergency care procedures. Unlike other chapters in this book that address anesthetic emergencies, this chapter focuses on methods for handling the potential repercussions of managing anesthetic emergencies in the presence of guests.

Every anesthesia provider must develop a practice model concerning guests. It is important that this model meet the needs of all "clients" (mothers-to-be, family and guests, the baby, the obstetrician, and the labor and delivery nurses) as well as his or her own needs. Fortunately, there is help available in handling these situations:

1) **Follow institution policies.** Hospital policies govern who can be in the delivery room or operating room (OR), and include processes of limiting access for medical cause as determined by the obstetric and anesthesia providers.

2) **Communicate with the labor nurses.** The nurses taking care of the patient often have a good understanding of the relationship dynamics of the patient's family and friends. Thus, the nurses can provide excellent advice on how to best broach the subject of presence during procedures. It is also important that the nurses, physicians, and other providers on the unit make a unified decision.

3) **Communicate with the obstetric provider.** The obstetric provider can be invaluable in helping the patient and her guests understand that the people she selected to be present at her delivery may be asked to leave the room if the care management plan necessitates it.

ⓒ 2006 Mayo Foundation for Medical Education and Research

4) **Communicate with the patient**. Discuss the potential of asking guests to leave the room if necessary during a procedure as part of the basic patient interview. It is the author's practice to *always* discuss this and to make sure the guests know that it is in the best interest of the patient.

5) **Always remain calm and professional**. Even in the midst of a real emergency or with an angry patient or guest, this is an important rule. If you must ask a guest to leave, try to frame it in terms of being able to best help the mom and the baby, rather than making it a contest of wills or control struggle.

6) **Use the institution's patient advocate**. Patient advocates are trained professionals who are invaluable in dealing with stressed and angry patients, family members, and health care providers. These advocates can be used if the previous strategies are ineffective. This step almost always works to avoid utilization of the last step, which is activation of the security team.

If all else fails, and if the anesthesia provider believes that guest presence puts the patient (or the provider) at risk, the last step is calling in the institution's security team to escort the guests from the scene. Proper preparation and utilization of the other techniques almost always solves the problem before the need for security.

HELPFUL HINTS FOR MANAGING GUESTS

These tips are considered reasonable by most obstetric anesthesia providers. Before the start of care:

- You MUST check privately with the mother-to-be regarding her desire for guests in general as well as individual guests in particular.

- Try to ascertain how much medical knowledge the guest has. Sometimes guests with a degree of medical knowledge may have control issues.

- In discussion with guests, always mention that the pace can quicken even in routine deliveries and find out how people will feel about being asked to step out.

- There are warning signs that may predict for a difficult or disruptive guest: confrontational and angry interactions with staff, poor interactions with the patient, and poor communication skills. Do not allow these people in the room.

- Exercise caution in allowing "guests to support guests." This situation sometimes arises with when the couple having the baby are themselves very young—for example, an older female family member might request to be in the room to support a teenaged father. This is felt by obstetric anesthesia providers to be a somewhat gray area. Allow it only if you feel the extra person(s) will help the care team better care for the patient.

For the labor and delivery rooms:

- There is no real limit on the number of support people except for space. The nurses will often help provide crowd control in the labor rooms so things do not get out of hand. Usually everyone except one person is asked to leave during procedures; however, anesthesia providers may reserve the right to have all guests leave the room if the epidural is anticipated to be difficult.

For the OR:

- Usually only one person is allowed in the OR for C sections, sometimes more if the anesthesia provider has met them and agreed beforehand to have them as guests.
- Guests may come and go from the OR only with an escort. Have a prearranged method to get a guest who gets woozy out of the delivery room.
- After the baby is delivered, guests may approach the baby warmer only if the okay is given by the delivery team (including the pediatric team, if they are there).
- Usually no guests are allowed in the OR until the block is in and working. However, a support person can occasionally be allowed into the room for the block, if the anesthesia providers believe that it may **help them** do their job more efficiently.

In general:

- Guests must be a minimum of 18 years of age to be in the room for C sections (unless the guest is the father of the baby). There is no age minimum for labor and delivery rooms.
- Expect as you gain experience that your practices will both loosen and tighten. This author has loosened up on the number of people in the OR, provided they do not interfere with the tasks of the anesthesia team, but tightened up about moving guests out if needed and *very* much tightened up about only one support person for labor epidurals and no videotaping of procedures.
- The doula is a member of the patient's care team and does not count as a guest.
- No cell phones are allowed in clinical areas.

    A final note from F. Jacob Seagull, PhD: Successful obstetrical anesthesia providers instinctively use a human factors approach for the management of guests in the obstetrical suite. In other words, you will do well to create an environment in which expectations are clear, and plans are discussed in advance. Doing this means that when the time comes, you will be activating an existing plan, not explaining a new plan, managing expectations, explaining your actions or trying to calm worried guests. By discussing the actions beforehand, you can address any questions while everyone is calm. You can effectively "offload" the bulk of the tasks involved in getting people out of the labor and delivery rooms to your low-workload times. This offloading is what experienced anesthesia providers do in planning any difficult case, by preparing in advance for contingencies.

Tell the guests that they may be asked to leave for a number of reasons pertaining to the ongoing management of the patient, (noise level too high, arrival of extra care team providers, need to treat the patient for non-lifethreatening events such as vomiting, a new peripheral IV, etc.) but that are not indicative of a true crisis. Guests will have a cognitive framework of the range of possible circumstances in which they might be asked to leave, and therefore may not assume the worst. They will be happy to "implement a plan" when the time comes; you will be happy that you don't have to explain the situation. The goal is to try to arrange a win-win situation.

SUGGESTED READINGS

Altendorf J, Klepacki L. Childbirth education for adolescents. *NAACOGS Clin Issu Perinat Womens Health Nurs*. 1991;2(2):229–243.

Move over, doc, the guests can't see the baby. September 11, 2005, New York Times. www.nytimes.com/2005/09/11/national/11birth.html?.

152

"I WANT MY EPIDURAL NOW!" THE EFFECTS OF EPIDURAL ANALGESIA ON PROGRESS OF LABOR AND DELIVERY

PATRICK G. BAKKE, MD AND JENNIFER COZZENS, MD, MPH

It is common on the labor and delivery ward to hear the nurses and doctors tell patients that they cannot have an epidural until cervical dilation reaches 4 cm. The reasons given for this include that labor will be prolonged, cesarean section rates increased, or that pain relief is just not needed before that point. In stark contrast is the American College of Obstetrician and Gynecologists (ACOG) recommendations that timing of epidural analgesia for labor and delivery is when the patient asks. That said, what are the impacts of epidural analgesia on labor and delivery?

The stages of labor are typically divided into the first, second, and third stages of labor. The first stage of labor can be separated into the early and active phases. Traditionally, early labor involves the onset of contractions and cervical dilation until 4 cm. The next portion of the first stage is known as the active phase and involves the cervix dilating from 4 to 10 cm. The second stage of labor is from complete cervical dilation until birth. The third stage of labor is from the time of birth until delivery of the placenta. In 1993, Thorpe published a paper stating that there was an increased risk of dystocia in nulliparous women who had epidural analgesia for labor prior to cervical dilation of 4 cm. This is where the "no epidural until after 4 cm" idea originated. Subsequently, in several well-designed randomized clinical trials, Chestnut showed this not to be the case. Since the 1990s, clinical studies have not shown that epidurals increase the cesarean section rate, so we can reassure our patients that the available evidence does not support delaying pain relief due to fear of increasing a woman's risk of cesarean section.

However, epidurals may affect the duration of labor. That is, the placement and use of an epidural for labor and delivery may prolong the first and second stages of labor. Typically, the first stage may be prolonged up to 40 minutes. Failure to progress should not be defined until the patient has achieved the active stage of labor. During the active stage, a number of indices are used to define failure to progress; however, epidural analgesia has not been associated with failure to progress to the second stage of labor. The second stage of labor has been reported to be 15 to 36 minutes longer with the use of epidural analgesia. The ACOG suggests that a prolonged second stage of labor should be considered when the second stage exceeds 3 hours

© 2006 Mayo Foundation for Medical Education and Research

if regional anesthesia is administered or 2 hours in the absence of regional anesthesia in nulliparous women. In multiparous women, such a diagnosis can be made if the second stage of labor exceeds 2 hours with regional anesthesia or 1 hour without. There is no significant prolongation of the third stage of labor with epidural analgesia.

Because use of an epidural in labor can prolong the first and second stages of labor, does this have an impact on instrument delivery or cesarean section? There may be an increased incidence of forceps- or suction-assisted delivery in patients who use epidural analgesia during labor. This is believed to be due to decreased maternal efforts at expulsion during delivery and not dystocia. For cesarean sections, populationwide studies have shown that the use of epidural analgesia for labor and delivery does *not* increase the rate of cesarean deliveries.

Most important, patients have lower pain scores and higher patient satisfaction with an epidural for labor and delivery compared with other forms of analgesia. When you couple these facts with the findings of neonatal Apgar scores, which are higher in infants born to mothers who used an epidural versus intravenous analgesia during labor, it is hard to argue against the use of epidurals for pain control during labor and delivery.

TAKE HOME POINTS

- The proper timing of an epidural is when the patients request the epidural and the obstetric providers are committed to delivery.
- The first stage of labor can be prolonged by as much as 40 minutes.
- The second stage of labor can be prolonged by 15 to 36 minutes.
- Neither failure to progress nor second stage arrest is increased by the use of an epidural.
- Instrumented delivery for dystocia is not increased.
- Cesarean section rates are not increased.
- Patients have lower pain scores and higher satisfaction.

SUGGESTED READINGS

Chestnut DH. Epidural analgesia and the incidence of cesarean section: time for another close look. *Anesthesiology.* 1997;87(3);472–476.

Leighton BL, Halpern SH. The effects of epidural analgesia on labor, maternal, and neonatal outcomes: a systematic review. *Am J Obstet Gynecol.* 2002;186(5 suppl Nature):S69–S77.

Sharma SK, Leveno KJ. Regional analgesia and progress of labor. *Clin Obstet Gynecol.* 2003;46(3):633–645.

Thorpe JA, Hu DH, Albin RM, et al. The effect of intrapartum epidural analgesia on nulliparous labor: a randomized controlled, prospective trial. *Am J Obstet Gynecol.* 1993;169(4):851–858.

Vahratian A, Zhang J, Hasling J, et al. The effect of early epidural versus early intravenous analgesia use on labor progression: a natural experiment. *Am J Obstet Gynecol.* 2004;191(1):259–265.

Wong CA, Scavone BM, Peaceman AM, et al. The risk of cesarean delivery with neuraxial analgesia given early versus late in labor. *N Engl J Med.* 2005;352(7):655–665.

153

IF CAREFULLY SELECTED, PATIENTS IN LABOR CAN AMBULATE SAFELY—THE KEY IS THE USE OF LOW-DOSE EPIDURAL ANALGESIA

CHRISTOPHER M. COLVILLE, MD AND
CHRISTOPHER E. SWIDE, MD

Effective analgesia for women in labor has become a reality since the 1950s. Labor suites have progressed from the time of sedated mothers and babies to modern central neuraxial techniques managed by professional anesthesia providers. Women can now enjoy a comfortable labor with safe, effective pain control. Many women and their obstetric providers believe that walking during labor can speed progress and provide comfort to the parturient. We can now provide effective pain control while preserving motor function, so the question becomes "does ambulation play a role for those patients with labor epidurals?"

What does ambulation do for mothers? The medical literature is unclear as to whether ambulation truly helps with the outcome of labor despite the common wisdom that this is true. Ambulation for the laboring patient theoretically can result in fairly substantive benefits. Faster labors, fewer instrumental and operative deliveries, and better maternal and infant outcomes are some of the alleged advantages to having the parturient walking early and often. Decreases of up to 2 hours in the first stage of labor, decreased requests for analgesia, lower rates for instrumental deliveries, and improved Apgar scores have all been reported in patients who walked after placement of the labor epidural. However, other studies have not found statistically significant changes in length of labor (from epidural insertion), Apgar scores, or cesarean delivery rate for these walking patients. The current literature has not revealed evidence of harm to the mother or baby if ambulation is allowed in the properly selected laboring patient. Patient satisfaction seems markedly improved because the majority of women who did ambulate in labor with analgesia reported that they would do so again for future pregnancies. Implicit in this satisfaction may be the decreased motor block that allows ambulation in the first place. With increased lower extremity mobility, parturients seem to feel greater independence from the labor bed. The low-dose epidural dosing studied (and used in many centers) also allows patients to void with greater autonomy. Patients have reported a somewhat greater satisfaction of the entire laboring experience when being allowed to walk, even if that ambulation is of short duration (e.g., walking across the room

© 2006 Mayo Foundation for Medical Education and Research

to the toilet). What is clear is that women like to walk in labor, and they particularly like to walk with adequate pain control, so patient satisfaction can be improved even if we cannot prove any medical benefits of ambulation.

Is it safe for laboring patients with epidural analgesia to ambulate? Safety concerns can be separated into two main classes: maternal safety and fetal safety. Maternal safety depends on having a protocol in place that addresses the main safety concerns in ambulatory epidurals, which are patient falls and hemodynamic stability. Patients who are allowed to ambulate with neuraxial labor analgesia need to be carefully selected and approved by the attending obstetrician or midwife and anesthesia provider after careful review of the patient's medical and obstetric history. In addition, this "freedom from the bed" should only be permitted with close ambulation supervision and with appropriate equipment (e.g., portable pumps, easily mobile intravenous [IV] stands). If medically dictated, at the discretion of the attending obstetrician or midwife, fetal heart rate monitoring will need to be portable, with mechanisms in place for remote monitoring units. Also, having a "rest" area at the nurses' station where the mom can have her blood pressure, heart rate, and fetal heart rate measured every 15 minutes facilitates nursing efficiency. A standard protocol is waiting 30 to 45 minutes after initial dosing, and then having the anesthesia provider examine the patient for signs of motor weakness and hemodynamic instability. A simple test is the modified Bromage score. If the patient can flex the leg at the hip and resist the examiners hand, then she is given a score of 5, and if she can stand from the bed with minimal assistance (deep knee bend), then she is given a score of 6 and is cleared to ambulate. To test hemodynamics, the patient is asked to stand, and both systolic blood pressure and fetal heart rate are measured to look for significant changes. Ambulation is then allowed using the patient's support person or designated helper to walk with her for assistance. The use of appropriate IV poles can help facilitate walking. Fetal safety depends on maintaining adequate perfusion of the placenta by ensuring maternal safety. For properly selected patients, there is no evidence in the literature of fetal/maternal harm from walking in labor.

How do we provide labor analgesia and ambulation? The key is in the use of epidural solutions using low concentrations of local anesthetic with narcotics. Examples of effective solutions are 1/16% to 1/20% bupivacaine or ropivacaine, with 0.5 to 1 mcg/cc sufentanil, or 1 to 2 mcg/cc fentanyl, which can provide effective analgesia without motor blockade. Techniques using low-dose combined spinal-epidural analgesia (2.5 mg plain bupivacaine, 5 μg fentanyl for the spinal with epidural dosing 40 minutes later with 0.1% or 0.05% bupivacaine and 2 μg/mL fentanyl) have been shown to allow for effective ambulation. In addition, earlier ambulation of the laboring patient can be obtained by omitting the lidocaine-epinephrine test dose and replacing it with an epidural bolus of 12 mL of 0.125% bupivacaine or using one of the dilute local anesthetic/narcotic solutions. The attending anesthesiologist needs to weigh the benefits of a test dose against the benefits of ambulation in this patient population.

Is ambulation with analgesia (primarily epidural based) the best solution for every laboring patient? As with everything in medicine, there are no absolutes. However, it is clear that there seems to be little harm in allowing selected patients to ambulate if the appropriate analgesic technique is chosen. Finally, the patient and her family, as well as the entire labor and delivery staff (obstetricians, family medicine physicians, midwives, nurses, certified registered nurse anesthetists, and anesthesiologists), need to be educated on the benefit of ambulation with analgesia.

TAKE HOME POINTS

- Patients can walk in labor with analgesia.
- Patients generally like this option to be available to them (even if they choose not to ambulate).
- Patient selection is a key to success. The obstetric provider needs to evaluate the patient and approve ambulation with analgesia.
- Epidural and Combined Spinal Epidural (CSE) solutions must be chosen to allow minimal motor block (all use combinations of dilute local anesthetics with narcotics).
- Proper monitoring must be available.
- Patients, nursing staff, and obstetric providers must be educated on the benefits of ambulation, and a proper protocol must be in place for all to follow.

SUGGESTED READINGS

Cohen SE, Yeh JY, Riley ED, et al. Walking with labor epidural analgesia. *Anesthesiology.* 2000;92:387–392.

Flynn AM, Kelly J, Hollins G, et al. Ambulation in labour. *Br Med J.* 1978;2(6137):591–593.

Frenea S, Chirossel C, Rodriguez R, et al. The effects of prolonged ambulation on labor with epidural analgesia. *Anesth Analg.* 2004;98:224–229.

Pickering AE, Parry MG, Ousta B, et al. Effect of combined spinal-epidural ambulatory labor analgesia on balance. *Anesthesiology.* 1999;91:436–441.

Roberts CL, Algert CS, Olive E. Impact of first-stage ambulation on mode of delivery among women with epidural analgesia. *Austr N Z J Ob Gynaecol.* 2004;44:489–494.

Vallejo MC, Firestone LL, Mandell GL, et al. Effect of epidural analgesia with ambulation on labor duration. *Anesthesiology.* 2001;95:857–861.

NOTHING BY MOUTH GUIDELINES DURING LABOR—"CAN I PLEASE JUST HAVE SOME WATER?"

PATRICK G. BAKKE, MD

There has been increasing pressure to liberalize oral intake during the active stage of labor. This has potentially disastrous consequences for patients with comorbid disease or those needing an emergent general anesthetic. Nothing by mouth (NPO) policies were first introduced on labor and delivery wards in the late 1940s and early 1950s. The hope was that by making patients NPO, the devastating consequences of pulmonary aspiration of gastric contents could be avoided if general anesthesia becomes necessary. Curtis Mendelson, MD (who was actually an obstetrician, not an anesthesiologist), first illustrated the dire consequences of aspiration in 1946. In his study of more than 44,000 pregnancies, 66 women experienced pulmonary aspiration of gastric contents. Of these 66, only 2 died, and the suggested cause of death was asphyxiation by solid food. Those who developed aspiration pneumonitis survived. This may be a good point to emphasize—volume, pH, and particulate matter are the main determinates of pulmonary injury and outcome following aspiration.

Factors that increase the risk of aspiration for the laboring woman can be broken down into two broad categories. First are the physiological changes due to pregnancy. These changes start in the second trimester. Increasing intragastric pressure is due to the expanding uterus. At the same time, the lower esophageal sphincter is pushed up and to the left, a similar situation to a hiatal hernia. Sphincter tone is decreased due to circulating hormones, mainly progesterone. This leads to an incredibly high incidence of gastric reflux in pregnant women, even if asymptomatic. Gastric pH becomes more acidic as the placenta begins to produce gastrin. The active phase of labor slows gastric emptying. It should be noted, however, that pregnancy, by itself, appears to have no effect on gastric emptying.

Second are the difficulties that laboring women present in airway management. It is well known that the morbidity and mortality associated with anesthesia in pregnant women are primarily related to difficulties in controlling the airway and intubation. The airway is more edematous with increased vascularity and friability. Young women tend to have intact dentition. Increase in breast size during pregnancy and the gravid abdomen make positioning of the laryngoscope difficult at best.

© 2006 Mayo Foundation for Medical Education and Research

So, we have a situation in which there is an increased gastric volume, decreased pH, and delayed gastric emptying during the active phase of labor. The good news is that there have been advances in anesthetic techniques since 1946. The advent of rapid sequence intubation with cricoid pressure in the 1970s and the more heavy reliance on regional techniques may have played a role in the decline seen in maternal deaths since Mendelson's study. In addition, treatment with H_2 blockers and nonparticulate antacids may have helped. There has been increased training of anesthesiologists since that time as well. If we couple these with NPO guidelines, it would seem that we are following the Hippocratic Oath to do no harm. Or are we?

In the 1960s, a body of literature began to emerge regarding maternal ketosis in the third trimester of labor. The increased metabolic demands of labor only serve to increase the production of ketones. These concerns led to the use of dextrose-containing intravenous solutions. However, the downsides of this practice quickly led to its discontinuation. One of the best studies of eating during labor came from Scrutton et al. in 1999. This prospective randomized study compared water, light diet, or low-fat diet on labor outcome; aspiration risk; and metabolic profile. Although the numbers were small, they found no difference on length or outcome of labor or fetal outcome. The water-only diet had higher ketone levels, while the fed groups had higher glucose levels. Ultrasound was used to evaluate gastric volumes. The fed groups were found to have significantly higher residual gastric volumes. It is interesting to note that many studies, including the previously mentioned one, found that women were less interested in eating as labor progressed.

Current recommendations from the American College of Obstetricians and Gynecologists are for a laboring patient to be on clear liquids during the active phase of labor or NPO if a surgical delivery is anticipated or likely. Current midwifery guidelines stress that the risk of aspiration is almost exclusively anesthesia related. As such, self-determination is advocated regarding eating during labor with consideration of limiting solid or liquid oral intake with increasing risk of operative delivery. Recommendations are as follows:

- Clear liquids during the active phase of labor
- NPO for patients with additional reasons for slowed gastric emptying
- NPO for patients with an increased risk for operative delivery
- Nonparticulate antacids with H_2 blockers prior to all operative deliveries
- NPO for 8 hours prior to elective operative delivery, clear liquids for 2 hours

---

TAKE HOME POINTS

- Aspiration of gastric contents has long been recognized as a rare but potentially devastating complication in the obstetrics suite.

- Aspiration risks occur both as the result of the physiological changes of pregnancy and as the need to manage the more difficult airway of the pregnant patient.

- There has been and continues to be increased pressure on anesthesiologists to allow relaxed NPO standards.

- It has been documented that ketosis increases in the fasting parturient.

- Practical guidelines are suggested that allow a moderate amount of clear liquids in the "uncomplicated" laboring patient but maintain stricter limits for complicated, high-risk, or possible surgical patients.

- The editor recommends that anesthesia providers read Mendelson's classic 1946 study. It is one of the most influential papers in the field of anesthesia. A synopsis can be found in the September 1999 ASA newsletter at www.asahq.org that includes the following passage:

> Dr. Mendelson argued quite aggressively for better-trained personnel in the administration of anesthesia to his patients. He clearly was not happy regarding the poor, inexperienced anesthesia support his specialty was receiving at this time and suggested methods by which obstetricians could overcome this problem. In the discussion section of his 1946 article, Mendelson stated, "The anesthetic deserves special consideration." He further goes on to address several important issues in the anesthetic care of the obstetrical patient, suggesting that local anesthesia would eliminate the dangers of "incompetently administered general anesthesia." Dr. Mendelson also listed several important skills in airway management in which he believed that individuals administering an anesthetic should become proficient (e.g., skill in laryngoscopy).

SUGGESTED READINGS

American College of Nurse-Midwives. Intrapartum nutrition—clinical bulletin #3. *J Nurse Midwifery.* 1999;44(2):124–128.

American College of Obstetricians and Gynecologists. *American College of Obstetricians and Gynecologists Guidelines for Perinatal Care.* 3rd ed. Washington, DC: American College of Obstetricians and Gynecologists, 1992.

Camann WR. "Can I please have something to drink?" Perioperative intake of clear liquids. Highlights of the 35th annual meeting of the Society for Obstetric Anesthesia and Perinatology; Phoenix, AZ: May 2003.

Mendelson CL. The aspiration of stomach contents into the lungs during obstetric anesthesia. *Am J Obstet Gynecol.* 1946;52:191–205.

O'Sullivan G, Scrutton M. NPO during labor: is there any scientific validation? *Anesthesiol Clin North Am.* 2003;21(1):87–98.

Scrutton MJ, Metcalfe GA, Lowy C, Seed PT, O'Sullivan G. Eating in labour: a randomised controlled trial assessing the risks and benefits. *Anaesthesia.* 1999;54(4):329–334.

155

BE PREPARED FOR THE PRESENCE OF A DOULA IN BOTH THE LABOR AND DELIVERY ROOM

CHRISTOPHER E. SWIDE, MD

Doulas are becoming increasingly popular in the United States and are active on many labor suites across the country. DONA International is the oldest and largest of the doula organizations in the United States. It has more than 5,800 members, including 2,300 certified birth doulas in all 50 states. Many hospitals and health systems hire doulas directly, but it is also common for doulas to contract separately with the patient. The term *doula* is derived from Greek and refers to the most important female servant in the ancient Greek household. Today's doulas are caregivers whose primary role is the emotional support of the mother during labor and delivery. Anesthesiologists and nurse anesthetists working on labor units will encounter doulas but are often confused about their role in the birth experience. It is important for them to have a general understanding of this caregiver's role to facilitate optimal care for obstetric patients.

Doulas are not licensed providers; therefore, there are no state requirements for doula education. However, DONA International offers a certification program that consists of completing a reading list; completing a workshop of a minimum of 16 hours; and documentation of previous experience in childbirth care by training in childbirth education or midwifery, work experience as a labor nurse, or observation of a childbirth preparation series. After completion of this program, the new doula must provide service to at least three clients and document the births with a 500- to 700-word firsthand account of each experience. In addition, the new doula must provide evaluations from three clients, three primary care providers, and three nurses or midwives.

Doulas do not provide clinical care to the mother. They do not make clinical decisions or offer opinions that might influence their clients' decisions. A doula that is also a midwife, nurse, or other care provider cannot function in those roles while serving as a client's doula. Their primary role is emotional support of the mother, and facilitating positive communication between the mother, her nurses, midwives, and physicians. They maintain continuous presence during labor and help the mother's partner be part of the experience. Although many doula clients do not want regional anesthesia for labor, a significant number of patients still expect or decide to receive a

© 2006 Mayo Foundation for Medical Education and Research

labor epidural for pain relief. It is important for the anesthesia provider taking care of these patients to interact with the patient and the doula. Patients with doulas must consent to having the doula present for confidential medical discussions. The doula will expect to be in continuous attendance with the mother, and this should be respected unless there are medical or hospital policy rules that do not allow it. Doulas can be helpful to the anesthesiologists and nurse anesthetists, often comforting the mother during the placement of the regional block and maintaining communication patterns between the patient, the nurses, physicians, other caregivers, and the partner during labor. If a patient needs cesarean section, the doula should be included in the discussion and planning made to accommodate the doula in the operating room if feasible. In the case of urgent cesarean section requiring a general anesthetic that precludes doula presence, the situation should be discussed with patient and doula, and all efforts made to preserve the team approach for delivery of the baby and to maintain respectful interactions.

In summary, doulas can provide obstetric patients with excellent emotional support and increase the mother's satisfaction with her birth experience. It is important for anesthesia providers to understand the doula's role and incorporate the doula into the overall care plan so patients who choose doulas can have an optimal birth experience.

TAKE HOME POINTS

- Take the time to understand the doula's role in childbirth.
- Respect the mother's choice in choosing a doula to participate.
- Introduce yourself to both the patient and the doula.
- Maintain respectful and professional interactions throughout the care of the patient.
- Learn the policy of your labor unit concerning doulas.
- Make patient care decisions and recommendations as you would with any patient in labor. Your standard of care does not change with patients using doulas.

SUGGESTED READINGS

Camann, WA. Doulas—who are they and how might they affect obstetrical anesthesia practices? *Society of Anesthesiologists Newsletter.* 2000;64:11–12.
DONA International website. Available at: www.dona.org. Accessed March 29, 2007.
Meyer BA, Arnold JA, Pascali-Bonaro D. Social support by doulas during labor and the early post partum period. *Hosp Physician.* 2001;Sept:57–65.

156

URGENT CESAREAN SECTION: WHAT'S GOOD FOR BABY IS GOOD FOR MOMMY?

NATHAN J. HESS, DO AND KAREN HAND, MD

Nearly one fourth of all births in the United States today are via cesarean section, a dramatic increase from the 5.5% of births in 1970. A considerable number of these fall into the classification of urgent, nonelective cesarean. In some cases (i.e., massive maternal hemorrhage, dystocia), both the mother and the baby are in jeopardy. Quite commonly, however, there is nonreassuring fetal status without concomitant maternal distress. The parturient presenting for urgent cesarean section brings with her unique anesthetic challenges, and anesthesia-related complications in this setting can be associated with considerable maternal morbidity and mortality. Indeed, anesthesia is the seventh leading cause of maternal mortality in the United States.

PHYSIOLOGICAL CHANGES ASSOCIATED WITH PREGNANCY

There are numerous physiological changes that occur by the third trimester of pregnancy, many of which potentially make anesthesia more hazardous. The anesthesiologist must be familiar with the major physiological changes that occur with pregnancy and the potential anesthetic implications (*Table 156.1*).

INDICATIONS FOR URGENT CESAREAN SECTION

The anesthesiologist must be in close communication with the obstetrician in determining the indication and true urgency for cesarean section. A distinction must be made between *urgent* and *emergent or stat* section, as those in the former category may allow time for regional anesthesia, while those in the latter nearly always require general anesthesia in the absence of a functioning epidural catheter. Although each individual case must be considered in consultation with the obstetrician, those falling in the **urgent but not emergent** category generally include (a) variable decelerations with prompt recovery of fetal heart rate (FHR), (b) dystocia, (c) previous classic cesarean and active labor, (d) active genital herpes and ruptured membranes, (e) ruptured membranes and abnormal fetal presentation (i.e., transverse, breech, multiple gestation), and (f) rapidly deteriorating maternal illness (pre-eclampsia, cardiac, pulmonary). Conversely, those indications generally falling into the **emergent or stat** category include (a) prolonged fetal bradycardia or persistent late decelerations (rule of 60s = FHR <60/minute **or** deceleration

© 2006 Mayo Foundation for Medical Education and Research

TABLE 156.1	**PHYSIOLOGICAL CHANGES ASSOCIATED WITH PREGNANCY**	
SYSTEM	**PHYSIOLOGICAL CHANGES AT TERM GESTATION (COMPARED WITH PREPREGNANT VALUES)**	**ANESTHETIC IMPLICATIONS**
Respiratory	30%–40% increase in oxygen consumption 20% decrease in FRC 45% increase in minute ventilation Increased airway edema and mucosal friability	Rapid development of hypoxemia during apnea, potentially difficult intubation
Cardiovascular	50% increase in cardiac output 20% decrease in SVR Possible aortocaval compression by gravid uterus 55% increase in plasma volume 45% increase in blood volume	Aortocaval compression→decreased preload→hypotension in supine parturient→uteroplacental insufficiency
Gastrointestinal	Anatomic displacement of stomach cephalad and left Decreased lower esophageal sphincter tone Delayed gastric emptying? Increased gastric acid secretion?	Increased risk for aspiration (Mendelson syndrome)
Nervous	Increased sensitivity to IV anesthetics MAC of volatile agents reduced 15%–40%	Adjust doses accordingly
Miscellaneous	Engorged breasts Increased sensitivity to nondepolarizing MR	Difficult laryngoscope insertion, reduce dosages of NDMR

FRC, functional residual capacity; SVR, systemic vascular resistance; IV, intravenous; MAC, minimum alveolar concentration; MR, muscle relaxant; NDMR, non depolarizing muscle relaxant.

lasting longer than 60 seconds), (b) massive maternal hemorrhage (placenta previa, placental abruption), (c) prolapsed umbilical cord, and (d) uterine rupture.

APPROACH TO THE URGENT CESAREAN SECTION

Ideally, the obstetric anesthesiologist should be familiar, at least superficially, with all patients present in the labor and delivery suite. Practically speaking, however, this is difficult on a busy service. Therefore, it is imperative that an attempt be made to identify those patients at increased risk for cesarean section (see Indications for Urgent Cesarean Section section). **Once again, a good working relationship with the obstetrician will facilitate this process. At the first sign of trouble, the obstetrician should contact the anesthesiologist to allow the maximum amount of time possible** for evaluation and formulation of an anesthetic plan. Once identified, a thorough pre-operative evaluation should be performed on each patient deemed to be at risk.

An aggressive approach should be taken in managing potentially confounding factors in each patient's anesthetic management. In those patients where difficult airway management is anticipated (i.e., excessive pharyngeal edema, obesity, short thyromental distance, poor mouth opening, poor neck extension), early placement and testing of an epidural catheter should be strongly considered. This will allow prompt initiation of regional anesthesia in the event that cesarean becomes necessary. Similarly, those patients presenting with hypertensive disorders of pregnancy (pre-eclampsia, HELLP [Hemolysis, Elevated Liver Enzymes, and Low Platelets] syndrome) in whom coagulopathy is developing (increasing international normalized ratio, falling platelet count) are candidates for prompt placement and testing of an epidural catheter before coagulation parameters deteriorate to a level deemed unsafe for regional anesthesia.

All patients presenting for cesarean section should have at least one well-functioning 18-gauge or larger intravenous (IV) catheter in place. Each patient should also have a current type and screen. If atypical antibodies or other factors are present that will make cross-matching difficult, 2 to 4 U of cross-matched blood should be made available in the operating room prior to proceeding. In those patients deemed to be at increased risk for peripartum hemorrhage, it is recommended that at least one additional large-bore IV catheter be placed and that blood be available for rapid administration.

Standard American Society of Anesthesiologists (ASA) monitors are required for each cesarean section. Additional monitoring may be necessary and should be considered on a case-by-case basis. Supplemental oxygen should be administered to all patients. Left uterine displacement should be performed in all parturients to decrease the likelihood of aortocaval compression and the accompanying hemodynamic compromise to mother and fetus.

A nonparticulate antacid should be administered to **all** patients shortly prior to or on arrival to the operating room. We commonly administer an H_2-blocker and metoclopramide at the same time. Although current data are conflicting, conventional teaching states that a gastric pH of <2.5 and gastric volume of >25 mL places patients at increased risk for aspiration pneumonitis.

Frequent reassurance and comfort given to the expectant mother is paramount prior to/during the urgent cesarean section. The anesthesiologist is frequently in the best position to do this and should become adept at doing so. Otherwise, unoccupied personnel should also tend to the expectant father and other family members because this can be a time of great confusion and emotional distress for all involved.

REGIONAL ANESTHESIA

Consideration should be given to the use of regional anesthesia, even in the face of urgent cesarean. Clearly, if a functional epidural catheter is in place, this will often provide the quickest and safest route to surgical anesthesia. For the emergent cesarean section in our practice, we dose the epidural catheter initially with 15 to 20 mL of 3% 2-chloroprocaine. Because of the low potential for systemic toxicity due 2-chloroprocaine's rapid clearance by plasma esterases, this large dose can be administered safely as a bolus or incrementally with very short dosing intervals. Adequate anesthesia generally develops within 3 to 5 minutes. It is important to remember that due to 2-chloroprocaine's short duration of action, the catheter must be redosed in approximately 25 to 35 minutes to prevent regression of the block to an unacceptable level. This is most often done with a longer-acting agent, such as 2% lidocaine with 1:200,000 epinephrine, 0.5% ropivacaine, or 0.5% bupivacaine.

Many **experienced** practitioners believe that they can successfully place a spinal anesthetic in the same amount of time it takes to induce general anesthesia. Communication with the obstetric team regarding this plan can allow the spinal to be placed while the team prepares for surgery. A sufficient block will generally have time to develop while the abdomen is prepped and draped. If complicating factors are present that may make placement of a spinal anesthetic difficult (i.e., obesity, scoliosis, previous lumbar spinal surgery), then it is best to not waste time trying to place a regional block and proceed directly to a general anesthetic. Regional anesthesia is best avoided in the face of significant bleeding/hypovolemia because the accompanying sympathectomy can cause catastrophic hemodynamic collapse.

Regardless of the type of anesthetic planned, each patient's position on the operating table should be optimized for airway management, and the proper equipment and drugs necessary for general anesthesia should be prepared in advance.

GENERAL ANESTHESIA

As mentioned previously, prior to induction of general anesthesia, a non-particulate antacid (i.e., Bicitra) should be administered, a well-functioning IV catheter and appropriate monitors should be in place, and the patient's position should be optimized for airway management. Depending on the patient's body habitus, this may involve placing a "ramp" of towels or sheets or placement of a commercially available intubating wedge under the patient's shoulders to facilitate intubation. Several small endotracheal tubes (6.0–6.5 mm cuffed) and a variety of laryngoscope blades should be available. It is often helpful to have a short-handled laryngoscope because engorged breasts can interfere with insertion of the blade into the patient's mouth. An intubating stylet may also be helpful and should be at hand. Finally, backup airway equipment, including laryngeal mask airways (LMAs) of different sizes, intubating LMAs, Combitube or other airway devices, and the ability to provide jet ventilation should be immediately available.

Preoxygenation is mandatory prior to induction of anesthesia. Full denitrogenation takes approximately 3 to 5 minutes of normal tidal volume breathing with 100% oxygen. However, some studies have demonstrated four to six vital capacity breaths to be nearly as effective as the traditional method. The urgency of the situation and clinical judgment should dictate which method is undertaken. **It should be emphasized that the anesthesiologist must take control of the situation and should not proceed until the previous criteria are met. With proper training and direction of operating room personnel, adequate preparation can be carried out in a very short period of time. The mother's life should not be placed in jeopardy if the anesthesiologist deems the situation unacceptably risky.** As the situation and urgency dictate, possible alternatives include awake intubation or, on rare occasions, local infiltration by the obstetrician, although the block achieved in this instance is generally not ideal.

Prior to induction, the abdomen should be prepped and draped, and the surgical team should be ready to proceed. Rapid sequence induction with properly administered cricoid pressure by an assistant is the usual method indicated for cesarean general anesthesia (GA). Depending on the situation, any of the available induction agents, including propofol (2 to 3 mg/kg), sodium thiopental (3 to 4 mg/kg), etomidate (0.2 to 0.3 mg/ kg), or ketamine (1 to 2 mg/kg) may be indicated. Succinylcholine (1 mg/kg) is administered immediately after the induction agent. If succinylcholine is contraindicated, rocuronium is an acceptable alternative (rapid sequence dosage should be reduced 30% to 50% from nonpregnant values). As soon as anesthesia is induced, the surgical team is allowed to proceed. Anesthesia is generally maintained with a low concentration (i.e., 0.5 MAC) of volatile agent in 50% to 60% nitrous oxide. Opioids are generally minimized until after delivery of the fetus to minimize respiratory depression in the neonate. If poor uterine tone is of concern after delivery of the fetus, the concentration of volatile agent may be further reduced. Extubation is carried out awake, assuring that airway reflexes are intact.

TAKE HOME POINTS

- Physiological changes of pregnancy potentially make anesthesia for urgent cesarean section hazardous.

- Communication with the obstetric team, early identification and evaluation of potential candidates, and proper anesthetic planning can greatly reduce anxiety surrounding an urgent cesarean section and may be life-saving.

- Early placement and testing of an epidural catheter should be considered in at-risk parturients.

- Preparation for general endotracheal anesthesia for cesarean section includes, at a minimum, administration of a nonparticulate antacid, placement of a well-functioning 18-gauge or larger IV catheter, application of standard ASA monitors, optimizing position for intubation, and adequate preoxygenation prior to induction.

The key to managing these patients is to remember that you have an obligation to both mom and baby, and a "nonreassuring" tracing for the baby should not trigger an unsafe situation for mom. With proper planning, communication, and teamwork, these difficult situations can be managed to provide the best possible outcomes for both the mother and her child.

SUGGESTED READINGS

Chestnut DH. *Obstetric Anesthesia Principles and Practice*. 3rd ed. Philadelphia, PA: Mosby; 2004:421–459.

Hawkins JL, Koonin LM, Palmer SK, et al. Anesthesia-related deaths during obstetric delivery in the United States, 1979–1990 [Clinical Investigation]. *Anesthesiology*. 1997;86(2): 277–284.

Munnur U, de Boisblanc B, Suresh M. Airway problems in pregnancy. *Crit Care Med.* 2005;33(10):s259–s268.

Santos AC. Anesthetic management of the preeclamptic parturient. *ASA Refresher Courses in Anesthesiology*. 2004;32(1):197–209.

Wickwire JC, Gross JB. From preop to postop: cesarean delivery from the anesthesiologist's point of view. *Clin Obstet Gynecol*. 2004;47(2):299–316.

157

PAIN CONTROL AFTER CESAREAN SECTION—"HOW CAN I TAKE CARE OF MY BABY IF I JUST HAD SURGERY?"

PATRICK G. BAKKE, MD

Pain control after cesarean section (C section) is crucial for the comfort of the new mother. In addition, poor pain control on postoperative day 1 when the mother is mobilizing can hinder her ability to care for her child. The discomfort results from two distinct pathways of nociception: (i) the somatic component derived from the surgical wound, and (ii) a visceral component derived from the ongoing contractions of the uterus. There are also concerns about the development of residual pain after C section. The most commonly used routes for delivering analgesics for postoperative pain control following C section are systemic and neuraxial. Commonly employed medications are opiates, nonsteroidal anti-inflammatory drugs (NSAIDs), and local anesthetics.

Systemic delivery of analgesics traditionally involved intravenous (IV) or intermuscular injection of opiates. It is now clear that the use of the IV route results in more patient satisfaction, overall lowered pain scores, and decreased nursing workload. IV patient-controlled analgesia (IVPCA) results in even higher patient satisfaction scores due to the availability of a more consistent level of analgesia and a greater measure of patient control. Opiate side effects of pruritus, nausea and vomiting, urinary retention, constipation, sedation, and respiratory depression must be monitored and treated accordingly. Although all opiates are present to some degree in breast milk, they have not been shown to be a problem with neonatal sedation. Morphine has the least presence in breast milk. Meperidine, however, is best avoided due to accumulation of its active metabolite in breast milk. It is interesting to note that patients with epidural opiate/local anesthetic infusions had lower pain scores than those with an IVPCA; however, patient satisfaction is still reported to be greater in the IVPCA group.

Neuraxial delivery of opiate analgesics has become more common with the use of spinal or epidural anesthesia for C section. Using neuraxial techniques for the primary anesthetic may help prevent central sensitization with resulting hyperalgesia and allodynia. In fact, residual pain is more prevalent in patients after C section who have had a general anesthetic than those receiving a neuraxial technique. Certain patient factors such as pre-eclampsia, low platelet count, or anticoagulation must be kept in mind when planning a

© 2006 Mayo Foundation for Medical Education and Research

neuraxial technique. In addition, there is a subset of patients who will refuse neuraxial techniques, and their wishes need to be respected.

When given intrathecally, preservative-free morphine can give excellent pain control up to 24 hours. There seems to be little effect on pain scores with doses above 0.1 to 0.2 mg. However, with escalating doses, the side effects of pruritus, nausea and vomiting, urinary retention, and respiratory depression increase. Of these side effects, the most feared is delayed respiratory depression, which can occur 12 to 14 hours after administration. Abouleish et al. studied 856 patients who had spinals for elective C section—0.2 mg of preservative-free morphine was included, and <1% (all of whom were morbidly obese) met the criteria for respiratory depression. Clearly, this route and dose can be used with safety. (*Note:* Most obstetrics units will discharge a **low-dose** "Duramorph mom" to the floor with the caveat that no IV narcotics can be prescribed in the first 12 hours without assessment from the anesthesia service—generally, this is not an issue because most moms can be transitioned directly from Duramorph to oral pain medication.) Fentanyl or sufentanil can also be used for analgesia in the intrathecal space. These drugs have fewer propensities for nausea, vomiting, or itching. They are faster in onset and have a shorter duration of action, likely due to their greater lipid solubility. Respiratory depression, if it is to occur, usually does so within 30 minutes.

Epidural solutions containing both local anesthetics and opiates provide excellent analgesia. The presence of local anesthetics reduces the opiate requirements. However, the solution must be dilute enough not to cause significant motor or sensory weakness to the lower extremities. A commonly employed strategy is to remove the epidural catheter on postoperative day 1 when the patient is expected to ambulate. Plus, bowel function has usually returned by then, allowing oral administration of medications for pain relief.

Although opiates are excellent at treating the somatic portion of pain, they are somewhat inadequate with visceral pain. NSAIDs play their biggest role here. NSAIDs have a well-documented opiate-sparing effect. What is commonly overlooked, however, is the role NSAIDs play centrally by inhibiting production of prostaglandins in the spinal cord. Prostaglandins are pronociceptive in central sensitization. Diclofenac and ketorolac have both been shown to be particularly effective. It must be noted that even though the American Academy of Pediatricians regards ketorolac as safe for use in breastfeeding women, the manufacturer states that its use is contraindicated during labor and delivery or by nursing mothers, and the U.S. Food and Drug Administration has a black box warning because of the possible effects on fetal circulation and uterine contractions.

Last, we should not overlook the role of the surgeon. Local infiltration of the wound has marked immediate postoperative effects on pain reduction.

Some advocate the silo elastic "pain balls" hooked to a subdermal catheter for postoperative pain control.

In summary, there are a number of modalities for pain relief following C section. Opiates may be given either systemically or by intrathecal route. Local anesthetics mixed with opiates in the epidural space are very effective. NSAIDs have opiate-sparing effects and help prevent central sensitization that can lead to residual pain. Our surgical colleagues can help by using local injections or infusions in the surgical wound.

TAKE HOME POINTS

- IVPCA results in the highest patient satisfaction scores after C section.
- Epidural solutions with mixed local anesthetics and opiates result in the lowest pain scores after C section.
- Neuraxial techniques for the primary anesthetic may lead to less residual pain after C section.
- Preservativefree morphine given via the intrathecal route is safe up to 0.2 mg and is not more effective for pain relief beyond that dose.
- NSAIDs have an opiate-sparing effect.
- NSAIDs also help prevent central sensitization.
- Surgeons should use local anesthesia in the wound.

SUGGESTED READINGS

Gadsden J, Hart S, Santos AC. Post-cesarean delivery analgesia. *Anesth Analg.* 2005; 101(5 suppl);S62–S69.

Lavand'homme P. Postcesarean analgesia: effective strategies and association with chronic pain. *Curr Opin Anaesthesiol.* 2006;19(3):244–248.

Abouleish E, Rawal N, Rashad MN. The addition of 0.2mg subarachnoid morphine to hyperbaric bupivacaine for cesarean delivery: a prospective study of 856 cases. *Reg Anesth.* 1991;16(3):137–140.

158

BE AWARE OF THE CONSEQUENCES OF AORTOCAVAL COMPRESSION AND THE SUPINE HYPOTENSIVE SYNDROME WHEN CARING FOR A PREGNANT PATIENT

THOMAS M. CHALIFOUX, MD AND RYAN C. ROMEO, MD

Positioning in the pregnant patient is very important. About 10% of women at term experience the supine hypotensive syndrome caused by complete or near-complete occlusion of the inferior vena cava (IVC) by the gravid uterus. A resultant drop in venous return decreases cardiac output (CO), leading to systemic hypotension for which the cardiovascular system cannot compensate. The nature and severity of symptoms range from unspecific symptoms such as pallor, sweating, nausea, and vomiting, to severe maternal hypotension, loss of consciousness, cardiovascular collapse, and consecutive fetal depression. Inferior vena caval compression can begin to occur in pregnant women as early as 13 weeks' gestation and may be exaggerated by multiple gestations (twins) and obesity.

Complete or near-complete obstruction of the IVC can occur when the parturient is supine. Collateral circulation can allow for some venous return, but the result is a decrease in right atrial filling pressure. This drop in preload leads to a decrease in CO. The lateral decubitus position causes partial caval obstruction, but the right ventricular filling pressure is unaltered due to collateral circulation, and there is little effect on the CO.

Aortic compression also occurs. There is little aortic compression at term in the lateral position. In the lateral tilt position, 40% of patients will have a fall in femoral artery pressure, indicating a compression of the aorta. In the supine position, the fall is even greater and inversely proportional to arterial pressure. Thus, there is enhanced compression of the aorta when the patient is hypotensive.

Objective parameters of fetal well-being deteriorate in the supine position compared to the lateral or tilted position. Neonatal outcome, as accessed by umbilical cord pH and Apgar scores, is also compromised in the supine position. These effects are explained by aortocaval compression and the resulting impairment in uteroplacental blood flow.

CARDIOVASCULAR SYSTEM ADAPTATION TO PREGNANCY

Table 158.1 summarizes the body's cardiovascular adaptation to pregnancy. Labor augments CO. Uterine contractions add 300 mL to the central

© 2006 Mayo Foundation for Medical Education and Research

TABLE 158.1	SUMMARY OF THE BODY'S CARDIOVASCULAR ADAPTATION TO PREGNANCY
Maternal oxygen consumption	Increased
Heart rate	Increased
Cardiac output	Increased
Stroke volume	Increased
Peripheral vascular resistance	Decreased
Mean arterial pressure	Decreased
Central venous pressure	Unchanged
Blood volume	Increased
Plasma volume	Increased
Erythrocyte volume	Increased
Hemoglobin	Decreased

circulating volume and relieve the degree of vena caval compression. CO, heart rate, and stroke volume all increase substantially shortly after delivery. The maximum rise in CO is coincident with the autotransfusion of blood from the evacuated uterus. There is a decline in aortocaval compression, and the loss of the placental shunt. The cardiovascular changes and parameters return to prelabor values within an hour after delivery. They gradually return to prepregnant values within 2 to 4 weeks postdelivery.

POSITIONING THE PREGNANT PATIENT

Aortocaval compression and the supine hypotensive syndrome can be minimized by having the parturient lie in the lateral position. For cesarean section or when the lateral position is not practical, left uterine displacement using the lateral tilt position should be employed. Place a wedge under the patient's right hip to elevate the hip 10 to 15 cm and displace the uterus to the left, away from the IVC. This should be done from 20 weeks' gestation to term.

When placing an epidural catheter or performing a spinal anesthetic, the sitting position may be preferred because it has been shown to be associated with less decrease in CO than the maximal lateral flexed position when placing an epidural in laboring women.

Cardiopulmonary resuscitation in the parturient is complicated by vena caval compression. The patient should be placed in the lateral tilt position and an assistant should move the uterus further off the IVC by lifting it with two hands to the left and toward the patient's head. Cesarean section plays an important role in the resuscitation of the mother in cardiopulmonary arrest and is advocated if the resuscitation is not successful within 5 minutes. It is believed that occlusion of the IVC is relieved completely by emptying the uterus, whereas it is only partially relieved by manual uterine displacement or an inclined position.

DETERMINANTS OF UTERINE BLOOD FLOW

Uterine blood flow (UBF) represents about 10% of the CO at term, which is about 500 to 700 mL/minute. In comparison, the nonpregnant uterus sees about 50 mL/minute. UBF is directly related to perfusion pressure and inversely related to vascular resistance.

$$UBF = \frac{\text{Uterine arterial} - \text{Uterine venous pressure}}{\text{Uterine vascular resistance}}$$

Thus, UBF decreases when perfusion pressure decreases or when vascular resistance increases.

UBF may decline when the perfusion pressure decreases because of decreased uterine arterial pressure, which occurs during systemic hypotension. Not only will UBF decrease because of the decline in perfusion pressure, but uterine vascular resistance also increases because of increased concentrations of vasopressin and angiotensin II, which are secreted in an attempt to maintain systemic blood pressure.

UBF may decline when perfusion pressure decreases because of increased uterine venous pressure. This typically occurs with vena caval compression, during uterine contraction, and during the Valsalva maneuver that accompanies pushing during the second stage of labor.

UBF may decline because of increased uterine vascular resistance. This may occur secondary to endogenous catecholamines (stress) or exogenous vasoconstrictors such as phenylephrine administration. However during pregnancy, anatomical adaptations result in near maximal vasodilation of the uterine arteries, resulting in a low-resistance pathway for delivery of blood to the placenta. Therefore, adequate uteroplacental blood flow depends on the maintenance of a normal maternal perfusion pressure.

There is little evidence available for supporting autoregulation of blood flow in the placenta, and the circuit mainly depends on maternal blood pressure.

EFFECTS OF ANESTHESIA ON UTERINE BLOOD FLOW

Regional anesthesia has the following effects on UBF. It can increase UBF by causing pain relief, decreased sympathetic activity and decreased maternal hyperventilation. It can decrease UBF by causing hypotension, unintentional intravenous injection of local anesthetic and/or epinephrine, and absorbed local anesthetic (little effect). Adjuvant drugs used in regional anesthesia can have varying effects on UBF, and these effects can be found in more comprehensive texts.

General anesthesia has minimal effects on UBF. The drugs used to induce general anesthesia such as barbiturates and propofol may decrease UBF by causing a degree of hypotension. Usual clinical doses of inhalation agents have little or no effect on UBF. Noxious stimuli secondary to light anesthesia may cause the release of catecholamines and thereby decrease UBF.

TAKE HOME POINTS

- The supine hypotension syndrome can be life threatening to both the mother and the fetus.
- Aortic compression in the supine position is actually a separate but related phenomenon.
- The detrimental effects to the fetus when the mother is allowed to assume the supine position are well documented.
- Left uterine displacement should be used once the patient is past 20 weeks' gestation, regardless of whether she experiences symptoms in the prone position.
- There is little if any autoregulation of UBF, the main determinant is maternal blood pressure.
- If the mother is undergoing cardiopulmonary resuscitation, she should be placed in the left uterine displacement position and the uterus should be manually lifted off the vena cava.

SUGGESTED READINGS

Chestnut DH. *Obstetric Anesthesia: Principles and Practice.* 3rd ed. St. Louis, Mo.: Mosby; 2004.
Kiefer RT, Ploppa A, Dieterich HJ. Aortocaval compression syndrome. *Anaesthesist.* 2003;52(11):1073–1083.
Morris S, Stacey M. Resuscitation in pregnancy. *BMJ* 2003;327:1277–1279.
Ramanathan S, Mandell G, eds. *Obstetric Anesthesia Web Manual: A Semi-Comprehensive Web Text Book.* Available at: www.ramanathans.com. Accessed March 29, 2007.

159

HEADACHES AND HYPERTENSION: MANAGEMENT OF PRE-ECLAMPSIA IN THE OBESE PATIENT

PATRICK G. BAKKE, MD

The incidence of hypertensive disorders of pregnancy is 2% to 8%. These disorders can be thought of as a continuum from gestational hypertension to eclampsia. Pre-eclampsia is defined as systolic blood pressure (SBP) ≥ 140 and diastolic blood pressure (DBP) ≥ 90, diagnosed after 20 weeks' gestation and accompanied by proteinuria >300 mg/24 hours. Severe pre-eclampsia is defined as SBP ≥ 160, DBP ≥ 110, proteinuria >5 g/24 hours. In addition, signs of end-organ dysfunction (oliguria, elevated serum creatinine, pulmonary edema, visual disturbances, headaches, epigastric pain), fetal growth restriction, oligohydramnios, or HELLP syndrome (Hemolysis, Elevated Liver Enzymes, and Low Platelets) make the diagnosis of severe pre-eclampsia. Eclampsia is diagnosed by the presence of seizures.

The etiology of pre-eclampsia is poorly understood. Currently, it is believed that initially there is abnormal trophoblastic invasion during placental implantation. Trophoblastic invasion of the decidual and myometrial portions of the spiral arteries results in an increase in diameter of these arteries. In pre-eclampsia, only the decidual portions change; the myometrial segments remain small and exceptionally responsive to vasomotor stimuli. This abnormality explains the drop in placental perfusion and the predisposition to uterine growth retardation. In turn, this leads to the changes that characterize the systemic maternal disease. There is endothelial dysfunction that can cause platelet aggregation, downregulation of circulating anticoagulants, and capillary leaks. In addition, an imbalance between decreased prostacyclin I_2 and increased thromboxane A_2 exists. Prostacyclin I_2 is a potent vasodilator and activator of platelets. Thromboxane A_2 is a potent vasoconstrictor and promoter of platelet aggregation. Endothelial dysfunction may impair nitric oxide and increase endothelin-1. Endothelin-1 is also a potent vasoconstrictor and platelet aggregator. These changes result in generalized vasospasm, reduced intravascular volume, decreased glomerular filtration rate, generalized edema, and a hypercoagulable state.

Obesity, among others, is an independent risk factor for developing pre-eclampsia. When the two entities are combined, anesthetic management can be quite challenging. Current obstetric management involves treating elevated blood pressure with labetalol first, then using oral nifedipine. These

© 2006 Mayo Foundation for Medical Education and Research

patients will likely be receiving magnesium sulfate for seizure prophylaxis. It is crucial to have open and complete communication with the obstetricians regarding these patients. The only definitive treatment is delivery of the fetus.

The anesthetic management of labor should involve the early placement of a continuous lumber epidural catheter. Given the obese body habitus and generalized edema, intravenous line placement may be difficult at best. Next, it is important to check a platelet count and prothrombin time/international normalized ratio prior to proceeding. Early involvement of anesthesia can allow placement before platelet counts fall to an unacceptable level. Most obstetric anesthesiologists are comfortable placing an epidural with platelet counts >80,000. Obesity increases the technical difficulty of placing an epidural catheter. Help should be recruited to ensure optimal positioning. Early placement of an epidural has benefits besides patient comfort. Controlling the pre-eclamptic patient's pain can blunt the hypertensive response to pain, decrease circulating catechols, and improve uteroplacental blood flow. In addition, early epidural catheter placement may avoid a general anesthetic in case of a C section. Fluid bolus must be done with some caution because too much fluid may result in pulmonary edema. If there is presence or suspicion of pulmonary issues, boluses of 250 mL at a time may be wise. Vasoactive medications such as ephedrine or phenylephrine may have a much greater effect than anticipated on the already exceptionally responsive vascular system.

In the event of an operative delivery, the combination of pregnancy, pre-eclampsia, and obesity all conspire against us. The method of choice is still an epidural for C section. If the catheter has been placed early, you are in luck. If not, refer to the previous paragraphs for consideration of placing the epidural. In the past, spinal anesthesia was a relative contraindication in the pre-eclamptic. It was believed that the drop in blood pressure sometimes seen with a spinal would be extreme given the vasoconstricted and volume depleted state of the pre-eclamptic. A body of evidence now exists that shows that a spinal can be used safely. Combined spinal epidural may be a wise choice given the increased operative difficulties obesity may present. Fluid boluses and support with vasopressors should be done cautiously as previously mentioned. SBP should be maintained at no less than 20% of baseline values in order to maintain placental perfusion.

If general anesthesia is required, there are a few extra considerations for the obese pre-eclamptic above and beyond the healthy obstetric patient. Again, communication with the nurses, obstetricians, and patient must be clear. For example, a patient with a terrible airway and extremely low platelets may benefit from a controlled C section instead of an emergent procedure. Next, careful consideration must be given to the overall medical condition of the patient. During the history and physical, extra attention should be paid to the airway, cardiac, pulmonary, abdominal, and neurologic systems. The airway may be even more edematous. Signs of heart failure should be explored. If the patient requires oxygen to maintain oxygen saturation or if there are rales on auscultation, pulmonary edema is likely. Complaints of right upper quadrant pain or a tender enlarged liver on abdominal examination may herald impending Glisson capsule rupture. Headache or visual changes are especially worrisome on neurologic exam. Labs should be recent with complete blood count, metabolic panel, liver function tests, and a coagulation panel at the least. Two large-bore intravenous (IV) catheters should be in place. The medications that the patient is receiving for blood pressure control and seizure prophylaxis must be noted. The anesthesiologist must also check the fetus by way of prenatal records and fetal heart tracing. This is also a time to decide on monitors. A mild pre-eclamptic will likely need no more than American Society for Anesthesiologists' standard monitoring. However, in the case of the severe pre-eclamptic, presence of pulmonary edema, renal insufficiency, or inability to obtain adequate venous access, invasive monitoring in the form of an arterial line, central line, or even pulmonary artery catheter may be necessary. A difficult airway cart should be present given the likelihood of airway difficulties. On induction, the response to direct laryngoscopy needs to be sufficiently blunted to prevent intracranial bleed. Besides the usual induction agent, lidocaine and opiates, it may be necessary to use esmolol, nitroglycerine, or even nitroprusside to control the hypertensive response. Magnesium sulfate should be continued in the perioperative period. When it is time to extubate, a leak test should be performed to ensure that airway edema has not increased with intraoperative fluid administration to a point that compromises airway patency. The obese patient should be awake, following commands, fully reversed, and seated upright prior to extubation.

Postoperatively or postpartum, laboratory values should be checked prior to removing the epidural catheter. The nadir of the platelet count can be 2 to 3 days postpartum, and it may take 5 to 6 days to reach an acceptable level for epidural removal. Pulmonary edema risk is greatest 2 to 3 days postoperatively when fluid is mobilized. Magnesium should be continued for 24 hours because the risk of seizure is greatest in the postpartum period.

TAKE HOME POINTS

- Clear and early communication among the obstetrician, nursing staff, and anesthesiologist is crucial.
- The airway may be even more challenging in the obese pre-eclamptic.

- Be involved with the IV access—most experienced obstetric anesthesia providers will try for at least one decently running 18g peripheral line with these patients.
- Pay close attention to the platelet count and laboratory values before epidural placement and before epidural catheter removal.
- Place the epidural catheter early.
- A spinal is acceptable for a C section.
- Do not hesitate to place invasive lines.
- Continue the magnesium; seizure risk is greatest postpartum. Despite therapy, patients may become eclamptic. Therapy to treat the acute onset of seizures and airway support should be immediately available. Historically, thiopental was used to good effect—50 mg (or 2 cc) will stop the seizures. Because thiopental is now not always immediately available, propofol 20 to 120 mg can be used for seizure control, with succinylcholine 80 mg used for emergency airway control and intubation.
- Be careful with fluid administration; pulmonary edema is most likely 2 to 3 days postoperatively.
- Patients will likely be sensitive to vasopressors.
- Prevent hyperdynamic responses during direct laryngoscopy.
- Early regional anesthesia for labor can prevent the need for general anesthesia and the potential airway issues.

One final note (and a common folklore saying in the labor and delivery suite): Do NOT let a pre-eclamptic patient "get away from you," or you will be the one with the headaches and hypertension!

SUGGESTED READINGS

Duley L, Meher S, Abalos E. Management of pre-eclampsia. *BMJ.* 2006;332(7539):463–468.

Polley LS. Anesthetic management of hypertension in pregnancy. *Clin Obstet Gynecol.* 2003;46(3):688–699.

Sibai BM. Diagnosis and management of gestational hypertension and preeclampsia. *Obstet Gynecol.* 2003;102(1):181–192.

160

ACUPUNCTURE HAS SIGNIFICANT EFFICACY FOR THE TREATMENT OF THE PREGNANT OR LABORING PATIENT

LEENA MATHEW, MD

The perception of acupuncture as a complementary medical modality (as opposed to an *alternative* therapy) has grown a lot in the last ten years, as the integration of complementary and conventional medicine continues to take root in the Western world. This is reflected by the surge of scientific studies and increasing evidence that establishes acupuncture as an accepted modality in Western medicine. Approximately 1 million U.S. consumers use acupuncture annually, primarily seeking relief of pain, and acupuncture is now available as a treatment option in most chronic pain clinics.

At present, the research data on acupuncture are mixed. Most trials on the efficacy of acupuncture are equivocal or contradictory. The randomized controlled trials using acupuncture to treat addictions and tinnitus have been predominantly negative. Multiple reviews of identical conditions such as asthma, depression, and bronchitis use overlapping studies and have conflicting interpretations.

However, notable exceptions are randomized controlled trials of acupuncture for emesis, labor pain, and dental pain, which have been overwhelmingly positive. The World Health Organization mentions acupuncture as a nonpharmacologic method to be used in the obstetric population, especially during labor, and emphasizes the necessity of clinical studies to further validate the role of acupuncture. Theoretically, acupuncture is an ideal adjunct for the obstetrics population because it poses a low risk to the mother and fetus and is relatively free of side effects.

The term *acupuncture* comes from the Latin words *acus* meaning needle and *punctura* meaning puncture. It is an ancient science dating back almost 5,000 years. It relies on the stimulation of well-demarcated points situated along set meridians. It is a concept of medicine, which in simple terms suggests that internal homeostasis depends on the unobstructed flow of *Qi* (chee) through these meridians.

A thorough understanding of surface anatomy is essential to the practice of acupuncture, which involves the placement of fine disposable stainless steel needles at select acupuncture points. There are 365 acupuncture points that lie along 14 meridians, which correspond to organ systems. Acupuncture

ⓒ 2006 Mayo Foundation for Medical Education and Research

needles are inserted at these points and stimulated by various techniques (similarly, acupressure involves holding pressure over the acupoint). These needles range from 1/4 in. to several inches in length and a few thousandths to several thousandths of an inch in diameter. One inch to 1.5 in. is the most commonly used length of needle. Longer needles are used in certain specialized therapies. After needle placement, manual twirling of the needle is performed to elicit a characteristic sensation called *De Qi*. Other methods used include electrical stimulation, laser, and moxibustion.

The mechanism of action of acupuncture is not completely understood, but it is hypothesized that it involves the rhythmic discharge of nerve fibers that can cause the release of endorphins and oxytocin. One popular theory explaining how acupuncture modulates pain is the neurohumoral hypothesis of acupuncture analgesia. The neurohumoral hypothesis, based on more than 100 scientific papers, states that the pain-relieving properties of acupuncture are partly mediated by a cascade of endorphins and monoamines that are activated by stimulating De Qi, a sensation of numbness and fullness. De Qi is associated with the stimulation of A-delta afferents, which set the cascade in motion. It is interesting that different manners of needle manipulation are known to produce different therapeutic effects.

Although the exact scientific mechanisms remain largely unknown, the analgesia produced by electroacupuncture of different frequencies may be mediated by different endogenous opioids. It is suggested that at low-frequency (2-Hz) electroacupuncture analgesia is mediated by enkephalin, whereas dynorphins play a role at high-frequency (100-Hz) electroacupuncture analgesia. Among the endorphins, enkephalin and beta-endorphin act at mu and delta receptors. The endomorphins act at the mu receptors alone. Dynorphins are purely kappa receptor agonists. Some studies have suggested that analgesia induced by 2-Hz electroacupuncture is mediated by the m receptor and that of 100-Hz electroacupuncture by k opioid receptors, and that this analgesia is reversible by naloxone. With 2-Hz stimulation electroacupuncture, the release of beta-endorphins into the peripheral blood improves pain, modulates stress, and coordinates contraction of the uterus caused by oxytocin. In animal studies, beta-endorphin levels have been observed to rise in the brain tissue of animals after both acupuncture and exercise. Acupuncture may also decrease sympathetic discharge by the inhibitory effects that the hypothalamic beta-endorphinergic system has on the vasomotor center.

Acupuncture-mediated analgesia is further modulated through neurohumoral pathways. The stimulation of the acupuncture point by needling selectively activates myelinated nerve fibers, and there is neuronal activation at the level of dorsal horn, nucleus raphe magnus in the brainstem, hypothalamus, and thalamus. Subsequently, there is inhibition of the small unmyelinated pain-carrying fibers. The endorphins also allow for a sense of well-being and relaxation.

In the obstetric population, acupuncture may be used effectively in the treatment of first-trimester nausea and vomiting or hyperemesis, carpal tunnel syndrome, headaches, migraine, backache, sciatica, and other chronic pain syndromes. Acupuncture has also been used to aid in the correction of malpresentation, induction of labor, and pain relief in labor. In the postpartum period, acupuncture has been used to treat postpartum depression and pain from breast engorgement. To date, the evidence about acupuncture for labor analgesia is quite encouraging, and the data available from scientific studies suggests that the analgesic effect is superior to placebo. However, the data are limited, and elegant studies are few.

BRIEF OVERVIEW OF THE COMMON ACUPUNCTURE POINTS USED IN OBSTETRICS

Nausea and Vomiting. Hyperemesis occurs in 1% to 2% of pregnancies. Acupressure or acupuncture done at P6 point has been shown to be efficacious in the treatment of nausea and vomiting. The P6 point/Neiguan point lies on the pericardial (P) meridian. It is located between the tendons of the flexor carpi radialis and the palmaris longus 2 cun (pronounced as "soon") proximal to the distal wrist crease. One cun is the interphalangeal distance on the third finger (*Fig. 113.2*).

Acupressure may be self-administered by using a finger to hold pressure over this point for 15 to 20 minutes. Acupressure is not as efficacious as acupuncture. With placement of the acupuncture needle at this point, the patient may report a sense of heaviness or warmth in the hand, which is called De Qi. If the patient reports continuous sharp pain, the position of the needle must be readjusted. A randomized blind crossover comparison of P6 acupuncture versus placebo showed a significant decrease in the resolution of nausea and decreased episodes of emesis.

Labor Analgesia. Although acupuncture may not be a complete analgesic, it may act to provide some analgesia and relaxation. One study comparing acupuncture with conventional care showed that women receiving acupuncture requested significantly fewer pain-relieving interventions than the women not receiving acupuncture. Among the women who received acupuncture, 86% said they would use it again for childbirth, although the results concerning the analgesic effects of acupuncture were not always successful. There were no differences in labor outcomes between the two groups, including the duration of labor, cesarean section rates, and measures of infant wellness.

Acupuncture during labor provides relaxation. It has been suggested that if the parturient is more relaxed, she is likely to have more control and consequently cope better with the pain. Some studies suggest decreased requirement for epidural analgesia in patients treated with acupuncture; however, other studies suggest that acupuncture did not decrease the need for additional analgesics during labor. Although many points are used, there are two classic points that may be beneficial in labor:

- **LI 4 (Hegu):** This point is located at the base of the anatomical snuff box—on the dorsum of the hand, between the first and second metacarpals, approximately in the middle of the second metacarpal bone on the radial side (*Fig. 160.1*). The needle is inserted to a depth of 0.5 cm.
- **SP 6:** This point is located on the spleen meridian and is an empirical point located 3 cun above the medial malleolus (*Fig. 160.2*). It is especially useful in difficult labor. It may also aid in cervical dilatation. It is needled with a perpendicular or oblique proximal insertion to a depth of 1 cm.

Another point that is quite useful is the DU 20 (Baihui). It is located at the top of the scalp equidistant from both pinnae (*Fig. 160.3*). It is needled with perpendicular insertion 0.5 to 1 cm using a 0.25-mm diameter needle. It allows for intense relaxation and mild sedation. It is never subjected to electroacupuncture stimulation.

For labor analgesia, LI 4 and SP 6 are stimulated bilaterally. Ideally, the treatment should be started at the beginning of the active phase in the first stage of labor. Fine 0.25-mm diameter stainless steel filiform needles

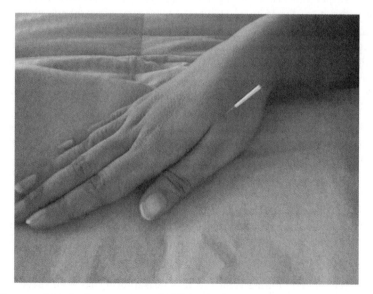

Figure 160.1. Acupuncture at the LI 4 point.

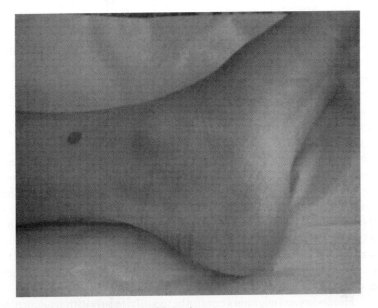

FIGURE 160.2. Marking of the SP 6 point.

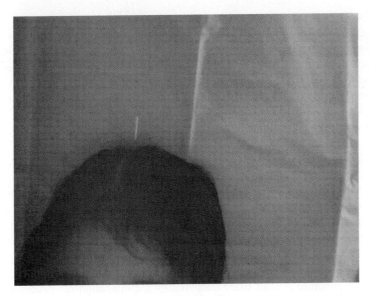

FIGURE 160.3. Acupuncture at the DU 20 point.

are inserted into the acupoints to a depth of 10 mm at LI 4 and 15 mm at SP 6. Once the patient reports a De Qi sensation, which is basically a sore and distending sensation, the needles are retained for 2 minutes. At this time, the free end of the needles can be connected to the electroacupuncture apparatus and stimulation set at a frequency of 2 to 100 Hz and electric current of 14 to 30 mA. Gradually, the stimulation strength can be increased. The needles can be removed after 15 to 30 minutes. This can be repeated as needed during the course of labor. It is recommended that when 7 to 8 cm of cervical dilatation is achieved, the procedure can be repeated.

Chronic Pain During Pregnancy. Acupuncture can also be used to relieve chronic pain syndromes such as low back and neck pain, carpal tunnel syndrome, headaches, migraines, and sciatica. Acupuncture decreases pain and has been shown to diminish disability in low back pain better than physiotherapy during pregnancy. The insertion of needles at points LI 4 and DU 20, along with other points as prescribed as per the patient's needs, is of benefit. For carpal tunnel syndrome, bilateral needles are placed in the SP 6 and LI 4 points, and either left in place or stimulated with low-frequency stimulation for 30 minutes.

Headaches and migraines can also be treated similarly with acupuncture treatment. Adequate acupuncture can avoid the risk of side effects, but more important reduced the intensity and frequency of muscle pain, the degree of headaches, and decreased tenderness over trigger points.

POSTPARTUM DEPRESSION

Comparison of the current randomized controlled trials suggests some evidence for the utility of acupuncture in depression. Acupuncture modalities were as effective as antidepressants employed for treatment of depression in the limited studies available for comparison. However, placebo acupuncture treatment was often no different from intended verum acupuncture. Efforts are now being made to standardize complementary approaches to treat depression, and further research is warranted.

TAKE HOME POINTS

- Acupuncture is an increasingly common therapeutic modality in Western medicine.
- The efficacy of acupuncture for the treatment of some disorders has not been clearly established; however, the results of randomized controlled trials for the treatment of obstetric patients have been overwhelmingly positive.
- Acupuncture is most likely mediated by a combination of endogenous opioids and neurohumoral pathways.

- In the obstetric population, acupuncture may be used effectively in the treatment of first-trimester nausea and vomiting or hyperemesis, carpal tunnel syndrome, headaches, migraine, backache, sciatica, and other chronic pain syndromes.

- Studies (to date) have not shown improvement in several key obstetric outcomes, but parturients overwhelmingly report that they would request it for a subsequent labor.

SUGGESTED READINGS

Brinkhaus B, Witt CM, Jena S, et al. Acupuncture in patients with chronic low back pain: a randomized controlled trial. *Arch Intern Med.* 2006;166:450–457.

Carlsson CP, Axemo P, Bodin A, et al. Manual acupuncture reduces hyperemesis gravidarum: a placebo-controlled, randomized, single-blind, crossover study. *J Pain Symptom Manage.* 2000;20(4):273–279.

He D, Veiersted KB, Hostmark AT, et al. Effect of acupuncture treatment on chronic neck and shoulder pain in sedentary female workers: a 6-month and 3-year follow-up study. *Pain.* 2004;109(3):299–307.

Lyrenäs S, Lutsch H, Hetta J, et al. Acupuncture before delivery: effect on pain perception and the need for analgesics. *Gynecol Obstet Invest.* 1990;29(2):118–124.

Nesheim BI, Kinge R, Berg B, et al. Acupuncture during labor can reduce the use of meperidine: a controlled clinical study. *Clin J Pain.* 2003;19(3):187–191.

161

ALWAYS BE PREPARED FOR EMERGENT DELIVERY AS A CONSEQUENCE OF EXTERNAL CEPHALIC VERSION

ANGELA M. PENNELL, MD

Breech presentation affects 3% to 4% of term pregnancies. Because a fetus is more likely to be safely delivered vaginally from the vertex position, external cephalic version is a technique used by obstetricians to change the presentation of the fetus from breech to vertex. The obstetrician is balancing the risks of the version (umbilical cord compression, and fetal and/or maternal hemorrhage leading to urgent or emergent delivery) against the risks of a potentially difficult breech vaginal delivery (leading to urgent or emergent delivery). The procedure is typically scheduled after 38 weeks' gestational to decrease the possibility of the fetus reverting back to a breech position and is sometimes performed with the adjunctive use of tocolytics.

Overall, external cephalic version is successful in 35% to 86% of nonlaboring, term parturients. Maternal and fetal factors that increase the chance of successful external cephalic version include that the patient is not obese, the cervix is not fully dilated, amniotic membranes are intact, the fetus is in a frank breech or transverse lie, there is normal amniotic fluid volume, the presenting part of the fetus has not entered the pelvis, and there is posterior positioning of the fetal back. Both obstetric and anesthesia staff also generally acknowledge that the success of external cephalic version may depend to a considerable degree on the skill and experience level of the obstetrician combined with the level of pain tolerated by the patient.

The question of whether the use of neuraxial anesthesia (spinal or epidural) facilitates successful external version and improves outcomes is an interesting and unanswered one. There is also the dilemma of what drug to use and how much to give. Most anesthesiologists tend to use "labor doses" for version, and because labor epidurals are quite routine in current anesthetic practice, the matter seems a simple one. When giving anesthesia for external version, however, for every pro there is a con. Patients are sometimes quite anxious about the procedure and fearful of the pain. Assuring the patient that she will have little, if any, pain, and then providing her with a painfree experience, can help the obstetrician perform the version with fewer maneuvers by providing a relaxed and reassured patient. However, removing pain as a limiting factor in the procedure may also *increase* the potential for a greater number of maneuvers and more aggressive attempts.

© 2006 Mayo Foundation for Medical Education and Research

This may in turn increase the potential for significant complications, such as placental abruption. This is equally true if the patient is unable to feel pain from a resulting abruption or uterine rupture *after* the trial of external version is complete. Also, the risks of neuraxial anesthesia, including hypotension, infection, paresthesias, bleeding/epidural hematoma, subdural puncture headache, and, most important, fetal distress, are incurred by the patient in addition to the risks of the version. If the attempted version does result in a call for urgent or emergent delivery, it is advantageous for the patient, anesthesiologist, and obstetrician to have the block already in place and working, unless, of course, it is determined that the block contributed significantly to the inability to monitor the maternal vital signs or to the fetal difficulties. It is incumbent on the anesthesia provider to document **before the version is attempted** that the block is stable and the mother and fetus are at baseline.

Currently, there is not a plethora of data available on the safety of neuraxial anesthesia for external version. There have been several trials and retrospective studies on the success rate of external cephalic version with adjuvant neuraxial techniques. According to a search of the Cochrane Pregnancy and Childbirth Group trials register, three randomized trials were analyzed with patients receiving spinal or epidural anesthesia versus no analgesia. In summary, two of the trials revealed a decrease in external cephalic version failure, noncephalic births, and cesarean section, with one trial showing no benefit. However, the differences among the conflicting trials were not statistically significant. The retrospective reviews of neuraxial anesthesia for external cephalic version have shown overall success but suggest further studies to evaluate maternal and fetal safety related to its use. Finally, the American College of Obstetricians and Gynecologists indicates that there is not enough consistent evidence to recommend either spinal or epidural anesthesia for external cephalic version.

Of course, any anesthesia professional providing neuraxial anesthesia for external cephalic version must be prepared for emergent cesarean section (it is wise to be prepared for a call for emergent delivery even if the anesthesia team has *not* provided a block for the procedure). Prior preparations in the operating room should include a recent anesthesia machine check; intravenous fluids; emergency syringes of succinylcholine, atropine, lidocaine, epinephrine, ephedrine, and/or phenylephrine; uterotonics, including oxytocin and methergine; spinal anesthesia kits; and intubating equipment. For a patient who has an existing epidural, use a bolus of 15 to 20 mL of 3% chloroprocaine or 15 to 20 mL of 2% lidocaine with 1:200,000 epinephrine plus or minus fentanyl. An urgent cesarean section or a poor candidate for general anesthesia may permit time for the placement of spinal anesthesia using 12 mg of 0.75% bupivacaine. An emergent surgical intervention or failure of neuraxial analgesia will require general anesthesia with a rapid sequence induction using thiopental 3 to 4 mg/kg or ketamine 0.5 to 1 mg/kg plus succinylcholine 1 to 1.5 mg/kg to facilitate intubation. Maintenance of anesthesia can be accomplished with 50% nitrous oxide plus 0.75 MAC volatile anesthetic prior to umbilical cord clamping and 70% nitrous oxide plus <0.50 MAC volatile anesthetic post cord clamping with the addition of morphine or midazolam as indicated.

TAKE HOME POINTS

- External cephalic version is typically performed in near term patients and has a highly variable success rate.
- Be aware when a version is imminent or underway on the labor unit—this is not a good time to go down to the lobby to pick up the food.
- Many factors influence the success of the attempted version, including skill of the obstetrician.
- There are significant pros and cons to providing analgesia for the version—anxiety and pain may hinder the version but also act as a harbinger of impending trouble.
- Anesthesia providers will typically place peripheral access, even if no analgesia is requested.

SUGGESTED READINGS

American College of Obstetricians and Gynecologists (ACOG). *External Cephalic Version.* ACOG Practice Bulletin No. 13. *Obstetrics & Gynecology.* 2000;95(2):1–7.

Birnbach DJ, Matut J, Stein DJ, et al. The effect of intrathecal analgesia on the success of external cephalic version. *Anesth Analg.* 2001;93:410–413.

Carlan SJ, Dent JM, Huckaby T, Whittington EC, Shaefer D. The effect of epidural anesthesia on safety and success of external cephalic version at term. *Anesth Anal.* 1994;79(3):525–528.

Cherayil G, Feinberg B, Robinson J, et al. Central neuraxial blockade promotes external cephalic version success after a failed attempt. *Anesth Analg.* 2002;94:1589.

Chestnut D. *Obstetric Anesthesia: Principles and Practice.* 3rd ed. Philadelphia, PA: Mosby; 2004:634–636.

Dugoff L, Stamm CA, Jones OW III, et al. The effect of spinal anesthesia on the success rate of external cephalic version: a randomized trial. *Obstet Gynecol.* 1991;93:345–349.

Hofmeyr GJ. Interventions to help external cephalic version for breech presentation at term. *Cochrane Database Syst Rev.* 2004;(1):CD 000184.

Macarthur AJ, Gagnon S, Tureanu LM, Downey KN. Anesthesia facilitation of external cephalic version: a meta-analysis. *Am J Obstet Gynecol.* 2004;191(4):1219–1224.

Neiger R, Hennessy MD, Patel M. Reattempting failed external cephalic version under epidural anesthesia. *Am J Obstet Gynecol.* 1998;179(5):1136–1139.

Schorr SJ, Speights SE, Ross EL, et al. A randomized trial of epidural anesthesia to improve external cephalic version success. *Am J Obstet Gynecol.* 1997;177:1133–1137.

162

OBSTETRIC ANESTHESIA/ANALGESIA *CAN* WORK IN A SMALL HOSPITAL: THE KEY PRINCIPLES ARE COMMITMENT, FLEXIBILITY, AND PLANNING

JAMES S. HICKS, MD, MM

The ability to offer obstetric (OB) conduction anesthesia to laboring patients in a small hospital where 24-hour in-house anesthesia coverage is not available or feasible is both a challenge and an opportunity to provide excellent service both to patients and obstetric colleagues. To be successful, interposing obstetric conduction anesthesia services within a surgical schedule and managing the same service after usual operating room hours require careful planning, interdisciplinary cooperation, and ongoing continuous quality improvement.

Among the challenges that must be addressed to provide satisfactory small hospital OB services are the following:

- Recognize and minimize the potential delay in the elective surgical schedule required to perform epidurals
- Recognize and minimize the delay in responding to requests for epidural anesthesia due to the unavailability or on-call status of the anesthesia provider
- Manage the potential inability to provide timely emergency cesarean section anesthesia
- Recognize the need for obstetric nurses to assist with management of epidural infusions and provide them with appropriate education and experience
- Meet regulatory requirements

Surmounting these obstacles requires a commitment on the part of the anesthesiology service that obstetric anesthesia is no less of a priority than surgical anesthesia. This does not imply that obstetric anesthesia will take priority on the surgical schedule, but simply that the efforts to meet the needs of obstetric patients are genuine, compassionate, and equivalent to our efforts to provide excellent surgical anesthesia.

Successful rural OB service is achievable. The American Society of Anesthesiologists' (ASA) Consultation Program has provided hospitals with the expertise of board-certified anesthesiologists who are specially trained in assessing anesthesia practices and in providing recommendations for

---

ⓒ 2006 Mayo Foundation for Medical Education and Research

improvement. The program also provides ASA with a multiple-exposure snapshot of many anesthesia practices, many of which involve rural anesthesia coverage. The following recommendations are the result of experiences drawn from observations gained from this program throughout the United States:

1) Convene a "council of stakeholders" composed of anesthesia providers, obstetricians (and, if applicable, family practitioner and certified nurse-midwife obstetric providers), surgeons, emergency physicians, obstetric nurses, pharmacy, and hospital administration. Obtain consensus from this group that labor epidural analgesia for all patients desiring such is a worthwhile and desirable goal. To gain this consensus, council members must acknowledge that the needs of the patients may require customization of policies that would, if otherwise applied, preclude the ability to have labor analgesia coverage. For example, pharmacists need to acknowledge the need to maintain adequate supplies of premixed epidural solutions, even if this results in occasional outdates of solutions. Obstetric nurses must be willing to titrate epidural anesthesia infusions (given clear parameters and orders) in the face of a national organization's recommendations to the contrary. Surgeons must acknowledge the occasional delay between cases for the anesthesia provider to place an epidural catheter. None of these roadblocks has proven to be an obstruction to the small hospital and anesthesia service that are determined to offer comprehensive OB anesthesia, however.

2) Meet as an anesthesia service and adopt standardized processes for epidural and cesarean section techniques and procedures so anesthesia providers can easily manage blocks, surgical anesthetics, and postoperative patients of colleagues. Ideally, this should include standardization of
   - Labor epidural agent mixture
   - Order sheet, anesthesia record (if different from the surgical record), billing forms and practices
   - Cesarean section techniques and preferences (opioid mixtures and local anesthetic mixtures for both elective cesarean section spinals and labor epidurals used for cesarean section)

3) Perform a task analysis of all tasks necessary to accomplish a labor epidural (e.g., examining the chart; taking history and performing physical examination; obtaining pump, infusion bag, gloves, epidural tray and anesthesia cart, placing, test dosing, and securing catheter and beginning infusion).

4) Prepare an educational course for obstetric nursing staff that can be recorded for future additions to the staff. This should include anatomy, physiology, pharmacology, and practical work with the technique of epidural placement, dosage management, and management of known complications. Request that nursing staff complete all possible steps in

the task analysis (step 3) that can be safely accomplished by them prior to your arrival. This step is vital to your ability to place an epidural quickly during a break in a busy surgical schedule.

5) Certify the competence of nurses successfully completing the labor analgesic course after observing them manage a given number of epidurals. (This will give them increased assurance in managing epidural infusions in the face of contradictory information from national organization recommendations.)

6) Inform surgical colleagues of your intent to provide labor epidural services with the minimal interruption of the surgical schedule and request their cooperation.

7) Plan in advance for labor epidurals whenever possible. This means contacting the labor floor early in the morning for patients who will likely need an epidural during the morning, as well as inserting and testing a catheter before the beginning of the surgical schedule. As soon as the patient then requires pain relief, the infusion may begin without a bolus dose at the usual rate. This results in an effective dose being achieved in approximately the same time frame as would have occurred had the usual sequence of notify-attend-insert-test-bolus taken place.

8) An anesthesia provider's rest *is* important when he or she is on call for the operating room and/or is expected to provide anesthesia the following day, as is often the case at smaller hospitals. By maintaining frequent communication with obstetric nursing staff, checking the labor floor before departing for the day or after an on-call surgical case, and encouraging nurses to call sooner rather than later for patients who require epidurals, return trips to the hospital or loss of sleep can be minimized.

9) Obtain assurance from emergency department physicians that they will respond to the extremely rare instance of adverse reaction to an established epidural analgesic, and educate them on the possible complications. The use of a test dose coupled with an extremely low local anesthetic concentration (the author's department uses 0.055% bupivacaine with 1 mcg of sufentanil and 1.7 mcg of epinephrine per mL) make the possibility of such complications almost nonexistent.

One final note: The question is often asked, "Do I have to remain in the hospital during the entire course of a labor epidural?" According to ASA, the answer appears in the introduction to the *Guidelines for Regional Anesthesia in Obstetrics*: "Because the availability of anesthesia resources may vary, members are responsible for interpreting and establishing the guidelines for their own institutions and practices. . . ." Thus, ASA acknowledges that local convention based on capability and personnel are determining factors in obstetric anesthesia services and allows hospitals to meet their standards in ways that are best for patients.

- The first step in providing OB services in a small or rural hospital is recognizing the challenges.
- There must be commitment to the idea that obstetric analgesia/anesthesia is no less important than surgical anesthesia.
- The consensus must be across a wide range of medical and administrative staff.
- Standardization of anesthetic techniques for labor epidurals and cesarean sections is of paramount importance.
- Labor nurses must willingly accept training in certain aspects of the setup and management of labor epidurals.
- Complications due to labor epidurals can be minimized by standardized, careful test dosing of catheters and very low-dose epidural infusions.

SUGGESTED READINGS

American Society of Anesthesiologists Optimal Goals for Anesthesia Care in Obstetrics; Approved by ASA House of Delegates October 28, 2000; American Society of Anesthesiology, Park Ridge, IL, 2000.

Practice Guidelines for Obstetrical Anesthesia: A Report by the American Society of Anesthesiologists Task Force on Obstetrical Anesthesia; Anesthesiology 1999;90:600–611.

American Society of Anesthesiologists Guidelines for Regional Anesthesia in Obstetrics; Approved by ASA House of Delegates October, 2000; American Society of Anesthesiologists, Park Ridge, IL, 2000.

Manual for Anesthesiology Department Organization and Management, American Society of Anesthesiologists, American Society of Anesthesiologists, Park Ridge, IL, 2005.

163

REMEMBER THAT ANESTHESIA FOR THE PREGNANT PATIENT HAVING NONOBSTETRIC SURGERY IS NOT LIMITED TO ANY PARTICULAR AGENTS OR TECHNIQUES

L. MICHELE NOLES, MD

The primary goals in the anesthetic management of patients undergoing nonobstetric surgery during pregnancy (NOSP) are to ensure maternal safety, avoid intrauterine fetal hypoxia and acidosis, know the implications of fetal exposure to anesthetic agents, and avoid preterm labor (PTL). Also, it is fairly common for these patients to experience severe anxiety over possible injurious effects to their pregnancies from both anesthesia and surgery—the anesthesia provider must maintain a working knowledge of the pertinent issues and be able to maintain a calm and reassuring demeanor.

NOSP is fairly common, involving approximately 75,000 patients per year or 1% to 2% of pregnant women, and has specific implications for anesthetic management based on the physiologic changes in the pregnant woman and the presence of a live fetus. The most common nonobstetric surgeries performed on pregnant women include appendectomy, cholecystectomy or biliary tract procedures, breast surgeries, ovarian surgeries, procedures related to carrying a pregnancy to term (i.e., cervical cerclage), and the range of trauma-related procedures. Emergent surgical procedures should proceed as the mother's medical condition warrants. Elective surgery should be postponed until 6 weeks postpartum when the physiological changes of pregnancy have resolved and fetal exposure can be avoided. It is advantageous to proceed with necessary surgery during the second trimester if possible, when organogenesis has been completed and the higher myometrial irritability of the third trimester has not yet begun. The American College of Obstetricians and Gynecologists (ACOG) recommends an obstetrics consultation prior to surgery on any pregnant patient undergoing nonobstetric surgery.

ANESTHETIC IMPLICATIONS OF MATERNAL PHYSIOLOGICAL CHANGES DURING PREGNANCY

Pregnant women have a decreased respiratory reserve due to their increased oxygen consumption (15% to 20%) coupled with decreased functional residual capacity (15% to 20%). Thus, they develop hypoxemia and hypercapnia more rapidly than a nonpregnant patient during hypoventilation or apnea. Due to laryngeal edema, engorged and friable oronasopharyngeal

© 2006 Mayo Foundation for Medical Education and Research

mucosa, weight gain affecting the tissues of the neck, and increased breast size, they also have an increased likelihood of difficult airway management and intubation.

Pregnant women are at increased risk of regurgitation of gastric contents and aspiration pneumonitis due to impaired lower esophageal sphincter tone. Both hormonal and mechanical factors contribute as the pregnancy progresses. There are conflicting data regarding whether pregnant women have slower gastric emptying, increased gastric volume, and/or decreased pH of gastric contents. However, a pregnant patient should be considered at significant risk for aspiration after 18 weeks' gestation or earlier if symptoms of gastroesophageal reflux exist.

An airway plan for a pregnant patient should include aspiration prophylaxis premedication with at least a nonparticulate antacid (Bicitra); addition of an H_2 blocker and/or metoclopramide is at the anesthesiologist's discretion. Use supplemental oxygen during sedation, and for general anesthetics, plan a full 5-minute preoxygenation, a classic rapid sequence induction, and oral intubation with an endotracheal tube that is one size smaller than usual. If difficult intubation is anticipated, opt for awake oral fiber-optic intubation.

During pregnancy, cardiovascular changes include an increased cardiac output, dilutional anemia, decreased vascular responsiveness, an increased risk of thromboembolism, and, after 20 weeks' gestation, a risk of aortocaval compression by the gravid uterus leading to supine hypotension syndrome. Even normal physiological compensation for aortocaval compression can be blunted by general and regional anesthetics that interfere with sympathetic nervous system responses to hypotension. The result is a profound decrease in venous return and cardiac output, leading to impressive maternal hypotension and significantly decreased placental perfusion. Uterine blood vessels are maximally dilated at term, leaving no reserve for vascular autoregulation with perfusion pressure changes. Positioning with left uterine displacement by placing a wedge under the right hip, adequate hydration, and judicious use of pressors can help maintain maternal normotension. Ephedrine has long been the initial pharmacologic agent of choice in hypotensive pregnant women. To minimize risk of thromboembolism, thromboprophylaxis including preinduction placement and activation of pneumatic compression stockings is recommended.

The central nervous system changes in the pregnant patient include a 30% decrease in MAC of volatile anesthetics even in early pregnancy. An engorged epidural venous plexus leads to a one-third decrease in the local anesthetic volume needed for neuraxial anesthetics and an increased risk of inadvertent intravascular injection.

OPTIMIZATION OF THE FETAL ENVIRONMENT

Optimization of the fetal environment follows from preserving uterine blood flow and fetal oxygen delivery, which are directly dependent on maintaining maternal oxygenation, normocapnia, and normotension. Maternal hyperventilation and overly aggressive positive-pressure ventilation lead to uterine artery constriction and decreased venous return, respectively, thereby causing decreased uterine blood flow. Faced with hypoxia, the fetus is unable to significantly increase its oxygen extraction because it is already near maximum.

The extent of fetal and uterine activity monitoring should be decided on with a consultant obstetrician. Personnel trained in the interpretation of fetal heart rate (FHR), and uterine activity tracings should be involved perioperatively. In general, fetal monitoring in pregnancies less than 24 weeks should include, at minimum, documentation of presence of FHR pre- and postoperatively with or without uterine activity monitoring. After 24 weeks, continuous perioperative FHR and uterine activity monitoring is ideal. Loss of beat-to-beat variability under general anesthesia is typical, but persistent fetal bradycardia is almost always an indication of fetal distress. The anesthesiologist may benefit from this indirect measure of fetal well-being to respond with changes in maternal oxygenation, blood pressure, fluid load, positioning, and/or recommendations for altering the placement of surgical retraction instruments.

TERATOGENICITY AND IMPLICATIONS OF FETAL EXPOSURE TO ANESTHETIC AGENTS

Although maternal hypoxia, hypotension and acidosis pose a greater risk to the fetus, considerable concern exists regarding the potential harmful effects of anesthetic agents on the fetus. There is wide consensus that no anesthetic agent in common use, including induction agents, volatile agents, anxiolytics, muscle relaxants, or opioids, appears to be teratogenic or safer than other agents. The known association between NOSP and an increased risk of fetal loss, growth restriction, and an increased frequency of low-birth-weight neonates is generally attributable to the patient's underlying medical condition, site of surgery, or surgical procedure. No drug or anesthetic technique has been shown to impact the onset of preterm labor (PTL). Some anesthesiologists prefer to use "tried and true" drugs such as morphine because patients may be somewhat reassured by the fact that a drug has been used with hundreds of thousands of pregnant women over a period of decades without incremental ill effect.

Numerous studies have failed to show the association once believed to exist between benzodiazepines, specifically diazepam, and cleft lip and palate abnormalities. Nitrous oxide (N_2O) is known to interfere with methionine synthase activity and DNA synthesis. These known cellular effects have not been shown to lead to adverse effects in human pregnancy. However, a cautious approach advocated by some experts in the field includes limiting N_2O to 50% or less and limiting its use in lengthy operations. Volatile agents may provide a margin of safety from the point of view of protection from PTL due to their depressant effect on myometrial contractility.

Neuromuscular blocking agents do not cross the placenta in clinically significant amounts and thus fetal exposure is minimal. Maternal plasma cholinesterase concentration is decreased; however, the impact on succinylcholine use is usually clinically negligible.

REGIONAL ANESTHETIC TECHNIQUES

Many anesthesiologists prefer to use regional techniques whenever possible during NOSP. Although evidence is lacking to support that this approach is safer for the mother and baby, there certainly is strong theoretical reasoning to support this, particularly for extremity surgeries for which regional techniques such as subarachnoid blocks, epidural blocks, and peripheral nerve blocks can provide complete surgical anesthesia. It is important to remember that pregnant patients are more sensitive to local anesthetics, so techniques should be employed that reduce the total volume of local anesthetic solution required for anesthesia. In our practice, we use spinal and epidural anesthesia in lower extremity surgery, and brachial plexus blocks in upper extremity surgery, in pregnant patients agreeable to regional anesthesia. We also consider the use of the Bier block when appropriate. Although there are no published studies on peripheral nerve blocks in pregnant patients, we find that reducing the local anesthetic concentration by 20% to 30% while maintaining the same volume as a nonpregnant patient works to give effective anesthesia and reduces local anesthetic toxicity. Similarly, we reduce the amount of local anesthetic used for spinal anesthesia—7.5 mg of hyperbaric bupivacaine generally provides an adequate level for lower extremity surgery.

LAPAROSCOPIC SURGERY

Laparoscopic surgery has become an acceptable safe alternative to open procedures in the pregnant patient. The physiological changes of pneumoperitoneum are magnified in the pregnant patient, thus pneumoperitoneum pressures should be minimized (8–12 mm Hg) not to exceed 15 mm Hg. Fetal $paCO_2$ correlates directly with maternal $paCO_2$ such that maternal hypercapnia results in fetal acidosis and potential myocardial depression and hypotension. The resultant need for hyperventilation and increased ventilatory pressures can lead to decreased venous return, cardiac output, and ureteroplacental perfusion.

TAKE HOME POINTS

- Nonobstetric surgery for the pregnant patient is actually fairly common.
- Obtain an obstetrics consult before initiating the anesthetic if clinical urgency permits; if not, obtain it as soon as the mother's condition permits.
- Remember that the status of the fetus is optimized by optimizing the status of the mother—this may involve a light sedative to control hyperventilation in an anxious patient having elective surgery all the way to an arterial blood gas to direct resuscitation if the mother has sustained trauma.
- Be especially careful and conservative with airway management!
- Remember that fetal outcome depends much more on the condition of the mother and the nature of the surgical case than the type of anesthesia or the specific anesthetic agents.

SUGGESTED READINGS

ACOG Committee Opinion Number 284, Committee on Obstetric Practice, August 2003: nonobstetric surgery in pregnancy. *Obstet Gynecol.* 2003;102(2):431.

Cohen SE. Nonobstetric surgery during pregnancy. In: Chestnut DH, ed. *Obstetric Anesthesia: Principles and Practice.* 2nd ed. St. Louis, Mo.: Mosby–Year Book; 1999:279–298.

Hawkins J. Anesthesia in the pregnant patient undergoing nonobstetric surgery. *ASA Annual Meeting Refresher Course Lectures.* 2004;302:1–4.

Hong J, Park JW, Oh JI. Comparison of preoperative gastric contents and serum gastrin concentrations in pregnant and nonpregnant women. *J Clin Anesth.* 2005;17(6):451–455.

Melnick DM, Wahl WL, Dalton VK. Management of general surgical problems in the pregnant patient. *Am J Surg.* 2004;187(2):170–180.

Rosen MA. Management of anesthesia for the pregnant surgical patient. *Anesthesiology.* 1999;91(4):1159.

164

DO NOT GUESS AT THE EQUIVALENT DOSE WHEN DETERMINING AN OPIOID CONVERSION

AMIT SHARMA, MD

Opioids are robust analgesic medications that have played a core role in the management of acute and chronic pain for decades. The term *opioid* is used for drugs that are derived from the opium plant *Papaver somniferum*. The term *narcotic* is derived from the Greek word "narcosis" (meaning stupor), which, in legal context, includes opium derivatives, their semisynthetic substitutes, and certain stimulants such as cocaine. Thus, all opioid medications are narcotics, but all narcotics are not opioids. Anesthesiologists constantly deal with opioid management for their patients in the perioperative setting. This frequently involves changing one opioid to another or changing the delivery route of a given opioid. The complex pharmacology of these drugs, coupled with significant interpersonal variation seen clinically with these medications, often makes this job cumbersome. Mastering the art of these challenging conversions requires understanding some of the basic pharmacology of these drugs.

Opioid medications are delivered by all possible routes: topical, transdermal, transmucosal, oral, rectal, and parenteral (subcutaneous, intramuscular, or intravenous [IV]). They bind to *Mu, Delta,* and *Kappa* types of opioid receptors in central and peripheral nervous system to cause analgesia or certain untoward side effects. Based on their affinity to *Mu*-receptors, there is a considerable divergence among these medications. Fentanyl, for instance, is almost 15 times as potent as hydrocodone, which in turn is 4 to 5 times stronger than morphine for its analgesic properties. Moreover, there is a significant degree of interpersonal variability for any given opioid, depending on the type of pain, psychological factors, therapeutic drug interactions with other medications, age (elderly are considered to be more sensitive), certain pathophysiological states (increased sensitivity with central nervous system comorbidity), hepatic and renal dysfunction, and even genetic variations. Thus, 2 to 4 mg of IV morphine may not provide adequate pain control in a young patient after shoulder arthroscopy but may produce sedation and respiratory depression in an elderly man with arthritis pain. A brief outline of pharmacokinetic properties of commonly used opioids is given in *Table 164.1.*

To resolve some of these complex issues, Houde et al. and Bruera et al. performed single-dose relative potency studies on opioid medications. Based

© 2006 Mayo Foundation for Medical Education and Research

TABLE 164.1	OPIOID ANALGESIC GUIDE				
	ORAL (MG)	PARENTERAL (MG)	DURATION (H)	PEAK EFFECT (H)	$T_{1/2}$ (H)
MSO4	30	10	3–6 (O) 3–4 (P)	1–2 (O) 0.5–1 (P)	1.5–2
Hydromorphone	7.5	1.5	3–6 (O) 3–4 (P)	1–2 (O) 0.5–1 (P)	2–3
Sustained release oxycodone	20	—	8–12	3–4	4–6
Oxycodone	30	—	3–6	1–2	2–3
Hydrocodone	30	—	4–8	1–2	3.5–4.5
Methadone	10[a] 2–4[b]	5[a] 2–4[b]	4–6	1–2	15–30
Levorphanol	4[a] 1[b]	2[a] 1[b]	6–8	1–2 (O) 0.5–1 (P)	12–16
Fentanyl	—	0.1	1–2	<10 min	1.5–6
Oxymorphone	15	1	4–6 (O) 3–4 (P)	1.5–3 (O) 0.5–1 (P)	NA
Codeine	200	130	4–6		3
Meperidine	300	75	2–4		3–4

$T_{1/2}$, elimination half-life; O, oral; P, parenteral; NA, not applicable.
[a] For acute pain management purposes.
[b] For chronic pain management purposes.

on these relevant studies, an equianalgesic dose table (*Table 164.2*) has subsequently been formulated that describes relative potencies between these diverse opioids for both oral and parenteral routes of administration. The term *equianalgesic* is used for two doses with comparable pharmacologic analgesic effects, either of different drugs or of the same drug but with different routes of delivery. Thus, the first two columns of *Table 164.2* list the oral and parenteral doses of opioids that are equivalent to 10 mg of parenteral morphine. These values essentially account for pharmacodynamic and pharmacokinetic differences among these drugs. *Table 164.2* is a stepping stone in solving complicated issues related to opioid management.

OPIOID CONVERSIONS IN PERIOPERATIVE SETTING

Opioids are the analgesic agents of choice in intra- and postoperative setting. Patients are often given these drugs via IV route using a microprocessor-controlled infusion pump (patient-controlled analgesia or PCA). The patient can activate a button (demand) to deliver a specified amount of drug (demand dose) into their IV line. Once the microprocessor is activated, it is programmed to go into dormant (or sleep) mode for a specified time during which no further demand doses are delivered (lockout interval). Physicians can also program a maximum 1-hour cumulative dose that serves as an

TABLE 164.2 PHARMACOKINETICS OF COMMONLY USED OPIOIDS

MEDICATION	ABSORPTION	DISTRIBUTION	METABOLISM	ELIMINATION
Morphine	40% GI tract[a] T_{max} = 30 min	25%–30% reversibly PPB	Liver: <5% demethylation >95% glucuronidation to M3G 50% (inactive) and M6G 15% (active but does not cross BBB)	Renal—Mainly as M3G/M6G and 10% unchanged Feces—7%–10% $T_{1/2}$ = varies
Hydromorphone	24% GI tract[a] T_{max} = 30–60 min	8%–19% PPB	Liver: Glucuronidation >95% to H3G <5% to 6-hydroxy reduced metabolites	Renal—Mostly as inactive metabolites $T_{1/2}$ = 2.6 h
Oxycodone	60%–87% GI tract[a] T_{max} = 1.6–3.2 h[b]	45% PPB	Liver: Noroxycodone (weak analgesic) Oxymorphone (analgesic) via CYP450 2D6	Renal: 50% Conjugated oxycodone 19% Free oxycodone 14% Conjugated oxymorphone $T_{1/2}$ = 3.2–4.5 h[b]
Fentanyl transmucosal	25% buccal mucosa (rapid) 25% GI tract[a] T_{max} = 20–40 min	Highly lipophilic PPB = 80%–85% α-1 AG> Alb> Lipo	Liver and intestinal mucosa by CYP450 3A4 isoform to norfentanyl (inactive)	Renal (>90% inactive metabolites, 7% unchanged) Feces (1% unchanged) $T_{1/2}$ = 40–50 min
Fentanyl transdermal	92% skin 13%–21% unbound fraction in plasma are finally achieved T_{max} = 12–24 h	Highly lipophilic PPB = 80%–85% α-1 AG> Alb> Lipo	Liver CYP450 3A4 isoform to norfentanyl (inactive) by oxidative N-dealkylation	Renal (75% inactive metabolites, <10% unchanged) Feces (9% metabolites) $T_{1/2}$ = 17 h (13–22)
Methadone	Excellent GI absorption T_{max} = 2–3 h	PPB = major site: alpha 1-acid glycoprotein	Liver CYP3A4	Renal and feces pH-dependent urinary excretion $T_{1/2}$ = 8–59 h

T_{max}, peak plasma concentration time; PPB, plasma protein bound; M3G, morphine-3-glucuronide; M6G, morphine-6-glucuronide; BBB, blood–brain barrier; $T_{1/2}$, plasma half-life; H3G, hydromorphone-3-glucuronide; α-1 AG, α-1 acid glycoproten; Alb, albumin; Lipo, lipoprotein.
[a]Drug that escapes hepatic and first-pass elimination.
[b]Depending on type of preparation, such as immediate release, or sustained or controlled release.
Modified from Sharma A, Raja SN. Assessment and management of chronic pain and palliative care. In: Sieber FE, ed. *Geriatric Anesthesia.* The McGraw-Hill Companies, Inc. 2007;319–336.

TABLE 164.3 INTRAVENOUS OPIOID PATIENT-CONTROLLED ANALGESIA GUIDELINES FOR OPIOID-NAIVE ADULTS WITH ACUTE PAIN

DRUG (USUAL STANDARD CONCENTRATIONS)	USUAL STARTING DEMAND DOSE	USUAL DOSE RANGE	USUAL STARTING LOCKOUT (MIN)	USUAL LOCKOUT RANGE (MIN)
Morphine (1.0 mg/mL)	1.0 mg	0.5–2.5 mg	10	6–10
Hydromorphone (0.2 mg/dL)	0.2 mg	0.05–0.4 mg	10	6–10
Fentanyl (10 mcg/mL)	10 μg	10–50 μg	6	6–8

From American Pain Society. *Principles of Analgesic Use in the Treatment of Acute Pain and Cancer Pain.* 5th ed. Glenview, Ill.: American Pain Society; 2003;20.

additional line of safety. Standard PCA guidelines for opioid-naive patients are described in *Table 164.3*. Furthermore, a continuous infusion mode can be added to this program to deliver a specified dose on a baseline (basal infusion). Although basal infusion is avoided in opioid-naive patients, they are often a helpful tool in managing acute-on-chronic or cancer-related pain issues.

Opioid conversions in perioperative setting are required in many different scenarios. Some of the patients undergoing surgical procedures are already on opioid medications for their pain management. These medications need to be taken into consideration when planning for postoperative PCA pain regimen. Similarly, PCA can be used in any setting where oral pain management becomes impossible. Prior to calculating the new dose of any alternate opioid, it is recommended to note the average 12- to 24-hour usage of current opioid medications. Subsequently, the equianalgesic conversion can be done by using the following formula:

Dose of alternate opioid drug or route in a given period

$$= \frac{\text{Dose of current opioid drug (s)}}{\text{EAN of current opioid drug (s)}}$$

$$\times \text{EAN of alternate opioid drug or route}$$

where EAN is the equianalgesic number of an opioid given by a specific route (*Table 164.2*). For instance, a patient who takes 30 mg of long-acting morphine preparation twice a day along with three to four tablets of short-acting morphine for his or her chronic back pain takes approximately 180 mg of oral morphine. For any PCA orders to be written in this situation requires correction for this additional morphine. Calculation of equianalgesic dose (EAD) for IV morphine can be done as

$$24\text{-hour dose of IV morphine} = \frac{180}{30} \times 10$$

$$= 60 \text{ mg or 2.5 mg of morphine per hour } (60/24)$$

Thus, 2.5 mg of IV morphine per hour is added to the PCA orders. An increase in the total dose by 25% to 50% is recommended for treating moderate to severe pain in patients who are on opioid therapy for longer than 5 days. Subsequent changes in PCA orders should only be made after five half-life ($T_{1/2}$) periods. Thus, treatment of postoperative pain following a spine surgery in the previously mentioned patient would require approximately 3 to 3.75 mg of IV morphine per hour. Half of this dose can be safely administered as basal infusion, with the remaining provided as demand doses with suitable lockout interval. Only 10% to 20% increment is recommended for an opioid-naive patient (therapy less than 5 days) under analogous circumstances.

Following repeated usage, the rotation of one *Mu*-opioid receptor agonist to another often results in evidence of pharmacologic supersensitivity toward the new agent, a concept known as *incomplete cross-tolerance*. Thus, conversion of one opioid to another requires a reduction in the total dose of new opiate by 25% to 50% to compensate for incomplete cross-tolerance and to avoid overdose. For example, if the aforementioned patient was on 20 mg of sustained-released oxycodone and five to six doses of 10 mg of short-acting oxycodone for breakthrough pain, the EAD calculations would suggest changing it to roughly 40 mg of IV morphine. In practice, though, this dose of morphine is likely to cause overdose or side effects in this particular patient. If pain had been adequately controlled on previous regimen, then this dose should be reduced by 25% to 50% (0.8- to 1.2 mg of IV morphine per hour). Again, half of this dose can be given as basal infusion and the remainder as demand doses. It is important to understand that due to significant interpersonal variations, a "one size fits all" technique would lead to both physician and patient dissatisfaction. After a therapy is initiated, regular pain assessments should be made, and treatment should be titrated accordingly.

$$24\text{-hour dose of IV morphine} = \left\{ \frac{40}{20} + \frac{60}{30} \right\} \times 10$$

$$= 40 \text{ mg}/24 \text{ hours or 1.67 mg of morphine per hour}$$

Conversion of transdermal fentanyl to other opioid drugs is slightly intricate. Rather than using the EAD formula, it is probably safer and easier to

TABLE 164.4	**RECOMMENDED IINITIAL TRANSDERMAL FENTANYL DOSE BASED ON DAILY ORAL MORPHINE DOSE**
ORAL 24-H MORPHINE DOSE (MG/D)	**TRANSDERMAL FENTANYL DOSE (μG/H)**
60–134	25
135–224	50
225–314	75
315–404	100
405–494	125
495–584	150
585–674	175
675–764	200
765–854	225
855–944	250
945–1034	275
1035–1124	300

use a separate transdermal fentanyl table as recommended by the manufacturer (*Table 164.4*). For example, a patient receiving 50 μg/hour of transdermal fentanyl corresponds to 135 to 224 mg of oral morphine (mean = 180 mg). This range can now be used to convert to any other opioid drug or route using the standard method, as previously described. A conservative estimate would mean that it is equivalent to the lower end of this range and vice versa. In our practice, we often accept the mean of this range (180 mg in this case) and adjust the dose further based on the patient's response. In short, to accommodate 50 μg/hour of transdermal fentanyl into IV morphine PCA, we need to add 60 mg morphine/24 hours.

$$24\text{-hour dose of IV morphine} = \frac{180}{30} \times 10$$

$$= 60 \text{ mg or } 2.5 \text{ mg of morphine per hour } (60/24)$$

OPIOID CONVERSIONS FROM INTRAVENOUS TO ORAL FORM

Conversion of parenteral opioids to oral formulation is based on similar principles but may pose certain unique problems. Often, these calculations are requested by the surgical team at the time of the patient's discharge. Any overestimation with these calculations may impose unwanted side effects on the patient. It is essential to teach the surgical teams in your hospital that these steps should be taken at least 24 to 48 hours prior to the patient's discharge, which is usually a sufficient time to assess the patient's response to the new medical regimen. A basic guide for these conversions is shown in

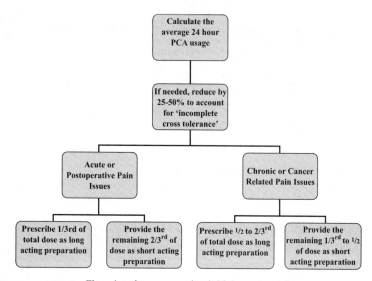

FIGURE 164.1. Changing the parenteral opioid dose to oral form.

Fig. 164.1. For acute pain management, a smaller proportion of total drug should be prescribed as a long-acting formulation. As the pain-inducing injury (or postsurgical inflammation) heals, lesser amounts of short-acting medications will be used by the patient. Based on this response, the long-acting preparations can be reduced afterward and eventually discontinued. On the contrary, more aggressive conversions should be reserved for cancer pain, where as much as half to two-thirds of total dose can be given as long-acting preparation, and dose can be escalated further based on breakthrough drug usage (*Fig. 164.1*).

TAKE HOME POINTS

- The use of opioid medications in the perioperative setting is increasing.
- Equianalgesic opioid drug conversions are easy to perform and give a reasonable estimation of the initial dose.
- Common errors in these conversions can be avoided by following the described method.
- The safety of these calculations can be enhanced by initially accepting the conservative side of dose range and later adjusting the dose according to the patient's response.
- When in doubt, always err on using smaller doses of basal infusion or long-acting preparations.

■ Physicians should also be prepared to recognize and manage any possible side effects or add adjuvant medications to the regimen when needed. Compassion and diligence eventually lead to smooth transitions, which is often a gratifying experience for both the physician and their patients.

SUGGESTED READINGS

American Pain Society. In: Ashbum MA, Lipman AG, Carr D, et al., eds. *Principles of Analgesic Use in the Treatment of Acute Pain and Cancer Pain*. 5th ed. Glenview, Ill.: American Pain Society; 2003;13–41.

Bruera E, Belzile M, Pituskin E, et al. Randomized, double-blind, cross-over trial comparing safety and efficacy of oral controlled-release oxycodone with controlled-release morphine in patients with cancer pain. *J Clin Oncol.* 1998;16(10):3222–3229.

Fine PG, Portenoy RK. Overview of clinical pharmacology. In: *A Clinical Guide to Opioid Analgesia*. McGraw-Hill Companies, Minneapolis, MN, 2004;16–27.

Houde R. Wallenstein S, Beaver W. Evaluation of analgesics in patients with cancer pain. In: Lasagna, ed. *International Encyclopedia of Pharmacology and Therapeutics, Section 6, Clinical Pharmacology, Vol. 1*. Oxford, UK: Pergamon Press; 1966:59–98.

Pasternak GW. Incomplete cross tolerance and multiple mu opioid peptide receptors. *Trends Pharmacol Sci.* 2001;22(2):67–70.

Stein C, Rosow CE. Receptor ligands and opiate narcotics. In: Evers AS, Maze M, eds. *Anesthetic Pharmacology: Physiological Principles and Clinical Practice*. Churchill Livingstone/Elsevier; 2004.

165

CONSIDER DISCUSSING THE USE OF KETOROLAC (TORADOL) WITH YOUR SURGICAL TEAM BEFORE THE NEED ARISES

AMIT SHARMA, MD

"In a fight between an anesthesiologist and a surgeon, the patient is always defeated."

It was another fine morning. We were finishing our first scheduled laparoscopic urologic surgery case when I received a Stat page to the operating room (OR). As I was reaching the OR, I could hear our famous urologist roaring at my resident. Apparently, my patient-compassionate resident had used ketorolac (Toradol; 30 mg IV) for postoperative pain control, and our surgical friend firmly believed that it would lead to renal failure or postsurgical bleed. I tried dodging his logic of so-called experience with my shield of scientific data leading to more noise pollution in the OR. The end result of our *battle for Middle Earth* was the formulation of the Eleventh Commandment by our respected colleague: "NO TORADOL for any of my patients EVER." Currently, ketorolac is perhaps one of the leading causes of tense anesthesiologist–surgeon relationships, and it is briefly discussed in this chapter.

Ketorolac tromethamine (commercially available as Toradol) is a member of the pyrrole-pyrrole group of nonsteroidal anti-inflammatory drugs (NSAIDs). It is available for intravenous (IV) or intramuscular (IM) administration as 15 mg in 1 mL and 30 mg in 1 mL (60 mg in 2 mL) solution. It is also available in tablets of 10 mg for oral use. It is a peripherally acting analgesic agent that inhibits prostaglandin synthesis. The drug possesses no sedative properties, making it a good agent in the perioperative setting. The bioavailability with oral, IM, or IV use is 100%, with peak analgesic activity time of 2 to 3 hours via oral route and 1 to 2 hours when used parenterally. Ketorolac is highly protein bound; metabolized in the liver via hydroxylation and conjugation, and eliminated by the kidneys (60% metabolites, 40% parent drug). It has a half-life of about 5 to 6 hours. The drug half-life is prolonged and unpredictable in the elderly and in the presence of renal impairment, having poor correlation with creatinine clearance values. Its pharmacokinetics are relatively unchanged in the presence of mild to moderate hepatic dysfunction. Thirty milligrams of IV ketorolac provide similar

© 2006 Mayo Foundation for Medical Education and Research

analgesic results as 4 mg of IV morphine, but a similar dose via IM route is equivalent to 6 to 8 mg of IM morphine. When used with opioids for postoperative pain management, ketorolac reduces opioid requirements, lowering their potential side effects.

Currently, ketorolac is indicated for short-term (≤ 5 days) management of moderately severe pain in the postoperative setting. It may be given as a single or multiple dose on a regular or as needed schedule up to a maximum of 5 days. Its frequently used dose profile is depicted in *Table 165.1*. IV injection is recommended to be given over at least 15 seconds, while the IM dose must be given slowly and deeply into the muscle. The time of onset of ketorolac is roughly 30 minutes. Peak effects are seen in 1 to 2 hours via either route, and clinical effects last for 4 to 6 hours. Mixing parenteral formulations with morphine, meperidine, promethazine, or hydroxyzine in the same syringe leads to precipitation and should be avoided.

Despite these desirable attributes, use of ketorolac comes with its own set of problems. Its relevant side effects and absolute contraindications are described in *Table 165.2*. Prostaglandins play a positive role in maintenance of platelet function and renal perfusion. The potent inhibitory effects of ketorolac on prostaglandin synthesis might jeopardize either of these vital phenomenons. Ketorolac use should be avoided in patients on therapeutic doses of anticoagulants, including prophylactic low-dose heparin therapy. It should also be avoided preoperatively, in any major surgical case, or when hemostasis is critical. It should be kept in mind that ketorolac-induced increased risk of bleeding cannot be detected on routine testing, via platelet count, prothrombin time, or activated partial thromboplastin time. It should also be used with extreme caution, if at all, in patients with impaired renal function. Ketorolac may cause dose-dependent reduction in renal prostaglandin formation and may precipitate acute renal failure. This is more likely to occur in patients with impaired hepatic or renal functions, dehydration, heart failure, concomitant use of diuretics, and advanced age. It is, therefore, not surprising that our surgical colleagues get really nervous with ketorolac use.

Regardless of these intimidating concerns, ketorolac use has been shown to be relatively safe in innumerable studies. A recent meta-analysis showed that NSAIDs caused a clinically unimportant transient reduction in renal function in the early postoperative period in patients with normal preoperative renal function. The authors concluded that NSAIDs should not be withheld from adults with normal preoperative renal function because of concerns about postoperative renal impairment. Ketorolac has been shown to effectively control postoperative pain after major abdominal, orthopedic, or gynecologic surgery, or after ambulatory laparoscopic procedures. Simultaneous use of ketorolac with opioids results in a 25% to 50% reduction in

TABLE 165.1 RECOMMENDED DOSE OF KETOROLAC IN PERIOPERATIVE SETTING

	INTRAMUSCULAR (IM)		INTRAVENOUS (IV)		ORAL (PO)[†]
	SINGLE DOSE SCHEDULE	MULTIPLE DOSE SCHEDULE	SINGLE DOSE SCHEDULE	MULTIPLE DOSE SCHEDULE	
Age 2–16 years	1 mg/kg Max = 30 mg	NR	0.5 mg/kg Max = 15 mg	NR	NR
Age >16 but <65 and BW ≥110 lbs	60 mg	30 mg Q6° Max = 120 mg	30 mg	30 mg Q6° Max = 120 mg	1st Dose = 2 tabs followed by 1 tab Q4–6° Max = 40 mg/d
Age ≥65 Or BW <110 lbs Or Renal Impairment	30 mg	15mg/kg Q6° Max = 60 mg	15 mg	15 mg Q6° Max = 60 mg	1st Dose = 1 tab followed by 1 tab Q4–6° Max = 40 mg/d

NR = not recommended; BW = body weight; Q = every; ° = hours; lbs = pounds; mg = miligrams.
[†] = Recommended ONLY as a continuation therapy of IM or IV ketorolac therapy.

TABLE 165.2   COMMON CONCERNS WITH KETOROLAC USE

RELEVANT SIDE EFFECTS	CONTRAINDICATIONS
■ Headache (17%) ■ Nausea (12%) ■ Drowsiness or dizziness (6%–7% each) ■ Dyspepsia (12%) ■ GI pain (13%) ■ Peptic ulceration ■ GI bleeding and/or perforation ■ Platelet function inhibition ■ Hypersensitivity reactions: range from bronchospasm to anaphylactic shock ■ Acute renal failure ■ Interstitial nephritis ■ Nephrotic syndrome ■ Fluid retention and edema (4%) ■ Oliguria, elevated BUN and creatinine ■ Elevated liver enzymes	■ Active peptic ulcer disease ■ Recent GI bleeding or perforation ■ H/O peptic ulcer disease or GI bleeding ■ Advanced renal impairment ■ Renal failure risk due to volume depletion ■ Suspected or confirmed cerebrovascular bleeding ■ Hemorrhagic diathesis ■ Incomplete hemostasis ■ High risk of bleeding ■ Prophylactic use before any *major* surgery ■ Intraoperative use when hemostasis is critical ■ H/O hypersensitivity reaction to ketorolac ■ H/O allergic reaction to aspirin or other NSAIDs ■ Concurrent use with aspirin or other NSAIDs ■ Intrathecal or epidural use ■ In labor and delivery

GI, gastrointestinal; BUN, blood urea nitrogen; H/O, history of; NSAIDs, nonsteroidal anti-inflammatory drugs.

opioid requirement, resulting in reduction of side effects, more rapid return to normal gastrointestinal (GI) function, and a shorter in-hospital stay. Although many published case reports and case series have shown an increase in intra- and postoperative bleeding following tonsillectomy in children after ketorolac use, such findings have not been reproduced in adults. Ketorolac does increase bleeding time to some extent, but its actual contribution to surgical site bleeding is perhaps inconsequential. Besides, these risks can be reduced to minimal by adhering to its strict treatment guidelines.

It is imperative for anesthesiologists to be aware of issues related to ketorolac prior to its use. Thorough knowledge would help us enhance the pleasant nature of the "Toradol conversation" with our surgical associates. No textbook can teach us communication skills, which would certainly come in handy during these intricate dialogues. Surgeons do have the right to know the anesthetic management and our plans for postoperative pain control. A formal discussion would help them understand the benefits of ketorolac and would also help their patients in the long run.

- Ketorolac tromethamine is a nonselective NSAID available in both parenteral and oral formulations for the management of moderately severe pain in the postoperative setting for ≤5 days.
- Administering 30 mg of IV ketorolac has the same equivalent analgesic effect as 4 mg of IV morphine, with much lower incidence of nausea.
- Ketorolac is contraindicated in patients with a history of peptic ulcer disease, bleeding problems, and advanced renal impairment, or in patients at risk for renal failure due to volume depletion, prior to major surgery, in the presence of uncertain hemostasis.
- Ketorolac has been shown to be a safe and effective analgesic agent in the postoperative setting.
- A mutual agreement between the anesthesiologist and the surgeon prior to the use of ketorolac would result in a more cordial atmosphere and better patient outcomes.

SUGGESTED READINGS

Bourne MH. Analgesics for orthopedic postoperative pain. *Am J Orthop.* 2004;33(3):128–135.

DeAndrade JR, Maslanka M, Maneatis T, et al. The use of ketorolac in the management of postoperative pain. *Orthopedics.* 1994;17(2):157–166.

Eger EI, White PF, Bogetz MS. Clinical and economic factors important to anaesthetic choice for day-case surgery. *Pharmacoeconomics.* 2000;7(3):245–262.

Gillis JC, Brogden RN. Ketorolac: a reappraisal of its pharmacodynamic and pharmacokinetic properties and therapeutic use in pain management. *Drugs.* 1997;53(1):139–188.

Lee A, Cooper MC, Craig JC, et al. Effects of nonsteroidal anti-inflammatory drugs on postoperative renal function in normal adults. *Cochrane Database Syst Rev.* 2001;(2):CD002765.

166

THE BASAL INFUSION MODE IN PATIENT-CONTROLLED ANALGESIA IS BOTH FRIEND AND FOE

AMIT SHARMA, MD

Patient-controlled analgesia (PCA) is the core therapeutic drug delivery system in acute and acute-on-chronic pain settings. Historically, in 1971, Sechzer published the first report showing the safety and efficacy of delivering small incremental doses of opioids using a machine. Since his initial description, this novel technique of analgesic drug delivery has been enormously refined and widely accepted. It emanated from the basic pharmacologic principle that a given analgesic medication needs to attain a specific serum concentration to produce analgesia. The lowest drug levels at which this is accomplished is the minimum effective analgesic concentration (MEAC) of that particular drug. Maintaining a constant serum drug concentration above MEAC would thus result in sustained analgesia. It is almost impossible to achieve stable serum drug levels with intermittent oral and intramuscular drug delivery methods. They often result in *peaks* of high drug concentrations that cause side effects and *troughs* of lower drug levels leading to inadequate analgesia (*Fig. 166.1*). These variations in drug levels can be avoided with the use of intermittent small intravenous (IV) doses or a continuous infusion.

Using these principles, opioids are now often delivered intravenously using highly sophisticated microprocessor-controlled units (e.g., PCA machine) in numerous acute and certain selected chronic pain settings. These machines allow several modes of drug administration, some of which are as follows:

1) **Demand-Only Mode (DOM):** This is the most commonly used method. The patient can self-administer a fixed dose (demand dose) into their IV.

2) **Continuous Plus Demand Mode (CDM):** A fixed baseline (basal or background) dose is infused intravenously every hour in addition to demand dosing.

3) **Variable-Rate Infusion Plus Demand Mode (VID):** In addition to patient dosing, continuous basal rate is preprogrammed on an internal clock to vary, turn on, or turn off during specified hours of the day.

© 2006 Mayo Foundation for Medical Education and Research

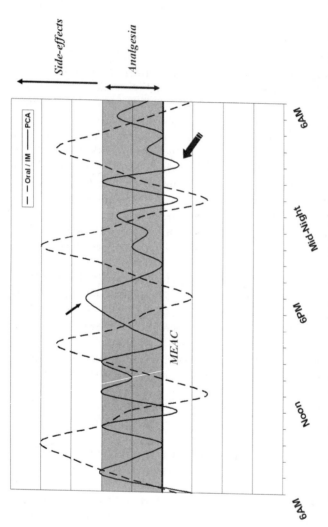

FIGURE 166.1. Comparison of systemic drug concentrations (*y* axis) during conventional oral or intramuscular (IM) opioid drug delivery system and during patient-controlled analgesia (PCA) use. The dark line demonstrates the minimally effective analgesic concentration (MEAC), and the shaded area represents the analgesic window. Serum drug concentrations above the analgesic window (*thin arrow*) result in clinically relevant side effects, while those below (*bold arrow*) cause poor pain control.

4) **Variable-Rate Feedback Infusion Plus Demand Mode (VFID):**
Basal infusion rate is varied by the PCA machine's microprocessor and
is based on patient's usage.

Given the widespread use of PCA in postoperative settings, it is imperative for all anesthesiologists to have a precise understanding of their functioning. Although standard PCA guidelines exist for postoperative analgesia
(*Table 164.3*), confusion often prevails with regard to basal infusion. Propo-
nents of basal infusion claim that it allows better patient satisfaction because
the demand frequency with CDM is lower than in DOM. It seems that the
constant IV infusion of opioid would maintain a certain level of serum drug
levels and would then be easier to reach the MEAC using fewer demand
doses (*Fig. 166.2*). In reality, this perception is oversimplistic and does not
account for multiple variables on which drug pharmacokinetics actually depends. For instance, the serum drug concentration required to reach MEAC
varies from one individual to the next. This situation is further complicated
by the fact that significant interpersonal variability exists for the safe *analgesic window*, which is defined as the serum drug concentrations that are
associated with clinically relevant analgesia without any side effects (shaded
area in *Fig. 166.1*). Certain individuals, such as elderly people, have relatively
narrow analgesic windows, and use of basal infusion would pose undue risks
for side effects in these patients.

The futility and risks of basal infusion, especially in opioid-naïve patients, has been shown in multiple studies (*Table 166.1*). Guler et al. showed
significant improvement in pain scores with the use of CDM technique in
the postoperative pain setting, but most other studies have failed to replicate
those results. Even with similar analgesic response, opioid consumption has
been shown to be higher with CDM than with DOM in numerous studies.
Moreover, the low-dose continuous nighttime-only infusion (VID mode)
failed to show any improvement in patients' sleep or comfort in most studies
(*Table 166.1*). CDM technique in these studies failed to show any major increase in the incidence of severe side effects. Other studies and case series, in
contrast, have frequently linked the additional background opioid infusion
to myriad side effects. Some of the feared complications include respiratory
depression and higher chances of programming errors.

Despite additional risks, use of continuous basal infusion is recommended for opioid-tolerant patients by some authors and is frequently used
in cancer patients in clinical practice. It can also be a handy tool in the
presence of certain personality traits and some neurologic disorders. One
of the important prerequisites of PCA usage is the patient's willingness
and capacity to self-administer demand doses at appropriate times. Patients
with external locus of control, severe depression, and learned helplessness
are often unable to use the demand doses adequately. Also, patients with

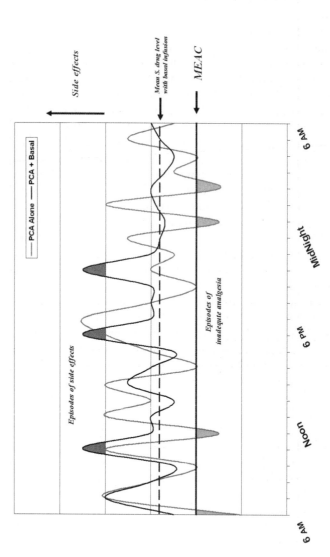

FIGURE 166.2. Optimum use of basal infusion during opioid drug delivery using a patient–controlled analgesia (PCA) system. Under ideal situations, continuous basal infusion raises serum drug concentrations closer to or above minimally effective analgesic concentration (MEAC) (*dotted line*). This may reduce the number of demand doses required to stay in the analgesic window and may reduce the episodes of inadequate analgesia. As evident, it may also increase the chances to develop clinically relevant side effects.

TABLE 166.1	RELEVANT TRIALS COMPARING IV PCA DEMAND-ONLY AND CONTINUOUS PLUS DEMAND MODE	

STUDY, YEAR	TYPE OF STUDY METHOD	RESULTS
Guler 2004	Randomized controlled trial 60 adults undergoing elective CABG surgery IV morphine PCA: DOM vs. CDM Follow up: 24 h postoperative	Similar sedation scores in both groups CDM group had √ Significantly lower VRS scores after first hour √ Greater cumulative morphine consumption √ No episodes of hypoxemia or hypertension
Dal 2003	Randomized double-blind trial 35 adults patients undergoing elective open heart surgery IV morphine PCA: DOM vs. CDM Follow up: 44 h postoperatively	√ Less morphine consumption at 44 h in DOM ($P = 0.0006$) √ No significant difference between two groups in VAS scores, blood levels of morphine, and adverse effects
Russell 1993	Controlled trial 62 patients undergoing gynecologic surgery IV morphine PCA: DOM vs. CDM (1 mg/h) Follow-up: VAS scores and SpO_2 for 24 h postoperatively	√ Significant increase in total morphine consumption in CDM √ Similar pain scores in both groups √ No difference in severity of postoperative desaturation between two groups
Parker 1992	Randomized controlled trial 156 adult women undergoing elective abdominal hysterectomy IV morphine PCA: DOM vs. CDM (POD 0—continuous infusion of 1 mg/h, POD 1-2—nighttime infusion, 10 PM-8 AM)	√ No improvement in patient's ability to sleep or to rest comfortably at night √ Similar numbers of patient demands and supplemental bolus doses, opioid usage, and recovery parameters in the two treatment groups √ CDM group had six programming errors; in addition, therapy was discontinued in three patients due to hemoglobin oxygen desaturation

CABG, coronary artery bypass grafting; IV, intravenous; PCA, patient-controlled analgesia; DOM, demand-only mode; CDM, continuous plus demand mode; VRS, verbal rating scale; VAS, visual analog scale; SpO_2, oxyhemoglobin saturation.

neurologic problems such as Parkinson disease or motor neuron diseases might find the use of the demand button challenging. A low-dose basal infusion can be slowly titrated in these subgroups with improved results. Caution is certainly advised in all patients whenever basal infusion is being considered. Risk factors for respiratory depression with IV PCA usage include age older than 70 years; presence of renal, hepatic, pulmonary, or cardiac impairment; obesity and sleep apnea (suspected or history); use of concurrent central nervous system depressants; and upper abdominal or thoracic surgery. Basal infusion should be avoided in these patients, whenever possible.

The concept of PCA involves the administration of drug based on the patient's demand. It also applies to alternative routes of drug delivery, such as transdermal, subcutaneous, oral transmucosal, epidural (patient-controlled epidural analgesia [PCEA]), intrathecal, and regional (patient-controlled regional analgesia [PCRA]). Although this chapter mainly focuses on IV PCA basal infusion, similar notions can be extrapolated to these alternative modes of drug delivery, with few exceptions. In general, for postoperative pain control, demand dose systems using local anesthetic and an opioid combination (PCEA and PCRA alone) provide similar analgesic response with superior patient satisfaction rates when compared to continuous infusion techniques. They also require fewer interventions by nursing staff and acute pain team members. However, addition of a small-dose continuous infusion along with demand boluses has been shown to reduce total anesthetic consumption with similar analgesic results. It is thus recommended that PCEA and PCRA management should be optimized with the addition of a low-dose basal infusion on a routine basis.

TAKE HOME POINTS

- PCA is being universally employed to enhance analgesia in acute and certain chronic pain conditions.
- Overall, PCA with DOM provides better pain control with no worsening of side effects when compared to intermittent intramuscular or oral regimen.
- In opioid-naive patients, use of background or basal infusion leads to increase in opioid consumption with no significant improvement in pain control.
- Basal infusion can be effectively used in the presence of opioid tolerance, certain complex personality traits, and neuromuscular diseases, as well as in cancer-related pain states.

SUGGESTED READINGS

Dal D, Kanbak M, Caglar M, et al. A background infusion of morphine does not enhance postoperative analgesia after cardiac surgery. *Can J Anaesth.* 2003;50(5):476–479.

Grass JA. Patient-controlled analgesia. *Anesth Analg.* 2005;101(5 suppl):S44–S61.

Guler T, Unlugenc H, Gundogan Z, et al. A background infusion of morphine enhances patient-controlled analgesia after cardiac surgery. *Can J Anaesth.* 2004;51(7):718–722.

Hagle ME, Lehr VT, Brubakken K, et al. Respiratory depression in adult patients with intravenous patient-controlled analgesia. *Orthop Nurs.* 2004;23(1):18–27.

Notcutt WG, Morgan RJ. Introducing patient-controlled analgesia for postoperative pain control into a district general hospital. *Anaesthesia* 1990;45(5):401–406.

Parker RK, Holtmann B, White PF. Effects of a nighttime opioid infusion with PCA therapy on patient comfort and analgesic requirements after abdominal hysterectomy. *Anesthesiology.* 1992;76(3):362–367.

Russell AW, Owen H, Ilsley AH, et al. Background infusion with patient-controlled analgesia: effect on postoperative oxyhaemoglobin saturation and pain control. *Anaesth Intensive Care.* 1993;21(2):174–179.

Schug SA, Torrie JJ. Safety assessment of postoperative pain management by an acute pain service. *Pain.* 1993;55(3):387–391.

Sechzer PH. Studies in pain with the analgesic-demand system. *Anesth Analg.* 1971;50(1):1–10.

167

MANAGEMENT OF PERIOPERATIVE PAIN IN OPIOID DEPENDENT PATIENT—OUT OF THE FRYING PAN, INTO THE FIRE

AMIT SHARMA, MD

"To be conscious that you are ignorant is a great step to knowledge."
-Benjamin Disraeli

Medical science has witnessed a dramatic shift in the awareness and treatment of chronic pain over the past few decades. Numerous organizational and regulatory bodies have declared pain as the fifth vital sign to encourage physicians to actively pursue and treat pain problems. Moreover, expansion in life expectancy has caused a relative increase in the elderly population, which carries the brunt of chronic pain problems. Given this scenario, it is not uncommon for anesthesiologists to encounter patients who are taking opioids. Some of them are on certain colossal doses that widen our eyes. Lack of knowledge on our behalf, bundled with uncertainty about opioid dose requirements and expectations of a smooth perioperative course by family and the surgical team, certainly make these cases challenging. These difficult situations can be handled with poise by knowing some fundamental principles related to the perioperative care of chronic opioid-dependent patients.

Anesthetic care of these intricate cases begins with early recognition of opioid-tolerance issues (*Table 167.1*) and formulation of a clear plan. A preoperative visit allows the anesthesiologist to perform a thorough medical evaluation, outline a postoperative pain management plan, and advise on therapeutic options. Information about the patient's opioid and adjuvant medication doses should be gathered. An electrocardiogram should be obtained to look for any QT interval prolongation, which is sometimes seen with the use of high doses of methadone. Prolongation of the QT interval is also seen with tricyclic antidepressant medications, which are frequently used as adjuvant drugs in chronic pain patients. A prolonged QT interval can predispose a patient to ventricular tachycardia, ventricular fibrillation, or torsades de pointes, and must be identified. A detailed discussion should be had with the patient to address his or her anxieties and fears. Patients are often worried about excessive pain following the surgery, which is frequently a reflection of their previous experiences. Anesthetic management options should be discussed. Whenever possible, a regional anesthetic technique should be chosen and explained to the patient.

© 2006 Mayo Foundation for Medical Education and Research

TABLE 167.1	PERIOPERATIVE ISSUES IN OPIOID-DEPENDENT PATIENTS

- Tolerance or increased analgesic requirements
- Poor pain control
- Opioid-induced hyperalgesia
- Opioid withdrawal
- Excessive anxiety
- Gastric aspiration
- Cardiac arrhythmias
- Physician's biases

There have been numerous studies indicating delayed gastric emptying in opioid-tolerant patients. Delayed gastric emptying is presumably related to an increase in pyloric sphincter tone associated with prolonged opioid use. Thus, opioid-dependent patients should be encouraged to stay "nothing by mouth" for longer durations to reduce the aspiration risk. They should also be advised to continue their analgesic regimen until the day of surgery to prevent any withdrawal or falling behind on opioid requirements. The only analgesic medication that should be reduced during the perioperative period is intrathecal baclofen, which has been suggested to enhance the effects of neuromuscular-blocking drugs and increase the incidence of hypotension and excessive sedation. Any such decision must be made after talking to the patient's pain physician.

Patients should be advised to arrive early on the day of surgery. Appropriate pre-emptive analgesia should be given in the preoperative period. Oral acetaminophen (1 g orally 1–2 hours preop) and certain nonsteroidal anti-inflammatory drugs (NSAIDs) (piroxicam 20 mg oral or Celebrex 200 mg oral—2 hours preop), with or without antiepileptic drugs (gabapentin 600 mg oral—2 hours preop), should be given. The anesthetic plan should again be discussed in detail with the patient, and regional anesthesia should be considered, whenever feasible. Recent reports have indicated that erroneous doses of fentanyl can be delivered from the transdermal system (fentanyl patch) when a warming blanket is placed on or near the patient. Transdermal fentanyl patches should be removed prior to taking the patient to the operating room. Furthermore, every effort should be made to avoid placing warming devices at the site from where fentanyl patches have been removed because similar effects can be seen with an increased uptake from the dermal fentanyl "depot."

If opioid medications have been discontinued preoperatively for any reason, a long-acting opioid should be titrated intravenously at the time of induction to achieve a spontaneous respiratory rate of 14 to 16/minute. An intravenous (IV) bolus of ketamine (0.5 mg/kg) should also be administered intraoperatively and then followed with an infusion of 4 μg/kg/minute. Ketamine is an NMDA receptor antagonist drug that has been shown to reduce the postoperative opioid usage in opioid-dependent patients. Clonidine and dexmedetomidine (α 2-adrenergic agonists) have also been shown to have similar effects. If pre-emptive analgesia was not begun preoperatively, then 1 g of acetaminophen (per rectal) and IV ketorolac (30 mg) or flurbiprofen should be considered at the time of (or following) induction. Last, but not least, the surgical team should be encouraged to infiltrate a long-acting local anesthetic solution at the site of incision. Intraoperative pain management often requires as much as 50% to 300% higher doses of opioids in an opioid-dependent patient, than in an opioid-naive patient for a similar surgical procedure. If general anesthesia is required, these patients should be reversed early and allowed to return to spontaneous ventilation. IV opioids should then be titrated to achieve a respiratory rate of 12 to 14/minute prior to extubation.

As expected, postoperative pain management is equally difficult in these patients. Unfortunately, intraoperative opioid usage does not help in estimating postoperative opioid requirements. Therefore, continuous regional techniques certainly come in handy under these circumstances. If epidural technique is used, a local anesthetic, in combination with a potent lipophilic opioid drug (e.g., fentanyl or sufentanil), should be used. Even when regional techniques are used, a patient-controlled analgesia (PCA) with a moderate demand-only dose should be used for supplemental analgesia. When regional techniques are not an option, PCA (with basal infusion and a moderately higher demand dose) should be considered as a second choice. Patient's preoperative total opioid usage should be taken into account while prescribing PCA basal infusion. These oral-to-IV opioid conversions are discussed in Chapter 164. A two- to four-fold increment in opioid requirement should be expected in the postoperative period than those used by an opioid-naive patient. The patient should be monitored in a postanesthetic care unit for oversedation or respiratory depression, and frequent evaluations should be done to ensure timely adjustments in PCA settings. If ketamine was begun during the intraoperative course, it should be at least resumed for 24 to 48 hours postoperatively. Acetaminophen and NSAIDs should also be continued during the postoperative period, with hepatic and renal function monitoring. The patient should be subsequently referred to the chronic pain management service of the hospital for a close follow-up.

TAKE HOME POINTS

- Perioperative pain management in opioid-dependent patients is demanding.

- A preoperative visit certainly helps address many issues, including patient's concerns.
- Pre-emptive analgesia is the most important step leading to reduction in postoperative opioid requirements.
- Whenever possible, regional techniques should be used for intraoperative and postoperative management.
- Adjuvant medications such as acetaminophen, NSAIDs, ketamine, and α 2-adrenergic agonists also help reduce opioid requirement in this difficult population.
- A close follow-up by acute and chronic pain management teams is warranted to ensure best postoperative care in opioid-dependent patients.

SUGGESTED READINGS

Brill S, Ginosar Y, Davidson EM. Perioperative management of chronic pain patients with opioid dependency. *Curr Opin Anaesthesiol.* 2006;19(3):325–331.

Carroll IR, Angst MS, Clark JD. Management of perioperative pain in patients chronically consuming opioids. *Reg Anesth Pain Med.* 2004;29(6):576–591.

Hadi I, Morley-Forster PK, Dain S, et al. Brief review: perioperative management of the patient with chronic non-cancer pain. *Can J Anaesth.* 2006;53(12):1190–1199.

Rozen D, Grass GW. Perioperative and intraoperative pain and anesthetic care of the chronic pain and cancer pain patient receiving chronic opioid therapy. *Pain Pract.* 2005;5(1): 18–32.

168

DO PATIENTS WITH CONGENITAL INSENSITIVITY TO PAIN NEED ANESTHETICS AND POSTOPERATIVE OPIOIDS?

KATARINA BOJANIC, MD, TOBY N. WEINGARTEN, MD, AND JURAJ SPRUNG, MD, PhD

HEREDITARY SENSORY AND AUTONOMIC NEUROPATHY

Congenital hyposensitivity to pain, hereditary sensory and autonomic neuropathy (HSAN), is a group of rare genetic disorders characterized by varying degrees of sensory loss, including nociceptive hyposensitivity, loss of other types of sensation, and various degrees of autonomic dysfunction. Sensory loss, especially the loss of pain sensation, is associated with self-mutilation that may require frequent surgery (*Fig. 168.1*). Little is known regarding whether or how much these patients require anesthesia for surgery or opioids postoperatively. Furthermore, because of various degrees of autonomic dysfunction, these patients may be at increased risk of perioperative anesthetic complications.

CLASSIFICATION OF CONGENITAL HYPOSENSITIVITY TO PAIN

Congenital hyposensitivity to pain disorders were categorized by Dyck et al. into five different types of HSANs (I–V). Different expressions of sensory loss are possible within each HSAN category, and some patients may have variable pain sensation. The types of HSAN are distinguished by the mode of inheritance, clinical features, degree of autonomic nervous system abnormalities, loss or degeneration of sensory fibers, and increasingly specific molecular genetic abnormalities:

- **HSAN I** is the only autosomal dominant disorder. It is characterized by onset later in life and a sensory deficit that is more pronounced in the legs than in the hands. In HSAN I, sensory deficits overshadow autonomic dysfunction.

- **HSAN II** patients tend to have pain hyposensitivity of the upper and lower limbs. Many have defective tactile sensation, whereas a minority may have areas of normal trunk sensation. Relevant autonomic dysfunction may include episodic hyperthermia and swallowing deficiencies.

- **HSAN III**, also known as Riley-Day syndrome or familial dysautonomia, has a higher prevalence in Ashkenazi Jews. These patients typically present in infancy with a profound dysautonomia (poor feeding with repeated vomiting, failure to thrive, and temperature and vasomotor dysregulation

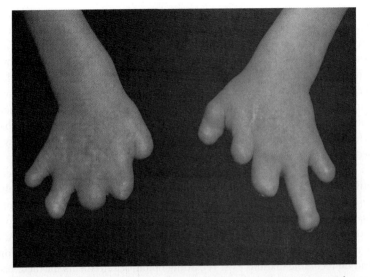

FIGURE 168.1. The hands of a 12-year-old boy with hereditary sensory and autonomic neuropathy (HSAN) II showing acromutilation. This type of self-mutilation may be found in all types of recessively inherited HSANs and is attributed to loss of pain sensation, neglect of injury, excessive surgery, and indifferent personality. (From Weingarten TN, Sprung J, Ackerman JD, et al. Anesthesia and patients with congenital hyposensitivity to pain. *Anesthesiology.* 2006;105:338–345. Used with permission.)

associated with hypertension or hypotension), recurrent pulmonary infections, diminished peripheral pain and temperature sensation, and absence of vibratory perception.

- **HSAN IV**, also known as congenital insensitivity to pain *with* anhidrosis, is characterized by hyposensitivity to superficial and deep visceral pain, mild to moderate mental retardation, and recurrent episodes of hyperpyrexia due to absence of sweating (no innervation of sweat glands).
- **HSAN V**, also known as congenital insensitivity to pain *without* anhidrosis, resembles HSAN IV but is associated with a selective absence of small sensory myelinated fibers (Aδ fibers), which are important for sensing the sharp, well-localized, and prickling sensations of pain. These patients typically respond to tactile, vibratory, and thermal stimuli.

ANESTHESIA AND HEREDITARY SENSORY AND AUTONOMIC NEUROPATHY DISORDERS

No consensus exists regarding the intraoperative analgesic needs of HSAN patients. Some patients with HSAN have tactile hyperesthesia, and some may have partially preserved pain sensation; therefore, most reports have described the use of volatile anesthetics in standard concentrations. In addition, anesthetics are necessary to ensure cooperation and immobility during surgery for pediatric patients, especially for those with mental retardation. The optimal dose of anesthetics for patients with HSAN has yet to be determined. At present, inhalational anesthetics should be titrated in accordance with the patient's hemodynamic response. A case reported by Layman showed that, in a 30-year-old man with congenital insensitivity to pain, bilateral lower extremity amputation could be performed by using only heavy sedation, without opioids or general anesthesia.

Most reports have documented minimal or no use of opioids postoperatively in patients with HSAN IV. When opioids were used perioperatively, no reasoning for their use was offered. The use of opioids in these patients may have followed the anesthesiologists' daily practice of administering opioids with every anesthetic. This "automatism" may occur because HSAN is rarely encountered by anesthesiologists, and because scarce information and no recommendations exist regarding opioid requirements for these patients. Furthermore, some patients with HSAN may have partially preserved nociception, and others may have preserved mechanoreceptor, cooling and warming sensations; therefore, they may sense some aspects of intense surgical stimulation.

Despite decreased pain perception in patients with HSANs, anesthetic administration for these patients has generally been similar to that for patients with normal pain perception. Postoperatively, these patients have minimal or no pain, and most did not require opioid medications.

PERIOPERATIVE MANAGEMENT OF BODY TEMPERATURE

Besides hyposensitivity to pain, patients with HSAN have various degrees of autonomic dysfunction that may affect the course of anesthesia. An important element of anesthesia is prevention of autonomic reflexes. Because patients with HSAN IV have anhidrosis, management of temperature homeostasis in daily life may be difficult. One study indicated that almost 20% of these patients died of hyperpyrexia during the first 3 years of life. Thus, perioperative thermoregulation is a concern, and continuous temperature monitoring is of great importance in these patients. Only one report has documented intraoperative hyperthermia in a patient with hyposensitivity to pain; in general, normothermia can be easily maintained with alterations of environmental temperature. Atropine inhibits the activity of the sweat glands and, in healthy children, may cause hyperthermia. However, because children with HSAN IV lack innervation of sweat glands, the use of atropine should not be associated with hyperthermia. Of note, malignant hyperthermia is not associated with HSAN IV; the genetic mechanisms for precipitating hyperpyrexia in malignant hyperthermia and HSAN IV are fundamentally different. All triggering agents associated with malignant hyperthermia (succinylcholine, halogenated agents, and others) have been used without any complications in HSAN patients.

TAKE HOME POINTS

- Knowledge regarding the safety of anesthesia in patients with HSAN II, IV, and V is scarce. To date, anesthesia has not been associated with any major adverse events in patients with HSAN disorders.

- Although patients with profound congenital insensitivity to pain may undergo major surgery without general anesthesia, most reports indicate that these patients received standard doses of anesthesia for operations.

- Factors other than analgesia, such as immobilization, prevention of autonomic reflexes, anxiolysis, and sedation, are equally important aspects of these patients' anesthetic management.

- Generally, patients with HSAN II, IV, and V do not need opioids postoperatively, even after major operations.

SUGGESTED READINGS

Dyck PJ. Inherited neuronal degeneration and atrophy affecting peripheral motor, sensory, and autonomic neurons. In: Dyck PJ, Thomas PK, Lambert EH, eds. *Peripheral Neuropathy.* Vol 2. Philadelphia, Pa.: WB Saunders; 1975:825–867.

Hilz MJ. Assessment and evaluation of hereditary sensory and autonomic neuropathies with autonomic and neurophysiological examinations. *Clin Auton Res.* 2002;12(suppl 1): 133–143.

Karkashan EM, Joharji HS, Al-Harbi NN. Congenital insensitivity to pain in four related Saudi families. *Pediatr Dermatol.* 2002;19:333–335.

Kawata K, Nishitaneno K, Kemi C, et al. Anesthesia in congenital analgesia [Japanese]. *Masui.* 1975;24:820–824.

Klein CJ, Dyck PJ. HSANs: clinical features, pathologic classification, and molecular genetics. In: Dyck PJ, Thomas PK, eds. *Peripheral Neuropathy.* 4th ed. Philadelphia, Pa.: Elsevier/Saunders; 2005:1809–1844.

Layman PR. Anaesthesia for congenital analgesia: a case report. *Anaesthesia* 1986;41:395–397.

Malan MD, Crago RR. Anaesthetic considerations in idiopathic orthostatic hypotension and the Shy-Drager syndrome. *Can Anaesth Soc J.* 1979;26:322–327.

Mori S, Yamashita S, Takasaki M. Anesthesia for a child with congenital sensory neuropathy with anhydrosis [Japanese]. *Masui.* 1998;47:356–358.

Nolano M, Crisci C, Santoro L, et al. Absent innervation of skin and sweat glands in congenital insensitivity to pain with anhydrosis. *Clin Neurophysiol.* 2000;111:1596–1601.

Okuda K, Arai T, Miwa T, et al. Anaesthetic management of children with congenital insensitivity to pain with anhydrosis. *Paediatr Anaesth.* 2000;10:545–548.

Rosemberg S, Marie SK, Kliemann S. Congenital insensitivity to pain with anhidrosis (hereditary sensory and autonomic neuropathy type IV). *Pediatr Neurol.* 1994;11:50–56.

Rozentsveig V, Katz A, Weksler N, et al. The anaesthetic management of patients with congenital insensitivity to pain with anhidrosis. *Paediatr Anaesth.* 2004;14:344–348.

Sweeney BP, Jones S, Langford RM. Anaesthesia in dysautonomia: further complications. *Anaesthesia* 1985;40:783–786.

Tomioka T, Awaya Y, Nihei K, et al. Anesthesia for patients with congenital insensitivity to pain and anhidrosis: a questionnaire study in Japan. *Anesth Analg.* 2002;94:271–274.

Yoshitake S, Matsumoto K, Miyagawa A, et al. Anesthetic consideration of a patient with congenital insensitivity to pain with anhidrosis [Japanese]. *Masui.* 1993;42:1233–1236.

169

RULE OUT FACET ARTHROPATHY BEFORE INITIATING EXPENSIVE AND INVASIVE MANEUVERS FOR BACK AND SPINE PAIN

AMIT SHARMA, MD

Spinal pain is one of most common and most intricate problems faced by physicians today. Pain of just the lumbar back alone is believed to be the most common etiology of chronic pain syndrome. In addition to the significant personal morbidity, spine-related pain has an enormous economic impact on society—the total cost of low back pain exceeds $100 billion per year in the United States alone. About one third of the overall costs are direct health care expenditures due to overuse of unnecessary diagnostic modalities and therapeutic maneuvers with unproven benefits. The remaining two thirds of the cost are indirect, due to lost wages and reduced productivity. Given this scenario, it is important to formulate precise evidence-based diagnostic and therapeutic plans for patients with spinal pain.

Facet arthropathy has been implicated as the etiology in 67% of patients with chronic neck pain, 48% of patients with chronic thoracic pain, and as many as 40% of patients with chronic lumbar pain. Thus, the high prevalence of facet arthropathy makes it a leading differential cause of almost all spinal pain issues. The facet (or zygapophyseal) joints are true synovial joints connecting the adjacent vertebra posteriorly. They are formed by the inferior articular process of superior vertebra and the superior articular process of inferior vertebra. Two adjacent vertebral bodies thus have a pair of facet joints preventing axial movements of one vertebra over another. The articular surfaces of each facet joint are covered with cartilage, and its edges are covered with synovial membrane and fibrous capsule. Primary dorsal rami of spinal nerves exit from the neural foramen just above and medial to the facet joints and send off medial and lateral branches. This medial branch, in turn, supplies corresponding facet joint and paraspinous muscles. Each facet joint receives innervation from the medial branch of exiting nerve root of corresponding vertebral level and from the level above. Facet joints can develop degenerative changes under certain circumstances (trauma, osteoarthritis, inflammation of synovial capsule, or joint subluxation) and can become quite painful. This painful degeneration of facet joints is known as *facet syndrome* or *arthropathy*.

© 2006 Mayo Foundation for Medical Education and Research

PRESENTATION

Cervical facet arthropathy pain presents as pain involving the head, neck, shoulder, suprascapular and scapular area, and upper arm. Distribution of pain varies, depending on the specific facet joint involved. For instance, involvement of the C2-3 joint leads to pain in the occipital area, C3-4 in the neck, and C4-5 along the lateral aspect of the nape of the neck and shoulder area. The associated physical findings may include decreased range of movements at the neck, exacerbation of pain with neck extension, and some degree of alleviation with flexion. Palpation over the specific facet joint may also aggravate pain. Thoracic facet arthropathy presents mainly as thoracic pain along with paraspinous tenderness. The presentation of lumbar facet arthropathy is often as axial lumbar back pain with stiffness, especially in the morning. Pain also involves the hips, buttocks, or thighs and is often exacerbated by prolonged sitting or standing. Similar to cervical facet syndrome, paraspinous tenderness over the affected joint may be elicited. Movements such as hyperextension and lateral rotation over the spine (facet loading maneuver) that stress the facet joints will also aggravate the pain.

DIAGNOSIS

The differential diagnosis for pain that mimics facet arthropathy includes migraine and tension headaches, degenerative disc disease (discogenic pain), spondylosis, spondylolysis, spondylolisthesis, myofascial pain, and sacroiliitis. Unfortunately, the clinical picture is similar in most of these conditions, and it is difficult to distinguish between them by symptomatology or physical signs alone. Laboratory data and imaging studies are not helpful in diagnosing facet arthropathy because degenerative changes of the facet joints are seen on the plain films and on the computed tomography and magnetic resonance imaging scans in asymptomatic subjects. The only reliable way to identify the presence of facet arthropathy is if amelioration of symptoms occurs after local anesthetic blockade of the facet joint's nerve supply. Historically, this was done by injecting the local anesthetic solution inside the facet joint itself under fluoroscopic guidance. In current practice, the same effect is achieved by injecting the anesthetic solution adjacent to the nerve branches (medial branches) supplying these joints.

This catch-22 situation involving a high prevalence of facet arthropathy and only a single invasive mode of diagnosis would seem to indicate that all patients with spinal pain should be subjected to the intervention of facet block. In fact, this scenario is probably too aggressive and would cause discomfort in many patients with other etiologies of spine pain. Hence, identification of the predictive factors for facet arthropathy became imperative to avoid imposing this rather uncomfortable testing on every patient. In 1998,

Helbig and Lee formulated a scoring system to predict a positive response to facet joint injection. Based on a limited study on 12 subjects, 30 points were allocated to back pain associated with groin or thigh pain, and to the reproduction of pain with extension-rotation at spine (positive facet loading). Similarly, 20 points were given to the presence of well-localized paraspinal tenderness and to corresponding positive radiographic changes, while a negative score of 10 was assigned to the existence of pain below the knee. Using this system, a score of 60 points or more was shown to indicate a very high probability of satisfactory response to facet injections. This scoring system can be used as a clinical guide to decide whether diagnostic facet injections are indicated for any given patient.

Diagnostic nerve blocks have limitations. Single diagnostic facet injections or medial branch blocks have been shown to have a high sensitivity but a low specificity. False-positive results have been shown in 63% of single local anesthetic blocks at cervical level, and these numbers are as high as 62% and 30% at thoracic and lumbar levels, respectively. Presence of placebo response and spread of local anesthetic solution in the adjacent epidural space have been reasoned as the probable causes of these high numbers. Many authors thus recommend double diagnostic blocks using different local anesthetic solutions such as lidocaine and bupivacaine. A differential duration response (lidocaine block being short lasting and vice versa) is taken as dual confirmation before aggressive therapeutic options are exercised.

The blocks are always done under fluoroscopic guidance. Because every facet joint has a dual innervation, it is crucial to block both nerves. At cervical level, C2-3 facet joint is supplied predominantly by the medial branch of C3 dorsal ramus (also called the third occipital nerve). The remaining joints are supplied by medial branches of the dorsal rami exiting at that vertebral level and from the level above. Thus, C4-5 facet joint is supplied by medial branches of C4 and C5 dorsal rami (C4 being exiting from C3-4 neural foramen). Likewise, at lumbar levels, each facet receives nerve supply from the dorsal rami of the same level and from the level above. Because L4 dorsal ramus exit from L4-5 neural foramen, medial branches of L3 and L4 dorsal rami need to be blocked to achieve L4-5 facet block. The interventional pain physician should also be aware of the correct positions of these medical branches to optimally perform these blocks. At cervical level, the target area is the central part or "waist" of the articular pillar on the A-P view (*Fig. 169.1*) and the midpoint of articular pillar projection on the lateral view (*Fig. 169.2*). At the lumbar levels, the target area is the junction of superior articular process and superior border of transverse process of the level below (*Fig. 169.3*) for L1-4 medial branches. The L5 medial branch lies at the junction of the sacral ala and superior articular process of S1.

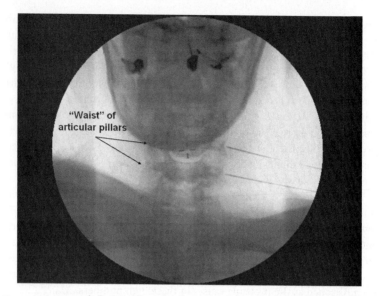

FIGURE 169.1. A-P view of needle placement for cervical medial branch blocks. The needle tip is positioned at the midpoint of articular pillar of corresponding cervical vertebral body (*arrows*).

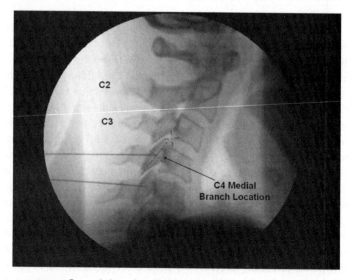

FIGURE 169.2. Lateral view of needle placement for cervical medial branch blocks. The needle tip is positioned at the midpoint of articular pillar of corresponding cervical vertebral body.

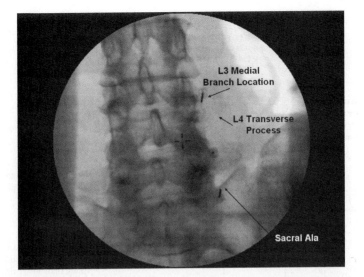

FIGURE 169.3. Placement of needle under fluoroscopic guidance for diagnostic (or therapeutic) medial branch blocks. Note that the L3 nerve root exits below the L3 transverse process and sends a medial branch (L3 MB) that runs along the junction of the superior articular process of the L4 vertebral body and the L4 transverse process.

MANAGEMENT

After the diagnosis of facet arthropathy has been made, patients are often offered therapeutic interventions with relatively long-term pain relief. Previously, this was achieved by intra-articular injection of steroids. With the advancement of radiofrequency technique, better results can be achieved by radiofrequency neurotomy (rhizotomy) or denervation (ablation) of corresponding medial branches. A detailed description of the mechanism of action of radiofrequency or pulsed-radiofrequency is beyond the scope of this chapter. The technique is similar to the diagnostic blocks, wherein radiofrequency probes are positioned at the specified sites of medial branches using 22-gauge spinal needles as introducers. After positive sensory testing (50 Hz) at <0.5 V and negative motor testing (contraction of ipsilateral paraspinal muscles but not lower extremity musculature) at 2 V, ablation is carried out for 90 to 120 seconds. Outcome results of radiofrequency techniques vary, depending on the inclusion criteria and level of blockade (*Table 169.1*). In general, radiofrequency procedure is relatively safe, gives a prolonged pain relief, and can be safely repeated with similar results.

TABLE 169.1 SELECTED OUTCOME STUDIES FOR RADIOFREQUENCY ABLATION OF MEDIAL BRANCHES FOR FACET ARTHROPATHY RELATED PAIN

Author (Year)	Level Type	Nᵃ	Diagnostic Block(s) Therapy Follow-up	Response
Lord (1996)	Cervical Randomized, double-blind, placebo-controlled trial (rhizotomy vs. sham procedure)	24	Dual double-blind, placebo-controlled local anesthetic block *90 s RF lesion at 80°C* 12 mo	Median time before return of preprocedure pain = 263 d in study group (8 d in sham group).
Stolker (1993)	Thoracic Prospective study	36	Single local anesthetic block *RF lesion at thoracic MBs* 18–54 mo	After a median follow-up of 31 mo, 16 patients (44%) were pain free and 14 patients (39%) had more than 50% pain relief.
Van Kleef (1999)	Lumbar Randomized, double-blind, placebo-controlled trial (rhizotomy vs. sham procedure)	31	Single local anesthetic block *60 s RF lesion at 80°C* 12 mo	Statistically significant differences in effect on the VAS scores, global perceived effect, and the Oswestry disability scale. 3, 6, and 12 mo after treatment, there were significantly more success patients in the RF group compared with the sham group.
Dreyfuss (2000)	Lumbar Prospective audit	15	Double local anesthetic block *2 lesions, 90 s RF lesion at 85°C* 12 mo	60% of the patients obtained at least 90% relief of pain at 12 mo while 87% obtained at least 60% relief.

RF, radiofrequency; MB, medial branch; VAS, visual analog scale.
ᵃNumber of patients included in study.

TAKE HOME POINTS

- Facet arthropathy is a leading cause of spinal pain.
- Clinical and radiographic analysis helps little in its diagnosis.
- Diagnostic local anesthetic blocks are the only method to identify this disease and should be considered early, if the clinical picture (based on a rigorous epidemiologic evaluation) is suggestive.

- Therapeutic radiofrequency ablation of medical branches innervating the specific facet joint gives relatively long-term pain relief.

SUGGESTED READINGS

Dreyfuss P, Halbrook B, Pauza K, et al. Efficacy and validity of radiofrequency neurotomy for chronic lumbar zygapophysial joint pain. *Spine*. 2000;25(10):1270–1277.

Frymoyer JW. Back pain and sciatica. *N Engl J Med*. 1998;318(5):291–300.

Helbig T, Lee CK. The lumbar facet syndrome. *Spine*. 1988;13(1):61–64.

Katz JN. Lumbar disc disorders and low-back pain: socioeconomic factors and consequences. *J Bone Joint Surg Am*. 2006;88(suppl 2):21–24.

Lord SM, Barnsley L, Wallis BJ, et al. Percutaneous radio-frequency neurotomy for chronic cervical zygapophyseal-joint pain. *N Engl J Med*. 1996;335(23):1721–1726.

Manchikanti L, Singh V, Pampati V, et al. Evaluation of the prevalence of facet joint pain in chronic thoracic pain. *Pain Physician*. 2002;5(4):354–359.

Manchikanti L, Singh V, Pampati V, et al. Is there correlation of facet joint pain in lumbar and cervical spine? An evaluation of prevalence in combined chronic low back and neck pain. *Pain Physician*. 2002;5(4):365–371.

Stolker RJ, Vervest AC, Groen GJ. Percutaneous facet denervation in chronic thoracic spinal pain. Acta Neurochir (Wien). 1993;122(1-2):82–90.

van Kleef M, Barendse GA, Kessels A, et al. Randomized trial of radiofrequency lumbar facet denervation for chronic low back pain. *Spine*. 1999;24(18):1937–1942.

Weiner DK, Kim YS, Bonino P, et al. Low back pain in older adults: are we utilizing healthcare resources wisely? *Pain Med*. 2006;7(2):143–150.

170

WHEN EVALUATING BACK PAIN, ALWAYS EXAMINE FOR TRIGGER POINTS BEFORE ORDERING EXPENSIVE IMAGING STUDIES

LEENA MATHEW, MD

A 45-year-old patient presents to the pain clinic complaining of lower back pain and insisting that he needs to be "run through the CT scanner." He was in his usual state of health until experiencing back pain 6 weeks ago when he spent a weekend planting trees at his mother-in-law's house (in other words, seriously overdoing it). Although the initial pain subsided after 2 weeks, he had recurrence of the same pain 2 weeks ago when he slipped and fell on the sidewalk. Since then, the pain has steadily escalated in intensity to its current level. It is a constant nonradicular pain that he describes as tightness and an aching sensation mostly localized in the left low back. There is no sensory or motor deficit associated with this. He denies any bowel or bladder dysfunction. He also denies any constitutional symptoms such as fever, night sweats, chills, and loss of weight or appetite. There is no increase of pain with Valsalva maneuver. Pain worsens with increased levels of activity, especially with lateral flexion, extension, and rotation at the lumbar spine. His physical exam was within normal limits, except for left paraspinal muscle spasm associated with a trigger point.

When a patient presents with low back pain, there is often immediate focus on obtaining imaging studies to establish a diagnosis. However, indiscriminate expensive imaging studies can add greatly to total health care expenses both in terms of the acute episode of back pain and in the long-term management of a chronic condition. A careful history and physical exam will usually exclude diagnoses that may require immediate operative treatment from those that can be safely and efficiently managed with other modalities. If imaging is sought, many practitioners advocate just a basic x-ray (if low back, flexion and extension are also recommended).

It is crucial to remember that myofascial pain is one of the most common reasons for low back pain. There is a primary or idiopathic etiology, as well as a secondary etiology, stemming from radiculopathy, disc or facet syndrome, dystonia, or postural imbalance such as a leg length discrepancy. The failure to recognize this can result in apparent treatment failures.

The presence of trigger points is the classic hallmark of myofascial pain. Because trigger points are not visualized on any imaging studies or laboratory

© 2006 Mayo Foundation for Medical Education and Research

tests, they are identified only by careful palpation. Trigger points may be appreciated as bands or knots within involved muscles. Palpation of trigger points produces pain concordant with the patients' usual pain. The pain from the trigger point is centrifugally referred in the affected muscle along the myofascial plane. The most common muscles affected are those in the neck, shoulder girdle, and low back.

Muscles are sprained when placed under constant stress. A sprain usually affects a few fibers in the body of the muscle. The initial inflammation settles within 1 to 2 weeks. If sensitization of the dorsal horn occurs at the corresponding level in the spinal cord, there is an increase in tone within the whole muscle. Chronically, the taut band remains as a painless "latent" trigger point. This makes the muscle vulnerable to further injury because the latent trigger point makes the muscle less pliable. In some patients, the sensitization leads to a self-perpetuating loop that keeps the trigger points active for many months after the original injury.

Treatment of myofascial pain syndrome varies. It includes trigger point injections, spray and stretch, transcutaneous electrical nerve stimulation, ultrasound therapy, dry needling, massage therapy, and elimination of causative and perpetuating factors. The major goal of trigger point therapy is to relieve both pain and the tightness of the involved muscles. An interesting feature of trigger point injections is that they are useful as both a diagnostic *and* a therapeutic tool.

Trigger point injections should always be done in conjunction with a physical therapy program that focuses on stretching, strengthening, and improving the range of motion. The mechanism of trigger point inactivation by injection is unknown. Simons and Travell suggested several possible mechanisms: (i) mechanical disruption of the trigger point, (ii) depolarization block of the nerve fibers by the released intracellular potassium, (iii) washout of the neurosensitizing inflammatory mediators by injected fluid or local hemorrhage, (iv) interruption of the central feedback mechanism, and (v) focal necrosis of the trigger point by the injected drug.

Trigger point injection is contraindicated for patients with a fear of needles, as well as for patients that are pregnant, exhibit signs of infection, have bleeding disorders, or have allergies to anesthetic agents. Although some practitioners like to document that aspirinlike pharmaceuticals have been avoided 1 week before trigger point injection, American Society of Regional Anesthesia currently does not require that the patient be off of aspirin for 1 week prior (in fact, it is likely that most of these patients will actually be on some anti-inflammatories for musculoskeletal pain).

Injecting the trigger points may provide the patient with symptom relief while the primary disease pathology is being addressed. It is a simple, low-risk procedure, which if done correctly decreases the need for aggressive and expensive interventions. Myofascial trigger points are eliminated by infiltration with a local anesthetic, which in turn blocks the reflex mechanisms perpetuating the syndrome and allowing the taut muscle fibers to relax. This action provides relief of the referred pain syndrome.

Trigger point therapy begins with accurate identification of the point. After palpation, these points are marked. Using sterile preparation and technique throughout, the needle is introduced at a 30- to 60-degree angle, just beyond the dermis into the myofascial plane. When the myofascial plane is entered, a gritty sand paper sensation or crackling sound is appreciated. The length of the needle depends on the muscle being accessed. For superficial muscles, a 25- to 27-gauge 1-in. needle is used. For deeper muscles such as the gluteus maximus or quadratus lumborum, a 25-gauge 5-cm needle may be needed. The point is then injected with a local anesthetic with or without steroid. The local anesthetic injected may be 1% to 2% lidocaine or 0.125% to 0.5% bupivacaine. Although 0.5% bupivacaine is used by some practitioners, caution must be exercised when injecting over the site of major nerves. Remember that longer-acting local anesthetics are more mycotoxic. One milliliter of local anesthetic is sufficient at each trigger point because larger volumes decrease the specificity of the block and may be ultimately mycotoxic. Although multiple trigger points may be injected simultaneously; it must be kept in mind that the more points that are injected, the less specific the trigger point injection would be for diagnostic purposes. The most symptomatic points are targeted first. One to 10 trigger points can be injected at a visit. When multiple points are injected, care should be exercised not to exceed toxic doses of the local anesthetic. Although it is believed that the addition of steroids to the local anesthetic may increase the duration of analgesia and also act as a local anti-inflammatory agent, there is little evidence to support any beneficial effect of adding corticosteroid to the injection. If the practitioner so chooses, a total of 10 to 40 mg of triamcinolone or methylprednisolone or 2 to 8 mg of dexamethasone may be used in divided doses. Repeated trigger point injections with corticosteroids may cause local myofibrillar scarring and suppression of the pituitary adrenal axis, resulting in a poor long-term functional outcome. Epinephrine should never be used in the local anesthetic injectate mixture. The injection may be repeated in 1 to 2 weeks along with a program of physical therapy focusing on stretching, strengthening, and improving range of motion.

Some practitioners will place the needle in the marked point and "dry needle" it by moving the needle back and forth horizontally in the plane of the trigger point. Saline has also been used as an injectate. Most of the studies seem to suggest that the injection of saline or local anesthetic is not as important as the act of needling itself. There is a paucity of good studies stating superiority of one technique over the other. The efficacy of needling techniques compared to placebo is not supported or refuted by the evidence suggested from clinical trials.

Botox A injections may be considered in resistant cases after successful treatment with local anesthetic with or without steroid injection has been documented. In this event, trigger points are deactivated by injecting with botulinum toxin A (Botox A). Botox blocks motor nerve impulses from reaching the injected muscle fiber, producing pain relief because of intense relaxation. Botox binds irreversibly to specific receptors, producing muscle relaxation, which lasts up to 3 months. Muscle tone slowly returns as new receptors are produced.

Long-term outcomes of Botox use in myofascial pain syndrome have not been published. In fact, no study of myofascial, lumbar, or generalized neck pain have described more than two injections, with the second injection usually 3 months post the first injection. Long-term adverse effects, such as development of antibodies to the toxin or muscle weakness/atrophy, have not been described but remain a theoretical concern.

TAKE HOME POINTS

- The diagnosis of myofascial pain depends on careful history and physical exam to identify trigger points.
- Again, it is important to make sure that there are no radicular symptoms or red flags/constitutional symptoms prior to forgoing the "expensive imaging/workup." Many practitioners are advocating a basic x-ray (if low back, flexion and extension are also recommended). The thinking behind this is that a bone-involving process (i.e., a vertebral compression fracture) will have point tenderness, and this can often mimic a trigger point in presentation.
- Trigger points may represent a feedback loop involving dorsal horn cells in the spinal cord.
- Trigger point injections have *both* a diagnostic and a therapeutic value.
- The mechanism of trigger point deactivation by injection is not known, but because it is a simple, low-risk procedure, it should be considered when appropriate.
- Lidocaine or bupivacaine *without* epinephrine is typically used. Multiple trigger points can be injected per treatment, but exercise caution not to exceed the toxic dose.
- Addressing trigger points early may obviate the need for expensive imaging studies and restore early functionality.
- Botox A injections have been used in resistant cases. However, there are no long-term studies to date that examine outcomes pertaining to this practice.

SUGGESTED READINGS

Alvarez DJ, Rockwell PG. Trigger points: diagnosis and management. *Am Fam Physician.* 2002;65:653–660.

Borg-Stein J, Simons DG. Myofascial pain. *Arch Phys Med Rehabil.* 2002;83:S40–S47.

Cheshire WP, Abashian SW, Mann JD. Botulinum toxin in the treatment of myofascial pain syndrome. *Pain.* 1994;59(1):65–69.

Garvey TA, Marks MR, Wiesel SW. A prospective randomized double-blind evaluation of trigger point injection therapy for low-back pain. *Spine.* 1989;14:962–964.

Parris WC. Nerve block therapy for myofascial pain management. In: Rachlin ES, Rachlin IS, eds. *Myofascial Pain and Fibromyalgia.* 2nd ed. St. Louis, Mo.: Mosby; 2002:421–433.

Rachlin ES, Rachlin I. Trigger point management. In: Rachlin ES, Rachlin IS, eds. *Myofascial Pain and Fibromyalgia.* 2nd ed. St. Louis, Mo.: Mosby; 2002:231–258.

Raj PP, Paradise LA. Myofascial pain syndrome and its treatment in low back pain. *Semin Pain Med.* 2004;2(3):167–174.

Simons DG, Travell JG, Simons LS. *Travel & Simons' Myofascial Pain and Dysfunction: The Trigger Point Manual.* 2nd ed. Vol 1. Baltimore, Md.: Williams & Wilkins; 1999.

Sola AE, Bonica JJ. Myofascial pain syndromes. In: Bonica JJ, ed. *The Management of Pain.* Vol 1. Philadelphia, Pa.: JB Lippincott; 1990:352–367.

171

KNOW THE COMPLICATIONS OF EPIDURAL CORTICOSTEROID INJECTIONS

ANNE E. PTASZYNSKI, MD AND TOBY N. WEINGARTEN, MD

Epidural corticosteroid injections for back and radicular pain have been performed since the 1950s. Although these injections are generally considered safe, several important complications can occur.

Corticosteroids may be injected epidurally via the interlaminar, transforaminal, and caudal approaches. Common corticosteroids used include betamethasone, methylprednisolone, triamcinolone, and dexamethasone. These vary in potency, duration of action, preparation (solution or suspension), and additives (benzyl alcohol or polyethylene glycol). These factors may have a role in potential complications.

Most complications are relatively mild and include headache, vasovagal reactions, transient increase in pain, dural puncture, and systemic effects such as hyperglycemia. Serious complications are rare. Arachnoiditis is inflammation of the arachnoid mater, which leads to painful paresthesias and weakness. Infectious complications, such as meningitis or epidural abscess, can be devastating or fatal. Paralysis can also occur. Careful and thoughtful performance of epidural corticosteroid injections can reduce the rate of these complications.

ARACHNOIDITIS

Adhesive arachnoiditis can occur after intrathecal administration of corticosteroids. The cause of arachnoiditis is unknown, but particulate corticosteroids in suspension and additives used as preservatives have been implicated. Arachnoiditis can occur if a portion of an epidural corticosteroid injection is delivered to the intrathecal space. Negative aspiration, however, does not guarantee that inadvertent partial injection into the intrathecal space will be prevented.

Administration of a contrast agent under fluoroscopy before injection of a corticosteroid can localize the needle in the epidural space. Use of a microbore attachment ("pigtail") limits movement of the needle during syringe changes, thereby limiting the chance of needle migration into the intrathecal space. Attention must be paid to the contents of the epidural kit and injectant to ensure that they do not contain neurotoxic agents or preservatives. Antimicrobial skin preparations should be allowed to dry before needle placement because these agents may be neurotoxic.

PARALYSIS

Paralysis after epidural corticosteroid injection can have immediate or late onset. In cases of immediate-onset paralysis, a vascular source is usually suspected, such as vascular trauma or embolism from intravascular injection. The vessels of particular concern are radicular arteries feeding the spinal cord and, at the cervical level, the ascending cervical, deep cervical, and vertebral arteries. The anterior two-thirds of the cord is supplied by the anterior spinal artery. At the cervical level, the radicular and segmental medullary arteries are fed by the ascending cervical and deep cervical arteries. A recent cadaveric study demonstrated that 22% of the posterior portion of the cervical vertebral foramina, once considered the "safe" location for needle placement, contained radicular cervical or segmental medullary arteries.

In the thoracic and lumbar spine, the anterior spinal artery is fed by radicular arteries from the lumbar and intercostal arteries. Of particular concern is the artery of Adamkiewicz, typically located between T5 and L2 on the left. Its origin has considerable anatomic variability. Radicular arteries enter the spinal column through the foramen, putting them at risk during transforaminal injections. Previous spine surgery appears to be a risk factor for anterior spinal cord infarctions associated with epidural injections.

To limit the possibility of intravascular injection, needle placement should be confirmed by administering contrast agent under fluoroscopic imaging. Digital subtraction angiography provides increased sensitivity in detecting intravascular injections. A test dose of local anesthetic can confirm intravascular needle placement by resulting in temporary paralysis, or, in cases of cervical injections, seizures. Use of a microbore attachment limits needle movement while syringes are changed between injections. A pencil-point spinal needle may decrease the risk of vascular cannulation. Corticosteroid solutions rather than particulate formulations may decrease the possibility of embolism during inadvertent intravascular injection. Cases of cervical anterior cord syndrome and cerebellar injury have occurred after cervical transforaminal epidural injections, despite needle placement using fluoroscopy and real-time computed tomography (CT). We recommend that such injections be performed only with extreme caution and after careful consideration of the risks and benefits.

Late onset paralysis may be due to several complications, including compression of the spinal cord from hematoma or epidural abscess; thrombosis due to vascular trauma may also be a source. A preprocedural history should be taken to exclude the use of anticoagulant or antiplatelet medication or an underlying bleeding disorder. Screening laboratory tests on all patients are not indicated. Minimizing needle manipulation in the epidural space further decreases the risk of vascular trauma. Because spinal cord compression can be such a devastating complication, it is important to keep a high index of suspicion for epidural hematoma and abscess. Magnetic resonance imaging (MRI) is becoming the gold standard for diagnosis of these lesions, although CT with or without myelography is also useful.

INFECTIONS

Infections due to epidural injections are rare but include meningitis, epidural abscess, and soft tissue or skin infections. Risk factors appear to include remote extraspinal infections and an immunocompromised state, including that resulting from diabetes mellitus, chronic corticosteroid use, and cancer. *Fig. 171.1* shows MRI findings for a patient in whom discitis developed after an intralaminar epidural corticosteroid injection.

Several precautions should minimize the risk of infection. Strict adherence to sterile technique is an absolute. Skin preparation with 10% povidone

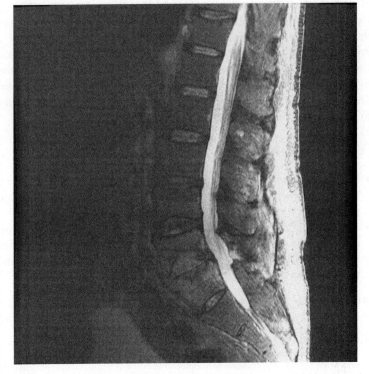

FIGURE 171.1. A T2 sagittal magnetic resonance imaging scan of the lumbar spine showing evidence of discitis after an intralaminar epidural corticosteroid injection at the L5/S1 interspace. The patient had a history of prior empyema and recurrent pulmonary infections

iodine was found to leave 35% of epidural needles contaminated with *Staphylococcus epidermidis* or *Staphylococcus aureus*; therefore, use of chlorhexidine should be strongly considered. Administration of antibiotics active against *S. aureus* and *S. epidermidis* to patients with risk factors has also been advocated. Needle passage should avoid superficial skin infections. The classic triad of fever, back pain or tenderness to palpation, and focal neurologic signs does not appear in all patients with epidural abscess. Most patients present with worsening back pain only, making a delay in diagnosis common. The clinician must maintain a high degree of suspicion in any patient complaining of back pain after an injection. Measurement of nonspecific markers of inflammation, such as sedimentation rate and C-reactive protein, are highly sensitive in identifying spinal infections. If epidural abscess is suspected, it is necessary to immediately perform MRI, CT, or CT myelography. These patients frequently need surgical intervention.

SYSTEMIC EFFECTS

Exposure to corticosteroids has both transient and long-term effects. Facial flushing and hyperglycemia have been reported after epidural corticosteroid injections. Long-term exposure to corticosteroids can result in more serious complications such as depression of the immune system, osteoporosis, and hypertension. Using the lowest dose that is likely to be effective should minimize systemic adverse effects. Corticosteroid injections should be limited to a reasonable number per patient per year.

TAKE HOME POINTS

- Epidural steroid injection is an established technique for the treatment of back and radicular pain. A variety of steroid agents and anatomic approaches are used.
- Mild complications include headache, vasovagal reactions, transient increase in pain, dural puncture, and systemic effects such as hyperglycemia.
- More serious complications include arachnoiditis, paralysis, infection, and the long-term systemic sequelae of steroid use.

SUGGESTED READINGS

Abram SE, O'Connor TC. Complications associated with epidural steroid injections. *Reg Anesth.* 1996;21:149–162.

Botwin KP, Gruber RD, Bouchlas CG, et al. Complications of fluoroscopically guided transforaminal lumbar epidural injections. *Arch Phys Med Rehabil.* 2000;81:1045–1050.

Hooten WM, Kinney MO, Huntoon MA. Epidural abscess and meningitis after epidural corticosteroid injection. *Mayo Clin Proc.* 2004;79:682–686.

Huntoon MA. Anatomy of the cervical intervertebral foramina: vulnerable arteries and ischemic neurologic injuries after transforaminal epidural injections. *Pain.* 2005;117:104–111.

Huntoon MA, Martin DP. Paralysis after transforaminal epidural injection and previous spinal surgery. *Reg Anesth Pain Med.* 2004;29:494–495.

Latham JM, Fraser RD, Moore RJ, et al. The pathologic effects of intrathecal betamethasone. *Spine.* 1997;22:1558–1562.

Manchikanti L. The value and safety of steroids in neural blockade, part 1. *Am J Pain Manage.* 2000;10:69–78.

Nelson D. Arachnoiditis from intrathecally given corticosteroids in the treatment of multiple sclerosis [letter]. *Arch Neurol.* 1976;33:373.

Tiso RL, Cutler T, Catania JA, et al. Adverse central nervous system sequelae after selective transforaminal block: the role of corticosteroids. *Spine. J* 2004;4:468–474.

Weingarten TN, Hooten WM, Huntoon MA. Septic facet joint arthritis after a corticosteroid facet injection. *Pain Med.* 2006;7:52–56.

Yentur EA, Luleci N, Topcu I, et al. Is skin disinfection with 10% povidone iodine sufficient to prevent epidural needle and catheter contamination? *Reg Anesth Pain Med.* 2003;28: 389–393.

172

CHEMICAL NEUROLYSIS HAS GOOD EFFICACY IN THE TREATMENT OF INTRACTABLE AND TERMINAL CANCER PAIN, BUT PRECISE ADMINISTRATION OF THE APPROPRIATE ANESTHETIC AND LYTIC AGENTS IS IMPERATIVE

LEENA MATHEW, MD

Chemical neurolysis involves the administration of a chemical agent that destroys nociceptive neural structures to create long-lasting analgesia. Neurolytic blocks are most often done in the setting of intractable pain due to cancer and inoperable chronic illnesses with a short life expectancy.

These agents may be used at peripheral nerves, paravertebral somatic nerves, along the sympathetic chain, or at various epidural or intrathecal levels. The rationale for choosing an agent is based on patient positioning factors. A diagnostic block using local anesthetic with amelioration of symptoms is essential prior to proceeding with neurolytic blocks. The success and duration of the block can vary anywhere from partial to excellent pain relief lasting from weeks to months, depending on the type of block, agent used, and the skill of the physician. The most common cause of an unsuccessful block is incorrect placement of the neurolytic agent.

Alcohol and phenol are the most commonly used neurolytic agents. Other agents, such as hypertonic saline, have also been tried with varying degrees of success.

PHENOL

Phenol is also known as carbolic acid. It is an aromatic compound with the chemical formula C6H5OH. It is comprised of a hydroxyl group bonded to a phenyl ring. It is prepared as a sterile, commercial-grade phenol in a maximum concentration of 6.7% solution in water. Although it has poor solubility in water, it is highly soluble in organic solvents such as alcohol and glycerol. The addition of small amounts of glycerol may increase its concentration to 15%. The shelf-life of phenol exceeds 1 year when the solution is refrigerated and not exposed to light. Phenol turns red on exposure to sunlight and air because of oxidation.

Phenol can be diluted with saline and is compatible when mixed with radiocontrast dye to allow fluoroscopic guidance during injection of the agent

ⓒ 2006 Mayo Foundation for Medical Education and Research

and to monitor spread of the solution. When mixed with glycerol, it slowly diffuses from the solution. With glycerol, phenol forms an extremely viscous hyperbaric solution from 4% to 10%. This is an advantage when injected intrathecally because it allows for limited spread localized in a small target area. For the injection of intrathecal phenol, the patient is placed in lateral decubitus position with the painful side down. When mixed with water, concentrations of 3% to 10% are possible. However, in this formulation, it is a more potent neurolytic with a wider spread.

The choice of diluents depends on the extent of neurolysis desired. At low concentrations, phenol has local anesthetic properties (the use of higher concentrations of phenol also predisposes to a higher incidence of vascular injury). With increasing concentrations, phenol causes increasing neural damage. At concentrations >5%, there is protein coagulation with segmental demyelination and Wallerian degeneration. At 6%, nociceptive fibers are lysed. With higher concentration, axonal abnormalities and nerve root damage are seen. Concentrations <5% may only provide a sensory block. Some studies have shown that 5% phenol is equipotent to 40% alcohol. Degeneration takes 14 days, and regeneration is complete in 14 weeks. Effects of the block cannot be evaluated until after 24 to 48 hours, to allow time for the local anesthetic effect of phenol to dissipate. The neurolytic effect may be clinically evident only after 3 to 7 days. If inadequate pain relief is obtained after 2 weeks, this may indicate incomplete neurolysis and require repetition of the procedure.

The subsequent fibrosis that occurs following phenol injection makes nerve regeneration more difficult, but not impossible. Nerve regeneration can occur as long as the nerve cell body is intact, at a rate of 1 to 3 mm/day. Nerve arborization and neuroma formation can occur at the site of nerve disruption and can be a focus of a neuropathic type of pain.

A wedge pillow is used to help roll the patient 45 degrees posteriorly so the dorsal column of the effected side is most inferior, or the painful side down. The bevel should face down and the injection must be done slowly because of the high viscosity of the drug. Warming the phenol can make it easier to inject. Phenol has systemic side effects, including central nervous system (CNS) stimulation, cardiovascular depression, nausea, and vomiting. Systemic doses of >600 mg can cause convulsive seizures and CNS depression. Doses <100 mg are less likely to cause serious side effects. Accidental intravascular injection causes tinnitus and flushing. Chronic toxicity can cause hepatic and renal damage. Phenol is metabolized in the liver by conjugation to glucuronides and oxidation to equinol compounds or to carbon dioxide and water. Excretion of metabolites is via the kidneys.

ALCOHOL

Ethyl alcohol has a destructive effect similar to phenol. In 1933, Labat and Greene noted that 33.3% alcohol injection produced satisfactory analgesia in the treatment of painful disorders. Alcohol is primarily used for intrathecal neurolysis, sympathetic blockade, celiac plexus block, and chemical hypophysectomy for patients with diffuse pain secondary to metastatic disease.

Its mechanism of nerve destruction is similar to phenol. Alcohol causes dehydration; extraction of phospholipids, cholesterol, and cerebrosides; and precipitation of mucoprotein and lipoprotein. This causes sclerosis, demyelination, and Wallerian degeneration of nociceptive structures.

Alcohol is available commercially as a 95% solution. Although 50% to 100% alcohol is used as a neurolytic agent, the minimum concentration required for neurolysis has not been established. A local anesthetic is commonly used as a diluent. Following its injection, the patient complains of severe burning pain along the nerve's distribution, which may last for a minute and is subsequently replaced by a warm, numb sensation.

It is hypobaric relative to cerebrospinal fluid. The patient is kept in the lateral decubitus position with the painful side up, and the patient is rolled forward by 45 degrees so the dorsal horn of the effected side is the most superior part of the spinal column. A tuberculin syringe is then used to inject alcohol in 0.1-mL increments. Each segment needs at least 0.3 mL per segment, is readily soluble in body tissues, and produces severe burning pain on injection. A maximum volume of 0.7 mL can be used at one session for intrathecal neurolysis. For the lysis of the sympathetic chain, more dilute concentration may be used, but larger volumes may be needed and up to 20 cc may be used.

It spreads quite rapidly from the injection site and requires 12 to 24 hours before the effects of the injection can be assessed. Similar to phenol, if inadequate pain relief is achieved after 2 weeks, the block should be repeated.

A concentration of 95% will reliably lyse sympathetic, sensory, and motor components of the nerve. Ninety to 98% of the injected alcohol is rapidly metabolized by oxidation in the liver principally by the enzyme alcohol dehydrogenase.

HYPERTONIC SALINE

The use of hypertonic saline by intrathecal injection to treat intractable pain was first reported by Hitchcock in 1967. The most commonly used solution is the 10% aqueous solution, and this is available as a pharmaceutical preparation. The mechanism of neurolysis is not well elaborated. It causes severe pain on injection, and local anesthetic is first injected before the saline solution. When administered intrathecally, hypertonic saline can cause an increase in intracranial pressure, increase in blood pressure, heart rate, and respiratory rate.

MISCELLANEOUS AGENTS

In the past, other agents have been used to promote neurolysis, including ammonium salt solutions, chlorocresol, and distilled water. However, their neurolytic effect is unpredictable, and their use is now relegated to history. Butyl aminobenzoate (Butamben) is a substance that has been reported to cause neurolysis and is under investigation.

INDICATIONS FOR CHRONIC NEUROLYSIS

- Management of chronic, intractable, nonterminal pain that is not responsive to other modalities
- Treatment of pain in patients who have short life expectancy (<1 year)
- Alternative management to treat spasticity in order to improve balance, gait, self-care, and global rehabilitation

SELECTION CRITERIA FOR INTRATHECAL NEUROLYSIS

- Well-established diagnosis
- Life expectancy: <12 months
- No response to conservative therapies
- Pain localized to two to three dermatomes
- Somatic pain
- Unilateral symptoms—if bilateral symptoms exist, then the intrathecal block should be staggered

Psychological evaluation is also important in completely evaluating the patient before neurolysis is considered. Extensive communication with the patient is necessary, and the risks and benefits of the procedure should be explained before proceeding. Understanding and acceptance of complications by the patient and the family is essential.

An important difference between neurolytic blocks for pain relief versus spasticity is that motor or mixed nerves are targeted preferentially in the management of spastic disorders.

COMPLICATIONS OF CHEMICAL NEUROLYSIS

Skin and Other Nontarget Tissue Necrosis and Sloughing. This is due to damage of the vascular supply to the skin, causing ischemia, and chronic trauma to denervated tissue. Necrosis of muscles, blood vessels, and other soft tissues has also been reported. Flush the needle with 0.2 mL of air prior to removal.

Neuritis. Partial destruction of the somatic nerve followed by its regeneration is responsible for neuritis. This complication has been reported as frequently as up to 10%. Neuritis is less likely to occur with a subarachnoid or ganglion neurolytic block. The symptoms of neuritis present as hyperesthesia and dysesthesia. Some patients may perceive the postneurolytic neuritis to be worse than the original pain problem. It is one of the limiting factors in the use of chemical neurolysis.

Anesthesia Dolorosa. Pain may persist in an area of anesthesia. The symptom is a poorly understood but well-established complication that patients must be warned of prior to proceeding with neurolytic blocks. It is probably a result of an imbalance in afferent input and the resultant central nervous system changes. A local anesthetic block done a few hours prior to the performance of the neurolytic block seems to prevent the development of this complication. The pain from this condition may be treated by the adjuvant analgesics such as tricyclic antidepressants, membrane stabilizing agents, and anticonvulsants.

Paralysis. This is the most feared major complication. It occurs infrequently and is usually temporary.

Perineal and Sexual Dysfunction. About 1.4% and 0.2% of patients will have bowel or bladder dysfunction at 1 week and 1 month, respectively. Usually, there is return of function.

Systemic Complications. Hypotension occurs secondary to vasodilatation after a sympathetic block. Thrombosis of vascular structures can occur if injected into or around major vessels. Hypertonic saline when administered intrathecally, causes an increase in the intracranial pressure, hypertension, tachycardia, and tachypnea.

TAKE HOME POINTS

- Chemical neurolysis is considered in patients with intractable pain refractory to other therapies.
- It is a useful analgesic modality in terminally ill patients with a life expectancy of <1 year.
- Alcohol and phenol are the most commonly used agents for neurolysis. The choice of agent depends largely on patient positioning factors.
- Prior to performing a neurolytic block, a diagnostic block should be done to demonstrate efficacy and symptomatic improvement.
- Phenol is hyperbaric, and alcohol is hypobaric.
- Phenol has intrinsic local anesthetic properties that render it painless during injection, unlike alcohol, which burns during injection.

■ The side effects can be varied and serious, ranging from skin necrosis and sloughing, vascular thrombosis, hypotension, neuritis to paraplegia, and loss of bowel and bladder function.

SUGGESTED READINGS

Bonica JJ. *Management of Pain.* 2nd ed. Philadelphia, Pa.: Lea & Febiger; 1990:1980–2039.
Candido K, Stevens RA. Intrathecal neurolytic blocks for the relief of cancer pain. *Best Pract Res Clin Anaesthesiol.* 2003;17(3):407–428.
de Leon-Casasola OA. Critical evaluation of chemical neurolysis of the sympathetic axis for cancer pain. *Cancer Control.* 2000;7(2):142–148.

173

UNDERSTANDING THE HUMAN FACTOR

F. Jacob Seagull, PhD

Have you ever accidentally poured orange juice in your cereal instead of milk? Have you ever tried to drive from work to the store and ended up driving home by accident? Most likely you have. Have you ever accidentally put sugar into your shoes instead of talcum powder? Probably not. Why not? Because "mistakes" do not happen randomly when humans are involved—they occur in systematic patterns. Some are likely, some are not.

Understanding how people think allows us to understand the types of mistakes that they might make and the types that they are unlikely to make. The study of how people act in the context of work—including the mistakes that they make—is known as "human factors."

Applying the principles of "human factors psychology" to the domain of anesthesia can create an environment in which a serious mistake is much less likely to occur. Giving the wrong drug should be like putting sugar in your shoes, not like putting juice in your cornflakes. Anesthesia has been at the forefront of human factors in the medical domain for a number of years, adopting safety initiatives, making continuous process improvements, and attaining advances that significantly reduced the likelihood of adverse events. Anesthesia has been singled out by the Institute of Medicine as the medical discipline that can serve as a model of "safety culture."

The concept of human factors has its roots in aviation. It was first used by the U.S. Air Force to help push human performance to the limit in order to beat the enemy. The fighter pilots in World War II were surrounded by advanced cockpit technology in life or death situations—not entirely unlike an anesthesiologist in an operating room. By designing the pilots' environment to support the task at hand, human factors helped give them the edge they needed.

The field of human factors is multidisciplinary, encompassing domains from psychology to engineering to anthropology to computer science and more. Many different aspects of human activity relevant to anesthesiology fall under the scope of human factors. A few of the more relevant aspects are described briefly in this chapter.

DECISION MAKING

People make decisions in a very different manner than computers. Instead of using precise calculations, people often use heuristics, or rules of thumb,

© 2006 Mayo Foundation for Medical Education and Research

to decide what to do. Heuristics can be a powerful tool that lets a person make quick decisions when relevant information is incomplete or unavailable. Unfortunately, there are times when using heuristics may lead to systematic biases in decision making, or put more simply, can make a mistake more likely. Human factors psychology has examined a wide array of decision-making aspects, including heuristics and biases. Through the application of human factors principles, one can remediate many common biases, leading to better, safer decisions in critical anesthesia situations.

TECHNOLOGY DESIGN AND COGNITIVE ERGONOMICS

In a fighter jet, well-designed avionics displays can mean the difference between a kill and a crash. In anesthesia, clear monitoring displays, easy-to-program infusion pumps, and clearly identifiable syringes and drugs can have a similar effect. Technology designed with human factors' "cognitive ergonomics" considerations can reduce the likelihood of making an error and improve the odds of recovering from adverse events.

COMMUNICATION

Human perceptual abilities have their limits and weaknesses. Whether interacting with a piece of technology or with another human, people must take in and make sense of information in the environment and convert the perceptual signals into concepts and knowledge about the world. Application of the principles of human factors can cater to human perception's strengths and compensate for perceptual weaknesses, facilitating clear, concise, and error free communication.

ENVIRONMENTAL DESIGN

It is easier to place a central line in a quiet, calm, well-lit room than in the shadow of a noisy code team during an emergency resuscitation. Environmental factors such as noise, lighting, and work space layout can influence the margin of safety in which care is provided.

COMPLEX SYSTEMS

Each individual artifact with which we interact undoubtedly influences the ultimate success or failure of our endeavors. However, beyond these individual influences, there is an overarching interaction among the multitude of systems, artifacts, and people that can have an influence greater than the sum of the parts. Ultimately, it is most often a system failure, and not a failure in the function or design of an individual artifact, that leads to catastrophic failure and adverse events in anesthesia. Human factors addresses issues arising from the complexity of highly coupled technical systems, and can help offer effective system design, or even impart effective strategies for interacting with flawed systems.

Understanding some key aspects of human factors can provide you with points of leverage in critical situations, and perhaps more importantly, can help you prepare yourself properly to avoid critical situations before they arise. The chapters in this unit touch on a small selection of relevant topic areas where consideration of human factors can contribute to safe and effective practice of anesthesia care.

TAKE HOME POINTS

- Mistakes do not happen randomly but rather in systematic patterns.
- The Institute of Medicine paper that singled out anesthesia as the medical discipline that can serve as a model of "safety culture" is an important document that is now driving much of the pay-for-performance/quality movement.
- Anesthesia providers at all levels will increasingly be called on to understand, master, and integrate the basic principles of human factors psychology into the delivery of anesthetic care.

SUGGESTED READINGS

Botney R, Gaba DM. Human factors issues in monitoring. In: Blitt C, ed. *Monitoring in Anesthesia and Intensive Care*. New York, NY: Churchill-Livingstone; 1994:23–54.

Kohn L, Corrigan J, Donaldson M, eds. *To Err Is Human: Building a Safer Health System*. Washington, DC: Committee on Quality of Health Care in America, Institute of Medicine, National Academy Press; 2000.

Norman DA. *The Design of Everyday Things*. New York, NY: Currency/Doubleday; 1988.

Reason J. *Human Error*. Cambridge, UK: Cambridge University Press; 1990.

174

LEARN FROM THE PILOTS TO MINIMIZE ERRORS IN ANESTHESIA MANAGEMENT: RECOGNITION AND PREVENTION

STEPHEN J. GLEICH, BS (MSIII) AND
JURAJ SPRUNG, MD, PHD

Crew resource management (CRM), also known as crisis resource management, emphasizes a team approach to managing a situation in which the role of human factors is considered. Included in the CRM model are the effects of fatigue, predictable perceptual errors (e.g., misreading monitors or mishearing instructions), and the effects of various management and organizational styles in high-stress, high-risk environments. Originally developed in the aviation industry, CRM training fosters a unified environment with effective communication in which junior personnel are unconstrained about alerting others when something is amiss. If an error occurs, the goal of the team is to capture the error before it progresses and causes an adverse event.[1]

APPLICATION OF AVIATION-ADOPTED CREW RESOURCE MANAGEMENT TO ANESTHESIA PRACTICE

The practice of anesthesiology and the operation of commercial aircraft share some key characteristics: interaction with team members, continuous monitoring, and standard operating procedures (SOPs). The aviation industry has taken great strides in enhancing safety by adopting and implementing CRM in the 1980s. Likewise, these safety procedures captured interest in the anesthesia community as a method for decreasing risk to patients.

In 1978, a commercial airliner experienced a minor landing gear indicator malfunction, which required the crew to troubleshoot the problem before landing. The aircraft was low on fuel, and even with the installation of new digital fuel gauges and warnings, the three-person crew did not realize the low fuel situation until the engines began to flame out. The flight circled the airport until the plane ran out of fuel and crashed. The experienced crew was focused on resolving the landing gear problem, did not coordinate their actions, and did not identify another developing adverse event, even in the presence of modern technology.

The widespread adoption of CRM principles can decrease adverse events in aviation and in the perioperative setting. Adverse events are rarely

---

[1]Data from Helmreich RL. On error management: lessons from aviation. *BMJ* 2000;320:781–785; Gaba DM. Anaesthesiology as a model for patient safety in health care. *BMJ* 2000;320:785–788.

caused by a single factor and typically occur when a number of conditions are met. According to Rampersad and Rampersad, adverse events often occur along the following trajectory of adversity:

1) A catalyst event (e.g., landing gear malfunction vs. patient oxyhemoglobin desaturation).
2) A system fault (e.g., failure of the new digital fuel gauges to alert the crew to a low fuel situation vs. failure of the pulse oximete. alarm to alert the anesthesiologist of the desaturation).
3) Loss of situational awareness (e.g., cockpit crew was focused on the landing gear problem vs. anesthesiologist preoccupied with charting and does not recognize the desaturation).
4) Human error (e.g., lack of recognition of the low fuel situation vs. lack of continuous monitoring of the vital signs by the anesthesiologist).

Barriers to adverse events that exist in the operating room include technology, SOPs, proficiency, and judgment. An adverse event can be thought of as a ball rolling down a hill. Technology, SOP, proficiency, and judgment represent barriers to stop the ball (*Fig. 174.1*). At any time, the ball can be stopped by recognition and resolution of the event by one of the four barriers. If the ball continues to roll past the barriers, an adverse event occurs. The angle of the hill (steepness) can also be modified. Anesthesiologist

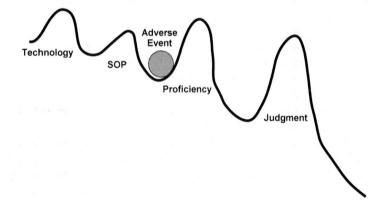

FIGURE 174.1. Dynamic error model. The ball represents an adverse event. Any one of the four barriers (peaks) can prevent the ball from rolling down the hill. If the ball rolls over all four hills, an adverse event occurs. (From Rampersad C, Rampersad SE. Crew resource management for people who don't fly the airplane. Presented at the Society for Pediatric Anesthesia winter meeting; Fort Myers, Fla.; February 17, 2006. Available at: http://www.pedsanesthesia.org/meetings/2006winter/pdfs/Friday_Rampersad_Crew%20Resources.pdf. Accessed March 30, 2007. Used with permission.)

fatigue increases the slope of the hill, allowing the ball to more easily pass through the four barriers. Higher patient acuity, such as elevated American Society of Anesthesiologists physical status, similarly increases the slope because the higher acuity of disease makes these patients less able to tolerate errors.

Certain behaviors in the operating room increase risk to patients. According to Helmreich, failures of CRM can be divided into four categories: communication, leadership, conflict, and vigilance.

Communication

■ Failure to inform the team of the patient's problem (e.g., surgeon fails to inform anesthesiologist of surgical bleeding before a decrease in blood pressure is observed).

■ Failure to discuss alternative procedures (e.g., patient is high risk for the selected procedure, and an alternative, less-invasive approach could be performed).

Leadership

■ Failure to establish leadership in the operating room team (e.g., anesthesiologist does not direct the actions of other team members during an intraoperative cardiac arrest).

Conflict

■ Overt hostility and frustration (e.g., patient deteriorates while surgeon and anesthesiologist argue over who is responsible for newly developed tension pneumothorax).

Vigilance

■ Failure to monitor situation and other team member activities (e.g., distracted anesthesiologist fails to detect decrease in blood pressure after a monitor power failure; anesthesiologist treats hypertension while the transducer is "sitting" on the floor).

■ Failure to plan for lapsed vigilance (e.g., anesthesiologist does not have appropriate resuscitation drugs ready).

CRM applied to the anesthesia and operating room team encompasses the effective integration and practice of these components. The practice of anesthesiology is amenable to improvement, and many elements of safety enhancements in the aviation industry are applicable. Integration of CRM practices in every operating room is vital to ensure prevention and effective management of adverse events.

SUGGESTED READINGS

Agency for Healthcare Research and Quality, U.S. Department of Health & Human Services. PSNet Patient Safety Network: A National Patient Safety Resource. Available at: http://psnet.ahrq.gov/glossary.aspx. Accessed March 30, 2007.

Gaba DM, Fish KJ, Howard SK. *Crisis Management in Anesthesiology*. New York, NY: Churchill Livingstone; 1994.

Helmreich RL. On error management: lessons from aviation. *BMJ*. 2000;320:781–785.

National Transportation Safety Board. Aircraft Accident Report, United Airlines, Inc., Douglas DC-8, N8082U, Portland, Oregon, 1978 Dec 28. NTSB Public Docket, 1979.

Rampersad C, Rampersad SE. Crew resource management for people who don't fly the airplane. Presented at the Society for Pediatric Anesthesia winter meeting; Fort Myers, Fla.; February 17, 2006. Available at: http://www.pedsanesthesia.org/meetings/2006winter/pdfs/Friday_Rampersad_Crew%20Resources.pdf. Accessed March 30, 2007.

175

IN A NOISY OPERATING ROOM, USE A "SPELLING ALPHABET" TO COMMUNICATE THE PATIENT'S NAME OR CHECK IN BLOOD PRODUCTS

CATHERINE MARCUCCI, MD, DANIEL T. MURRAY, CRNA, AND F. JACOB SEAGULL, PhD

You are about to deliver anesthesia in a chaotic emergency situation. The operating room (OR) desk paged you in the cafeteria to tell you that a patient is coming over from the floor with a carotid blowout. The surgical intern is riding on the stretcher to apply pressure to the bleeder. You are told that there are blood products in the blood bank but that you have to call down there stat and let them know what to pack in the cooler. The problem is, you don't know the name of the patient. You ask the person who is on the OR desk to identify the patient, but due to background noise in both the OR and the cafeteria, you cannot catch the name she says. It might be Atkins, it might be Adkins, or it might be Adams. You just can't hear. You ask several times, each time a little louder. She replies, each time a little louder. You still can't hear the name, and you feel yourself getting tachycardic. Suddenly, on the telephone, you hear the calm voice of your CRNA colleague (who served as a U.S. Air Force medic in Vietnam), saying slowly, "The patient is Alpha-Delta-Kilo-India-November-Sierra." Armed with the correct information, you place the appropriate call to the blood bank. Mr. Adkins does fine.

Spelling alphabets are also commonly called radio alphabets, telegraph alphabets, or police letters. There are a number of different versions, but each uses a single phonetically distinct word to replace the name of the letter with which it starts. Spelling alphabets have their origins deep in military and communications history, and have been used at least since the beginning of the 20th century. They arose because early aviation and military radios were plagued by static. Because so many letters in the English language are phonetically similar (e.g., *B, C, E, T, D, P*), a burst of static would have made it impossible to accurately transmit letter-based information. Thus, in World War II, the sequence *B-E-D* would have been "called" as Baker-Echo-Dog. Spelling alphabets are used in at least 30 languages (from Finnish to Urdu), and there is a numeric code as well. Spelling alphabets are often called phonetic alphabets, but this is actually a misnomer. Phonetic alphabets are written representations of spoken sound as opposed to spoken representations of written symbols.

ⓒ 2006 Mayo Foundation for Medical Education and Research

ORs are noisy places. Decibel levels have been measured under a variety of situations and for different types of procedures. The "average" noise in a routine case will approach 70 to 80 db. In certain orthopedic procedures, such as total joint replacement, noise levels are routinely 110 db, which is the same level of noise in some boiler rooms, and will intermittently approach 140 db, which is high enough to put the surgeons (and other OR staff) at risk for occupationally associated hearing loss.

Operating noise is known to have detrimental effects on anesthesia providers. In a study by Murthy et al., when anesthesia residents were exposed to a 90-minute cassette of OR noise at 77 db, they had lower scores on tests for mental efficiency and short-term memory. More important, the same noise level significantly affected both speech reception threshold and speech discrimination, which led researchers to conclude that there is a marked decrease in the ability to discriminate spoken words at ambient OR noise levels. The use of a spelling alphabet may, therefore, have the same efficacy for anesthesia providers as for the military and pilots.

TABLE 175.1	NATO SPELLING ALPHABET
A	**ALPHA**
A	Alpha
B	Bravo
C	Charlie
D	Delta
E	Echo
F	Foxtrot
G	Golf
H	Hotel
I	India
J	Juliet
K	Kilo
L	Lima
M	Mike
N	November
O	Oscar
P	Papa
Q	Quebec
R	Romeo
S	Sierra
T	Tango
U	Uniform
V	Victor
W	Whiskey
X	X-ray
Y	Yankee
Z	Zulu

The spelling alphabet used in World War II was modernized in the 1950s, as military pilots returned to their civilian careers. The most commonly used alphabet today is known as the international radiotelephony or NATO spelling alphabet (*Table 175.1*). It is simple to memorize and easy to use.

TAKE HOME POINTS

- The noisy OR introduces the possibility of verbal miscommunication and is a cause of errors and breaches in patient safety.
- The spelling alphabet is a time-tested method of more accurately transmitting letter-based information.
- If you ever check in blood with a veteran (especially one who has been in a combat area), he or she will use it automatically.

SUGGESTED READINGS

Lingard L, Espin S, Whyte S, et al. Communication failures in the operating room: an observational classification of recurrent types and effects. *Qual Saf Health Care.* 2004;13(5): 330-334.

Love H. Noise exposure in the orthopaedic operating theatre: a significant health hazard. *Aust N Z J Surg.* 2003;73(10):836-838.

Murthy VS, Malhotra SK, Bala I, et al. Auditory functions in anaesthesia residents during exposure to operating room noise. *Indian J Med Res.* 1995;101:213–216.

Murthy VS, Malhotra SK, Bala I, et al. Detrimental effects of noise on anaesthetists. *Can J Anaesth.* 1995;42(7):608–711.

176

KNOW WHEN TO STOP—PATIENTS CAN BE SERIOUSLY INJURED NOT BECAUSE THE ANESTHESIA PROVIDERS CAN'T DO SOMETHING BUT BECAUSE THEY CAN'T STOP TRYING

F. JACOB SEAGULL, PhD AND CATHERINE MARCUCCI, MD

Here is a situation that must be avoided at all costs: An anesthesia team is genuinely surprised and has unexpected difficulty intubating a patient. A mask airway is established, and one more attempt is made to intubate the patient. A reasonable safety limit is set—the team members say to each other, "Okay, you are going to try once more and I am going to try once more and then we are going to stop." However, by this time, there are several other providers in the room who have brought additional airway equipment. When the two additional attempts are unsuccessful, the safety limit is disregarded in order to keep trying. Later, albeit with great difficulty, the airway is managed by mask and the patient is awakened. Unfortunately, such difficulty and violation of safety limits can occur with airway attempts, regional block techniques, and invasive line placements. The question is why? Why do high-skilled practitioners who know the risks set a limit and then go over it?

There are two central explanations for this phenomenon, both of which deal with people's tendency to consistently make decisions that are not rational. There is a whole field of psychology, formally called the psychology of decision making, that explores the consistent ways in which people's minds are irrational. Here are two examples, both of which are classics in decision making.

The first is the concept of "sunk cost." Sunk cost is the initial investment in an endeavor—the cost can sometimes be financial, but it can also consist of effort or time invested. Having invested in something, people are much less willing to walk away from it, even if the gain from further investment is not worth the risk. The process is sometimes called "throwing good money after bad." Once a bad investment is made, extreme (often futile) measures will be undertaken to turn the loss into a gain. The proper strategy is to cut one's losses. It is much easier for a second anesthesiologist to enter a room after someone else has given three attempts and say, "Okay, let's change tactics," than it is for an individual who has made attempts to "admit defeat."

© 2006 Mayo Foundation for Medical Education and Research

Second, a more global theory of decision making under uncertainty is prospect theory, which generally revolutionized decision-making theory. One tenet of prospect theory is that people are much more willing to gamble and take chances to avoid loss than they are to gamble to reap gains. The idea is that "losses hurt more than gains comfort." People are actually quite sensitive to their perception of whether something is a loss or a gain. One way of countering this tendency to be biased is to "reframe" the decision (e.g., "You aren't losing a daughter, you are gaining a son-in-law."). So, think of framing the failed intubation as a "gain" of a preserved airway instead of a "loss" of the previous efforts; you are more likely to get someone to change his or her mind and abandon the risky persistence. "Putting the patient first" may help.

What can you do? Think of the patient. Avoid the failure of creating injury or bodily insult. Bring in a fresh pair of eyes—someone who has not "invested" in the situation and who can think in an unbiased manner. Last, understand that futile persistence is itself a loss of good practice.

TAKE HOME POINTS

- Practitioners in all fields, including anesthesia, will have a tendency to consistently make decisions that are not rational.
- Be aware and understand the concept of sunk cost—having invested in something, people are much less willing to walk away from it, even if the gain from further investment is not worth the risk.
- Prospect theory states that people are much more willing to gamble and take chances to avoid loss than they are to gamble to reap gains. The idea is that "losses hurt more than gains comfort."
- When you find yourself in a difficult clinical situation that involves failed attempts at a procedure, including intubation, keep these principles in mind. Bring in unbiased practitioners to help you make the decision to stop if necessary.

SUGGESTED READINGS

Arkes H, Blumer C. The psychology of sunk cost. *Organ Behav Hum Decis Process.* 1985;35: 124–140.
Kahneman D, Tversky A. Prospect theory: an analysis of decision under risk. *Econometrica.* 1979;47(2):263–292.
Tversky A, Kahneman D. Advances in prospect theory: cumulative representation of uncertainty. *J Risk Uncertainty.* 1992;5:297–323.

177

FOLKLORE CAN BE A POWERFUL ALLY—SHARE STORIES AND DON'T FORGET TO LISTEN

F. JACOB SEAGULL, PHD, DEBORAH DLUGOSE, RN, CCRN, CRNA, AND CATHERINE MARCUCCI, MD

People may understand statistics, but they believe stories. Imagine you are supervising a junior resident during an eye procedure and the patient exhibits a significant oculocardiac reflex with a heart rate of 17 bpm that is unresponsive to atropine. It is your practice to have a syringe of epinephrine 10 mcg/cc available on your cart, and the patient responds to a 2-cc bolus. The next day in a vascular bypass operation, you are supervising another junior resident, and give epinephrine 20 mcg to good result for a near "flat line" of the electrocardiogram and arterial line tracings after reperfusion of the lower extremities. The resident (who heard stories about the previous case) asks whether you always have low-dose epinephrine available and, if so, why. You reply that when you were in training, one of your favorite faculty members said to you, "Always be able to get your hands on 20 mcg of epinephrine within 2 seconds. You may only need it twice in 5 years, but when you need it, you need that and only that, and you need it fast."

The stories that we tell, or folklore, can be an indispensable part of our clinical practice. Cultural scientists and sociologists actually recognize several types of folklore; the subset most relevant to the field of anesthesia is known by the scientific term of "institutional memory." *Institutional memory* is defined as a collective of facts, concepts, experiences, and plain old-fashioned know-how held by a group of people. It is transmitted (often orally) by senior members of the group to junior members, but just as often it is transmitted through the stories shared among veteran care providers around the water cooler or in the anesthesia break room. Institutional memory can be facilitative to a group's "way of work," preserve a desired ideology, or be maladaptive—if too heavily established, it can make change difficult in the face of new information and input to the system.

The value of institutional memory and the importance of lore in maintaining patient safety have been established in anesthetic practice on many levels. Although morbidity and mortality seminars are one type of story, they often leave out an essential narrative that carries value: the personal experience. Pearls of wisdom that have been developed through folk tales and anesthesia "mythology" can be a source of useful information. In this raw

© 2006 Mayo Foundation for Medical Education and Research

form of folklore, the information distilled through the experience of others is concentrated and often powerful. Telling co-workers a personal story of a specific patient "going south" in a narrative can provide the valuable context that will help that person recognize the diagnosis when they encounter it themselves.

Stories can have an effect beyond conveying the clinical facts. Stories of an attending thanking the nurse that stopped a procedure when the nurse noticed the attending's breach of sterile practice send a powerful message that patient safety is more important than the caregiver's ego. Stories of the nurse being recognized for excellence by the institution create a folklore about the values of the institution, promulgating the values of the workplace.

Although institutional memory and folklore are frequently based on factual information, almost by definition they are anecdotally based and not outcomes based or verified by rigorous trials. The advantages of this are that the information is often vividly presented and therefore quite memorable— the human mind is wired to remember stories, not facts. Judgment is often biased by the "salience" heuristic, in which conspicuous or dramatic events are easily recalled. Use the bias to your advantage: By telling a compelling story, it becomes more likely that the story will be recalled when a person needs to retrieve relevant information. The disadvantages are that anesthesia providers must maintain an open but discerning mind and a healthy skepticism.

Sometimes the folklore even "turns out to be true." One interesting piece of folklore that crossed into the realm of the peer-reviewed literature in recent years involves the long-perceived difficulties in giving anesthesia to redheads. For years, the anecdotal tradition said that anesthetizing redheads was more challenging. In 2004, Liem et al. reported that desflurane requirements for noxious electrical stimulation were significantly higher in redheaded women as opposed to dark-haired women. They were able to establish that 9 of 10 redheaded women were either homozygous or compound heterozygotes for mutations on the melanocortin-1 receptor gene. They concluded that red hair appears to be a phenotype linked to increased anesthetic requirement that can also be traced to a specific genotype. It was also subsequently reported that redheaded women have increased sensitivity to thermal pain and manifest reduced subcutaneous lidocaine efficacy.

The value of folklore in the practice of anesthesia and the training of anesthesia providers should not be underestimated. The folklore you hear will depend on where you trained (*Table 177.1*). Gather as much as you can and remember that it is not all true, although there is frequently at least a kernel of truth. Try to always place it within proper and accepted practice parameters, and use whatever you can to make your practice safer and more consistent.

TABLE 177.1	FOLKLORE MAXIMS IN THE PRACTICE OF ANESTHESIA
TOPIC	**HELPFUL FOLKLORE**
Understanding patients	▪ Patients who go to sleep crying, wake up crying. ▪ Dads can cry just as much as moms. ▪ Make your pediatric patients as pristine as possible when wheeling by the parents' waiting room. ▪ Patients are heavily influenced by the prior anesthetic experiences of their friends and family.
Monitoring	▪ If you really want to know what is going on, look at the patient, not the monitor. ▪ If you cannot get the radial artery line, you are almost always too lateral. ▪ Follow urine output avidly–the Foley catheter is not just there to keep the urine off your shoes.
Going south	▪ If the acuity of the case starts to escalate, stand up. ▪ In a certain way, as the surgical case gets more acute, the anesthesia case gets simpler, until at the bottom of every algorithm are oxygen and epinephrine.
Managing cases	▪ There is a secret to making every case go well—your job is to find the secret and then not let go of it no matter what else is happening in the case. ▪ It is better to do a difficult case in a happy room than an easy case in an unhappy room. ▪ Make all parts of the anesthesia case "match" each other and always match the severity of the surgical case. ▪ Even if circumstances force you to "rush" on an aspect of a case, never rush on the airway. ▪ Patients will usually be okay if they do all right (meaning that some patients can pull through only if there are no complications). ▪ If you want train tracks, give your fluids and narcotics up front. ▪ Fentanyl is for tubes; morphine is for laryngeal mask airways.
Philosophy	▪ You do not work for the surgeon, you work for the patient. ▪ Do not put anything on the patient that you would not put on yourself. ▪ The only two drugs that are so good that every patient needs them are oxygen and ondansetron, and even they have contraindications. ▪ The reason an anesthesia provider goes to work is provide access, airway, and precise administration of dangerous drugs—focus your energies and efforts on making these aspects of the case go smoothly.

One final note: Here are two pieces of folklore that are *so true,* they deserve special mention:

■ "When you choose your anesthetic, you choose your complications." – Stephen Robinson, MD

■ "Never be scared alone; invite all your friends." –Kenneth R. Abbey, MD

SUGGESTED READINGS

Beyea SC, Killen A, Knox GE. Learning from stories—a pathway to patient safety. *AORN J.* 2004;79(1):224–226. (Republished: *AORN J* 2006;84[suppl 1]:S10–S12.)

Dawes R. A message from psychologists to economists: mere predictability doesn't matter like it should (without a good story appended to it). *J Econ Behav Organ.* 1999;39:29–40.

Liem EB, Lin CM, Suleman MI, et al. Anesthetic requirement is increased in redheads. *Anesthesiology.* 2004;101:279–283.

Newman TB. The power of stories over statistics. *BMJ.* 2003;327(7429):1424–1427.

Rooksby J, Gerry RM, Smith AF. Incident reporting schemes and the need for a good story. *Int J Med Inform.* 2007;76S1:205–211. Epub 2006 Sep 7.

Tversky A, Kahneman D. Judgment under uncertainty: heuristics and biases. *Science.* 1974;185: 1124–1131.

DON'T IGNORE YOUR INTUITION

F. JACOB SEAGULL, PHD AND CATHERINE MARCUCCI, MD

Something doesn't feel right. You can't put your finger on why, but something about the patient's status just seems wrong. You look at the monitors and there are no alarms going off, and the patient's vital signs appear to be normal... but things just don't feel right. What should you do?

The answer is that there is no one best answer.

When you are able to gather data and analyze your options, you can spend time seeking additional information, running tests, and using tools such as decision aids to help you. Using decision aids and standard protocols for treatment can avoid some of the common biases that plague human decision-making powers, as discussed in Chapter 177. Unless you have time, don't trust your gut.

However, anesthesiology often operates under time pressure and in situations where complete data are not available. When time is short and you suspect that a problem is developing, trusting your intuition may be the best option.

Intuition is increasingly recognized as an important component of decision making. But what is intuition, exactly? It is the ability to judge a situation on the basis of information that is activated in memory but not consciously retrieved. People making decisions often recognize patterns of information without consciously naming those patterns.

There is little or no information on intuition in the anesthesia peer-reviewed literature. However, since the 1990s, researchers have looked at its role in a number of other areas including firefighting, industrial and chemical processing plants, corporate and business planning, nursing units, and pilot and military situations (the nursing and military studies are perhaps the most relevant to anesthesia care). Gary Klein is one author in the field of recognition primed, or "naturalistic," decision making who has published a number of interesting recent studies. He estimates that as many as 95% of decisions in naval aviation (specifically those of the antiaircraft warfare operators in the AEGIS Cruiser) involve recognition of a specific situation, not a choice between alternative actions. He has also studied the phenomenon of neonatal intensive care nurses "sensing" when a baby's health was deteriorating before any tests or monitors picked up on the problems. Klein was actually able to determine what cues the nurses were subconsciously

© 2006 Mayo Foundation for Medical Education and Research

picking up on in making their "intuitive" diagnoses. Also, although the exact mechanisms underlying intuitive judgments are still under discussion, it has been established that study subjects can make intuitive judgments about linking coherent or disqualifying incoherent data triads in as little time as a few seconds.

Similarly, anesthesia providers should be aware of the role that intuition may play in the delivery of anesthesia care and the possible consequences of ignoring it. The authors suggest that there are several clinical situations where a flash of intuition commonly occurs.

The first of these involves assessment of the patient's overall health status. What you say to your anesthesia colleagues is important—a simple comment of "this guy doesn't look so perky" or "it's not going to be so easy to wake this lady up" probably reflects a set of subtle clinical signs, including the appearance of mucous membranes, skin turgor, mental status, and respiratory pattern. The second circumstance involves airway evaluation. Often, the first glimmer of an impression about an airway proves to be the most reliable, formed just in the instant when you catch a glimpse of the patient through an operating room window or as he or she comes into the room. Often, what you think seems ridiculously simple, such as "that's a really big tongue" or perhaps you feel a slight sense of anxiety. The third situation arises when you thought "this patient needs an arterial line, definitely" and then have trouble with placement. Sometimes, a surgeon will ask whether the patient really does need the arterial line and then a discussion begins that may end in changing the plan.

Trusting your intuition does not mean ignoring the data that you have, or data that are available to you. Intuition stems from information gathered, processing the right aspects of the data, and recognizing the pattern created. Intuition is not a magical gift of clairvoyance but rather a skill that can be developed through practice and experience. One way of developing intuition is by gaining a wide array of divergent experiences to foster recognition.

Certainly, intuition cannot and should never substitute completely for a carefully thought out and articulated anesthetic plan that is based on the available outcomes-based evidence. In fact, a part of intuition stems from having a good contingency plan for unexpected events—with a plan, you will be primed to look for relevant cues and able to respond by confirming your "gut" with data. Most experienced anesthesia providers, however, can relate cases and circumstances in which they ignored that first flash of intuition to their later regret.

TAKE HOME POINTS

■ Intuition is real and can be an important component of decision making.

- Intuition is not just guessing, it is based on subconscious pattern recognition.
- Trusting your gut is not the same as ignoring evidence—intuition can help you when no other data are available.
- Varied experiences and careful contingency plans help you use "intuition" to recognize situations correctly and respond to them appropriately.

SUGGESTED READINGS

Bolte A, Goschke T. On the speed of intuition: intuitive judgments of semantic coherence under different response deadlines. *Mem Cognit.* 2005;33(7):1248–1255.

Bonabeau E. Don't trust your gut. *Harvard Bus Rev.* 2003;May:116–123.

Dahlgren VA, Kaempf GL, Klein G, et al. Decision making in complex naval command-and-control environments. *Hum Factors.* 1996;38(2):220–231.

Klein G. *Intuition at Work: Why Developing Your Gut Instincts Will Make You Better at What You Do.* New York, NY: Doubleday/Currency Books; 2003.

Ruth-Sahd LA, Hendy HM. Predictors of novice nurses' use of intuition to guide patient care decisions. *J Nurs Educ.* 2005;44(10):450–458.

Zsambok CE, Klein G, eds. *Naturalistic Decision Making.* Mahwah, NJ: Lawrence Erlbaum; 1997.

179

DO NOT RELY ON ROTE MEMORIZATION OF CONTRAINDICATIONS

ERIK S. ECKMAN, MD, PETER ROCK, MD, MBA, AND
F. JACOB SEAGULL, PhD

Developing expertise in the practice of anesthesia, as with any other highly specialized field, involves memorizing facts and recognizing situations. It has long been recognized by educators and psychologists that memorizing facts is easier when the student or trainee has a cognitive framework into which the facts fit. This is nowhere more true than in the practice of medicine and the subspecialty of anesthesiology. Knowing the principles behind a physiological system will help the anesthesia practitioner not only remember but also understand the individual items that must be recalled. For example, knowing the anatomy of the subclavian vein and the fact that it would be difficult to apply direct pressure to it (or other reasons) will help you remember that coagulopathy is a contraindication to placing a central venous catheter in the subclavian site. Understanding why congestive heart failure (CHF) patients should not lie flat should prevent you from placing them in the Trendelenburg position, even if you do not initially remember that CHF can also be a contraindication for subclavian catheterization.

Recognition of a specific situation can be a powerful tool. Knowing what cues to look for in a situation is a major part of making good decisions. Knowing patient pathology, recognizing unusual circumstances, or even thinking that things that do not "feel" right could and should be hints to the junior anesthesia practitioner to slow down and actively search for reasons that something might be or go wrong. If you feel uncomfortable entering a situation (see Chapter 178), then it might be a good time to think about contingency plans. This feeling can be a signal that you should actively generate a list of contraindications to the procedure or therapy you are considering. Ask yourself what could go wrong, what you can do to prevent a problem, and how you can effectively respond to a problem when it arises. Generating "what could go wrong" scenarios can lead to better decision making and allow you to respond more gracefully to adverse events.

Fortunately, absolute contraindications in anesthetic practice are relatively few. They often involve either a commonly used drug, such as succinylcholine, or a rarely seen medical disease, such as scleroderma or acute intermittent porphyria. When confronted with an absolute contraindication

© 2006 Mayo Foundation for Medical Education and Research

in a clinical situation, the anesthesia practitioner should not only "know" the specifics of the contraindication but also take steps to "rule out" the contraindication, with the use of a forcing function. Several familiar examples of this involve the use of items on a "latexfree" cart for a patient with a latex allergy or the physical removal of all vials of succinylcholine from the anesthesia cart if there is a strong contraindication. Similarly, when caring for a patient with acute intermittent porphyria, consider writing out a list of medications considered safe or probably safe and then using only those drugs on the list.

Relative contraindications in the practice of anesthesia are much more common than the very strong or absolute contraindications. Usually, they involve the exercise of more judgment, and as such, must always be placed in the context of the appropriate risk–benefit analysis. If you are discussing a proposed anesthetic plan with a senior anesthesia provider and she says something to the effect of "Well, you *can* do that, but you don't want to if you don't have to and you must be very careful," take the time to discuss the pros, cons, risks, benefits, and factors that will ultimately determine the final decision.

Finally, remember that contraindicated medications and procedures for children and in the obstetrics suite can be *very different* from those for the general adult surgical population. Generally, the list of what should or must be avoided for these patient populations is more extensive. Again, simply knowing and regularly reviewing a few key facts, such as the anatomy and innervation of the pediatric airway or the physiological changes of pregnancy, will provide a good start to understanding what not to do.

ABSOLUTE OR STRONG CONTRAINDICATIONS IN ANESTHESIA PRACTICE

- The use of succinylcholine in a patient who has sustained a burn with a total body surface area >10% can lead to hyperkalemia if given between 24 hours and 1 year after the burn.
- In patients with known or suspected malignant hyperthermia (MH), or suspected myopathy, inhalation anesthetic agents and succinylcholine may precipitate MH.
- Because they are metabolized by pseudocholinesterase, succinylcholine and mivacurium are contraindicated in patients with pseudocholinesterase deficiency.
- The use of succinylcholine is contraindicated in patients with conditions that upregulate acetylcholine receptors, which can greatly increase sensitivity to depolarizing muscle relaxants and lead to life-threatening hyperkalemia. Conditions that can produce this receptor upregulation include

upper or lower motor neuron injuries, simple immobilization, infection (e.g., muscle paralysis from *Clostridium botulinum* toxin), and burns. This upregulation can cause hyperkalemia with succinylcholine administration in a dose-dependent fashion as early as 48 hours postinjury and may last 1 to 2 years after injury recovery.

- Barbiturates can precipitate porphyria in susceptible persons.
- The use of high-concentration oxygen delivered via face mask in a procedure with electrocautery around the face is contraindicated due to concern for ignition of electrocautery sparks.
- The use of naloxone in opioid-dependent patients can cause opioid withdrawal.
- The use of nitrous oxide is contraindicated in patients with known or suspected pneumothorax because nitrous oxide can cause expansion of an enclosed gas-filled space. Following is a personal anecdote from Dr. Norman Cohen, who is one of the editors of this book: In the only case of mine where I caused a pneumothorax during placement of an interscalene block, I didn't realize it until the end of the case when the patient had some dyspnea. I had used nitrous oxide, which probably turned a small pneumothorax into a clinically significant one. As a result, I don't use nitrous oxide anymore on any patient after any needle procedures in the neck or subclavian region.
- Ketamine is contraindicated in patients with increased intracranial pressure (ICP) because it increases cerebral metabolic rate of oxygen ($CMRO_2$), cerebral blood flow, and ICP.
- An absolute contraindication to neuraxial blockade is patient refusal. Relative contraindications include shock or hypovolemia (increases the risk of hypotension), increased ICP (increases the risk of brain herniation if cerebrospinal fluid is lost), coagulopathy or thrombocytopenia (increases the risk of epidural hematoma), sepsis (increases risk of meningitis), and infection at puncture site (increases risk of meningitis).
- In patients taking monamine oxidase inhibitors, meperidine and indirect-acting sympathomimetics (e.g., ephedrine) can produce an exaggerated response through the release of accumulated catecholamines.
- Arterial lines are contraindicated in patients with collagen vascular diseases (e.g., scleroderma and Raynaud phenomenon) because arterial catheterization increases the risk of severe ischemia to the hand.
- Inadequate anesthesia in patients with thoracic spinal cord lesions may cause autonomic hyperreflexia when stimulus is presented below the level of cord injury. This unopposed sympathetic activity is most commonly seen when any hollow viscus is distended, such as placement of bladder catheter or cystoscopy.

RELATIVE CONTRAINDICATIONS IN ANESTHESIA PRACTICE

- The use of naloxone in opioid-dependent patients can cause opioid withdrawal.

- Nasal intubation is contraindicated by factors that increase the risk of bleeding: coagulopathy or thrombocytopenia, pregnancy, basilar skull or severe facial fractures, hemangiomas, or congenital abnormalities of the nasal passage.

- The use of carboprost in patients with asthma may result in bronchospasm.

- The interscalene block is relatively contraindicated in a patient with respiratory insufficiency because of the predictable anesthetization of the ipsilateral phrenic nerve (and subsequent ipsilateral diaphragm paralysis) during an interscalene block. Based on the location of the area of the upper extremity needing a block, another technique may be appropriate.

- In patients with epidermolysis bullosa, trauma to the skin or mucous membranes should be avoided to prevent excessive bullae formation. Adhesive tapes, adhesive electrocardiogram electrodes, blood pressure cuffs without loose cotton padding, and unlubricated anesthetic face masks should be avoided.

- The placement of a pulmonary artery (PA) catheter is *relatively* contraindicated in patients with an existing left bundle branch block due to the possibility of the catheter inducing a right bundle branch block leading to complete heart block. If a PA catheter is placed in this situation, pacing equipment should be immediately at hand. Other contraindications to the PA catheter are tricuspid or pulmonary valve mechanical prosthesis, right heart mass (thrombus and/or tumor), and tricuspid or pulmonary valve endocarditis.

- Recurrent laryngeal nerve blockade, elective mask ventilation, or laryngeal mask airway usage is contraindicated in patients with risk of gastric contents aspiration (e.g., full stomach, hiatus hernia with significant gastroesophageal reflux disease, morbid obesity, intestinal obstruction, delayed gastric emptying, poor history).

SUGGESTED READINGS

Barash P, Cullen F, Stoelting R. *Clinical Anesthesia*. 3rd ed. Philadelphia, Pa.: Lippincott Williams & Wilkins; 1997.

Benumof JL, ed. *Anesthesia and Uncommon Diseases*. 4th ed. Philadelphia, Pa.: WB Saunders; 1998.

Chestnut DH, ed. *Obstetric Anesthesia: Principles and Practice*. 3rd ed. Philadelphia, Pa.: Mosby; 2004.

Gravenstein N, Kirby R, eds. *Complications in Anesthesiology*. 2nd ed. Philadelphia, Pa.: Lippincott Raven; 1996.

Martyn J, Richtsfeld M. Succinylcholine-induced hyperkalemia in acquired pathologic states. *Anesthesiology*. 2006;104(1):158–169.

180

BE AWARE OF THE INTERFACE BETWEEN SPIRITUALITY AND THE PRACTICE OF MEDICINE, AND NEVER INTERRUPT THE CHAPLAIN

ANGELA C. WOODITCH, MD AND
JOSEPH F. TALARICO, DO

Here is the editor's favorite *true* anecdote concerning spirituality in medicine: A patient was just going under anesthesia, when he waved the mask off his face, and asked to see the Catholic chaplain, as he had just heard God asking him to be blessed before surgery. The priest was paged, but unfortunately was still several miles from the hospital. A considerable delay ensued. As luck would have it, the eminent chief of surgery (Dr. John Cameron) was operating in the next room. His opinion was sought by the surgical residents as to whether the operating room (OR) schedule for that day could tolerate this disruption. Dr. Cameron (to his eternal credit) told the house staff to wait for the chaplain as long as necessary, be thoroughly blessed, and then send the father to his room to bless him and his operation as well!

Avoiding anesthesia errors is important because it promotes patient safety and physical well-being. As physicians, we have been trained to focus on the physical aspects of our patients' health, and we continually strive to improve their bodily condition. However, that is not the only component to our patients' general state of health. Multiple surveys have suggested that most patients have a spiritual life that is often equally as important as their physical well-being. In a 1998 study of alternative medicine, 35% of patients reported using prayer in relation to health problems. The same study found that 82% of Americans believe in the healing power of prayer. Physicians often fail to consider the patient's spirituality and its relationship to their general sense of well-being. Possible reasons for this failure are a lack of awareness of the importance of spirituality in many patients' lives, discomfort with religious beliefs of others, and the prominence of more scientific concepts in medical education.

In a meta-analysis of studies relating to spirituality, religion, and physical health, a correlation was found between patients with a religious/faith affiliation and better health outcomes, greater longevity, and improved coping skills. These patients also had a lower incidence of depression, anxiety, and suicide. Depression has been associated with poorer outcomes in surgical interventions, including cardiac, gynecologic, and orthopedic procedures.

© 2006 Mayo Foundation for Medical Education and Research

It could be concluded that if patients are allowed to practice their religion and express their faith preoperatively, a lower incidence of depression and, therefore, better surgical outcomes would result.

WHAT CAN WE DO?

It can be argued that the practice of medicine is not only the science of healing but also an art. In practicing the art of medicine, the physician must be cognizant of the importance of taking into account the patient's emotional well-being. This consideration is the essence of providing good customer service, a concept that is all too often neglected when practicing the science of medicine. This concept does not involve the indulgence of the patient's every demand, but we do have a responsibility to listen to our patients and honor requests within reason. This responsibility is paramount particularly when the request has a known association with better outcomes. Many patients express their desire to be prayed over preoperatively by a clergyman of their faith. Accommodating this request commonly results in delaying the start of surgery. Regardless of the inconvenience, this may impose on the surgical, anesthesiology, and OR staff, the patient's emotional well-being is of primary importance, and the patient's comfort level on entering the OR must be considered. This will enhance our ability as anesthesiologists to relax a patient and develop a healthy doctor-patient relationship. Also, if there is a true connection between the practice of faith and better outcomes, the time spent could make a difference in the patient's healing. Ultimately, patients have rights, and one of those rights is to be free to practice one's religion without restraint, regardless of whether those beliefs coincide with those of the physicians and the OR staff. As physicians, we are obligated to respect these rights and make any reasonable accommodation to preserve them.

THE POWER OF PRAYER: PRIVATE VERSUS INTERCESSORY PRAYER

There are few studies directly investigating prayer and outcomes in patient populations undergoing surgical interventions. Most of the studies attempting a randomized controlled design are focused on intercessory prayer (IP) for cardiac patients. IP is when one asks God, the universe, or some other higher power to intervene on behalf of an individual. Prior to the Study of the Therapeutic Effects of intercessory Prayer (STEP) trial published in 2006, there were four studies investigating IP in cardiac patients. The results were mixed. Two studies revealed a beneficial effect of prayer in coronary care unit (CCU) patients and two (one of CCU patients and the other of patients undergoing cardiac catheterization) showed no difference. The STEP trial studied approximately 1,800 patients in six U.S. hospitals undergoing coronary artery bypass grafting (CABG) surgery. There were three study groups: the first received prayer after being informed that they may or may

TABLE 180.1	PRIMARY BELIEFS OF THE WORLD'S MAJOR RELIGIONS
Buddhism	■ Accumulation of wisdom to which each generation adds its own understanding ■ Karma—for every action there is a consequence ■ Goal is achievement of Nirvana through continual reincarnation ■ Fate, inn, and ko determine health ■ Health practices include meditation, chanting, the four requisites, vegetarianism, no alcohol or tobacco, emetics/purging, oils, medicinal herbs, and surgery
Hinduism	■ Brahman is the supreme being ■ If prana (life force energy of humans) and chakras (energy centers) are in harmony, good health conditions result ■ Treatment may focus on balancing "humors" by diet, fasting, purging, enemas, and massage
Islam	■ Allah is God and teachings are provided in the Koran ■ Five pillars of faith include profession of faith, prayer, almsgiving, fasting, and pilgrimage ■ One main goal is to protect life, and this may contribute to certain health care decisions ■ Illness and death are met with patience, prayer, and meditation ■ Modesty is practiced, especially among women, and they may prefer female practitioners ■ Prayer is usually five times daily and must be done facing east
Judaism	■ The law of God is set forth in the commandments of the Torah (Old Testament of the Bible) ■ Saving human life takes precedence over all other laws ■ The family is the basic unit of society ■ Spirit and body are separated at death ■ Sabbath is regarded as the holy day of the week
Christianity	■ One God whose teachings are defined in the Bible (Old and New Testaments) ■ Salvation is a primary goal ■ Many different denominations each with slightly differing view points ■ Prayer used often to ask for healing
Magicoreligious	■ Supernatural forces influence health and illness ■ Examples include Christian Science and certain Hispanic/African/Caribbean healing practices
Holistic	■ Forces of nature should be kept in harmony, and these forces dictate health or illness ■ Examples include Chinese and Native American healing practices ■ Chinese medicine can include the balance of yin and yang; herbalists and shamans as healers; and the acts of massage, pinching, or cupping ■ Native Americans may seek a medicine man for folk healing who often leads large communal ceremonies

This table is not meant to be all inclusive or to stereotype any religions; rather, it is designed as a quick reference to broaden the health care provider's awareness of certain religious practices. Adapted from Young C, Koopsen C. *Spirituality, Health and Healing.* Thorofare, NJ: Slack; 2005;65–69, 80–81.

not receive prayer, the second did not receive prayer after being informed that they may or may not receive prayer, and the third group received IP after they were informed that they would receive prayer. The study concluded that IP had no effect on error-free recovery, and the certainty of receiving prayer was associated with a higher incidence of complications.

There are limitations of IP studies. They do not allow for the fact that study patients may also be praying private prayer as well as having close family, friends, and personal religious groups praying for them. Most of the studies do not allow those praying to interact with the patients or follow up with the patient's condition. Also, a contribution to the "power of prayer" may be the patient's own personal beliefs. These studies did not consider patient's thoughts on religion, healing, and prayer.

Even fewer studies have focused on private prayer and outcomes of surgery. One study in 1998 retrospectively studied patients and their use of private prayer as a coping mechanism for the difficulties related to CABG. The results suggested that private prayer might serve to facilitate psychosocial adjustment to the procedure. A more recent study of 246 patients awaiting cardiac surgery suggested private prayer predicted optimism, which implies that clinicians should attempt to provide a better spiritual assessment and care.

IN CONCLUSION... DO NOT INTERRUPT THE CHAPLAIN

As physicians, we may not always agree with our patient's religious beliefs. Sometimes we may find those beliefs difficult to respect, particularly if that respect leads to detrimental outcomes. However, it is well within patients' rights to practice their faith as they choose. Previously published studies on prayer are controversial and have produced mixed results. Certainly, more studies with improved methods are necessary before definite conclusions are made regarding prayer. Despite this, other studies show that faith and religious affiliation provides some patients with a sense of happiness and comfort that nothing else can provide. Prayer and other alternative healing methods may result in improved outcomes. For those reasons, next time a patient requests a chaplain, faith healer, or wants to participate in a religious ceremony prior to a surgical procedure, provide your patients with that opportunity by not interrupting the spiritual aspect of their healing process (*Table 180.1*).

SUGGESTED READINGS

Ai AL, Dunkle RE, Peterson C, et al. The role of private prayer in psychosocial recovery among midlife and aged patients following cardiac surgery. *Gerontologist.* 1998;38:591–601.

Ai AL, Peterson C, Bolling S, et al. Private prayer and optimism in middle-aged and older patients awaiting cardiac surgery. *Gerontologist.* 2002;42:70–81.

Astin J, Harkness E, Ernst E. The efficacy of "distant healing": a systematic review of randomized trials. *Ann Intern Med.* 2000;132:903–910.

Aviles J, Whelan E Sr., Hernke D, et al. Intercessory prayer and cardiovascular disease progression in a coronary care unit population: a randomized controlled trial. *Mayo Clin Proc.* 2001;76(12):1192–1198.

Benson H, Dusek J, Sherwood J, et al. Study of the Therapeutic Effects of intercessory Prayer (STEP) in cardiac bypass patients: a multicenter randomized trial of uncertainty and certainty of receiving intercessory prayer. *Am Heart J.* 2006;151:934–942.

Byrd RC. Positive therapeutic effects of intercessory prayer in a coronary care unit population. *South Med J.* 1988;81:826–829.

Harris W, Gowda M, Kolb J, et al. A randomized, controlled trial of effects of remote, intercessory prayer on outcomes in patients admitted to the coronary care unit. *Arch Intern Med.* 1999;159(19):2273–2278.

Krucoff M, Crater S, Gallup D, et al. Music, imagery, touch, and prayer as adjuncts to interventional cardiac care: the monitoring and actualization of noetic trainings (MANTRA) II randomized study. *Lancet.* 2005;366:211–217.

Mueller P, Plevak D, Rummans T. Religious involvement, spirituality, and medicine: implications for clinical practice. *Mayo Clin Proc.* 2001;76(12):1225–1235.

Rosenberger P, Jokl P, Ickovics J. Psychosocial factors and surgical outcomes: an evidence-based literature review. *J Am Acad Orthop Surg.* 2006;14:397–405.

Young C, Koopsen C. *Spirituality, Health, and Healing.* Thorofare, NJ: Slack; 2005.

181

HOW NOT TO END UP IN A CLOSED CLAIMS FILE: LESSONS EARNED FROM THE ASA CLOSED CLAIMS PROJECT

LORRI A. LEE, MD AND KAREN B. DOMINO, MD, MPH

OVERVIEW OF THE ASA CLOSED CLAIMS PROJECT

One of the best ways to avoid common anesthesia errors is to review cases in which patient injuries occurred, identify alternative practice management that might have avoided the adverse outcome, and incorporate those lessons into one's own practice. Quality assurance (QA) or continuous quality improvement (CQI) committees for anesthesiology departments and hospitals use this strategy to improve patient safety. However, some adverse outcomes will occur despite good medical management and may eventually result in lawsuits.

Similar to the QA or CQI committee review of adverse outcomes, review of claims or lawsuits filed against anesthesiologists may also identify factors associated with specific patient injuries, as well as factors associated with patients' decisions to file a lawsuit and unfavorable judgments against anesthesiologists. Recognizing the value of these claims, the American Society of Anesthesiologists (ASA) established the Closed Claims Project in 1985 to collect detailed information from these insurance company files from across the country by trained anesthesiologist reviewers.

For those unfamiliar with the medicolegal system, "closed claims" refer to claims that were filed by patients against doctors, allied health professionals, or hospitals for medical malpractice, and were dropped, settled, or proceeded to trial with a resulting judgment. The litigation phase is completed on these claims and thus they are considered "closed." Since its inception, the ASA Closed Claims Project and related Registries has published >100 articles describing factors associated with particular patient injuries, with a focus on improving patient safety. It was reported in the *Wall Street Journal* in 2005 as one of the leading causes of improved patient safety in anesthesiology over the last two decades, resulting in some of the lowest medical malpractice premiums for any specialty. It currently contains >7,000 closed claims in its database, spanning the last three decades. This chapter focuses on recurring themes that are associated with claims and with unfavorable judgments taken from the ASA Closed Claims Project to better inform the reader on how *not* to end up in a closed claim.

© 2006 Mayo Foundation for Medical Education and Research

I. CONSENT

Though consent is frequently an issue in medical malpractice claims, it is rarely the sole reason for the lawsuit, and when consent becomes a legal concern, it is usually associated with an adverse outcome. The consent issue has been likened to an anniversary card—"obtaining one does not guarantee you a good time, but you're asking for it if you don't get one." Consent issues may arise for a variety of reasons: (a) inadequate disclosure of the risks of a procedure—e.g., risk of postdural puncture headache after a subarachnoid block; (b) failure to obtain consent for a procedure—e.g., performance of a regional technique under general anesthesia; or (c) documentation of refusal of care when a patient refuses your recommendations—e.g., a patient with severe chronic obstructive pulmonary disease and congestive heart failure who refuses a regional technique for ankle surgery.

Items for consent discussion should include common complications, as well as any rare devastating complication that the typical patient would find important to decide on a particular treatment. However, these discussions should not be used to list all possible complications, as patients will lose sight of the major concerns. Documentation of the risks-and-benefits discussion with patients is key to minimizing medicolegal issues surrounding consent. Certain states and certain malpractice liability companies require a separate anesthesia consent form with a patient signature.

An approximately 60-year-old woman had an open urologic procedure under general anesthesia. As the surgeon left the operating room (OR), he asked the anesthesiologist to place an epidural catheter for postoperative pain management. This had not been discussed during the preoperative evaluation. While the patient was still anesthetized, the anesthesiologist attempted placement at two thoracic levels but was unsuccessful. In the postanesthesia care unit (PACU) the patient was noted to have a flaccid right leg and minimal movement of her left leg. Magnetic resonance imaging demonstrated a lesion in the thoracic spinal cord at the attempted epidural insertion sites, with edema above and below. Payment was approximately $350,000.

II. PREOPERATIVE EVALUATION

Issues surrounding preoperative evaluation in closed claims usually involve (a) lack of documentation of an airway examination in cases of unsuspected difficult intubation or (b) lack of follow-up on abnormal preoperative tests (frequently ordered by other health care providers) in cases in which the delay in diagnosis, treatment, or consultation resulted in harm to the patient (e.g.. chest radiograph with a new cancerous lesion or abnormal electrocardiogram (EKG) with a subsequent perioperative myocardial infarction). These issues emphasize the importance of performing and documenting a thorough preoperative evaluation and addressing any abnormal test results with appropriate treatment, consultation, or referral.

A 50ish-year-old man presented for a transurethral prostatic resection under spinal anesthesia. The patient's EKG showed "ischemic changes with possible myocardial infarct." The EKG was not reviewed by the anesthesiologist or the urologist before surgery. There was no medical or cardiology consult for the elective procedure. The patient developed chest pain on the first postoperative day and a diagnosed myocardial infarction on the second postoperative day. The patient eventually had coronary artery bypass graft surgery. A lawsuit was settled out of court for failure to diagnose the myocardial infarct before surgery and for the lack of consultation. Payment amount was approximately $200,000.

III. CHANGING OF THE GUARD OR "HANDOFFS" WITH POOR COMMUNICATION

In this age of same-day surgery admissions and outpatient surgery, the frequency of one anesthesia health care provider doing the history and physical and another providing the anesthetic is an everyday occurrence. Pertinent medical information may be lost or specific patient promises may not be honored when poor communication occurs. Thorough documentation of any discussions with patients regarding their health history or specific wishes regarding their anesthetic management should help to avoid this problem. Patients may assume that both parties communicated effectively with each other, and that they have no need to repeat their questions, concerns, or information provided to the first anesthesiologist. Any unusual issues should be communicated directly between health care providers. Similar strategies of good documentation and direct communication during "handoffs" should improve patient care and minimize liability exposure.

A 50-year-old woman presented for major reconstructive spine surgery with instrumentation. Two anesthesiologists and two certified registered nurse anesthetists (CRNAs) were involved throughout the course of this 8-hour surgery. The first anesthesiologist started the case with the first CRNA and then left the building to take care of personal matters because he was on call that evening. He assumed that the second anesthesiologist had assumed care of the patient, but the second anesthesiologist denied assuming care for the patient, except to approve an order for lasix by the first CRNA for low urine output (<200 mL urine was measured during the first 6 hours of surgery.) During the 5 hours the CRNA was left unsupervised, she failed to recognize hypovolemia, treated low urine output with furosemide, and allowed the patient's systolic blood pressure to run in the 80s for 5 hours in a normally hypertensive patient. (She said the surgeon requested deliberate hypotension, but the surgeon denied this allegation in deposition.) No arterial line was used and no blood gases were sent *for analysis. The patient awoke with permanent bilateral blindness secondary to posterior ischemic optic neuropathy. There was no documented preoperative plan and no anesthesiologist signature on either the preoperative form or the anesthetic record. Because of the concern that the jury would view abandonment of the patient by the anesthesiologists harshly, the case was settled for over $300,000 before going to trial.*

IV. DOCUMENTATION (OR LACK THEREOF)

Inadequate documentation of the preoperative history and physical and consent, intraoperative events, postoperative care and follow-up, and critical events are a common cause of lawsuits being settled in favor of the plaintiff. The medical record is your line of communication with other physicians and health care professionals, and it is also the legal record. Routine care such as a preoperative history and physical and intraoperative care should be documented on the standard forms provided by your hospital/anesthesia group with your signature and date, as this demonstrates good care. Although one may not have time to document during a crisis, a thorough, detailed description of the events and actions taken should be written at the first available opportunity. Although basic charting of vital signs and medications should be recorded on the anesthesia record for intraoperative critical events, additional documentation should also be done in the medical record in the progress note section, because most other specialists do not understand or feel comfortable with the anesthetic record, and it may be lost during storage. Electronic documentation has the added advantage of not being "thinned" from the chart. Only list the facts—events as they occurred—and do not speculate about etiology of the damaging event. As many claims are not filed until more than a year has passed since the event, the documentation also serves as a reminder to you regarding specific details that may otherwise be forgotten. If an event is not documented, the judge and/or jury, and possibly even you, will be less convinced that it ever occurred, and it leaves the impression that you were not careful.

A 30-year-old women has an emergency caesarean section under spinal anesthesia. She specified in her consent that no residents were to be involved in her care. An attending anesthesiologist and an obstetric anesthesia fellow handled the case, with the fellow actually placing the needle—despite the patient's objection. The first placement was blood-tinged and the needle was repositioned one space higher to get clear cerebrospinal fluid. There is no record of level testing in the anesthesia chart. After the baby was born and the cord cut, the patient was given valium 10 mg and fentanyl 200 mcg. The patient later stated that she felt the entire surgical procedure, was in excruciating pain, and had complained of this during the procedure. There is poor documentation on this point in the medical record. Payment amount was $305,100.

V. ALTERING THE MEDICAL RECORD

Perhaps one of the most damaging things a health care provider can do after an adverse outcome is to alter or falsify the medical record. Revelation of this behavior leaves the judge and/or jury with the impression of a dishonest and incompetent anesthesiologist/anesthetist whose medical record and testimony cannot be trusted. That impression combined with a significant patient injury leads the average person to assume fault on the part of the health care provider. Any additional information that the anesthesiologist wants to place in the chart should be done on progress notes, with entry date and time noted. Never cross out incorrect information after an adverse event—rather, note any pertinent corrections in the progress notes. Law firms may send the medical records for ink analysis to determine if alterations have been made.

A 60-year-old man had inguinal hernia repair under spinal anesthesia. The patient received large amounts of sedation. There was a hypertensive episode at the conclusion of the surgery. The patient did not regain consciousness in the recovery room and died 6 months later. The anesthesiologist submitted a second anesthesia record. He claimed the patient was awake in the PACU. The PACU nurse and surgeon claimed that the patient did not wake up in the PACU. The surgeon said the blood was dark (during surgery). Payment amount was $3,000,000!

VI. POOR FOLLOW-UP/COMMUNICATION AFTER AN ADVERSE OUTCOME

Poor follow-up and communication after an adverse outcome leaves patients with the impression that you do not care about their welfare, that your time is more important than their health, and that perhaps not everything possible was done on their behalf to treat the complication. Although anesthesiologists have very busy work schedules during these times of "high efficiency" and a focus on "decreased turnover times," follow-up of patients and their complications with appropriate referral should occur with proper documentation. Failure to recognize the deterioration in a patient's condition and investigate with appropriate intervention increases liability exposure. Follow-up demonstrates to patients and juries that you are a professional and care about the welfare of your patient. Even though it may be uncomfortable to see patients after an adverse occurrence, particularly when there was some potential inadequacy of care on your part, follow-up is an essential part of handling adverse outcomes. One study on medical malpractice of the reasons patients and/or their relatives file claims showed that only 15.6% to 37.1% of patients were satisfied with the amount of information provided about an adverse outcome, the clarity and accuracy of explanation, whether the explanation was delivered sympathetically, and with the overall view of the explanation. Similar results were found in a study of 45 plaintiffs' depositions of medical malpractice, in which 32% of the depositions contained statements concerning patient desertion by physician, 29% with devaluing patient and/or family views, 26% with delivering information poorly, and 13% with failing to understand the patient and/or family perspective.

What to Do

1) Provide regular follow-up on the patient and arrange appropriate referral care.
2) Notify your hospital risk management group and your malpractice insurance company.
3) Find a private, comfortable location for discussion in person and minimize interruptions (e.g., have a colleague carry your pager).
4) Use simple, direct language delivered in a warm, caring, and empathetic manner.
5) Demonstrate that you are actively listening by paraphrasing the patient/family's words and showing interest in the patient's welfare.
6) Let the family know that there is a plan for continued treatment.
7) Express concern for the patient.
8) Make yourself open and available to the patient/family.
9) After the adverse occurrence has been thoroughly reviewed by all parties, and if the adverse outcome was a result of a medical error, a statement of remorse or apology (after speaking with your risk management team), full disclosure of events, and corrective actions to be taken should be discussed. (Make sure that your state law allows apologies to patients without incrimination.)
10) Always be honest with the patient/family.
11) Document your conversations with the patient/family, including their responses and the plan of action.

What Not to Do

1) Do not profess guilt or blame other health care team members.
2) Do not avoid the patient, as feelings of abandonment are common among patients after adverse occurrences, and you may miss sequelae of the complication that require further intervention or referral.
3) Do not rush the discussion.
4) Avoid technical/medical language.
5) Do not coerce other health care professionals to "change their story" or lie.
6) Do not submit a bill if the event was related to the anesthetic or as a result of a medical error.

VII. MALIGNING BY OTHER HEALTH CARE PROVIDERS

One of the underappreciated but more common reasons for plaintiffs filing claims is the insinuation by other health care professionals that there was a maloccurrence. One study found that 17 of 31 plaintiffs reported that other health care professionals had either directly or indirectly suggested that the care provided by the defendant had caused the patient injury. Of these 17 claims, 71% of the "other health care professionals" alleging maloccurrence were the subsequent consultants who were brought into the case because of the adverse occurrence. For anesthesiologists, one of the potential avenues for miscommunication about an adverse occurrence is through the surgeon. Therefore, the anesthesiologist should always accompany the surgeon for any discussions with the patient/family. "Charting wars" with surgeons or other health care providers should be avoided, because this type of behavior makes everyone involved look incompetent and only weakens defense of a case should a claim be filed subsequently.

A patient in his mid-30s with a history of hypertension, with a preoperative blood pressure of 140/70, presented for extensive 3–4–level spinal fusion. The surgeon requested systolic blood pressure in the 90s on multiple occasions and insisted that the blood pressure was too high and that was the cause of the bleeding. The anesthesiologist asked the surgeon on several occasions to control the bleeding better with the Bovie. The case eventually ended after 9.5 hours prone time (scheduled for 5 hours) and estimated blood loss of 4,000 mL. The patient complained of blindness the first postoperative night in the intensive care unit (ICU). The surgeon's operative note and addendum, dictated 2 days postoperatively, was highly inflammatory and accusatory, and critical of the anesthesiologist's care. The surgeon said the anesthesiologist kept the blood pressure too high and caused excessive bleeding, and used too much crystalloid, which caused the patient's blindness. The jury ruled in favor of the defendant anesthesiologist, but the cost of defense was $139,707.56.

TAKE HOME POINTS

Although adequate medical knowledge is essential for good patient care and to avoid adverse outcomes, not all adverse outcomes can be prevented, and medical misadventures occur. Other factors, besides good clinical care, that are important to minimize your involvement in lawsuits include:

- Document patient discussion and consent.
- Carry out thorough preoperative evaluation and follow-up of abnormal test results.

- Maintain good communication with colleagues regarding any pertinent patient health issues or discussions.
- Thoroughly and legibly document all perioperative care, with special attention to critical events.
- Never alter the medical record.
- Engage in a thorough and open discussion with the patient and/or family regarding adverse outcomes and provide a plan of action with appropriate referral or consultation.
- Continue follow-up with the patient and family and make yourself available to avoid feelings of abandonment.
- Make every effort to be present for any discussions by other health care providers regarding the adverse outcome to avoid any miscommunication.

SUGGESTED READINGS

Bean RV. Altering records: discrediting your best witness. *J Med Assoc Ga*. 1998;82:63–64.

Beckman, HB, Markakis KM, Suchman AL, et al. The doctor-patient relationship and malpractice: lessons from plaintiff depositions. *Arch Intern Med*. 1994;154:1365–1370.

Cheney FW. The American Society of Anesthesiologists Closed Claims Project: what have we learned, how has it affected practice, and how will it affect practice in the future? *Anesthesiology*. 1999;91:552–556.

Gorney M, Martello J. The genesis of plastic surgeon claims. A review of recurring problems. *Clin Plast Surg*. 1999;26:123–131,ix.

Hallinan JT. *Heal thyself:* once seen as risky, one group of doctors changes its ways. *The Wall Street Journal Online*. www.WJS.com. June 21, 2005:1.

Hickson GB, Clayton EW, Githens PB, et al. Factors that prompted families to file medical malpractice claims following perinatal injuries. *JAMA*. 1992;267:1359–1363.

Huycke LI, Huycke MM. Characteristics of potential plaintiffs in malpractice litigation. *Ann Intern Med*. 1994;120:792–798.

Pennachio DL. Alter records, lose the case. *Med Econ*. 2003;80:40, 43–44.

Vincent C, Young M, Phillips A. Why do people sue doctors? A study of patients and relatives taking legal action. *Lancet*. 1994;343:1609–1613.

182

REFUSAL TO DO A CASE ON MORAL OR ETHICAL GROUNDS: PRACTICAL NAVIGATION THROUGH VERY TROUBLED WATERS

KENNETH R. ABBEY, MD, JD AND
MARCUS C. STEPANIAK, CRNA, MS, BSN

Imagine that you are assigned by your group to the ambulatory surgery center for the day. Your first patient is a 21-year-old college student for dilation and evacuation (D&E) to terminate a pregnancy. She is G1P0 at 8 weeks' gestation. She has decided to terminate the pregnancy because she has split up with the man with whom she was involved (the baby's father), and she does not feel prepared to raise the child on her own while dealing with the demands of college. Would you feel justified in refusing to perform anesthesia for this woman? What would you think if one of your colleagues refused the case? Is it ever appropriate to refuse anesthesia for a procedure that is legal?

Imagine now that your group has assigned you to perform anesthesia at the state penitentiary. The governor has asked your group to provide general anesthesia to a 38-year-old man who is a death-row inmate scheduled for execution by lethal injection. A recent execution by lethal injection went badly awry when the intravenous (IV) line infiltrated, and the prisoner was believed to have suffered while a second IV was placed and the lethal cocktail given again. To ensure pain-free execution to the current prisoner, the state would like you to induce general anesthesia. When you are satisfied that the prisoner is anesthetized, you will be escorted from the room, and an executioner will administer a large dose of potassium to stop the prisoner's heart and complete the execution. You are informed by legal counsel that your state has a statute making your participation legal and shielding you from any ethical or legal liability. Would you feel justified in refusing to perform anesthesia for this man? What would you think if one of your colleagues refused the case? Is it ever appropriate to refuse anesthesia for a procedure that is legal?

The issue of refusal of care in medicine is both intellectually difficult and emotionally troubling. To some extent, objective discourse on this topic has been made more difficult because refusal of care in anesthesia is closely associated with the deeply divisive issue of abortion. However, the issue is broader than that and deserves consideration in the context of other factual scenarios. Questions worth considering include: Is it ever appropriate to

© 2006 Mayo Foundation for Medical Education and Research

refuse anesthesia for a procedure that is legal? If so, who decides when it is appropriate? How should a refusal be invoked?

Arguments regarding the legal and ethical appropriateness of refusals run the gamut from supporting an absolute right of refusal to concluding that no such right exists for any procedure that is legal. The arguments for a right of refusal stem essentially from the American tradition of freedom. After all, this country set forth the right of freedom of expression and religion in its very first Amendment in the Bill of Rights: "Congress shall make no law respecting an establishment of religion, or prohibiting the free exercise thereof; or abridging the freedom of speech." Certainly, it is argued, if one has a right to freedom of religion, and if one's religious beliefs (or ethical principles) forbid participation in certain procedures, then no one should be able to force one's participation.

The opposing view is well framed by Dr. Julian Savulescu in a recent issue of the *British Medical Journal* (see Suggested Readings). In his article, Dr. Savulescu states that "[w]hat should be provided to patients is defined by the law and consideration of the just distribution of finite medical resources," and further, that "[i]f people are not prepared to offer legally permitted, efficient, and beneficial care to a patient because it conflicts with their values, they should not be doctors." He notes that it is inefficient and inequitable for a large percentage of doctors to refuse to participate in abortions, because patients are then required to "shop" for doctors who will perform a legal service. He further notes that inconsistent moral positions of physicians lead to inconsistent care and discrimination. It could be argued from Savulescu's thesis that cases of abortion and execution are distinguishable because the abortion is beneficial to the patient whereas execution is not. However, that distinction is likely to be lost on the death-row inmate, who would probably believe it beneficial to be anesthetized by a licensed anesthesia provider before being put to death rather than be sedated by an amateur. If doctors are required to provide any legal, beneficial service requested by patients, could anesthesia providers ethically refuse to provide anesthesia to a death-row inmate who requested to be properly anesthetized before being given a lethal injection? Would the same ethical considerations apply to assisted suicide in a state in which it was legal?

In the United States, refusal to do a case is legally permissible to some extent in most states. Legal support for refusal comes from multiple sources, is often specifically targeted at certain types of cases or objections, and, not surprisingly, is highly politicized. At the federal level, just months after the *Roe v. Wade* decision (which found a constitutional right to abortion), the Church Amendment, 42 USC Sec. 300a-7, was passed, which released individuals who refused to perform abortions or sterilizations on moral grounds from compulsion via certain federal funding. More recently, Title VII of the

Civil Rights Act mandated that employers accommodate religious beliefs of employees to the extent that such accommodation does not cause undue hardship.

Among the states, 49 provide for at least a limited right of refusal on ethical grounds for health care providers. Twenty-five of those states provide a right of refusal only with respect to performing abortions. In Oregon, for example, Or. Rev. Stat. Sec. 435.225 states that no hospital employee is required to participate in an abortion. In Mississippi, the Miss. Code Ann. Sec. 41-41-215 provides broadly that health care providers may decline to comply with health care decisions for reasons of conscience. Vermont alone offers no right of conscientious objection.

Because federal and state laws support some right of refusal to health care providers and in reaction to specific situations, some hospitals and professional organizations have developed policies regarding whether, when, and how health care providers may refuse to participate in care on moral or ethical grounds. At our institution, for example, hospital policy states that "When [a health care professional's] belief system prevents him/her from being directly involved in a legally available, medically recognized intervention, the [professional] will not be required to be directly involved in initiating such intervention."

Recently, the American Society of Anesthesiologists (ASA) was compelled to respond to the issue of lethal injection with a "Message from the President." The case set forth at the beginning of this chapter involving a request to provide anesthesia for lethal injection is not entirely hypothetical. In fact, in February 2006, a federal judge in California issued an order requiring that an anesthesiologist personally supervise lethal injections. The anesthesiologist would be present to assess depth of sedation before the lethal injection was given. The American Medical Association (AMA) and the ASA reacted, with the president of the ASA stating that "[p]hysicians are healers, not executioners." Subsequently, the ASA issued the "Message from the President" that reviews the state of affairs regarding execution and then notes that while the "ASA does not have a detailed position on anesthesiologist participation in lethal injection," it does support the AMA "position regarding physician nonparticipation in executions." The ASA president advised the membership to "be well informed on the subject and steer clear."

The challenge of conscientious objection does not end with an anesthesia provider's determination to refuse participation in a given procedure. Rather, the determination to refuse imposes both obligations and liabilities on the provider. At our institution, for example, hospital policy provides that a practitioner refusing involvement in an intervention must "refer the patient to other persons who will either provide the intervention or facilitate appropriate referral," and further, that "[t]his process must not create undue delay, inconvenience, or impediment to receiving requested services for the patient." When health care providers fail to inform patients about available interventions or refer them to providers who are willing to provide those interventions, they open themselves up to potential liability. Thus, for example, a religious hospital that did not inform a rape victim about the availability of emergency contraception was found liable. In another, a fertility clinic that refused to artificially inseminate a gay patient was sued for discrimination. In addition to legal ramifications, refusing to provide care carries its own set of social and professional fallout. Anesthesia providers may wonder: What will my colleagues think of me? Will the patient receive the services he or she desires/needs? Will I face disciplinary action?

Given the complexity of this issue, the authors recommend a pragmatic and careful approach. Here is some practical advice derived from the foregoing discussion and our experience.

TAKE HOME POINTS

- Read your institution's policy related to conscientious objection, if it has one.
- Take time to investigate your state's statutes or laws related to refusal of care.
- Think hard about your ethical limits and try to imagine situations that might require you to make a conscientious objection.
- If you know you possess a moral or ethical objection to certain procedures, inform your department chair or designated individual before an ethical dilemma arises. Your goal is to avoid assignment to cases that violate your principles in the first place, not to react once the assignment is made.
- If you object to a case that is thrust upon you, decline, but refer your patient to a colleague, making certain that you are not, in fact or in perception, an impediment to your patient's choice of care. If you are backed into a corner (e.g., on call at night), delay the case until a nonobjecting colleague can arrive, if possible; but if this is not possible, be prepared to choose between your principles and your obligation to your patient, and make sure you are willing to pay the price with your job or in court if your refusal results in irreversible consequences for your patient.

SUGGESTED READINGS

Brownfield v. Daniel Freeman Marina Hospital, 256 Cal. Rptr. 240 (Ca. Ct. App., 1989).
Gawande A. When law and ethics collide—why physicians participate in executions. *N Engl J Med.* 2006;354(12):1221–1229.

Guidry OF. Message from the president: observations regarding lethal injection. American Society of Anesthesiologists website. www.asahq.org/news/asanews063006.htm. June 30, 2006.

Miss. Code Ann. Sec. 41-41-215.

OHSU Health Care System Administrative Policy Manual, Chapter Seven: Personnel & Human Resources, Conscientious Objection, Adm. 07.05. August 30, 2006.

Or. Rev. Stat. Sec. 435.225.

Prepared Witness Testimony of Professor Lynn Wardle before The Committee on Energy and Commerce, Subcommittee on Health, July 11, 2002.

Roe v. Wade, 410 US 113 (1973).

Savulescu J. Conscientious objection in medicine. *Br Med J*. 2006;332:294–297.

Stein R. Seeking care, and refused. *washingpost.com*. July 16, 2006:A06. www.washingtonpost.com/wp-dyn/content/article/2006/07/15/AR2006071500787.html.

42 USC Sec. 300a-7.

42 USC Sec. 2000e[2].

183

GET INFORMED ABOUT "INFORMED CONSENT"

LYNN A. FENTON, MD

Suppose your next patient for elective outpatient surgery, a 15-year-old boy, ASA I, for an open reduction, internal fixation (ORIF) of a mandible fracture is all alone in the preop area. You complete your perioperative checklist and discuss the Procedure, Alternatives, Risks, and give the patient the opportunity to ask Questions about the proposed anesthesia plan. You then notice that the Consent for Surgery/Anesthesia Form on the patient's chart shows that only the patient signed the written consent form. Is this consent valid? Is it acceptable to continue with the anesthesia and surgery plans under these conditions? To answer these questions and others related to the topic of informed consent, learn and apply the mnemonic: "PTS.' CONSENT & WE SMILE."

P is for **PARQ**. These are the basic elements of medical informed consent. Keeping the patient's perspective in mind, you should present and review the following with them: the nature and purpose of the **P**rocedure/surgery or treatment, accepted **A**lternatives, potential benefits, and material **R**isks of the proposed treatment. Here, the anesthesiologist must disclose all information that a "reasonable person" would consider important in making a decision to undergo treatment. The patient may then ask **Q**uestions and, once satisfied, make a choice.

T is for **TESTS TOO**. Consent is also required for HIV tests, genetic tests, research studies, alternative treatments for breast cancer, and termination of pregnancy (TOP).

S is for **SEVERAL FORM TYPES**. There are three types of consent forms in common use: (i) the patient-signed consent form that the surgeon (or anesthesiologist if a separate anesthesia-specific consent form is available) is responsible for obtaining before surgery; (ii) the verbal agreement by the patient to the anesthesia care plan, usually part of the "Day of Surgery" section in most preoperative anesthesia evaluation forms; and (iii) a patient-signed consent form, which the anesthesiologist obtains for procedures performed by the anesthesiologist without a surgeon's assistance (i.e., epidural blood patches, catheter or line placements, and pain management procedures). Some hospitals also have separate consent forms for blood transfusions (i.e., for Jehovah's Witness patients).

C is for **COMPETENCE, CAPACITY AND COMING OF AGE.** Consent can be obtained only from a patient, legal guardian, or advocate

---

ⓒ 2006 Mayo Foundation for Medical Education and Research

who is "*competent.*" *Competency* is a legal matter. It is a determination made by a court of law that an individual has the requisite abilities to make certain decisions such as those pertaining to medical care, daily aspects of life, personal finances, etc. It follows that a patient who has taken or been given mind-altering drugs (i.e., anxiolytics or narcotics) *may* not be able to give a valid consent. If a patient is deemed incompetent, social workers or psychiatrists may be consulted to further evaluate the individual's competence and/or a guardian of person, or property, or both may be appointed for him or her. One common mistake in obtaining consent is to confuse competency with the capacity for decision making. *Capacity* for decision making, in contrast to competency, is a clinical determination. There are four recognized and legally validated components to decision-making capacity: understanding, appreciating, formulating or reasoning, and communicating a choice:

1) The patient must *understand* the known risks and benefits of the treatment and its alternatives.

2) The patient must be able to *appreciate* his or her clinical condition relative to the proposed treatment plan.

3) The patient must be able to *formulate* a plan for himself or herself, that is, have the intact ability to consider these factors appropriately in arriving at a reasonable decision.

4) The patient must be able to *communicate* his or her decision in a manner that demonstrates the ability to weigh appropriately the pertinent risk/benefit issues and his or her reasons for arriving at the decision. The patient must also demonstrate the ability to both ask and answer appropriate questions relating to his or her decision.

Coming of age refers to the minimum age requirement by law (18 years and older) that defines adulthood. In most states, individuals who become married or emancipated are also deemed to be "adults." Confusingly, some states do allow minors (15 years and older) to consent for general hospital, medical, surgical, or dental care. In this situation it is not required to inform a parent or guardian, but he or she may be informed against the wishes of the minor without liability to the hospital or the physician.

O is for the patient's **OPINION**. Basically, this is the important endpoint of the consent process, when the patient makes autonomous choices regarding the type of anesthesia care that he or she will receive.

N is for <u>NO</u> **FAILURE TO OBTAIN**. Performance of an invasive procedure on a patient after failure to obtain consent may constitute the tort of battery, defined as the "unauthorized and offensive touching of one individual by another." In other words, without consent, medical "touching" may be deemed a battery that creates both criminal and civil liability.

S is for **STATE-TO-STATE VARIATION.** Several issues pertaining to consent are subject to interstate variation (i.e., certain procedures, minor status, document forms, and duration of consent). Therefore, it is advised that you know how these kinds of issues are addressed by both hospital/institution policy and the laws specific to the state in which you are practicing.

E is for **EXIT AT ANY TIME.** The patient may withdraw his or her decision (also called "exit") at any time before or during the treatment, procedure, or surgery. This means that if a patient is in the operating room and states that she no longer wishes to have the procedure, everyone must STOP, and the procedure must be cancelled.

N is for **NO COERCION.** Consent must be knowing and voluntary—period. If it is coerced, then any procedures performed subject to that consent may constitute battery.

T is for **TIME FRAME.** In theory, consent is valid indefinitely unless there is a change in patient status, procedure, or treatment, or consent is withdrawn. In practice, however, time frames do vary from place to place. Usually, both hospital policy and state law set guidelines for timelines to follow.

& W is for **WRITTEN VERSUS ORAL.** Legally, consent does not have to be in writing. Oral or "implied consent" is equally valid. However, written documentation makes it easier for the hospital to furnish proof in the event of any questions. Most hospital policies dictate obtaining consent when possible (see the section on emergencies below and check with your hospital/facility about telephone consents). There are legal implications, however. If a hospital has a policy requiring written consent, a jury may infer that no consent was obtained if the policy was not followed.

E is for **EXCEPTIONS TO THE RULES.** Two particular areas, Minors and Incompetence (discussed below), contain some inherently confusing concepts pertaining to exceptions and special situations.

S is for **SPECIAL SITUATIONS.** These are described below in the last **MILE.**

M is for **MINORS.** Legally, a minor is anyone under 18 years of age. In most states, consent must be obtained from his or her parent (with court-ordered legal custody, if divorced) or legal guardian. Exceptions commonly include emancipated minors and unwed minor mothers as well as treatments involving birth control, sexually transmitted diseases, abortion, substance abuse, and mental health.

I is for **INCOMPETENCE.** In this situation, a guardian or advocate under durable power of attorney must be contacted. If no guardian is appointed, the patient's spouse, adult child, parent, and adult sibling must be contacted in that order. Social services may also appoint a temporary guardian from the probate court in the patient's county of residence.

L is for **LIMITED CONSENT**. An example is the case of a Jehovah's Witness patient who agrees to anesthesia with the understanding that blood products/transfusions will be withheld (or administered only in accordance with his or her specific wishes).

E is for **EMERGENCIES**. If there is imminent threat to life or limb, treatment may be given without consent. Also, consent may be obtained over the phone if a responsible family member is not available in the hospital and the patient is incompetent or a minor. Many hospitals use permission phone "hot lines" to request a phone consent. In these circumstances, the practitioner seeking consent by telephone must have a witness on the line to hear the consent; and the identity of the consenting person and his or her relationship to the patient must be specifically requested. An appropriate statement describing the conversation should be recorded and signed by both witnesses. If the consenting person is later available, he or she should be asked to affirm by co-signing and dating the telephone consent document.

TAKE HOME POINTS

- Informed consent is a required component of every preoperative assessment.
- Consent is a shared decision-making process with the patient and thus is an effective tool to establish good rapport with the patient, which may avert future complaints and reduce your medicolegal risk.
- Some concepts and definitions involved in informed consent are inherently complex. Therefore, to avoid common errors in the area of informed consent, it is important to have a solid grasp of the pertinent legal and medical definitions, guidelines of the hospital/institution, and the laws of your state.

SUGGESTED READINGS

Bierstein K. Informed consent is more than a signature. *ASA Newsl.* www.asahq.org/Newsletters/2002/12_02/pracMgmt12_02.html. December 12, 2002.

Cole DJ, Schlunt M. *Adult Perioperative Anesthesia: The Requisites in Anesthesiology.* Philadelphia: Elsevier Mosby; 2004.

Huford WE. *Clinical Anesthesia Procedures of the Massachusetts General Hospital.* 6th ed. Philadelphia: Lippincott Williams & Wilkins; 2002.

Miller RD: *Anesthesia.* 5th ed. Philadelphia: Churchill-Livingstone; 2000.

Sandson NB, Marcucci C, Loreck DJ, et al. Capacity to give surgical consent does not guarantee capacity to give anesthesia consent: implications for anesthesiologists.

Waisel DB, Truog RD. Informed consent. *Anesthesiology.* 1997;87(4):968–978.

184

THE ANESTHESIA RECORD
IS A LEGAL DOCUMENT

JOSEPH F. TALARICO, DO, DAVID G. METRO, MD, AND
RENEE A. METAL, JD

In the unfortunate event that you are named in a lawsuit, the anesthesia record can be your best friend—or your worst enemy. Because the anesthesia record is the only document that is continuously and concurrently recorded during the course of surgery, the anesthesia record is often considered the most important document detailing occurrences in the operating room. The anesthesia record is used not only as a record of anesthesia management but also as one of medical and, to a degree, surgical management. For this reason, anesthesia providers must give considerable thought to the development of the anesthesia record as well as to its utilization. It is imperative that the anesthesia record be accurate, clear, and comprehensive regardless of the complexity of the case and regardless of whether complications occurred during the course of the case.

COMPONENTS OF THE ANESTHESIA RECORD

The anesthesia and operative record is the medical and ultimately legal document that records an anesthetic procedure. This record becomes part of the patient's permanent medical record and should be as accurate and complete as possible. It provides information to other care providers that may influence the postoperative medical decision making for the management of the patient. All anesthesia providers involved in the delivery of care should sign the anesthesia record. All providers signing the chart should confirm the record's accuracy, and it should include the information identified in *Table 184.1.* The old adage, "If it's not on the chart, it never happened," is not necessarily true (i.e., intravenous placement procedure does not need to be routinely documented in the absence of complications). It is, however, imperative that all significant occurrences be appropriately documented on the chart.

Although the components of the anesthesia record are virtually universal, there is considerable variation among institutions regarding the information to be included in the record: some records are all-inclusive, attempting to cover every aspect of anesthesia care (e.g., type of laryngoscope blade used, amount of air in endotracheal tube cuff, etc.), whereas others include little more than the minimum. Although there are legitimate opinions that

© 2006 Mayo Foundation for Medical Education and Research

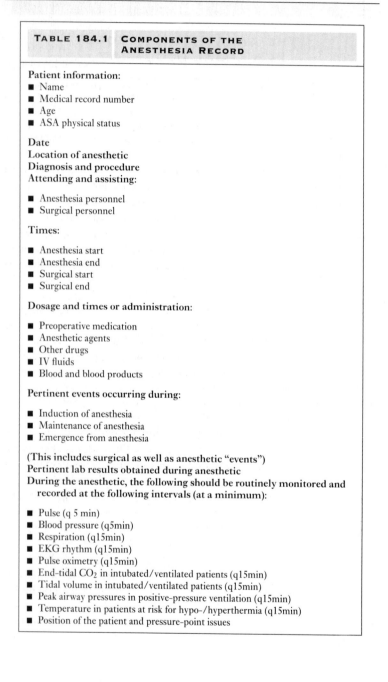

TABLE 184.1 COMPONENTS OF THE ANESTHESIA RECORD

Patient information:
- Name
- Medical record number
- Age
- ASA physical status

Date
Location of anesthetic
Diagnosis and procedure
Attending and assisting:

- Anesthesia personnel
- Surgical personnel

Times:

- Anesthesia start
- Anesthesia end
- Surgical start
- Surgical end

Dosage and times or administration:

- Preoperative medication
- Anesthetic agents
- Other drugs
- IV fluids
- Blood and blood products

Pertinent events occurring during:

- Induction of anesthesia
- Maintenance of anesthesia
- Emergence from anesthesia

(This includes surgical as well as anesthetic "events")
Pertinent lab results obtained during anesthetic
During the anesthetic, the following should be routinely monitored and recorded at the following intervals (at a minimum):

- Pulse (q 5 min)
- Blood pressure (q5min)
- Respiration (q15min)
- EKG rhythm (q15min)
- Pulse oximetry (q15min)
- End-tidal CO_2 in intubated/ventilated patients (q15min)
- Tidal volume in intubated/ventilated patients (q15min)
- Peak airway pressures in positive-pressure ventilation (q15min)
- Temperature in patients at risk for hypo-/hyperthermia (q15min)
- Position of the patient and pressure-point issues

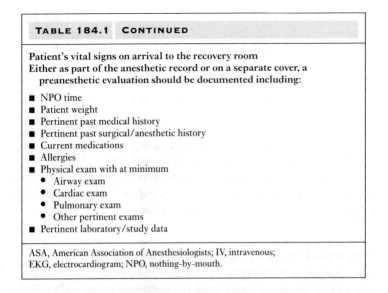

TABLE 184.1   CONTINUED

Patient's vital signs on arrival to the recovery room
Either as part of the anesthetic record or on a separate cover, a
  preanesthetic evaluation should be documented including:

- NPO time
- Patient weight
- Pertinent past medical history
- Pertinent past surgical/anesthetic history
- Current medications
- Allergies
- Physical exam with at minimum
  - Airway exam
  - Cardiac exam
  - Pulmonary exam
  - Other pertinent exams
- Pertinent laboratory/study data

ASA, American Association of Anesthesiologists; IV, intravenous;
EKG, electrocardiogram; NPO, nothing-by-mouth.

support both extremes, it is imperative that all sections of the anesthesia form that is in fact being utilized by the medical institution within which one is practicing be timely and entirely completed.

THE ANESTHESIA RECORD: FRIEND OR FOE

The anesthesia record, though not the exclusive record of occurrences in the operating room, is the most comprehensive real-time record of intraoperative events. Nursing notes primarily address statistical concerns for billing and equipment function and utilization. The surgeon's operative report, though it describes the procedure in detail, is not recorded in real time, and only superficially addresses medical management of the patient, if at all. For those reasons, the anesthesia record is often the primary document reviewed during intraoperative peer review and during the initial stages of litigation, including medical/legal expert review. It is therefore inevitable that, if one administers a considerable number of anesthetics, sooner or later one's anesthetic record will be examined in a legal setting.

A properly completed anesthesia record is the best defense in the event of involvement in medical malpractice litigation. Assuming one's actions are defensible, a clear record of these actions should establish practice within acceptable standards in the event of an adverse outcome. On the other hand, an incomplete or illegible record implies substandard care. As stated above, although there is considerable variation in the detail to be included in anesthesia records, it is critical to complete all main components listed in *Table 184.1*, as any incomplete section implies disregard. Essentially, if a component is deemed sufficiently important to warrant inclusion on the record, a legal assumption may be made that failure to complete that component, in and of itself, constitutes negligence. Or, perhaps more important, a legal assumption may be advocated whereby such a failure is proof that negligence occurred during the course of anesthesia management. An example of such an instance is the routine documentation of atraumatic intubation. If the anesthesia record requires documentation of, or if one routinely documents, atraumatic intubation, failure to address this component on the anesthesia record may imply that intubation was, in fact, traumatic. On the other hand, if this component is never documented, it would be reasonable to conclude that intubation is atraumatic unless documented otherwise. Without question, the vast majority of lawsuits involving anesthesia care include issues surrounding an incomplete or inadequate anesthesia record. Proper and timely completion of the record eliminates these issues.

POTENTIAL PITFALLS IN COMPLETION OF THE ANESTHESIA RECORD

Entries on the anesthesia record should be limited to a factual representation of intraoperative events rather than expressions of opinions. Implication of another practitioner in the event of a complication will not exonerate the anesthesia provider and may raise additional questions during litigation. An effort also must be made to limit the number of providers who write on the record; although changing providers is not always avoidable, excessive provider turnover raises questions as to continuity of care. In addition, the anesthesia record should be completed as if review is anticipated: in the event of litigation, it is expected that the record will be prominently displayed in court.

Although the anesthesia record is ideally a real-time record of intraoperative events, a complicated intraoperative course often makes timely record completion difficult at best. When faced with rapid blood loss, severe cardiovascular complications, or other critical events, patient care must take precedence over record completion. Although electronic record systems (discussed at length below) may be more beneficial than a manual anesthesia record in this scenario, if only a manual anesthesia record is available, the record *must* be reconstructed as promptly and accurately as possible after the event. In this case, the record must be exhaustively reviewed to ensure completion, especially in the event of an adverse outcome. Often, a poor outcome results in significant distress to the anesthesia provider. For this reason, it is beneficial in this scenario to have the record reviewed by an uninvolved peer before the record is finalized. An individual who is not emotionally involved will generally be better equipped to calmly inspect the record for key omissions. Such a scenario is best illustrated by the following case report.

A 50-year-old woman presented for removal of an infected pacemaker lead. During the course of the procedure, when the lead was extracted, ventricular injury occurred, leading to cardiac tamponade and death. Litigation was instituted against the surgeon, who alleged that the anesthetist was not monitoring the patient adequately and missed a prolonged period of cardiac arrest. The anesthetist testified that the patient was alert minutes before the fatal event. The circulating nurse corroborated this testimony. However, the anesthesia record failed to support their recollection of the events. Specifically, page one of the anesthesia record ended at 1730, and page two of the record began at 1800. The critical event occurred at approximately 1800. Although both the anesthetist and the anesthesiologist involved in the care of the patient, being appropriately distressed after the patient's death, reviewed the anesthesia record, they failed to note the gap between the pages. Following the initiation of litigation approximately 6 months later, the error was noted. Although anesthesia care in this patient was likely well within the standard of care, this documentation failure made the case much more difficult to defend. In the end, although the individual anesthesia practitioners were dropped from the suit, the anesthesia group, their employer, accepted some liability in settlement. It is doubtful that any liability would have been incurred if an uninvolved anesthesiologist had been asked to review the record immediately after the fact, as he or she would likely have discovered the error.

ELECTRONIC ANESTHESIA RECORDS

Although there is some controversy as to whether electronic anesthesia records are of benefit or instead create an increased medicolegal risk, the preponderance of opinion among those experienced in employing electronic records is that these systems are of significant advantage. Electronic records provide an accurate, real-time verification of vital signs, drug administration, and performance of procedures. The controversy arises when short-term abnormalities of vital signs are recorded, or when artifacts are recorded as real. Electronic record systems generally include a means of eliminating erroneous data, and some include algorithms that correct these anomalies.

Like any automated system, electronic record systems are only as reliable as the operator. One must carefully review the record for accuracy, correcting erroneous entries before the record is finalized. As with a manual anesthesia record, failure to review data and ensure accuracy upon finalization of the record may result in misrepresentation of intraoperative events, thereby resulting in a greater chance of being held liable for an adverse outcome. Additionally, it is much more difficult to dispute and/or disprove erroneous entries appearing on an electronic record after litigation has begun—timely review and correction is therefore imperative.

ADDITIONAL USES OF THE ANESTHESIA RECORD

Aside from the obvious legal use of the anesthesia record (i.e., medical malpractice litigation), components of the anesthesia record are often referenced for other purposes. Quality improvement programs make extensive use of anesthesia records in the tracking of anesthetic complications and the occurrences that most commonly precede these complications. The anesthesia record also serves as the primary billing document for the anesthesiologist. Anesthesia start and stop times, as well as the performance of special procedures, such as arterial and central lines, regional anesthetics, and transesophageal echocardiography, must be documented for proper billing and reimbursement to occur. To convey further relevant medical information that influenced decisions and therapy, pertinent lab studies such as hematocrit, blood gases, glucose, etc., that are obtained during surgery are documented, as well as resultant treatment of abnormalities. For the same reasons, surgical issues, including preoperative administration of antibiotics, administration of heparin for vascular procedures, and tourniquet times for orthopedic procedures are also documented on the anesthetic record.

The importance of the anesthesia record is certain to be enhanced in the future. Currently, Medicare is formulating a model that will determine reimbursement for anesthesia services based on "quality" indicators including administration of preoperative antibiotics within 60 minutes of surgery, maintenance of core temperature within specified limits, and other indicators that have not yet been determined. When this change occurs, the anesthesia record will be the exclusive reference in reviewing for specific outcomes. Failure to record these determinants of reimbursement effectively will have a direct effect on reimbursement for anesthesia services. Commercial insurance carriers, though not yet considering these changes, tend to follow Medicare's lead, especially when potential cost savings are involved.

TAKE HOME POINTS

- The anesthesia record is a legal document that contains vast amounts of legally relevant information.
- The importance of complete and accurate information entered on the anesthesia record cannot be overstated.
- The statement that "If it isn't written on the record, it didn't happen" is not necessarily true. Routine procedures (e.g., placement of intravenous lines) do not routinely warrant a procedure note in the absence of complication. Clearly, however, it is important to document all significant occurrences during anesthesia.
- The anesthesia record is also a quality improvement tool and serves as a guide for further and/or future medical therapy.

- The anesthesia record is also primary documentation for billing of services.
- An electronic anesthesia record may be helpful when it comes to verification of vital signs and completeness of these entries, but it is not without its own deficiencies (e.g., artifactual data appearing as "real").
- If a complication occurs, the anesthesia record should be reviewed by the care provider(s) as well as by an uninvolved party as soon as possible after the fact, to ensure completeness and accuracy. Although a contemporaneous record is preferable, documentation as to when and why a retrospective entry is included may be of considerable benefit in the event of litigation.

SUGGESTED READINGS

Gostt RK, Rathbone GD, Tucker AP. Real-time pulse oximetry artifact annotation on computerized anaesthetic records. *J Clin Monit Comput*. 2002;17(3–4):249–257.

Lanza V. Automatic record keeping in anesthesia—a nine-year Italian experience. *Int J Clin Monit Comput*. 1996;13(1):35–43.

Vigoda MM, Lubarsky DA. The medicolegal importance of enhancing timeliness of documentation when using an anesthesia information system and the response to automated feedback in an academic practice. *Anesth Analg*. 2006;103(1):131–136.

Yoder KS. Legal aspects of anesthesia charting. *AANA J*. 1979;47(1):47–54.

185

READING IN THE OPERATING ROOM—IS IT WORTH THE RISK?

MICHAEL AXLEY, MD, MS

Most anesthesiologists and anesthesia residents have heard the old truism that anesthesia is "95% routine and 5% terrifying." The problem, of course, is that the portions of an anesthetic procedure that can be dangerous for patients are often unannounced, or at least are heralded only by subtle signs. Further, they are often preceded by periods of relative calm, when, superficially at least, there is not much activity on our side of the curtain.

Imagine, then, that the anesthesiologist in charge of a case has settled in for one of those periods of calm. Confident that things are going smoothly, he or she reaches for a novel and quickly becomes engrossed in some very interesting reading. After about 5 minutes, the case suddenly and dramatically takes a serious and devastating turn for the worse. Things do not go well. The family is furious and hires legal representation. During deposition proceedings, their lawyer inquires exactly what book the anesthesiologist was reading at the time the patient experienced the critical event. Was it a mystery novel, perhaps? How long was the anesthesia provider reading while the patient was circling the drain?

Anesthesiologists have different opinions about reading in the operating room (OR), some of them quite firmly held. One camp feels that reading in the OR is absolutely a distraction. When reading, they say, the attention of the anesthesiologist is diverted from the patient. The anesthesiologist so engaged might miss some of the warning signs leading up to a critical event, possibly missing the window to intervene or losing valuable seconds of response time. Moreover, reading in the OR sends the wrong message to other members of the care team—if the anesthesiologist is obviously so bored that he or she has to read, how important can their task really be?

Others might counter that individual anesthesiologists are highly trained at multitasking, and when providing an anesthetic to an otherwise healthy patient there is no reason to prohibit a physician from spending time as he or she finds appropriate. Further, they note, there are no data available that suggest reading in the OR is contrary to our primary role as the guardians of patient safety.

Although it is true that there is not a great deal of data on this topic, there is a body of work assessing anesthesiologist vigilance, somnolence, and related matters that may allow reasoned, although non–evidence-based, conjecture.

© 2006 Mayo Foundation for Medical Education and Research

Anesthesia is often compared to other fields that demand high performance for long periods of time. The field of aviation, in particular, is often compared to anesthesia. In aviation, it has been noted that serious errors often occur because of minor distractions. This led to the adoption of a policy prohibiting conversations and distractions in the cockpits of commercial aircraft flying below 10,000 feet.

At the same time, some studies have found that a significant amount of the anesthesiologist's time in the OR is dedicated to tasks other than observing the patient—suggesting that there may be a certain, consistent amount of downtime during the provision of an anesthetic.

An article in the 1995 issue of the *Anesthesia Patient Safety Foundation* [APSF] *Newsletter* makes the following points:

1) Studies have suggested that the average anesthesiologist is "idle" during a case up to 40% of the time. This time serves as "spare capacity," that is, it is a reserve against moments when additional resources must be called into play rapidly.
2) Experienced providers are more efficient and have more spare capacity. In the absence of stimulation, they may become bored.
3) Boredom and low workload during the accomplishment of high-performance tasks may contribute to a low-arousal state that actually impairs performance.

The author of the article, Matthew Weinger, MD, performed a survey at his institution that included questions on boredom and reading. He found that almost 90% percent of responding providers experienced episodes of "extreme boredom" "occasionally." Twenty-nine percent read to relieve boredom. Nineteen percent read "frequently," 46% "sometimes" read, and 33% "rarely" read. Only one provider "never" read in the OR. Reading in the OR, suggested Weinger, "appears to be quite common." Further, he noted, to the extent that these secondary tasks prevent boredom, they could improve vigilance by maintaining arousal.

Weinger and others have commented on the type of reading material as a possible contributing factor to the debate. Reading materials related to the case at hand, for example, might actually improve outcomes. Reading novels, newspapers, or other absorbing but unrelated materials might prove deleterious as well as expose the anesthesiologist to substantial liability in the event of an acute critical event. The timing of reading may also be an important issue—it might be more appropriate, for example, to read while a patient is on cardiac bypass than during another part of the surgery.

It has been pointed out that reading during a case differs little from having conversations with OR staff, or playing music, or surfing the Internet. Although these practices do commonly occur, they all appear to fall under the category of external distractions. Insurance carriers appear to consider participating in activities that do not advance the patient's welfare while in the operating room as outside the standard of care. As a result, the medicolegal liability exposure sustained by anesthesiologists who read during a case can be considered quite high. Although lawsuits of this nature are not common, insurance companies have issued opinions suggesting that external distractions should be kept to a minimum during the operative period.

Another factor of importance is the culture at one's particular institution. Comments suggest that among some senior anesthesiologists in positions of authority, reading in the operating room is unacceptable. If the institutional culture at a medical center is such that reading is frowned upon, doing so would expose individual practitioners to a greater level of scrutiny and potential liability.

Of note, Dr. William Witt commented that a survey of anesthesia chairs was conducted, and of these, "90% of academic programs either forbid, strongly discourage, or otherwise limit reading in the OR during anesthetics."

Although overall debate on this issue remains inconclusive, it did generate a large number of comments in the APSF Newsletter—among these were reports of methods that experienced anesthesiologists utilize to reduce boredom in the OR other than reading:

1) Physically move around the room.
2) Observe the surgeon and the surgery. Surgeons will of course become fatigued and bored as well as anesthesiologists. Part of our job is to ensure that they are not missing an event that could become problematic, e.g., the compression of the vena cava with a pack, or a hidden bleeder dripping blood on the floor.
3) Review the surgery with the operating room staff.
4) Check the reserve equipment. Reassess the anesthesia machine and the monitoring equipment.
5) Examine the patient.

TAKE HOME POINTS

- Reading needs to be secondary to patient care; do not read during times in the case when you might be distracted from important events.
- If you are going to read, make sure your insurance and group do not prohibit that activity.
- Consider other activities to prevent boredom that do not distract your attention.
- Select appropriate reading materials.
- Do not: surf the Web, trade stocks, etc.

- If you read, imagine trying to explain to a jury why you were reading that material while your patient developed a complication. If you can't make it sound reasonable to yourself, it won't sound reasonable to a jury.

SUGGESTED READINGS

Howard SK, Rosekind MR, Katz JD, et al. Fatigue in anesthesia: implications and strategies for patient and provider safety. *Anesthesiology*. 2002;97(5):1281–1294.

McDonald JS, Peterson SF, Hansell J. Operating room event analysis. *Med Instrum*. 1983;17(2): 107–108.

Weinger MB. In my opinion: lack of outcome data makes reading a personal decision, states OR investigator. *Anesthesia Patient Safety Foundation Newsl*. 1995;10(2).

Weinger MB. Vigilance, boredom and sleepiness. *J Clin Monit Comput*. 1999;15:549–552.

186

ADEQUATE TREATMENT OF PAIN IS BOTH AN ETHICAL AND A LEGAL OBLIGATION. TREAT SEVERE PAIN SCORES LIKE UNSTABLE VITAL SIGNS: QUICKLY AND DECISIVELY

KENNETH R. ABBEY, MD, JD

Imagine that you are working in an ambulatory surgery center. You have just finished your last case of the day, a knee scope on a teenage soccer player, and he is now in the postanesthesia care unit (PACU) complaining to the nurse of 10/10 pain in his knee. The nurse states that he has been given the maximum PACU doses of pain medications, 15 mg of morphine and 250 mcg of fentanyl, on top of the 5 mg morphine, some fentanyl, and ketorolac that you gave in the operating room (OR). It is 6:00 P.M. You are supposed to be picking up your own kids from their soccer matches, and the surgeon has gone home. You examine your patient and find him to have otherwise stable vitals, and an exam of his surgical site is benign. He is alternating between dozing and whining tearfully about the pain. And now that you think about it, he was a bit whiny preop as well. How will you manage this patient? Send him home, assuring his mom that he'll feel better in front of the TV? Perform a block (if he'll let you)? Call the surgeon back (so that she can yell at you)? Admit your patient to the hospital across town?

It is obvious that physicians in general, and anesthesia providers in particular, have an ethical obligation to treat their patients' pain. Perhaps less obvious are the legal implications of the safety and adequacy of that treatment. A review of the legal literature and cases makes it clear that physicians will be held to a high standard of care with respect to pain management. Three cases are worth noting.

In *State of Kansas v. Naramore* (1998), an elderly woman with terminal cancer was suffering from intractable pain. Her physician admitted her to the hospital and gave escalating doses of opioids as her pain and tolerance increased. At some point, the doses required to relieve her pain began to compromise her respiration, and the doctor spoke with her family about the dilemma. Her son said, "Let me make one thing perfectly clear: I'd rather have my mother lay there and suffer for 10 more days than you do anything to speed up her death." She died in the hospital 3 days later. As if to prove that "no good deed goes unpunished," the doctor was later charged with

© 2006 Mayo Foundation for Medical Education and Research

and convicted of attempted murder. His conviction was later reversed on appeal. In the meantime, he spent 2 years in prison and lost his practice, his reputation, and his marriage.

While the *Naramore* case presents an extreme example of the legal risks of pain treatment, the bulk of recent cases, legislation, and regulation focuses on the legal implications of inadequate pain treatment. In *Bergman v. Chin* (2001), a California court considered the case of the pain management for a terminally ill cancer patient. William Bergman, suffering from back pain secondary to his lung cancer, was admitted to the hospital for pain management. He remained in the hospital for 6 days, with pain scores ranging from 7 to 10/10 throughout his stay. He was discharged with a pain score of 10/10 after he asked to be allowed to go home to die; and in fact, he died soon thereafter. His children, upset that his pain was not treated adequately, first complained to the California Medical Board about the treating physician. When that board refused to discipline the physician, the family sued. A jury awarded $1.5 million, concluding that the doctor had committed "elder abuse" in failing to treat Mr. Bergman's cancer pain adequately.

In 1999, an Oregon pulmonologist was disciplined for a series of incidents of inadequate treatment of pain. In one case, the doctor ordered "substantially inadequate amounts of pain medication" for a cancer patient and refused a hospice nurse's request for stronger medications. In another, he refused sedative or pain medications for a paralyzed and ventilated patient. In yet another, the physician performed a nasal intubation on an awake patient with no sedative or analgesic medications.

Government and regulatory bodies have taken an increased interest in the adequacy of pain management over the past decade. In 1999 the Veterans Health Administration declared that the pain score would be treated as a "fifth vital sign." The Joint Commission on Accreditation of Healthcare Organizations (JCAHO) followed suit, recommending that the simple 0-to-10 scale be used when possible to assess pain and that providers be vigilant in treating pain in noncommunicative patients as well. The JCAHO standards recognize the complex interaction of psychosocial, spiritual, and cultural values in modulating pain. The standards direct that patients and caregivers be educated regarding reasonable expectations for pain treatment and that the adequacy of pain management be assessed by data collection.

With respect to perioperative pain specifically, evidence-based guidelines are evolving and support mechanism-specific, multimodal approaches that are tailored specifically to particular surgical procedures. Thus, for example, evidence supports the use of acetaminophen for dental procedures but not for orthopedic procedures. Two organizations have begun to provide procedure-specific guidelines: the Veterans Health Administration (www.oqp.med.va.gov/cpg/cpg.htm) and the Prospect Working Group (www.postoppain.org). The guidelines of both organizations recognize that pain management techniques must be specific to both the patient and the procedure. The Veterans Health Administration also provides a "pocket guide" that includes a postoperative pain management algorithm requiring development and documentation of a pain management plan with re-evaluation and modification at designated intervals.

Perioperative pain management is a complex task under ever-increasing scrutiny by patients and regulatory bodies. To be successful, anesthesia providers must plan for pain management early and systematically. The plan should begin before surgery with assessment of the need for preoperative medications (e.g., nonsteroidal anti-inflammatory drugs, methadone) or anesthetizing procedures such as neuraxial or peripheral pain blocks. Any pain management plan should be specific to the surgical procedure, using drugs and techniques supported by best evidence. Finally, coordination of pain management with the surgeon is important to ensure optimal pain control and a smooth transition of pain management from the perioperative setting to the postoperative or postdischarge setting. When the pain management plan proves inadequate, providers are obligated to mobilize the resources necessary to manage the pain. This might include consulting the surgeon to determine whether a surgically correctable cause for the pain exists. It may also be necessary to consult pain specialists to assist in bringing intractable pain under control. Whatever additional intervention is used, reassessment at reasonable intervals and continued modification of the approach are required until the pain is well controlled.

TAKE HOME POINTS

- *Treatment of pain is a basic ethical obligation of all physicians.* Inadequate treatment of pain is not defensible on the grounds that "no one ever died from pain" nor that pain management involves some degree of risk.
- *Plan for postoperative pain management before surgery.* The plan should be specific to the patient and the procedure. It should involve the surgeon and be well documented. Postoperatively, reassess the pain management plan at reasonable intervals and modify it as needed to alleviate pain.
- *Treat pain as a vital sign.* Just as you would not discharge someone with unstable blood pressure or heart rate, do not discharge someone with unstable pain. Mobilize the resources needed to address the pain, including surgeons and pain/regional experts, and admit patients to an environment where their pain can be treated adequately with sufficient monitoring to ensure their safety.

SUGGESTED READINGS

Fleming RB, Curti TA. Oregon doctor disciplined for inadequate treatment of pain. *Elder Law Issues.* 1999;7(14). Available at www.elder-law.com.

Gray A, Kehlet H, Bonnet F, et al. Predicting postoperative analgesia outcomes: NNT league tables or procedure-specific evidence? *Br J Anaesth.* 2005;94:710–714.

Johnson SH. Relieving unnecessary, treatable pain for the sake of human dignity. *J Law Med Ethics.* 2001;29:11–12.

Joshi GP, Kehlet H. A procedure-specific approach to improve postoperative pain management. *ASA Newsl.* 2006;70(9). Available at www.asahq.org/newsletters.

King SA, JCAHO pain standards. *Geriatric Times.* 2000;I(4). Available at www.geriatrictimes.com.

Lewis T. Pain management for the elderly. *William Mitchell Law Rev.* 2002;29(1):223–244.

State v. Naramore. 965 P.2d 211 (Kan. Ct. App. 1998).

Yi M. Doctor found reckless for not relieving pain. *San Francisco Chronicle,* June 14, 2001.

187

HANDLE DENTAL INJURIES AS YOU HANDLE TEETH, WITH CARE

DOUGLAS W. ANDERSON, DMD AND
KENNETH R. ABBEY, MD, JD

Your first patient of the day is a middle-aged, morbidly obese man having an inguinal hernia repair, who happens to have the brightest, whitest smile you have ever seen. During his preoperative interview, he mentions that he used to have terrible teeth but has recently had a "major makeover" including the "caps" that give him his great smile. Of course, he turns out to be a difficult intubation; and while you are sneaking that bougie under an epiglottis you can only see the tip of, you hear the sharp crack of his front caps giving way to your Mac 4.

Injury to the teeth before anesthesia, during induction of or emergence from anesthesia, or under sedation is not common. *Nevertheless, such injuries represent the single largest source of claims against anesthesia providers.* The average payment for dental injury is only $1,700. However, because dental injuries constitute 29% of claims, total indemnity payments are substantial. In addition, administrative expenses associated with verifying and paying the claims add significantly to the cost.

Management of dental injuries begins before they occur. The first task for the anesthesia provider is to have a working knowledge of how dental injuries are handled in their institution. Be aware that there is a wide range out there! The editor has provided anesthesia care in hospital systems with policies that have ranged from providing no reimbursement for the repair of dental damage (on the advice of the institution's legal department, who feel that would represent a tacit admission of malpractice) to essentially providing free dental care for life. The second task for the anesthesia provider is to have a basic knowledge of dentition (if you can memorize the branches of the brachial plexus, you can master the simple numbering system of the teeth, *Fig. 187.1*). The third part of managing dental injuries before they happen involves discussion and documentation. Junior anesthesia providers who have never been involved in a dental complication often do not carefully document the exam of the teeth, whereas more experienced anesthesiologists and anesthetists who have seen complications do! Look closely at the teeth and take a minute to jot down the number of teeth that are missing or hanging by a thread (sometimes, it is more expedient to note where there *are* teeth, instead of where there aren't teeth). Also take notice of any open or fresh

ⓒ 2006 Mayo Foundation for Medical Education and Research

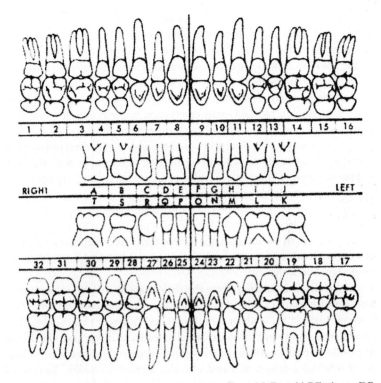

FIGURE 187.1. Number system of the teeth. (From McDonald RE, Avery DR. *Dentistry for the Child and Adolescence.* 3rd ed, St. Louis: Mosby; 1978:5.)

sockets. This documentation can seem costly in terms of time, and junior anesthesia providers are sometimes resistant to doing it. But consider the time required to bronch the patient while you are standing there thinking, "Did we bump that out, or was that the tooth the patient said fell out last night?"

The preoperative informed consent discussion is a key part of dental management and should *always* include information about the possibility of a dental injury. Here is one possible example:

> As you may know, I need to place a breathing device through your mouth so that I can use the anesthesia machine to keep you asleep and to breathe for you during your operation. It is uncommon, but it is possible to damage teeth or dental work when this breathing device is placed. For example, a crown or a bit of porcelain from your crown may come off, or a tooth may come out if it is extremely loose or if a filling breaks. You've shown me that number 30 is loose, that's one of your lower back molars on the right, so we'll be very careful about that one as well as the rest of your teeth, but I want you to know that damage can happen.

A number of routine circumstances should alert the anesthesiologist to the potential for dental injuries. Anatomic factors that contribute to dental injuries are primarily those that also make airway placement difficult—a large tongue, short neck, limited extension, limited flexion, micrognathia, anterior larynx, and certain pediatric syndromes such as Pierre-Robin syndrome.

Instruments may also cause injury, even those designed to prevent dental injury, e.g., hard bite blocks. During emergence, masseter muscle trismus can occur briefly before relaxation and awakening. Some devices such as folded gauze, an oral airway, or special props used specifically to protect teeth during emergence can actually contribute to damaging a filling or crown. Although nothing is foolproof, inexpensive folded gauze placed between the back teeth may be the most reliable preventative.

Special care should also be taken during intubation, extubation, mask ventilation, and laryngeal mask placement. In preparation for ENT or facial plastic procedures, for instance, the surgeon may tie the endotracheal tube to the front tooth with a suture, creating forces that dental restorations are not designed to withstand.

Generally, it is best to inform the patient about a dental injury during postoperative recovery. The patient probably already knows that something is wrong because his teeth or mouth may feel different than before. Have the patient seen by your in-house dental consultant, if you have one. If not, take time yourself to explain how the injury occurred and recommend that the patient visit a dentist or dental specialist as soon as possible. You should also report the injury to your liability carrier and risk management office right away (Do not reassure the patient that "everything will be paid for" unless you know for a fact that this is true!). Follow up with the patient by telephone in a day or two, express your concern, and remind the patient to seek treatment.

It has been customary for some anesthesiologists to pay for dental repairs when presented with a bill, even long after the incident. However, proper allocation of responsibility is more complex, because many factors apart from the anesthesia provider's actions may have contributed to the injury. Such factors include:

- Poor dentistry
- Restorations that are about to fail, particularly front tooth crowns with a crown-to-root ratio of 1:1
- Crowns that are too long
- Thin crown porcelain
- Dental neglect and poor oral hygiene

The patient's dentist may help him or her understand how the injury occurred and may discourage the patient from making a claim against the anesthesia provider. General anesthesia experience during training may temper the dentist's view regarding the cause of a restoration failure and the culpability of the anesthesia provider. Alternatively, an oral surgeon or an endodontist who has anesthesia experience may help to assess the cause of the injury. An endodontist or a prosthodontist will also be better equipped to evaluate how well a restoration should withstand anesthesia-related manipulations. Occasionally, a patient will call to report the development of a chronic pain syndrome due to restoration after a dental injury, and these have been known to result in tort claims, so maintain a file with as much detailed and complete information as possible.

Dental injuries happen. They are frequently the fault of no one. Weakened crowns on front teeth can sit for years waiting for the unsuspecting anesthesiologist/anesthetist. And yet, any dental injury makes a difference to the patient. Develop a mindset for prevention and know what to do if an injury occurs.

TAKE HOME POINTS

- Dental injuries are an occupational hazard for the anesthesiologist. Never act smugly or brag that you have never had a dental injury, because you will.
- The possibility of dental injury should be part of your informed consent discussion.
- If an injury occurs, tell the patient what happened.
- Report injuries early to your insurance carrier and risk management office.
- There are many reasons for dental injuries. Most are restoration failures that can result from normal manipulation of the airway.
- Develop professional relationships with general dentists, endodontists, or prosthodontists in your community who have anesthesia training.
- Recommend to the patient and his or her dentist that the injury be examined by one of these specialists.
- Also, recommend that no repairs be made by the patient's dentist until after an examination by an independent practitioner—and provide more than one choice. If the patient's dentist repairs the restoration quickly, no one will be able to evaluate the cause of the injury.

SUGGESTED READINGS

Anderson RE. *Medical Malpractice: A Physician's Sourcebook*. Totowa, NJ: Humana Press; 2005.

Cohen S, Hargraves KM. *Pathways of the Pulp e-edition*. 9th ed. Philadelphia: Mosby; 2006.

Shillingburgh HT, Sumiya H, Whitsett L, et al. *Fundamentals of Fixed Prosthodontics*. 3rd ed. Carol Stream IL: Quintessence; 1997.

Warner ME, Benenfeld SM, Warner MA, et al. Perianesthetic dental injuries: frequency, outcomes, and risk factors. *Anesthesiology*. 1999;90(5):1302–1305.

188

"DO NOT RESUSCITATE" ORDERS ARE NOT AUTOMATICALLY SUSPENDED IN THE OPERATING ROOM

KIRK LALWANI, MD, FRCA AND
VINCENT K. LEW, BA (MSII)

Cardiopulmonary resuscitation (CPR) is the only medical intervention that can be performed by a nonphysician without a physician's order or the patient's verbal consent. Consent to perform CPR is automatically presumed when the patient is unable to communicate his or her wish. Although CPR has the potential to reverse cardiac arrest, it may also unduly prolong life, cause unwarranted discomfort, and increase emotional distress.

Two central principles of medical ethics guide physicians in medicine: beneficence and nonmalfeasance. Though these tenets are instilled in all physicians, health care providers also have a duty to respect the wishes of the patient and his or her family. Patient autonomy reflects the right to self-governance and individuality. A provider may be forced to accept a patient's medical decision to refuse treatment, even if it results in the patient's death. Thus, the desire to preserve life without doing harm may conflict with the patient's wishes, and this is often encountered in patients with a "Do Not Resuscitate" (DNR) order.

THE DNR ORDER

DNR orders were created in the 1970s for terminally ill patients in order to prevent resuscitation from cardiac arrest resulting from the primary disease or its effects. Hospitals noticed a dramatic increase in DNR orders in 1988 following the Joint Commission on Accreditation of Healthcare Organization (JCAHO) mandate that all hospitals must develop formal policies regarding DNRs.

Unfortunately, DNR orders are often poorly worded. They can be vague ("treat me aggressively unless my condition is irreversible"), overly restrictive ("no life support desired"), or out of date. Documentation frequently omits the reason for the DNR order, how it applies, when it is valid, what procedures are covered, and what was discussed. This can be a problem when patients undergoing surgery have not indicated whether the DNR order applies in the operating room (OR). Legally, when documentation is unclear or unauthenticated, life-sustaining treatment is presumed and must be administered.

© 2006 Mayo Foundation for Medical Education and Research

DNR IN THE PERIOPERATIVE SETTING

Providers in the perioperative setting are often reluctant to adhere to DNR orders. The decision to suspend or uphold the DNR order has been the subject of much debate. There are three main issues that providers must confront with a DNR order in the OR.

First, by virtue of consenting to surgery, the patient expects to benefit either symptomatically or functionally from the procedure. Patients who undergo surgery have a reasonable expectation to survive the operation in order to obtain that benefit. The very objective of undergoing surgery would be redundant if the patient were allowed to die during the operation. Thus, the DNR order opposes the goal of surgery.

Second, the nature of anesthesia increases the chance of cardiac or respiratory arrest by producing profound disruption in normal physiologic functions such as consciousness, circulation, and breathing. Anesthesia frequently involves measures such as assisted ventilation, endotracheal intubation, and intravenous fluid resuscitation that are considered "resuscitative"; anesthesia may also induce cardiopulmonary arrest that may be readily reversible. Further, the survival rate of patients requiring CPR in the OR is very different from that of patients who have unwitnessed arrests; the difference may be attributed to the OR environment, in which patients are continuously monitored and physicians trained to administer CPR are always present. The overall recovery rate of CPR in anesthesia–related arrests is more than 90%. In contrast, cardiac arrests in patients elsewhere in the hospital have significantly lower survival rates (2% to 6% in general wards, 19% in intensive care units). Therefore, it is relevant to distinguish between arrests caused by the primary disease and those caused by anesthesia in the perioperative setting.

Finally, surgeons and anesthesiologists expect their patients to recover from surgery. No reasonable physician will operate on a patient with the knowledge that the patient will die in the OR. The goal of surgery is neither to kill nor expedite death, but rather to cure, improve, or palliate. In order to accomplish that goal, the patient must survive the operation.

ALTERNATIVE POLICIES FOR DNR ORDERS IN THE OR

Policies that automatically suspend or enforce the DNR order in the OR are not the ideal solution. Automatic suspension of DNR orders in the OR eliminates the opportunity for patients to make informed decisions about their care based on personal values and beliefs. It may also expose health care providers to medicolegal liability as a result of disregarding patient autonomy

On the other hand, automatic enforcement of DNR orders may have unintended effects on the patient. Certainly, a patient undergoing general anesthesia to improve his or her quality of life would not want a "do not intubate" order enforced during anesthesia. Automatic enforcement also may expose the health care provider to medicolegal liability, as the patient's family may hold the provider responsible for the patient's death.

GUIDELINES RELATED TO DNR ORDERS IN THE PERIOPERATIVE SETTING

The 1993 statement on ethical guidelines from the American Society of Anesthesiologists (ASA) and its subsequent amendment in 2001 is a useful guide to treating patients who have DNR orders. These guidelines have also been incorporated into the American College of Surgeons (ACS) "Statement on Advance Directives by Patients: Do Not Resuscitate in the Operating Room" and the American Academy of Pediatrics (AAP) guidelines for pediatric patients.

The guidelines discourage policies that automatically suspend or enforce DNR orders in the operating room, as either of these policies "may not sufficiently address a patient's right to self-determination." Instead, the ASA recommends that all physicians involved discuss with the patient or surrogate, before surgery, the appropriateness of upholding the DNR order during the operation. The ACP and AAP have termed this approach "required reconsideration." It is also recommended that the provider distinguish between full resuscitation, procedure-directed limited resuscitation, and goal-directed limited resuscitation. The procedure-directed approach focuses on careful consideration of specific interventions that are likely to be used during the operation. Goal-directed limited resuscitation focuses on the patient's goals, values, and preferences, rather than on specific procedures. This latter approach may allow the anesthesiologist and surgical team "to use clinical judgment in determining which resuscitation procedures are appropriate."

APPROACH TO THE PERIOPERATIVE PATIENT WITH A DNR ORDER ("REQUIRED RECONSIDERATION")

These guidelines provide the basis for an approach to the management of patients with DNR orders in the perioperative setting:

1) It is vital that in all cases the anesthesiologist and surgical team meet with the patient and/or surrogate preoperatively to discuss the roles of the anesthesiologist and the surgeon during the operation, and explain that some resuscitative measures are routine. Adequate time must be made available to address any ethical issues that may arise.

2) If the patient decides to suspend the DNR order, then the period for which it is suspended and the conditions for reinstatement should be specified.

3) Specific requests should adhere to institutional policy and professional society guidelines, and should be reviewed by the entire OR team before surgery.

4) It may be necessary to involve the institutional ethics committee for difficult situations.

5) It is essential to carefully document the preoperative discussion along with specific requests made by the patient in the medical record.

CONCLUSION

A well-informed patient or family will be better equipped to make decisions about their DNR order in the perioperative setting. Providers will be comfortable with the knowledge that due consideration has been afforded to patient autonomy without compromise of law, medical ethics, personal belief, or professional guidelines. Required reconsideration is a balanced approach to the management of the surgical patient with a DNR order.

SUGGESTED READINGS

Cohen CB, Cohen PJ. Required reconsideration of "do-not-resuscitate" orders in the operating room and certain other treatment settings. *Law Med Health Care.* 1992;20(4):354–363.

Ethical Guidelines for the Anesthesia Care of Patients with Do-Not-Resuscitate Orders or other directives that limit treatment. Available at www.asahq.org/publicationsAndServices/standards/09.html. Accessed August 23, 2006.

Ewanchuk M, Brindley PG. Ethics review: perioperative do–not–resuscitate orders—doing nothing when something can be done. *Crit Care.* 2006;10(4):219–222.

Fallat ME, Deshpande JK. Do-not-resuscitate orders for pediatric patients who require anesthesia and surgery. *Pediatrics.* 2004;114(6):1686–1692.

Lonchyna VA. To resuscitate or not in the operating room: the need for hospital policies for surgeons regarding DNR orders. *Ann Health Law.* 1997;6:209–227.

Statement on advance directives by patients: do not resuscitate in the operating room. Available at www.facs.org/fellows.info/statements/st-19.html. Accessed August 23, 2006.

189

INVOKE *PARENS PATRIAE* TO PROVIDE SAFE MEDICAL CARE TO A CHILD WHEN THE PARENTS CAN'T OR WON'T CONSENT

ANNE T. LUNNEY, MD

Parens patriae, Latin for "father of the people," was first instituted by King James I in England in the 1600s. At that time it was utilized to control the use of land by the state. Today, the doctrine of *parens patriae* is utilized when the state assumes decision-making authority for those not competent to make their own decisions. Although the scope of *parens patriae* encompasses incompetent adults as well as children, this chapter focuses on the authority of the state to make decisions regarding the medical care of children.

The state assumes medical decision-making authority on the child's behalf when the parental decisions are in conflict with the child's best interest or will result in harm, or when emergency medical care is required to prevent death or serious bodily harm and the parent is unavailable to provide consent.

ETHICAL DECISION MAKING

The ethical standards of beneficence and nonmalfeasance are preserved when parental decision-making authority is maintained. This outcome is based on the assumption that parents will act in the child's best interest. Furthermore, as the *best interest* of the child is complex and difficult to define, the parent is in the optimal position to make this determination. In 1976, the American Association of Pediatrics published a policy statement supporting parental authority and stated that only in cases of serious conflict should consultative and judicial assistance be sought to supercede parental decision-making authority.

Although it remains desirable to preserve parental decision-making authority, this authority is not absolute. When parental decisions will result in harm or death, the standards of beneficence and nonmalfeasence are not maintained. Under these circumstances the doctrine of *parens patriae* permits the state to assume decision-making authority.

As stated, the best interest of a child is difficult to define, and thus the best-interest standard (beneficence) is difficult to define and institute. Diekema suggests that the *do no harm* standard (nonmalfeasance) is more accurate and easily defined. A harm threshold is utilized to delineate this standard and is defined as the minimum standard of care tolerated by the community. Some clear examples of parental decisions trigger the harm

© 2006 Mayo Foundation for Medical Education and Research

threshold—including Jehovah's Witnesses (JW) who withhold a life-saving blood transfusion from their child, Christian Scientists who withhold insulin in the care of their diabetic child, and the situation when the parent is unavailable to provide consent for an emergency medical intervention.

The ethical framework of *do no harm* delineates the requirements that should be met before implementation of *parens patriae*. These requirements are the following: (a) there is a significant risk for serious harm; (b) harm is imminent and requires immediate action; (c) an intervention is required to prevent harm; (d) the refused intervention has proven efficacy; (e) the projected outcome outweighs harm; (f) there is not a more acceptable option; (g) the intervention is generalizable to similar situations; and (h) most parents would agree that the intervention is reasonable.

LEGAL PRECEDENTS

Common law supports self-determination, which includes the individual's right to make decisions regarding his or her own body. The seminal cases supporting self-determination are the 1767 decision in the United Kingdom of *Slater v. Baker and Stapleton,* in which physicians were charged with battery if they did not gain the consent of their patients before a surgery or procedure; and the 1914 United States decision of *Schloendorff v. Society of New York Hospital,* in which the justices determined that "every human being of adult years and sound mind has a right to determine what shall be done with his own body." In 1972, the American Medical Association included informed consent in the patient's bill of rights.

Legally, parents have medical decision-making authority on behalf of their child. Case law supports parental decision-making authority, provided that their decisions do not increase the likelihood of serious harm or death as compared with other options. In the case of *Newmark v. William,* the regional court decision to treat a 3-year-old boy with Burkitt lymphoma was reversed by the state supreme court. The high risk associated with chemotherapy coupled with the low probability of remission of this aggressive tumor made it difficult to clearly illustrate that the parent's decision to withhold treatment would result in harm, and thus the parent's decision-making authority was upheld.

In cases in which the harm threshold is met, religious beliefs are commonly the basis for the refusal of medical care. Case law consistently supports the position that freedom of religion does not include the right to act in a manner that will result in harm or death.

There are several pivotal legal decisions, both medical and nonmedical, that support *parens patriae*. In 1944, the decision of *Prince v. Massachusetts,* which addressed the general welfare of a 9-year-old selling JW magazines on the street, stated that "neither the rights of religion nor the rights of parenthood are beyond limitation" and that "parents may be free to make martyrs of themselves, but they are not free to make martyrs of their children before they have reached the age when they can make that choice for themselves." The decision in *Morrison v. State* (1952) stated that "the state has the power to preserve a child's life when medical treatment is necessary." The decision in *State v. Perricone* (1962) concluded that "it is unlawful to withhold blood when the child's life is in danger." Subsequent cases have consistently upheld the doctrine of *parens patriae,* supporting the state's obligation to protect those who are unable to protect themselves.

Under certain conditions, the state assumes decision-making authority for children when their parents are unavailable to do so. This most commonly occurs when emergency medical intervention is required to prevent death or serious bodily harm. Under these circumstances, parental consent is implied. Specifically, it is implied that the parents would make the best possible decision for their child if they were available to do so. In the instance of implied consent, it is important to make an aggressive attempt to contact the parents and to have a consensus from more than one physician that the medical intervention is required to prevent serious harm or death. It further is advised that one of the physicians making this declaration not be directly involved with the technical aspects of the proposed procedure.

Lastly, when invoking *parens patriae,* it is imperative to take the proper steps to assure that the ethical and legal tenets are fulfilled. Most institutions have established guidelines and corresponding documentation to safeguard the child, parent, and physician. Assuming medical decision-making authority for another individual is a profound responsibility, and every attempt should be made to assure that the individual's care meets the *do no harm* threshold.

TAKE HOME POINTS

- *Parens patriae* is a well-established legal principle permitting the state to act in the best interests of a child when the parents cannot or will not do so.
- *Parens patriae* should be applied in situations where the *do no harm* threshold is met.
- Invocation of the *parens patriae* prinicple requires the physician to follow the institution's policy for doing so.

SUGGESTED READINGS

American Academy of Pediatrics. Informed consent, parental permission, and assent in the pediatric practice. *Pediatrics.* 1995;95:314–317.

Diekema, DS. Parental refusals of medical treatment: the harm principle as the threshold for state intervention. *Theor Med.* 2004;25:243–264.

King James I on the Divine Right of Kings, A Speech to the Lords and Commons of the Parliament at Whitehall, March 1610.

Morrison v. State (1952).

Newmark v. Williams/DCPS (1991).

Prince v. Massechusetts (1944).

Schloendorff v. Society of New York Hospital (1914).

Sheldon, M. Ethical issues in the forced transfusion of Jehovah's Witness children. *J Emerg Med.* 1996;14:251–257.

Slater v. Baker and Stapleton (1767)

State v. Perricone (1962).

United States Department of Health and Human Services. *The Patients' Bill of Rights in Medicaid and Medicare.* HCFA Press Office. April 12, 1999.

AIRWAY AND VENTILATION

LINES AND ACCESS

FLUIDS, RESUSCITATION, AND TRANSFUSION

MEDICATIONS

INTRAOPERATIVE AND PERIOPERATIVE

EQUIPMENT

REGIONAL ANESTHESIA

PACU

PEDIATRIC ANESTHESIA

PROFESSIONAL PRACTICE

190

DON'T ASK THE OPERATING ROOM NURSE TO BE A SUPPLY TECHNICIAN, SECRETARY, OR MEDIATOR

CATHERINE MARCUCCI, MD, RALPH DIRADO, RN AND
PAMELA D. NICHOLS, RN

Operating room (OR) nurses (both the circulating nurse and the scrub person) have well-defined roles before, during, and after the surgical procedure. They assemble needed trays, instruments, and other supplies; count and set up the sterile tables; check in the patient; and complete the considerable preoperative and intraoperative paperwork. In smaller hospitals, they may be involved in transporting and checking in blood products, both before and during the surgery. Their duties intersect with but are not defined by the needs of the anesthesia team.

OR nurses will usually be able to provide valuable help during induction and intubation and will expect to leave their task at hand to assist with this. They are happy to deal with the dentures, jewelry, and religious items that come into the room with the patient. They will also deal with calls that come into the OR from the family waiting room. But they won't generally know where things are in the anesthesia workroom, so it is best not to ask them to run supplies for the anesthesia team, although they may be more than willing to try.

OR nurses are an independent, integral part of the OR team. Unfortunately, there can be attempts made to compromise their neutrality when disputes arise between the anesthesia and surgical teams. It is not necessarily true that they will "side" with the surgeons in a disagreement, but it is certain that they prefer not to be involved in disputes that don't really involve them.

Perhaps most unfair to OR nurses is to be used as a conduit for (usually bad) information to the surgeons. Good professional practice mandates that you keep the nurses informed in the preoperative period, but do not ask them to page the surgeons and give them a specific message, especially if it involves a delay, cancellation, or problem with starting the surgery. Unless it's an emergency and you absolutely cannot leave the patient, try to make the phone call yourself and do the negotiating. Similarly, the nurses in a room generally are not on the charge desk or running the board, so questions about why a case is being moved to a certain room can be frustrating and nonproductive.

© 2006 Mayo Foundation for Medical Education and Research

"Counting" is a fact of life for the OR staff. Since it has the indirect effect of diverting attention from other patient care issues at times that are some of the busiest for the anesthesia providers, it is also a fact of life for us as well. However, unless it is necessary for patient safety, do not interrupt the nurses when they are counting. It is best to call overhead for warm blankets, needed anesthesia supplies, and lifting help. Be willing to tolerate a slight delay on your side of things to avoid a possible long delay for the patient if the counts turn up incorrect.

There are really no legislative requirements for counting, other than "the law only requires that foreign bodies not be negligently left in patients." The Association of Operating Room Nurses (AORN) publishes general practice guidelines and each operating location will have its own policy. Depending on the case, sponges, sharps, and instruments must all be counted multiple times. For instance, the AORN recommends that sponge counts should be taken before the procedure to establish a baseline, before closure of a cavity within a cavity, before wound closure begins, at skin closure or end of procedure, and at the time of permanent relief of either the scrub person or the circulating nurse. Because there is a similar scheme for instruments, do not ask for clamps, etc. from the sterile trays and tables.

Finally, remember that the OR staff like to be called by their names, just as we do. Always introduce yourself to anyone in the room that you don't already know and say hello to those that you do.

SUGGESTED READING

Recommended practices for sponge, sharps, and instrument counts. *AORN J.* 2006 Feb;83(2): 418, 421–426, 429–433.

191

DO NOT ALLOW YOUR ADVANCED CARDIAC LIFE SUPPORT (ACLS) CERTIFICATION TO LAPSE

LISA MARCUCCI, MD AND SURJYA SEN, MD

To maintain a current Advanced Cardiac Life Support (ACLS) certification, health care providers are required to participate in a refresher course every 2 years. Because some hospitals do not require anesthesia staff to have ACLS certification to maintain hospital credentials, it is easy to let the recertification window elapse.

Resuscitation science continues to evolve, especially with the application of outcomes-based research methodology. In November 2005, the American Heart Association (AHA) published the most recent Guidelines for Cardiopulmonary Resuscitation and Emergency Cardiovascular Care in the journal *Circulation,* as well as on the AHA website at www.americanheart.org.

In 2001 the AHA revamped the ACLS guidelines and course to a case-based approach. The basic ACLS Provider course now provides the knowledge and tests the skills to manage the initial minutes of an adult ventricular fibrillation arrest. There are also 10 core cases covering the management of patients suffering respiratory arrests and acute ischemic strokes, as well as life-threatening cardiac arrhythmias. The Emergency Cardiovascular Care handbook is strongly recommended as an adjunctive text to the ACLS Provider manual.

Immediate postresuscitation care as well as ethical and legal issues have been added to the ACLS curriculum. The ACLS Experienced Provider Course "provides a stimulus for clinicians and scientists to identify areas in resuscitation that deal with special circumstances" and uses the ACLS Reference Textbook as the required course manual.

The ACLS course and recertification are now offered online as well as at hospital sites. Information on this, as well as the most recent changes to the ACLS protocols, are on the website.

TAKE HOME POINTS

- For those to have to pay for it out of pocket, ACLS certification is expensive and recertification usually costs less.

© 2006 Mayo Foundation for Medical Education and Research

- A certification (if one allows it to expire) will take 2 days whereas a certification is one day.
- An advanced providers course offers many challenging and interesting scenarios that many experienced practitioners may find valuable compared to having to redo an initial certification.
- Many anesthesia providers will find an existing certification necessary or helpful when applying for a new job (who wants to scramble around looking for a weekend course in order to complete credentials material)
- Losing ACLS certification means you'll have to redo certification in BLS as well.
- It is important to incorporate the changing ACLS guidelines into daily practice, both from a patient care perspective as well as a medicolegal (standard of care) viewpoint.

SUGGESTED READING

2005 American Heart Association guidelines for cardiopulmonary resuscitation and emergency cardiovascular care. *Circulation.* 2005;112(24)(suppl).

192

DO NOT ASK A FAMILY MEMBER TO TRANSLATE OR ASSIST WITH PROCEDURES

RANDAL O. DULL, MD, PHD

Family members sometimes ask (or are asked) to assist the anesthesia provider. This is understandable; most families genuinely wish to be helpful to the provider and attentive to and supportive of the patient. Remember, however, that during any kind of illness (and especially one requiring surgical intervention), family members often feel they have relinquished control of their loved one to a process that is both unfamiliar and threatening. Thus, the family may feel more stress and helplessness than the patient. Under these conditions, it is almost never a good idea to put the family "to work." It isn't fair to them and it creates both medical and legal problems. The primary role of the family should be to provide emotional support to the patient. The only exception occurs with the pediatric population, in whom the calming influence of parents can almost always be beneficial, and the parents may be asked (depending on the culture of the hospital) to carry the patient into the operating room (OR) and to provide "cradling" assistance during induction.

Today, virtually all hospitals serve a population that is culturally diverse. This has increased the frequency of non–English-speaking patients requiring anesthetic care. Often, a family member will volunteer to assist with translation and, given scheduling pressures in the operating room, it is common to allow this practice rather than waiting for an official hospital translator. This does not meet the standard for either informed consent or confidentiality requirements. Informed consent requires that the patient or his or her legal representative be presented the risks and benefits of anesthesia based on the patient's medical condition(s). Informed consent is more than a signature on a piece of paper; it is an actual exchange of information. When using a family member to translate, it is impossible to know that all information was adequately and, more important, accurately translated in a manner that would satisfy the legal requirements of the informed consent process. As such, having an official translator for the informed consent conversation is the best course of action. The anesthesia preoperative evaluation should clearly list the name of the hospital translator. If the situation is so urgent that it cannot be held until an official translator is present or the language is so obscure that a translator is not available, the official documentation

© 2006 Mayo Foundation for Medical Education and Research

should reflect this and the emergency/urgent nature of the impending surgery or procedure should be specifically noted. The hospital translator also serves the secondary purpose of ensuring that the patient is able to have a confidential (at least as far as the family is concerned) preoperative interview.

Family members also become involved in patient care during the placement of labor epidurals. Usually this involves the family member bracing himself against the table or Mayo stand on which the patient is leaning and assisting the patient to maintain proper body position. Although this allows the family member to have face-to -face contact with the patient, and that may be comforting to the patient, this situation is undesirable for several reasons. First, family members cannot be expected to know how to maintain best position for epidural insertion, which may prolong or impede the procedure. Second, the family member may herself faint or become light-headed at the sight of needles, blood, or the reaction of the patient to the needle sticks. Should the family member faint, he or she risks serious injury (a recent legal case involved a husband who fell backward and suffered a fatal brain hemorrhage). This also creates a situation that detracts from care of the primary patient. In general, it is always best to ask family members to leave the labor room during the placement of the epidural.

Similarly, family members are sometimes present when an intravenous (IV) line is placed preoperatively. The prudent anesthesiologist will ask if anyone is prone to fainting and take that opportunity to have susceptible family members or friends leave. If it is anticipated that the patient may be a difficult IV placement or the circumstances are such that family members are already stressed, it is again best to have them leave. If the IV placement requires more than one attempt, the family's protective instincts may result in unhelpful criticism or outright hostility toward the anesthesia provider(s). The goal is always to maintain a high level of trust between the anesthesia team and the patient and the family; anything that could undermine the anesthesiologist–patient relationship should be avoided.

TAKE HOME POINTS

- Remember that the family is there to support the patient, not the medical staff.
- Do not have the family translate—this does not meet criteria for informed consent or patient confidentiality.
- Do not have the family assist with procedures, including epidurals in the labor room.

- A widely recognized exception is the presence of a parent for induction in pediatric rooms.

SUGGESTED READINGS

Hoehner PJ. Ethical aspects of informed consent in obstetric anesthesia—new challenges and solutions. *J Clin Anesth.* 2003;15(8):587–600.

McDonough JP, McMullin P, Philipsen N. Informed consent: an essential element of safe anesthesia practice. *CRNA.* 1995;6(2):64–69.

193

TAKE STEPS TO SAFEGUARD YOURSELF IF YOU ARE PREGNANT, BUT TRY NOT TO WORRY EXCESSIVELY

ANGELA ZIMMERMAN, MD

You are giving a lunch break in an orthopedics case that is progressing along, when you hear the surgical resident say to no one in particular, "Is anyone in the room pregnant?" It so happens that you are 7 weeks pregnant. You haven't "announced" yet, and weren't planning to until about 12 weeks. Why is the resident asking, and what should you say?

When a female anesthesia provider becomes pregnant, she may develop a new concern that she has not experienced previously—what exactly are the potential hazards of working in the operating room for her baby? Unfortunately, this a difficult question because there are a number of potential hazards and there is really no definitive answer.

Historically, there was concern about the effects on the fetus from exposure to trace anesthetic gases. Studies dating back to the 1960s have attempted to analyze epidemiologic surveys to assess the effects of anesthetic gases on reproductive outcome. Conclusions showing that there was an increased risk of spontaneous abortion and congenital abnormalities in babies of operating room (OR) women have been countered by other reviews that reveal inconsistencies in the data. Also, there was no statistically significant difference between reproductive outcome from exposed and nonexposed groups. A later study in the 1980s did find a statistically significant relative risk of spontaneous abortion and congenital abnormalities due to trace anesthetic gases, but concluded the risk is very small compared to other, more documented environmental hazards. Essentially, pregnant OR staff have the same risk as women working in radiology, agriculture, and horticulture and do not incur meaningful additional risk to their pregnancies because of exposure to anesthetic gas.

Conflicting data exist regarding the implication that trace anesthetic gases may adversely affect any practitioner's vigilance and may decrease psychomotor function. So then the question becomes, is the mother's baseline health affected, apart from teratogenic effects? Review of articles from the 1990s to the early 2000s emphasized that with improvement of environmental conditions as required by modern occupational protection and

---

health care regulations, the use of inhalational anesthetics can be considered to pose no health risk. Some articles, however, do suggest that exposure of health care personnel may exceed recommended levels in poorly ventilated postanesthesia care units. In summary, no studies have demonstrated that trace concentrations of anesthetic waste gases adversely affect women in the OR. With routine use of scavenging techniques, environmental anesthetic levels have been lowered to the extent that proving any adverse outcomes using epidemiologic data will continue to be very difficult.

However, negative reproductive outcomes may be related to other job-associated factors, such as radiation exposure, fatigue, stress, infections, dehydration, and exposure to other toxic substances. Radiation exposure is probably the biggest concern to the anesthesia provider. The majority of pregnant anesthesiologists handles this issue by simply not working fluoroscopy cases in the OR or any type of case in the radiology suites. Modern OR fluoroscopy machines expose staff to much lower levels of radiation than previously, but there is no recommended safe level of radiation exposure for the developing fetus, especially during the first trimester when organogenesis is taking place. Most anesthesiologists and nurse anesthetists who have been pregnant will tell you that it's just not worth the anxiety, even with "double lead" and trying to stay a minimum of 6 to 10 feet away from the beam.

An example of a toxic substance to which pregnant women can be exposed in the OR is methyl methacrylate. Methyl methacrylate is a volatile compound that is used in the manufacture of resins and plastics. It is also mixed in the OR as a component of bone cement (it is the substance that has that distinctive, acrid odor). It is known to have adverse reproductive effects, and pregnant women are recommended to avoid exposure. The orthopedics resident in the above case was most likely getting ready to mix the bone cement and was giving the standard OR warning. The answer to the question is that you should leave the room quickly, even if it means "blowing your cover."

Infectious disease issues are also a problem for the pregnant anesthesia provider. AZT is not contraindicated in pregnancy (remember that its use during pregnancy can significantly decrease the chance of transmission of HIV/AIDS from mother to baby), but no woman who is pregnant or about to become pregnant would take much comfort in that thought. Therefore, it is of paramount importance to observe strict universal precautions, including gloves, handwashing, protective gowns, and eyewear) and impeccable sharps techniques. If you do have an exposure, call the "sticks" hotline immediately—you owe it to your baby. Also, if there is any thought that the patient may have active tuberculosis, request a respirator.

While dealing with all these "nervous-making" situations, remember that there is a large cohort of anesthesia providers who have had healthy babies with essentially zero problems. Pregnant anesthesia providers are often pleasantly surprised to find that their departments are supportive and flexible. It is generally the policy of training programs not to ask a woman to do a case she is not comfortable doing. Programs will also usually make allowances in the posting and call schedules to combat the ever-present fatigue problem. Expect that senior staff and colleagues will help you if you are forthright about your schedule, issues, and needs. Remember always that the key to being a successful anesthesia provider while pregnant is the same as for a "regular" anesthesia provider—use lots of common sense and don't forget to communicate!

TAKE HOME POINTS

- Trace anesthetic gases pose little or no incremental risk to the pregnant anesthesia provider.
- In general, women in stressful jobs may have poorer reproductive outcomes—this includes operating room personnel.
- A precedent exists for pregnant anesthesia providers to avoid radiation and/or methyl methacrylate cases.
- Pay scrupulous attention to universal precautions.
- Use the support that is extended to you.

SUGGESTED READINGS

Barash PG, Cullen BF, Stoelting RK, eds. *Clinical Anesthesia*. 4th ed. Philadelphia: Lippincott Williams & Wilkins; 2001.

Boivin JF. Risk of spontaneous abortion in women occupationally exposed to anaesthetic gases: a meta-analysis. *Occup Environ Med.* 1997;54(8):541–548.

Burm AG. Occupational hazards of inhalational anaesthetics. *Best Pract Res Clin Anaesthesiol.* 2003;17(1):147–161.

Byhahn C, Heller K, Lischke V, et al. Surgeon's occupational exposure to nitrous oxide and sevoflurane during pediatric surgery. *World J Surg.* 2001;25(9):1109–1112.

McGregor DG. Occupational exposure to trace concentration of waste anesthetic gases. *Mayo Clin Proc.* 2000;75(3):273–277.

Mehlman CT, DiPasquale TG. Radiation exposure to the orthopaedic surgical team during fluoroscopy: "how far away is far enough?" *J Orthop Trauma.* 1997;11(6):392–398.

Sessler DI, Badgwell JM. Exposure of postoperative nurses to exhaled anesthetic gases. *Anesth Analg.* 1998;87(5):1083–1088.

Tannenbaum TN, Goldberg RJ. Exposure to anesthetic gases and reproductive outcome. A review of the epidemiologic literature. *J Occup Med.* 1985;27(9):659–668.

U.S. Environmental Protection Agency. *Health and Environmental Effects Profile for Methyl Methacrylate.* EPA/600/x-85/364. Cincinnati, OH: Environmental Criteria and Assessment Office, Office of Health and Environmental Assessment, Office of Research and Development; 1985.

194

KNOW WHAT THE BASIC STATISTICAL TERMS MEAN

PETER F. CRONHOLM, MD, MSCE AND
JOSEPH B. STRATON, MD, MSCE

HOW CLINICIANS MAKE DECISIONS

In order to make informed, evidence-based decisions, providers need to have an understanding of several statistical concepts. The decision-making process begins by assessing information by means of a history and physical examination framed within an understanding of the relative probabilities of disease states. The next step is to determine the likelihood that the patient has the disease in question. If we have enough information at that time, no further testing is needed and we may move on to treatment. If not, more information is needed and further testing must be done to better determine whether the disease in question is in fact the underlying etiology. For each step of the decision-making process, we need to understand testing and disease characteristics.

Clinical decision making is based on an understanding of the incidence and prevalence of diseases considered in differential diagnoses for the types of patients considered. The *prevalence* of a disease tells you how many people at a given point or period of time have the disease in question. Prevalence combines people who already have the disease and those who will acquire the disease during that period of time. The *incidence* of a disease tells you how many new cases of a disease develop or are likely to develop over a period of time. Incidence is a measure of risk, whereas prevalence is more of a measure of the burden of disease for a given population. The process of developing a differential diagnosis is a ranking of etiologies based on our understanding of the incidence and prevalence of diseases for a given set of historical and physical data.

Decisions are made based on the likelihood of a disease for a given clinical situation. The likelihood of a disease ranges from nil (0%) to absolute (100%). There exists a range of likelihoods that vary depending on the balance of costs and benefits of provider decisions that determine what our next steps should be in terms of making choices to treat, not to treat, or to conduct diagnostic testing. Diagnostic testing should be considered when there is a difference between the likelihood that a patient has the disease and the threshold at which a provider chooses to move forward with treatment

© 2006 Mayo Foundation for Medical Education and Research

options. Two thresholds must be considered that determine the range over which diagnostic testing should be considered. The first is the testing threshold. The *testing threshold* is the likelihood below which providers consider the disease sufficiently rare a cause that they would not treat empirically for the disorder nor test for the presence of the condition. To make treatment decisions, providers need to have some point at which they will decide to treat a patient given the weight of the evidence with no further testing. This point is referred to as the *treatment threshold.*

Shaping a differential diagnosis is a process of categorizing the probabilities of various diseases associated with the patient history and exam. The probability that a patient has the disease before any diagnostic testing is done is known as the *prior probability* of disease. Diagnostic testing increases or decreases the likelihood that a person has the disease in question. The likelihood that person has the disease after diagnostic testing is known as the *posterior probability.* Diagnostic testing occurs along a continuum of likelihoods when the prior probability is lower than the treatment threshold but higher than the testing threshold (see *Fig. 194.1*). If the prior probability is above the treatment threshold, you would treat the patient without further testing. If the prior probability is below the treatment threshold, you require further testing, the results of which will either move you away from the treatment threshold if negative or closer or over the treatment threshold if positive. A series of tests may be necessary in order to move the posterior probability that a patient has the disease to the point of treatment. As an illustration, if you would operate on a person only if you were 70% sure that he had the disease, but after your history and physical you are only 40% sure, then you would need to do more testing to move your likelihood over 70%. There is no need to perform tests when you are already over the treatment threshold (although these are often done for "academic" reasons) or if the test will not provide enough evidence to move you over the treatment threshold if no other testing is linked or available. For example, if a febrile patient has tender anterior cervical anterior cervical adenopathy, with an exudative pharynx and the absence of cough by history, you should treat this patient for bacterial pharyngitis without further testing (*Fig. 194.1*).

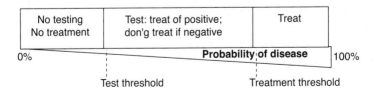

No testing No treatment	Test: treat of positive; don'g treat if negative	Treat

0%   **Probability of disease**   100%

Test threshold   Treatment threshold

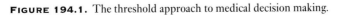

FIGURE 194.1. The threshold approach to medical decision making.

HOW CLINICIANS JUDGE A TEST

Sensitivity and specificity are characteristics of diagnostic tests. They inform the provider how the test will behave among people with or without disease. The *sensitivity* of a test is a measure of how often the test will be positive when testing people who have the disease. In contrast, the *specificity* of a test measures how often the test will be negative when testing patients who do not have the disease. Highly sensitive tests are used for screening because a highly sensitive test, when negative, rules out the disease (SeNsitive:OUT or SNOUT). A highly specific test, when positive, rules in the disease (SPecific:IN or SPIN).

As clinicians what we really want to know is if the test comes back positive or negative, what does this mean for the patient: does she have the disease or not? To answer this question you need to know the sensitivity and specificity of the tests used, but you also need to have a sense of the prevalence of the disease among people like the person you are testing so that measures known as positive and negative predictive values can be calculated. The *positive predictive value* of a test is the likelihood that a person has the disease if the test is positive. The *negative predictive value* is the likelihood that a patient does not have the disease if the test is negative. If a test comes back positive for a person who is very likely to have the disease (high prevalence), the result is likely to be a true positive. However, if the person is very unlikely to have the disease, the result is much more likely to be a false positive. Similar statements can be made for negative results for high- and low-prevalence conditions.

HOW CLINICIANS KNOW WHETHER THE TREATMENTS WILL WORK

Measures of association are means of estimating the strength of the relationship between observed outcomes and factors that may produce the outcome. Common measures of association are the odds ratio, relative risk, absolute risk reduction, and number needed to treat. Odds ratios are used in studies in which the incidence (or true risk) of disease cannot be assessed accurately (case series, case–control studies, and some retrospective study designs). *Odds ratios* are determined by calculating the ratio of the odds of exposure among the cases compared with the odds of exposure among the controls. For example, if the ratio of the odds of exposure to artificial tanning lamps among cases with melanoma and controls is 3 to 2, the resulting odds ratio is 1.5. *Relative risk* specifies the risk of developing the disease in the exposed group relative to those who are not exposed and can be reported from certain prospective study designs and clinical trials. Relative risk is the best measure of the association between exposure and disease. However, odds ratios can provide robust estimates of association and can approximate relative risk for outcomes that are rare.

The *absolute risk reduction* (ARR) is the difference in disease rates between the exposed and unexposed groups. It is important for clinicians to understand the difference between absolute and relative risk reductions. For uncommon diseases with high relative risks or common diseases with low or moderate relative risk reductions, the absolute risk reduction of an intervention may be quite low. An intervention may have a 10-fold relative risk reduction with rates of disease near 0.1 for those with the intervention and 1 for patients without (RR = 1%/0.1% = 10). However, the same study findings could be described as producing an absolute risk reduction of <1% (ARR = 1% − 0.1% = 0.99%) for those patients exposed to the intervention.

A clinical use of absolute risk reduction is to take its reciprocal, which is known as the *number needed to treat* (NNT). The NNT for an intervention is the number of people who would need to be exposed to the intervention in order to produce the desired outcome for one person. For example, if the ARR is 8% when giving clopidogrel to patients getting stents placed in the setting of symptomatic coronary artery disease with the intention of reducing myocardial infarction (MI), the NNT would be 12 (NNT = 1/ARR = 1/0.08 = 12). It follows that with a NNT of 12, you would need to give clopidogrel to 12 patients in order to prevent one MI. Although one MI was prevented, 11 of the 12 patients received no benefit from the intervention; however, all 12 patients needed to be treated, as you could not predict in advance which one would benefit. There is no single number that represents a "good" NNT. The clinical effect of NNT is based on the likelihood of the disease, the cost of the intervention (medications, procedures, harm associated with intervention) and the cost of not doing the intervention (rates and values assigned to patient morbidity and mortality associated with the disease).

When interpreting study results, it is important to understand what is referred to as power as well as types of errors that may be encountered. The *power* of a study, usually presented as a percentage, is a measure of the probability that the null hypothesis is rejected when it is false. That is to say that you will not find an association between the dependent and independent variables if there is no true relationship between them. If the measures of association (odds ratios, relative risk, etc.) of a study reach significance, then the power of the study is irrelevant and the findings stand as significant assuming the study methods are valid. However, results may not reach significance, either because there is no true relationship between the dependent and independent variables or because the study did not have enough power (usually an issue of sample size) to demonstrate the relationship.

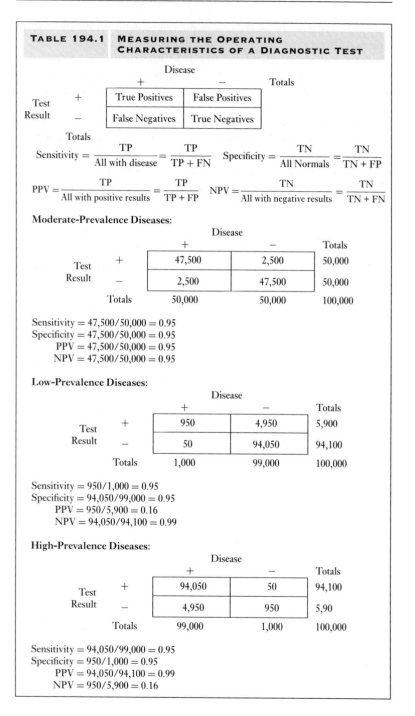

TABLE 194.1   **MEASURING THE OPERATING CHARACTERISTICS OF A DIAGNOSTIC TEST**

		Disease		Totals
		+	−	
Test Result	+	True Positives	False Positives	
	−	False Negatives	True Negatives	
	Totals			

$$\text{Sensitivity} = \frac{TP}{\text{All with disease}} = \frac{TP}{TP + FN} \qquad \text{Specificity} = \frac{TN}{\text{All Normals}} = \frac{TN}{TN + FP}$$

$$PPV = \frac{TP}{\text{All with positive results}} = \frac{TP}{TP + FP} \qquad NPV = \frac{TN}{\text{All with negative results}} = \frac{TN}{TN + FN}$$

Moderate-Prevalence Diseases:

		Disease		Totals
		+	−	
Test Result	+	47,500	2,500	50,000
	−	2,500	47,500	50,000
	Totals	50,000	50,000	100,000

Sensitivity = 47,500/50,000 = 0.95
Specificity = 47,500/50,000 = 0.95
PPV = 47,500/50,000 = 0.95
NPV = 47,500/50,000 = 0.95

Low-Prevalence Diseases:

		Disease		Totals
		+	−	
Test Result	+	950	4,950	5,900
	−	50	94,050	94,100
	Totals	1,000	99,000	100,000

Sensitivity = 950/1,000 = 0.95
Specificity = 94,050/99,000 = 0.95
PPV = 950/5,900 = 0.16
NPV = 94,050/94,100 = 0.99

High-Prevalence Diseases:

		Disease		Totals
		+	−	
Test Result	+	94,050	50	94,100
	−	4,950	950	5,90
	Totals	99,000	1,000	100,000

Sensitivity = 94,050/99,000 = 0.95
Specificity = 950/1,000 = 0.95
PPV = 94,050/94,100 = 0.99
NPV = 950/5,900 = 0.16

Type I errors represent the chance that the null hypothesis will be rejected when it is actually true, or that you will find a result that is significant by chance alone and there is no true underlying relationship between the dependent and independent variables. This is the rate of false alarms or false positives. Type I errors are the equivalent to the "significance" level reported in studies (e.g., p-values <0.05). Type II errors are the chance that you will not reject the null hypothesis when it is false. Type II errors are the complement of power (type II error rate $= 1 -$ power). Type II errors are the chance that you will miss an effect when it is really there. In other words, it is the rate of failed alarms or false negatives (*Table 194.1*).

SUGGESTED READINGS

Centre for Health Evidence. www.cche.net/usersguides/main.asp.

Hennekens CH, Buring JE, Mayrent SL. *Epidemiology in Medicine*. Boston: Little, Brown; 1987.

Rothman KJ, Greenland S. *Modern Epidemiology*. 2nd ed. Philadelphia: Lippincott-Raven; 1998.

Swinscow TDV, Campbell MJ. *Statistics at Square One*. 10th ed. London: BMJ Books; 2002.

195

ALWAYS AVOID THE BAD JOBS—KNOW THE ADVANTAGES AND DISADVANTAGES OF THE DIFFERENT TYPES OF PRACTICES

NORMAN A. COHEN, MD

One of the greatest challenges facing a physician at the end of residency is finding a "good" job. Although faculty at the resident's training program are great resources for training the young anesthesiologist about clinical matters, most academic anesthesiologists have little background in evaluating practices, understanding contracts, analyzing demographics, or the many other techniques necessary to properly vet a practice. This chapter provides the necessary background to help the reader avoid a most serious anesthesia complication: choosing the wrong practice.

TYPES OF PRACTICES

Anesthesia practices come in many flavors; however, just about all fall into one of six categories: solo practice, single-specialty group, multispecialty group, academic, government, and *locum tenens*. Each has unique strengths and weaknesses, and, as we will see, characteristics that may mesh better with the personality and goals of the job seeker.

SOLO PRACTICE

In a solo practice, the anesthesiologist is the only provider and has no associates. The anesthesiologist makes all the business decisions, and only external forces, such as medical staff bylaws, insurance contracts, facility agreements, and state medical practice regulations constrain the practice.

The solo practitioner's greater freedom compared to a member of a group practice is at least partially offset by the physician's lesser power to negotiate favorable agreements from payers and facilities. It is much easier for an insurer, hospital, or ambulatory surgical center (ASC) to replace a single doctor in their provider panel or medical staff than it is to do the same to a large group. On the other hand, not having to overcome a larger group's bureaucratic inertia affords the solo practitioner the flexibility to aggressively and quickly pursue new business opportunities.

SINGLE-SPECIALTY GROUP

A single-specialty anesthesia group can range in size from two physicians to hundreds. All the members practice anesthesiology or a recognized subspecialty. Larger groups have significant market clout and are often able to

© 2006 Mayo Foundation for Medical Education and Research

negotiate more favorable agreements with insurers and hospitals. However, there are risks in being large. Some dominant groups take advantage of their size to illegitimately raise prices. Such behavior can lead to exceptionally costly antitrust investigations and possible litigation by the Federal Trade Commission. Disgruntled competing anesthesiologists, who have been displaced from their jobs or seen their incomes reduced as a result of the large group exercising its market clout, may seek legal remedies. In addition, patients who believe that they have been financially harmed by excessive fees also have the option of creating a class-action lawsuit to recover overpayments. All of the risks lead responsible large groups to act conservatively in pricing and contracting.

Like the solo practitioner, smaller groups tend to be more nimble and flexible in taking advantage of business opportunities, but they may lack the resources and skills to implement their strategies effectively. They also do not have the economies of scale with regard to recruitment, benefits, and contract negotiations that a larger group can bring to bear on these matters. As groups increase in size, professional management and full-time office staff become a necessity. In addition, the breadth and scope of experience and knowledge that the physicians possess increases dramatically. Effective use of this resource often differentiates exceptional groups from average ones.

In large single-specialty groups, physician employees, even if they are shareholders in the group, may believe that their individual contributions to the group are limited. These physicians may assume an "employee" mentality, such that the motivation to attend to important matters such as group productivity and profitability, attention to customer satisfaction, and pursuit of new lines of business is no longer seen as a responsibility of the individual physician. In addition, this disengagement can lead to inadequate oversight of practice managers, billing vendors, and office staff, resulting in a range of problems including lost income, missed business opportunities, and even theft of funds. Well-run large groups have systems in place to help prevent these problems from occurring, which include careful oversight of employed managers, periodic audits, and mechanisms to encourage an "ownership" perspective for each physician in the group.

Because anesthesia practice is most commonly limited to a hospital or surgery center, fixed assets owned by the group and overhead expenses tend to be relatively limited. Medium to larger groups may own or lease office space and own office equipment; however, these groups do not usually have to hire clinical staff or own expensive medical equipment. A group that also offers chronic pain services may be an exception to this general rule. Because of these factors, group overhead expenses tend to be much smaller than seen for other medical specialties.

MULTISPECIALTY GROUP

A multispecialty group is a single entity that includes physicians from two or more recognized medical specialties. Multispecialty groups tend to be large in size and often possess significant market power. Because anesthesiology is a highly compensated specialty, a "Robin Hood" syndrome is often seen in multispecialty groups, whereby the practice redistributes revenues generated by anesthesiologists to physicians in lower-paid specialties. In addition, multispecialty groups have the overhead burden associated with medical, surgical, laboratory, and radiologic practices, and the anesthesiologists typically have higher overhead obligations than those in solo or single-specialty practices.

When negotiating with insurers, the multispecialty group negotiators may not adequately address the unique characteristics of the anesthesia payment system. The negotiators' goal may be to maximize revenue for the high-volume specialties such as internal medicine, pediatrics, or radiology. Although anesthesiology may account for a small volume of total revenue, mistakes at the negotiating table can and have transitioned anesthesia from a profit center to a cost center for the organization. When considering a multispecialty group practice setting, it is extremely important to make sure that the group negotiates effectively on behalf of all the specialties and that anesthesiology has representation on the contracting team. It is even better if one or more anesthesiologists have leadership roles in the organization.

Large multispecialty groups may have a monopoly or near-monopoly on medical care in their service area. Public perception of predatory pricing and restraint of competition may expose these large groups to the same antitrust issues as described for large single-specialty groups.

Despite the possible financial disadvantages for an anesthesiologist with a multispecialty group, this practice type may offer the anesthesiologist employee a few benefits. The surgeons are part of the same practice, providing the anesthesiologist a guaranteed referral stream. In a well-run organization, management will address behavioral issues and interpersonal conflicts internally. This avoids invoking hospital medical staff peer-review procedures. Because of their larger size, multispecialty groups may offer a more valuable benefits package. Both clinical and clerical support will typically be better in quality and quantity. Because the group is financially integrated, it is able to enter into more sophisticated risk-sharing arrangements with payers without running afoul of antitrust rules. This last advantage may be a double-edged sword, however, as poorly executed risk sharing can and has resulted in significant red ink. Investments in technologies such as electronic medical records and in coordinated health improvement initiatives are more likely in an integrated group practice. Lastly, the all-too-frequent attempts by a hospital CEO to try to "control" the anesthesia department is much less likely when such action may place the entire patient referral stream of a multispecialty group at risk.

ACADEMIC PRACTICE

An academic anesthesiology practice provides both clinical anesthesia care as well as teaching and research opportunities. Academic practices are in many ways similar to integrated multispecialty groups, with the added overlay of teaching responsibilities, research, and writing obligations. Newly minted anesthesiologists have more familiarity with this practice type than any other; however, in my brief experience with joining the academic practice where I trained, the amount that I did not know about the financial workings and interpersonal dynamics of the group still gives me pause.

As of the time of this writing, academic anesthesia practices are facing significant financing problems arising from three sources: a discriminatory Medicare payment policy that pays the teaching anesthesiologist only 50% of the usual fee when directing two residents, limitations on resident work hours, and less-than-proportional National Institutes of Health (NIH) research funding compared to other specialties. Without dwelling on the historical details of these three issues, the result is that a substantial proportion of academic anesthesia practices are receiving significant financial support from their institutions to maintain a compensation package that will allow for recruitment and retention of qualified anesthesiologists. Secondary effects include frequent tensions between the anesthesia chair and the dean over financial matters and reduced nonclinical time. The turnover rate in chairmanships recently has been around 20% a year, due in no small part to the difficulties and stresses associated with managing a financially troubled organization.

Funding for most nonclinical time comes from research grants. The relatively low prevalence of NIH grants for anesthesiologists limits opportunities for anesthesiologist/scientists to have the time away from clinical duties to allow pursuit of clinical interests, thus helping perpetuate reduced research activities.

Resident work-hour limitations have also placed increased clinical demands on academic faculty. Because there is a quota system for residency funding, academic departments are unable to easily increase the number of resident positions to offset the reduced work hours. The more financially solvent departments have been able to self-fund additional positions, but this is the exception, not the rule. Although work-hour rules apply to all residencies, anesthesiology department chairs facing the aforementioned funding problems often find themselves forced to increase the clinical obligations of their faculty to help meet operating room demand.

When considering an academic position, the job applicant needs to carefully assess the effects of these funding and staffing issues to determine whether the applicant's career goals will mesh with the opportunities a department offers and the clinical obligations he or she will be required to fulfill. If the applicant's reason for joining the department is tightly tied to the chairman, it is important to learn about the stability of the chairman's job.

GOVERNMENT/MILITARY PRACTICES

A relatively small number of anesthesiologists work directly for a government entity. These practice settings include the Veterans Administration (VA) hospital system, armed services hospitals, and public hospitals chartered to serve the economically disadvantaged. Each provides unique challenges and opportunities.

For example, during the time that I trained, the VA system was widely considered to be inefficient, costly, and a provider of relatively poor-quality care. Although they are by no means perfect, VA hospitals have had an enviable record in recent years of aggressively promoting and improving quality through such initiatives as the National Surgical Quality Improvement Project (NSQIP). The VA is also a leader in installing medical information systems to help optimize chronic disease management while simultaneously reducing medical error. A brief history of NSQIP can be found at http://acsnsqip.org/main/about_history.asp.

The Iraq war and U.S. efforts in Afghanistan have presented new challenges and opportunities for military anesthesiologists. Whether improving anesthetic management for multiple-trauma stabilization procedures in the field, employing continuous peripheral nerve blocks for pain control, or improving the continuity of patient medical information through application of modern devices such as the USB flash memory drive, our military anesthesiologists are playing a major role in helping our servicemen and -women in very challenging times.

Physicians working in publicly funded hospitals, often in inner cities or rural areas, fight a different type of war. They care for the poorest of the poor and must manage the medical products of poverty— malnutrition, drug abuse, teenage pregnancy, trauma, and noncompliance with chronic disease management. As perioperative physicians, anesthesiologists must deal with all these issues in the operating room, the labor suite, and the intensive care unit. A listing of many of these public hospitals can be found at the National Association of Public Hospitals and Health Systems website, http://www.naph.org/Content/NavigationMenu/About_ Our_Members/List_of_Members/List_of_Members_htm.

The financial rewards of working for a government entity pale in comparison to most other practice types; however, the satisfaction of reducing a soldier's pain, improving care for our veterans, or serving the underserved provides less tangible but equally significant rewards for this group of anesthesiologists.

LOCUM TENENS PRACTICE

A *locum tenens* physician is one who provides temporary coverage for another physician. Because of the ongoing shortage in the supply of anesthesiologists, local, regional, and national physician staffing companies have remained very busy in providing all types of anesthesia practices temporary personnel support.

What sort of physicians choose to be *locum tenens*? All types, actually. Some are early in their career and use the *locum* option to investigate and explore different practices and different parts of the country. Some *locum* physicians are "empty nesters" who, after practicing many years in their local community, now choose to travel around the country, often with a reduced workload. And some anesthesiologists, who enjoy the challenges and variety of working in new settings on a frequent basis, opt for a lifetime career as a *locum tenens* physician. It is certainly not easy to have to prove oneself to surgeons, nurses, and anesthesiologists every few weeks or few months!

As mentioned, the ongoing shortage of anesthesiologists, estimated to exceed 2,000 nationally, makes the supply–demand equation favor the temporary physician. Daily rates paid to the agency often exceed the revenues generated by the doctor. In addition, the group pays for travel, lodging, and often a per-diem for food and incidentals. Groups that have a service contract with their hospital and that have a personnel shortage are usually willing to suffer the loss associated with using a *locum* if it keeps the contract in force.

Although the staffing agency may get a reasonable rate for the temporary physician, the *locum tenens* anesthesiologist is most frequently an independent contractor to the agency, essentially a self-employed solo practitioner. These physicians are responsible for maintaining liability, health, and disability insurance, paying all taxes in all states in which they work, and covering all other business expenses. The staffing agency keeps a fee for serving as matchmaker and assisting in licensure and credentialing of the physician.

When considering the *locum* option, one must weigh lifestyle considerations, finances, and the uncertainty associated with never forming roots in a practice or never being certain about what problems and challenges might be associated with the next job.

196

ALWAYS AVOID THE BAD JOBS—KNOW YOURSELF

NORMAN A. COHEN, MD

SELF-ASSESSMENT

In trying to find the best practice type, self-assessment is absolutely essential. Depending on the individual's nature and personality, some practice types will work whereas others absolutely will not.

LONE RANGER OR COLLABORATOR

Are you a lone ranger, wanting to manage your life with the minimum of outside interference? Solo practice or *locum tenens* may fit you well, as these provide the individual the most freedom to choose one's destiny. If you are a team player, enjoy the camaraderie of others, and are willing to collaborate, then any of the group practice types might work for you.

FREE SPIRIT OR OBSESSIVE

Free-spirited types who "get along to go along" are much better suited to a group practice; however, if being a free spirit means a lackadaisical attitude toward your obligations, then a group may not enjoy working with you as much as you enjoy working with the group! Anesthesiologists are often detail-oriented and are somewhat obsessive about their practice. Within reason, obsessive behaviors can help an individual work well in either solo or group practice. When the obsessions start to create conflict with others, then solo practice may be preferable.

LEADER OR FOLLOWER

Every group needs leaders, but not every member of a group can be one. If you excel at leadership and enjoy the responsibilities that come with it, look for a group that offers a leadership track. Those groups that take professional development seriously will mentor you and allow you the opportunity to lead. One of the most difficult situations occurs when an anesthesiologist wants to lead but lacks the necessary interpersonal skills. These physicians often become dysfunctional group members, "stirring the pot" and creating havoc. Unless the group finds a productive outlet for these people, either the group will suffer or the individual will be let go. More often than not, groups choose to suffer and pay a significant price in lost goodwill with the surgeons, the operating room staff and the hospital administration.

© 2006 Mayo Foundation for Medical Education and Research

If, on the other hand, you are a follower, do not want to be bothered with leadership responsibilities, and want only to meet your daily clinical obligations, you are not a good candidate for solo practice. In fact, you might fit best with a large single- or multispecialty group that is professionally managed and already has a good leadership structure. Smaller groups often need everyone to chip in and help with medical staff and business responsibilities. A "seven-to-three" workday mindset is not a good fit, nor is an inability or refusal to participate in group management.

RISK TAKER OR RISK-AVERSE

Risk takers are often a better fit in a solo or small group practice. The bureaucracy and inertia found in larger organizations may frustrate the risk taker.

197

ALWAYS AVOID THE BAD JOBS—KNOW HOW TO ASSESS A PRACTICE

NORMAN A. COHEN, MD

In the sections immediately following, I will provide an overview of some of the key points to consider when evaluating a practice, both in general and for specific practice types.

ALL PRACTICE TYPES

All practice types have certain elements that must be carefully analyzed. The common factors include the practice's relationship to the facility, the payer environment, use of nonphysician anesthetists, and call and case assignments.

RELATIONSHIP TO FACILITY

When evaluating a practice, one of the most important questions to have answered is the nature of the relationship between the group and the hospitals or other facilities where service is provided. If the group has a contractual relationship, it is vital to assess the current status of the contract. Go beyond the group's description and check out alternative sources. The operating room (OR) manager, chief of surgery, or even the hospital administrator may be helpful in understanding the quality of the relationship. This suggestion applies whether or not the group has a formal contract with the facility.

When a group works at multiple sites, you will need to determine whether you will work at one, some, or all the group's sites. Depending on the answer, the amount of homework that needs to be done may increase significantly.

In the ideal situation, the facility has reasonable expectations of the anesthesiology staff and has good relations with the group and with the medical staff as a whole. Typically, groups that focus on the service aspect of their mission and on delivering safe and cost-effective care maintain enviable relationships with their facility(ies). On the other hand, groups that fail to manage problems (or problem employees) effectively often have tenuous relationships. Taking a job with such a group means that you are assuming significant risk that you will be looking for another job soon.

When I served as a consultant working with troubled anesthesia departments, the most common service problem involved obstetric anesthesia coverage. Many groups just refused to cover the service, and many hospitals refused to pay a subsidy to "those lazy good-for-nothing gas passers" without exacting a pound of flesh. And that pound of flesh was control—control

© 2006 Mayo Foundation for Medical Education and Research

over hiring, firing, and the group's obligation to the hospital. In most cases, if the group had focused on serving the needs of the community and had chosen to work with the hospital's leaders, they would have received some supplemental funding without giving up control of their group's destiny.

The second most common problem that I saw was not dealing effectively with problem physicians. The chronic "pot stirrer" can undermine the group, damage its credibility, and occasionally even lead to litigation or loss of a facility contract. Most reasonable individuals expect that anesthesiologists will show up to work on time, be courteous to their patients, and diligently complete required paperwork. This is *not* the case more often than one might imagine. The consequences include patient complaints, surgeon and OR staff dissatisfaction, and in some cases much more dire consequences such as government audits or potential loss of accreditation for the facility. The latter two outcomes are not appreciated at all by facility administrators!

THE MONEY GAME

For most physicians, compensation is *the* most important job characteristic. Although I disagree about priority, I do agree that money is an extremely important matter. Revenue derived from clinical practice depends on patient demographics (also known as "payer mix"), case volume, and average anesthesia units. A simple metric that is useful for comparison is the resulting "blended" conversion factor. Although all solo practices, many single-specialty group practices, some multispecialty practices, and few academic and governmental practices tie pay directly to the insurance status of your patients, following the money is exceptionally helpful in understanding the viability of your practice opportunity.

Patient Insurance Demographics. The key factor that determines payment for a given case is the patient's insurance status. Ranging from those who pay at your billed rate (rare) to patients with no insurance (who rarely pay full fare and often pay nothing), gaining an understanding of the breakdown by payer and frequency can help you validate whether the practice's estimates of your clinical income makes sense. When looking at an insurance demographic breakdown, pay particular attention to the self-insured, Medicare, and Medicaid groups. The larger their share, the smaller the group's net income. As of 2005, Medicare pays about a third as much as the average commercial payer for anesthesia services. In most states, Medicaid's rates are similar to Medicare's. Notable exceptions include New York and California, where Medicaid payments are far less than those for Medicare. On the other hand, Alaska's Medicaid rates have historically been near those of some private payers.

Other considerations include determining whether a particular payer has market dominance. If one does, then that payer has the ability, often exercised, to ratchet rates downward. On the other hand, having multiple payers competing for the practice's participation turns the tables and levels the playing field during rate negotiations.

Volume and Total Units. Once you have the insurance breakdown for the practice, the second key variable is case volume. It is fairly simple to take the insurance breakdown expressed as a percentage and multiply by total case volume to get volume by payer.

However, volume and insurance status is not enough information to calculate payments. The last element needed is average units per case. As will be explained in detail in the chapter on anesthesia coding and compliance, most payers value anesthesia services using the American Society of Anesthesiologist's (ASA) anesthesia relative value system. The ASA system rates each anesthetic by base units that value the complexity of the case and the pre- and postanesthetic work, and time units that value the time involved in direct anesthetic care. Most payers recognize one time unit for every 15 minutes, but pockets of the country may bill more than four time units each hour. The ASA system also includes modifiers that take patient condition, extremes of age, and special anesthetic techniques into account; however, some payers, most notably Medicare, do not recognize modifier units.

One calculates payment for an *individual* anesthetic by the sum of the base, time, and modifier units. This value is multiplied by the conversion factor to get the total charge. The conversion factor is the amount of money paid for each anesthesia unit.

When looking at the practice as a whole, one can take the average number of units per case multiplied by the product of the insurer's contribution to practice volume and the insurer's negotiated payment rate to determine income from a given insurer. Taking this a step further, one can divide this number by total group clinical income to determine the importance of a particular insurer to the practice. Case volume by insurer and case income by insurer can be dramatically different. In a hypothetical practice, Medicare patients may make up 40% of total units billed but account for only 20% of total revenue. On the other hand, a large private payer contributes 20% of the patients but 30% of total revenue. It doesn't take a rocket scientist to recognize the importance of this private payer to the group's financial health.

"Blended" Conversion Factor. Having all the insurance demographic, volume, and conversion factor data would be amazingly useful to an applicant trying to make a well-reasoned decision about a practice's income stream; however, it is rare that a group will share all or even most of the information needed to perform the analysis described above. Fortunately, a simple metric exists to allow one to make an "apples-to-apples" comparison of provider income between different practices. This metric is known as the "blended"

conversion factor and is a weighted average of the conversion factors of all the payers in a practice. It is calculated by dividing total clinical income by total units billed. Once you determine the average number of units generated by a full-time member of the practice and know the "blended" conversion factor, you can multiply the two values to determine estimated gross revenue generated by a physician in the group. Assuming equal case volume and units per case, the greater the "blended" rate, the greater the clinical income per provider.

Other Factors: Overhead Expenses and Nonclinical Income. In the discussion of demographics, volume, and "blended" units, I have spoken about gross clinical income. This is the revenue that an anesthesiologist generates from patient care. "Take-home" pay or net income is usually dependent on gross clinical income. However, before you get your paycheck as a member of your new group, "All-Star Anesthesiologists of Alcatraz, PC," the group has to pay for the expenses of doing business. For an anesthesia practice, these expenses often include billing and collection services, accounting and legal fees, corporate insurance, administrative and staff salaries and benefits, taxes, rent, equipment, supplies, pensions, and health insurance. In an academic practice, add the cost of the "dean's tax," otherwise unfunded research initiatives, and teaching and accreditation expenses, to name just a few. This "overhead," which separates your net income from the money you generate, varies from practice to practice but approaches 15% of gross clinical income in the average private practice.

What's nonclinical income? It is all the income your group generates outside of provision of clinical care and includes bank interest, realized investment gains, and any stipends paid to the group by a facility. Given that >50% of anesthesia groups currently receive some form of stipend from their hospital, that an even higher percentage of academic practices do so as well, and that some of these stipends can be quite large, this nonclinical income may be a substantial fraction of total group income, and ultimately your income, if you join the group. Assuring the viability of this income stream is extremely important when evaluating a group with such a dependence on nonclinical income.

As a new member of a group, the group may, and probably will, pay you less than an established member of the group. Just as you are taking a risk that the job will work out, the group is taking a risk on you as well. The group also needs to recoup the expenses involved in recruiting you, getting you on payer provider panels, privileging you with the facilities where you will be working, and all the other details involved in any new hire. Although a differential in pay is reasonable, it is vitally important to you that the duration is not unlimited and that you have a crystal-clear understanding of the requirements for you to achieve equal pay for equal work.

The Bottom Line. The ASA and the Medical Group Management Association (MGMA) recently completed a "Cost Survey for Anesthesia Practices." Practice administrators, physician leaders, and "number geeks" like me find the data fascinating and quite useful for benchmarking, negotiating, and payment policy development. The survey gathered data from >100 practices and provides exquisite detail on revenue and expenses for all practice types and sizes. If you have a head for numbers and want as much financial data as possible to use in your analysis of your practice opportunity, I think that this publication is the current "gold standard." If you have money burning a hole in your pocket, you can buy the 2005 edition   http://www5.mgma.com/ecom/Default.aspx?tabid=138&action=INVProductDetails&args=795. ASA members can get a discount on the book. If you are a resident, check with your department's practice manager, as the department is probably a member of MGMA and might have purchased a copy.

CASE DISTRIBUTION

Now that you know how to estimate the income-generating potential for the average member of the group, you need to understand how the group assigns physicians to cases. Methods for case assignments vary widely from group to group, and, depending on how income is allocated, can diverge significantly from the average in either direction. Unlike Lake Woebegone, not every anesthesiologist in a group is "above average"—in income, anyway.

"Gaming" of assignments is a well-honed practice with some physicians, leading to no end of discord within groups. No matter the system, if there are checks and balances to assure that case distribution is fair and equitable, consider this to be a positive characteristic of the prospective group; however, if the converse is true and your income is productivity-based, tread carefully. . . very, very carefully.

Although many methods exist to distribute cases, there are three common approaches. These include a pure surgeon request system, assignments based on estimated relative value units for the room, and assignments based on the estimated length of the day.

Surgeon Request. In a number of places, anesthesiologists get cases only when the surgeon specifically requests them. This sort of scheduling dance requires that the surgeon's office identify an anesthesiologist for each and every case. This system creates significant incentives for the anesthesiologists to pay exceptionally close attention to the needs of their primary customer, the surgeon. Efficiency and affability on the part of the anesthesiologist are commodities that are rewarded. Likewise, surgeons possessing a favorable patient mix (young, healthy, and well insured) with a decent average unit-per-case rate and who are efficient are often courted by the anesthesiologists.

The new kid in town gets the leftovers. Gaining credibility and respect in that marketplace is a long-term process and is very challenging.

When I was looking at jobs while still a resident, much of the Phoenix, Arizona, market operated this way. For me, one of the biggest negatives of the Phoenix approach was the need to drive from hospital to hospital in the course of a day to meet all of one's scheduling obligations. Having a habit of looking at potential problems in a system, I was concerned about the effect of longer-than-expected surgeries or postanesthesia management obligations on my ability to get to my next case across town. Despite these reservations, it is clear that the system seemed to work reasonably well in Phoenix at that time, as I was not aware of a disproportionate shortage of anesthesiologists in that market.

Unit-Based Distribution. A number of groups pool income but pay each member based on productivity. The conversion factor is the "blended" unit discussed above. For these groups, assigning cases based on the estimated number of units generated makes great sense. My last private practice uses a type of unit-based distribution system. Depending on the daily schedule, each anesthesiologist has a rank assigned that guides room assignment. In an effort to assure equity, the anesthesiologists rotate through the schedule in a well-defined pattern so that over any reasonable period of time, each anesthesiologist has each rank an equal number of times.

Confounding factors include inconsistency across anesthesiologists in estimating case unit values and the effects of vacations and personal time that lead to alterations in the schedule. Also, patient and surgeon requests can financially affect multiple providers whenever these requests occur and are honored. In settings where the anesthesiologists are not members of the same group, insurance status of the patients becomes very important. "Cherrypicking" of cases is a frequent cause of discord and dysfunctional behavior.

Although unit-based case allocation clearly pays people based on the relative value of the work they do, this system, by itself, values *only* work and does not account for other contributions to the practice, such as medical staff leadership, patient education, quality improvement efforts, and participation in local, state, and national medical organizations. Forward-thinking groups develop ways to also account for these very important activities. Approaches include assigning a unit value to each important nonclinical task, allocating bonus payments based on participation and citizenship, or paying separately for time spent at recognized activities.

Time Based Distribution. In time-based case distribution, anesthesiologists are assigned based on the length of time for which the room as scheduled. For example, the first call person may get the longest room, the post-call person the shortest room, and the rest of the anesthesiologists get a room assigned based on that day's pecking order. These groups typically pay their physicians based on a daily rate schedule—X dollars for a call, Y dollars for a day of work.

Although overall income to the group is still based on units generated, payer mix, and payer-specific conversion factors, the physicians in this group value their time far more than the complexity or intensity of the work that they do. Consequently, the physicians have an incentive to seek the least complex or shortest room, and may feel slighted if there seems to be a pattern of being assigned more complex rooms more frequently than average. Having a payment system in which at least part of total income is productivity-based addresses this concern, at least to some extent.

Call. Current residents and recent graduates of U.S. training programs have been subject to strict work-hour limits. Once you leave residency and get a job, those limits no longer apply—your practice may require you to work all day, all night, and a good part of the next day. You may be the only anesthesiologist available for 3 days in a row. If you are in solo practice at a small hospital, you may be responsible for all anesthetics $24 \times 7 \times 365$. It's a whole new, and perhaps unpleasant, world.

Ask a hundred anesthesiologists about their least favorite part of the job and you will hear an overwhelming consensus that night call wins that dubious honor hands down. The reasons are pretty obvious—fatigue, stress, challenging patients, poorer insurance status, and fewer resources available when the airway is unexpectedly difficult, the patient begins massively bleeding, or the anesthesiologist needs to take care of normal physiologic needs.

In evaluating call obligations at a practice, first ask yourself a few questions. Do you have the energy and stamina to potentially work 36 or 48 hours straight? Will you have that same stamina after 10 or 20 years in practice? Can you maintain good humor when exhausted? Do you have a spouse or children, and are you willing to spend the required numbers of days, nights, and weekends apart? Are your clinical skills sufficiently advanced to be able to manage very complicated patients with little if any backup?

The other part of evaluating call obligations is to make sure that the system is fair and equitable. Does everyone share equally in call? Groups may have a separate call rotation for cardiac, pediatrics, or pain management. Does the call burden appear reasonably equal across sections, keeping in mind the old saying that "the enemy of good is perfection"? Although senior members of a group are often granted a reduced call burden, determine if there is any quid pro quo, such as reduced pay, vacation, or mandated retirement after a defined period. If the group requires the employee to work the day after call, does this occur always or sometimes? Are efforts made to relieve the post-call person as early as possible?

Also consider how busy the hospital is after hours. A sleepy, community hospital setting with no obstetric service and a quiet emergency department is entirely different than a Level 1 trauma facility or a major teaching hospital. Get a sense for whether the surgical staff does only truly urgent or emergency surgeries after hours or whether the end of the office day is just the beginning of regular OR time in the eyes of the surgeons.

The prospective group may be helpful in answering these questions. However, if call is an important factor in your decision making about a practice, try to review surgical logs for the facility where you may be working and ask questions about after-hours cases with the nurse managers, OR, and postanesthesia care unit (PACU) nurses when you get the opportunity. And you should make sure that you get that opportunity! Understanding your tolerance for call and answering the questions in this section will go a long way in helping you make sure that the practice's call requirements are not deal breakers.

Care Team versus Physician Delivery. When looking for a job, you will see two specific types of practices—those with nonphysician anesthetists and those without. Nonphysician anesthetists come in two flavors, Certified Registered Nurse Anesthetists (CRNA) and Anesthesiologist Assistants (AA). Although CRNAs dominate in numbers, more and more states are permitting AAs to practice and an increasing number of AA programs are opening across the country. The differences in training and background between CRNAs and AAs is not particularly relevant to the issue of practice analysis, so will not be discussed here.

Residents in training spend almost all of their time in the hands-on delivery of anesthesia care. They may spend some time in the OR teaching junior residents, but rarely have any supervisory responsibilities for nonphysician anesthetists. Transitioning from residency to an all-physician practice may be relatively seamless, as it is the logical extension of the training continuum, in which the senior resident is given significant autonomy in patient evaluation, anesthetic plan development, and perioperative delivery of care. The difference is that you are now on your own, without an experienced anesthesiologist available to help when circumstances dictate.

Groups in which anesthesiologists work with CRNAs and AAs are known as "anesthesia care team" (ACT) practices. A newly minted anesthesiologist just entering practice will not only have to learn to operate independently but also how to manage other providers. Determining the skill levels of the other members of the care team and defining the division of labor takes some time. This is a two-way street. The CRNAs and AAs working with the newly trained anesthesiologist are on the line when they follow directions from the anesthesiologist. They want any and all recommendations to be sound and reasonable. They also want to be treated with respect. Only the passage of time will allow the two parties to gain confidence in each others' abilities.

Although anesthesiologists and nurse anesthetists have never seen eye to eye on all or even most issues on the political stage, and although a subset of anesthesiologists and CRNAs would never countenance working with the other provider group, a large number of anesthesiology practices work well in the ACT mode. For the physician members, having the ability to have a physician involved in the care of all patients, while not obligating a highly trained consultant to personally performing anesthesia in less challenging cases, is a distinct advantage. In these days of shortages among all anesthesia providers, this factor certainly has merit. Another less lofty but nonetheless relevant consideration is that net income is often higher in an ACT practice than in a physician-only practice. For nurse anesthetists, a substantial number enjoy working with physicians, appreciate the clinical expertise that anesthesiologists bring to the operating room, and also would rather be well-paid employees than independent entrepreneurs.

In looking at an ACT practice, pay particular attention to the interactions between the anesthesiologists and other anesthetists. Is it collegial or confrontational? Is there a well-defined delineation of responsibilities? Does the group employ the CRNAs, does the hospital, or do the anesthetists have their own group? Do the physicians ever personally deliver anesthesia, or is the practice mixed between medical direction and personal performance? Do the physicians who are medically directing actively participate in all the key parts of the anesthetic? Are all members of the group committed to correct coding? Working in an anesthesia care team entails additional and sometimes challenging obligations in correctly submitting claims to insurers for payments. Errors can be costly either monetarily or in possible decertification as a Medicare provider, which can lead to loss of facility contracts. The chapters on common errors in anesthesia coding will discuss some of the issues associated with anesthesia coding in an ACT practice.

COMPETITIVE THREATS

The health care marketplace is in constant flux. Anesthesiology practices are often dependent on the goodwill of the surgeons and hospital management at a single location. With the ongoing move to surgical care in the nonhospital setting, this dependence can quickly become a liability for an anesthesiology group.

Even groups with seemingly secure and long-standing relationships with their facilities may be faced with unexpected challenges. Perhaps a free-standing ambulatory surgical center (ASC) is being built by some of the group's most productive surgeons. Is the group planning to arrange anesthesia coverage at the ASC? How will the management of the group's primary hospital respond? Is there a noncompete agreement preventing the group from pursuing this line of business? If the group cannot or will not provide coverage, will the loss of business to the ASC affect the group's revenues substantively?

These are not hypothetical questions. Every day in every part of the country, anesthesia groups are facing these challenges. Mistakes and lost opportunities may make your new job a target of downsizing when group revenues become inadequate to maintain the partners in the lifestyle to which they have become accustomed.

198

ALWAYS AVOID THE BAD JOBS—UNDERSTANDING SOLO PRACTICE AND THE BASICS OF MEDICAL PRACTICE FINANCE AND LEGAL ORGANIZATION

NORMAN A. COHEN, MD

In addition to the issues discussed in previous chapters, the assessment of solo practice opportunities has some unique considerations.

CASE DISTRIBUTION

Unless you will be the sole practitioner for the facility, an admittedly rare circumstance, you will need to have an understanding of the case distribution model at your prospective facility. Make sure that the case assignment system has reasonable checks and balances to avoid abuse. This warning is particularly important when a large group has a significant presence.

The best case is having an independent party responsible for assignments. Also, if patient or surgeon requests are frequently made and honored, determine if there is any method to offset your lost income when one of "your" cases is taken from you. Without protection of some sort, lobbying of surgeons, direct advertising to patients, and other tactics have been known to result in an attempt to disproportionately direct patients to one of the competing anesthesiologists or anesthesia groups. This is a recipe for conflict, outlandish behavior, and dysfunctional anesthesia department function. I can hear the sound of consultants pounding on the door!

CALL DISTRIBUTION

As with case distribution, assuring fair distribution of call responsibilities is exceptionally important in a solo practice. Sometimes additional calls can be financially beneficial, particularly when starting out in practice and trying to create good relationships with surgeons. In other situations, additional calls may be a problem. In either case, make sure that the opportunities for gaming the system are at a minimum.

In addition to handling after-hours cases, those on call often must manage acute pain management issues such as epidurals and continuous nerve blocks, postanesthesia complications including postdural puncture headaches and persistent nausea or pain, and perhaps even calls from chronic pain patients for prescription refills, implantable pump issues, or other problems. Although many of these issues are common to all practices, as a solo practitioner you may find yourself saving patients from the misadventures of

ⓒ 2006 Mayo Foundation for Medical Education and Research

others or being forced to manage a treatment regimen far different from what you might have prescribed. At least in a group practice, you can weed out problem physicians and reduce your potential liability. You can also establish common protocols for managing specific issues.

Anesthesiologist Relationships

In a setting in which the anesthesiologists are in multiple practices and are competing with each other for business, relationships can easily become strained. Assess the history of these interactions carefully. Big warning signs include history of litigation between providers, hospitals threatening to enter into an exclusive contractual relationship, or a parade of consultants having visited the site in the recent past.

Meet with your competitors before applying for privileges to practice. There may be a significant shortage of providers and you will be welcomed with open arms; however, much of the time you will be seen as someone trying to steal food out of the mouths of the other physicians' children. If your competitors are hostile and you still want to practice, at least you will know the challenges you will be facing.

Control versus Responsibility

As a solo practitioner you will have maximum control over your business. However, with that control comes responsibility—responsibility to your patients, to any employees or vendors, to your surgeons, and to your facility. You will bear complete responsibility for *all* aspects of managing your business. As a busy practitioner, you may not have adequate time to fulfill all your obligations. In that case, you will need to vet any businesses to which you may want to outsource some of your business functions. Most anesthesiologists do not have any significant experience or training in running a business; however, in solo practice, you **are** a small businessman or woman. If you don't take this seriously, it may cost you far more than you can imagine. It is no wonder that so many physicians are the victims of scams, bad investments, or outright theft from those to whom they delegated financial control.

Finances/Accounting/Legal

Your net income will depend on having an effective billing and collection system. You can do billing yourself, hire a person to do it for you, or outsource. Given the complexities of billing and the significant financial risk if it is done incorrectly, I suggest outsourcing to a reputable firm. Even large practices outsource billing and collections; however, unlike the large practice, you will likely not get the volume discounts that they enjoy.

Consider hiring an accountant and a lawyer to assist you in establishing your business correctly, paying all the necessary fees, and obtaining all required licenses. You can choose to track your finances and pay all your bills yourself, using the accountant only for tax preparation and the occasional consult for a specific issue. To see if this makes sense to you, weigh the accounting fees for routine bookkeeping to your opportunity cost—reduced time available to practice and generate income as well as reduced time with your loved ones.

Check with your state's medical or anesthesiology associations. They may be able to refer you to attorneys and accountants with particular experience in health care. Just as you would likely not see a family practitioner to manage your brain tumor (even though this has occurred on numerous television series over the years), you probably would not have a patent attorney review your insurance agreements.

Once your business is established, you will probably want to have your lawyer review contracts for you. Insurance agreements and independent practice association contracts are two common reasons to consult a lawyer. I am not a lawyer, don't play one on TV, but I have read more than my share of contracts over the years. The language is often arcane, and definitions of terms may differ substantially from what one might expect. There is an old saying in the legal profession that a lawyer who uses himself as his attorney has a fool for a client. If this is true for a lawyer, it is doubly true for a physician. Legal advice may be expensive, but not understanding your obligations under a contract may cost you far more.

LEGAL STRUCTURE

When you establish your solo practice, you will need to set up the legal structure for your business. Your options depend on the laws in the state in which you will practice and include sole proprietorship, limited-liability company, partnership, and corporation. Corporations come in two varieties—Subchapter S and Subchapter C, referring to the section or "chapter" of the tax code in which they are defined.

When joining an existing group, decisions about legal structure will have already been made; however, you should still review the structure and understand the implications of the choices made before your arrival. In some cases, bad decisions on the part of the prospective practice may lead you to look for other opportunities.

The goals in choosing a legal structure are to minimize taxes, minimize administrative complexity, and maximize liability protection. I will provide a very brief overview, but I suggest that you research this issue further. As a starting point, you can find useful information at the following websites:

1) http://www.llcweb.com/struc.htm
2) http://www.selfemployedweb.com/corp-llc.htm
3) http://www.mycorporation.com/llc/

Sole Proprietorship. Sole proprietorships are the easiest to set up, requiring essentially no paperwork, but they provide no liability protection for your personal assets. Practice debts become your debts. Because of this lack of liability protection, this is rarely a choice that an anesthesiologist should make.

Limited-Liability Company (LLC). LLCs provide liability protection from the company's debts, contractual obligations, and legal entanglements for the owners (referred to as "members") of the LLC. A few exceptions do apply to these liability protections, though. LLCs are relatively simple to set up and have minimal reporting and administrative requirements. Also, income to the company passes through to the members, and the LLC is typically not subject to income tax. Most, but not all, states allow a single-member LLC. Also, in the past, at least, some states did not allow physicians to practice under an LLC. Where they are allowed, LLCs probably offer maximal protection with minimal administrative complexity of all the legal entities currently available.

Partnership. Although partnerships provide income pass-through, favorable tax treatment, and administrative simplicity, liability is joint and several. That means that if you subsequently bring in a new partner, you will be liable for any malfeasance performed or debt incurred by that partner. As with a sole proprietorship, partnerships are not a favored vehicle for physician practices because of the shared medical liability risk.

Corporation. A corporation provides liability protection for its owners/shareholders, but it has fairly strict administrative requirements, such as annual shareholder meetings, recording of minutes, and annual reports to the state. If these requirements are not met, the corporation could be considered invalid, the liability protections disappear, and the tax consequences could be extreme.

Subchapter C corporations, which are the standard, run-of-the-mill corporation (think Microsoft, Merck, or United Healthcare), may result in double taxation of profits. This means that corporate profits are taxed at the corporate tax rate and dividends to the shareholders are also taxed at the shareholders' tax rate. Careful accounting and distribution of income in the form of salaries to the employed shareholders can essentially eliminate double taxation for physician corporations, though.

Subchapter S corporations, which have limitations in number of shareholders (maximum of 75) and types of shareholders (no corporations, partnerships, resident aliens, and several other restrictions) do have the advantage of income pass-through to the shareholders, like LLCs and partnerships, without the risk of double taxation. However, in addition to the general risk of noncompliance with corporate requirements, failure to comply with specific Subchapter S reporting rules will risk losing the "S" status, with the potential for significant tax liability.

199

ALWAYS AVOID THE BAD JOBS—SPECIFIC CONSIDERATIONS FOR A GROUP PRACTICE

NORMAN A. COHEN, MD

For the purposes of this chapter, consider anything other than a solo practice as a group practice. Any unique issues related to a specific group practice type will be addressed within the following discussion.

MISSION STATEMENT AND GROUP PHILOSOPHY

A group's mission statement, if it has one, gives you an inkling of what is important to the organization. Although many mission statements are boiler plate—"We strive to provide quality, cost-effective care and serve our customers at the highest level. . . yada, yada, yada"—well-managed groups do use their mission statements as the foundation for all decision making. An example may be deciding not to enter into a business relationship with a facility that has a poor track record for quality or a history of confrontational relationships with providers. Although all groups should be able to address why they are in business, be particularly suspicious of intermediate-size or large groups that have not formally developed a group philosophy or mission. It might be a sign that the group places pecuniary interests above all else, a potential recipe for future problems.

Note that multispecialty groups will have a mission and focus that is much broader in scope than that of a single-specialty anesthesia group. For multispecialty groups, assuring a commitment to fair treatment of all physicians, regardless of specialty, is an important consideration. For academic practices, the mission will extend beyond delivery of anesthesia care and will address the research and teaching obligations of the organization.

STABILITY

Well-run groups are proactive in determining their needs and addressing challenges, have a well-defined plan to recruit new members as the practice grows or members retire, and have little turnover in established members. If you are looking at a group that demonstrates few or none of these characteristics, be very wary. You might be able to negotiate a better agreement initially because of the group's desperation to meet a significant shortfall in staffing; however, just as a leopard doesn't change its spots, a poorly run, unstable group rarely miraculously improves the quality of its decision making. Be sure to ask the group's representatives about turnover among the anesthesia

© 2006 Mayo Foundation for Medical Education and Research

staff and assess the longevity and quality of its relations with the facilities where the group practices.

NEW HIRE TURNOVER

As a new anesthesiologist in a group, you will likely be given a time-limited employment contract. Some groups promise new hires the moon—short time to partnership, astronomical income, and great benefits. But if you dig a little deeper, you might learn that the group has a long-standing history of bringing in "fresh meat," taking advantage of their lower pay and vacation allotment, and then letting them go before their probationary period is up.

Ask about the status of previous hires and follow up with nurses and surgeons at the hospital or facility. Also ask for contact information for those who have recently left the group. If there is a disconnect between the group's story and the other information gathered, the red lights should flash and the sirens should sound. Do remember to take the statements of those who have left with a grain (or more) of salt, as these individuals may have a personal axe to grind. The goal is to make an informed decision. If you know of problems but take the plunge anyway, that's your choice, but you will have no one else to blame if/when past history repeats.

BUY-IN AND PAY MECHANISM

As discussed in other chapters, groups have many ways to calculate compensation. When you join a group as a new member, the group may handle your pay differently than that of senior members or shareholders. In discussing these mechanisms, I will focus primarily on some of the implications, particularly for new graduates. I will also look at the cost of buying an ownership position in a practice.

Salary. Some practices may pay a new hire a guaranteed salary. For residents coming into practice, this may be a good deal, as they will not have to wait months to start collecting payments from insurance companies. Because the practice is paying the employee before the group collects from patients and payers, the group incurs a certain cost. For this reason, first-year salaries are often significantly discounted over what the new employee ultimately generates. When this discount seems too great, be concerned that the group may be looking at you as a potential profit center. Academic centers, military, and government-run hospitals frequently offer salary-based compensation, often with an overlay of production incentives.

Production. When your payments are all based on production, your income stream will be low until the billing department or service starts collecting money. You will see little if any income the first month, a moderate amount the second month, and then a more typical amount from the third month onward. If your new group proposes to pay this way, make sure that if you ultimately leave the group, you will still be paid the amount collected after your departure.

During the first year or two after joining a group that offers production-based payment, the group may charge a higher overhead expense to account for the costs incurred in hiring, privileging, and insuring you. Again, make sure that this amount is reasonable and justifiable; otherwise you may be funding someone's vacation home in the Cayman Islands.

Per Diem. "Per diem" means a payment made each day. A group may choose to pay its members for each day worked. There is often a differential amount paid for days on call. The advantage to this system is that if one doesn't work, one doesn't get paid, so there is a distinct incentive to show up to work; however, as mentioned elsewhere, there is also a disincentive to pick up extra cases or cover rooms with more complex cases.

For the new hire, a per-diem rate, like a salary, guarantees an earlier first paycheck. On the other hand, if you choose to leave the group or your contract is not renewed, you will have no cash flow subsequent to your departure. The group also may offer a lower per-diem rate for the new hire to recoup expenses. Differential per diems may also be used to provide incentives for accomplishments desired by the group, such as board certification.

Hybrid. Groups may combine any of these payment methods into a hybrid form in an attempt to maximize the advantages and minimize the disadvantages of each approach. Understanding the principles and caveats of each method will help you make sense of the particular method offered by your prospective practice.

Buy-in. Most private group practices offer the option for the new hire to advance to an ownership position in the organization. The advantage of ownership is that you will have a voice in group decision making. Also, if downsizing becomes necessary, the owners are the last ones to be let go.

Unlike many other medical specialties, anesthesiology practices typically do not have large investments in equipment or property. When you "buy in" to a practice, you are purchasing a share of the group's assets. The amount of money required should reasonably reflect the value of your share. Groups have many mechanisms to accomplish the buy-in. These include a one-time fee or reduced pay for a defined period (usually 1 to 3 years). A share of a typical anesthesia practice may be worth about 2 to 4 months of gross clinical income. In addition to assuming a share of the group's debt or liabilities, you are buying one or more of the following assets:

> *Goodwill.* Your new group has established relationships of value with facilities, payers, and surgeons. Unfortunately, quantifying that value is more art than science. Goodwill is not fungible and can devalue quickly.

Accounts receivable. If your group does not pay based purely on production, then the group owns the future income stream related to clinical activities already performed but for which payment has not been fully collected. Also, the group owns the income stream derived from contractual arrangements with hospitals such as stipends or administrative payments. The value of the accounts receivable can be calculated to a reasonable degree of accuracy.

Property and equipment. The group may own office space, part of an ambulatory surgery center, a fluoroscope used in a pain clinic, computers and software. These assets are measurable and have value, but they all decline in value or "depreciate" over time.

Buy-out. To maintain a karmic balance when looking at a practice, you should also discuss the "buy-out" of your share. At some point after purchasing an ownership interest, you may decide to leave the practice. A method for valuing the assets at time of separation should be well defined, as should be the period of time the group has to complete the repurchase of assets. Although the value of a group may increase over time, as with any investment, there is no guarantee that this will occur. For example, the group might experience a dramatic shift in payer demographics or might have obligations related to legal entanglements. In these circumstances, your investment in the business could show a loss, and possibly a large one.

MANAGEMENT

Medium-size to large groups usually employ professional administrators to see to the day-to-day operation of what is a fairly large business. Although the employee count may be small, anesthesiology groups can generate substantial clinical revenue, with medium-sized groups of 10 to 20 anesthesiologists having revenues of $5 million to $10 million a year and "megagroups" of more than 100 anesthesiologists generating $50 million, $100 million, or more each year. Given the large sums of money involved, professional management makes great sense.

From recent Medical Group Management Association (MGMA) cost survey data, a full-time anesthesiologist in a physician-only practice generates about $415,000 per year per full-time equivalent (FTE). When Certified Registered Nurse Anesthetists (CRNAs) are part of the practice, net clinical revenue increases to $467,000 if the practice has fewer than one CRNA per anesthesiologist and $749,000 if it has more than one per anesthesiologist.

Even smaller groups, which may not be able to support a full-time administrator, must have access to professional advice or choose to develop management expertise among the physician owners. Options include supporting a member in earning an advanced degree such as a Master of Business

Administration (MBA) or even the American Society of Anesthesiologists Certificate in Business Administration (http://www.asahq.org/conted/cba.htm).

Before joining a group, be sure to ask questions about group management, responsibilities, and involvement of physician owners in decision making. Ill-considered choices and poor attention to the business of medical practice have led to the financial ruin of many groups.

200

ALWAYS AVOID THE BAD JOBS—MAKE SURE YOU UNDERSTAND THE COMPLIANCE PLAN

NORMAN A. COHEN, MD

Being "compliant" with procedural coding conventions and payer policies and requirements means that the professional group makes every effort to bill correctly. A compliance plan is the practice's organized effort to assure correct coding, identify and correct errors, and address ambiguities in a consistent manner.

Why is billing compliance important? If auditors determine that a physician has systematically but innocently billed incorrectly, any overcharges must be paid back, interest may be applied, *and* the physician may be fined $10,000 for each incorrect claim, with the possibility of treble damages. If the physician "knowingly and willingly" submits fraudulent claims, the crime is a felony, with the potential for a $25,000 fine, 5 years in prison, or both. Decertification from Medicare is likely, making it exceptionally difficult for an anesthesiologist to be gainfully employed at any facility that accepts Medicare patients. Ignorance is no excuse when it comes to billing the federal government, as was well-outlined in the July 1997 issue of the http://www.asahq.org/Newsletters/1997/07_97/Pres_Pg0797.html.

Although a compliance plan does not protect a group or physician from having to repay overcharges or eliminate the chance for fines, a group that demonstrates commitment to being compliant through implementing and following a plan will be much more likely to reach a reasonable settlement with the government. I know of a number of groups, including my own, that identified problems through claims review, proactively addressed the problems with the government, and reached a fair settlement.

The Office of the Inspector General (OIG) has published a model compliance plan that includes these seven elements:
1) Auditing and monitoring
2) Implementing written standards and procedures
3) Designating a compliance officer/contact
4) Conducting training and education
5) Responding to detected violations
6) Developing open lines of communication
7) Enforcing disciplinary standards

© 2006 Mayo Foundation for Medical Education and Research

For those who like to go to the primary source, this link will take you to a reprint of the Federal Register issue where the OIG published the model plan:http://oig.hhs.gov/authorities/docs/physician.pdf.

The *ASA Newsletter* also includes a monthly column on practice management. Over the past 10 years, many columns have addressed compliance issues and creation of a compliance plan. For those with an interest, I suggest reviewing the many articles archived at the ASA site. Some of these articles appeared in the *ASA Newsletter* in October 1997, December 1999, November 2000, and August 2002, available at http://www.asahq.org.

For purposes of evaluating a practice, asking the following questions may prove helpful in determining the group's commitment to compliance.
1) Do you have a compliance officer?
2) Do you have a handbook of coding policies available for your physician employees?
3) Is there an ongoing process for reviewing codes submitted to assure accuracy?

The answers to all these questions should be a resounding "yes!" Although one can think of dozens of questions to ask about compliance, hearing any "no" answers to these very basic questions should be exceptionally worrisome. If you are an employee of a group that performs billing on your behalf, you are ultimately responsible that the billing is correct. Given your risk of monetary loss or even jail time, it is absolutely essential that you make sure your prospective employer takes compliance seriously.

BILLING AND COLLECTION SERVICES

Some groups perform billing in-house, but many groups outsource billing to a third party. In either circumstance, an understanding of how to measure the performance of a billing service and the division of responsibility between physician and billing department is an important factor in practice analysis. *Key Questions.* In evaluating a practice, at a minimum you should determine the following.
1) *Is the physician responsible for selecting the appropriate procedure code?* Ideally, the physician should select the procedure code, because the code determines payment and incorrect procedural coding exposes the physician to compliance risk as discussed above.
2) *What about diagnosis codes?* Many practices do not require the physicians to select diagnosis codes but do require thorough description of relevant diagnoses to support the anesthesia, monitoring, evaluation and management, and pain management codes submitted. If you are required to submit diagnosis codes, the current edition of the International Classification of Diseases (ICD) should be readily available to you.
3) *If the physicians do code their procedures, what resources do the practice or billing service provide to assist the physician in selecting the correct code?*

At a minimum, the current year's ASA Relative Value Guide should be available to each physician. If the group requires submission of surgical codes on billing forms, the current year's AMA Current Procedural Terminology (CPT) and ASA Crosswalk publications should be available as well.

4) *What process is followed if the billing clerk disagrees with the physician's choice of code or the supporting documents (anesthesia records, progress notes, dictations) are inadequate to support the choice?* The charge slip should be sent back to the physician with the reason for the discrepancy, a suggestion about alternative coding choices, and a request for additional supporting documentation when indicated.

5) *Are the billing coders certified by a coding certification body?* At least some of the billing staff should be professional coders. A number of organizations offer certification, such as the American Academy of Professional Coders and the American Health Information Management Association.

For more information on coding, see the chapters on common errors in anesthesia coding.

Assessment of Billing Service Effectiveness. Often, the only question that a naive applicant asks a prospective practice about billing is the cost charged to perform this task. Although this is important to know, it is also crucial to remember that a billing service that is more effective in collecting revenue may be worth a slightly higher rate. Typical rates for outsourced billing range from 4% to 7% of the amount collected. Although I have never worked in a practice with in-house billing, my understanding is that the cost to the group is usually about 2.5% to 3.5% of net collections. Being a larger group, having more favorable demographics, or not requiring supplemental services from the billing company all help the group negotiate a rate toward the lower end of the spectrum when dealing with an outsource organization.

A number of measures are available to assess the performance of a billing service. Some of the most important measures include the following.

Gross collection rate—dollars collected divided by amount charged at the group's standard rate. For anesthesia-only practices, the average was just under 50% in 2004. This measure is useful primarily as an indicator that further analysis may be necessary. In statistical terms, it is sensitive but not specific. Drift in the gross collection rate may be due to many factors, including changing performance of the billing service, changes in payer demographics, changes in payer contracts, changes in the overall economy, or a combination of factors.

Adjusted collection rate—dollars collected divided by expected collections. Because practices often have contracts with insurers that promise a discount over the usual fee and Medicare and Medicaid payments are substantially lower than most practices' normal rates, this metric estimates the amount of dollars collectible for each charge based on insurer agreements and uses this estimate of net expected collections to calculate the collection rate. The average adjusted collection rate based on ASA–MGMA 2004 data was just under 93%. The primary sources of variation in this measure are inability to collect the patient's share of the fee and failure of the insurer to meet its payment obligations.

Days fee-for-service charges in accounts receivable—accounts receivable is the amount of money charged but not yet collected. Conventional practice is to post the full fee amount to accounts receivable when the charge is entered. The accounts receivable total is reduced whenever patient or insurer payments are collected. It is also reduced by the amount of any negotiated discounts or "contractual adjustments." Although accounts receivable is considered a financial asset, this is an asset that is not equivalent to cash in the bank. Think of accounts receivable as a loan to the insurers and patients that is receiving no interest and that you cannot use for any other purpose. The group's goal should be to keep the size of accounts receivable as small as possible through efforts directed toward rapidly collecting money owed to the group.

If one divides the accounts receivable by the average dollars charged in a day, one has a measure known as "days fee-for-service charges in accounts receivable," more frequently known as "days in A/R." The smaller this number, the more efficient the billing operation is in collecting the group's money. The national average for anesthesia practices is about 47 days. Factors that can increase this number include delays in submitting charges for billing, delays in entering the charges, delays in filing claims with insurers or patients, delays in payment by insurers or patients, and denial of claims by insurers for not following billing requirements or meeting medical necessity requirements.

You should note that some insurers have a track record of blanket denial of claims when they are initially submitted, forcing the practice to resubmit and be delayed in payment. Surprisingly, some practices never resubmit a claim after the first rejection. Consider this a "win, win" for the insurer!

Several large insurers, including Aetna, United Healthcare, Wellpoint, and Health Net, recently settled class-action lawsuits related to a pattern of inappropriate delays and denials in payment of claims. As part of the settlement, these companies must establish physician advisory committees that will review revisions in payment policies and compliance with the terms of the settlement. This author was recently appointed to serve on the physician advisory committee for Health Net.

201

ALWAYS AVOID THE BAD JOBS—KNOW THE RISK-MANAGEMENT STRATEGIES OF THE PRACTICE

NORMAN A. COHEN, MD

Although improvements in the safety of anesthesia over the last several decades is nothing short of remarkable, anesthesia remains a high-risk endeavor. From the relatively frequent occurrence of dental injury to the lower-frequency but far more costly outcomes of permanent nerve injury, cardiac injury, lung damage, or death, practices should devote resources to risk reduction. Aggressive attention to risk management can lead to substantial reduction in medical liability insurance rates. Mandatory continuing education requirements, internal review of adverse outcomes, and requiring informed consent for all procedures are some of the characteristics you may look for in a risk-management program.

ADAPTABILITY TO CHANGE

The environment in which a practice operates is constantly changing. From recognizing and addressing new competitive threats to accommodating new payment initiatives such as "pay for performance," anesthesia groups must be able to adapt to and profit from change. To determine how your potential group manages change, you can ask open-ended questions about challenges facing the group and planned responses. If the group's leaders deny that any challenges exist or blame any and all problems on outside entities without offering any proposed solutions, dig deeper, as both are warning signs of possible problems. Although the group doesn't have to have a plan for every problem, it should have a well-defined process that will prioritize threats and lead to the development of a response. The process should be fairly inclusive, with input from all members of the group affected.

LIABILITIES

Although it is not typical, some anesthesia groups may have debts that may affect your potential income. Whether the group bought a share in an ambulatory surgical center or a medical office building, or borrowed money to pay for fines, overcharges, or back taxes, it is important for you to ask about liabilities before signing an agreement with the group. This is particularly important if you have an interest in buying a share of the group down the road, but it is also important because paying for or "servicing" these debts may affect the money available to pay employed physicians.

© 2006 Mayo Foundation for Medical Education and Research

OUTSTANDING LITIGATION

Anesthesia practices may be involved in litigation for a number of reasons. Examples include being a named co-defendant in a medical liability case, being the subject of a billing investigation, being accused of antitrust violations or violations of workplace rules such as the Americans with Disability Act or the Family Leave Act, or suing a facility for improper termination of a contract.

You should try to understand the potential loss or gain and ongoing costs if your practice is involved in one or more lawsuits. Consider the litigation as potential liabilities that need to be valued in evaluating your potential practice. The practice should be forthcoming in providing a reasonable amount of information when asked. Failure to disclose, unless under a court "gag" order, is a predictor of problems with trust and the group meeting its obligations to you.

202

ALWAYS AVOID THE BAD JOBS—REVIEW THE PRACTICE'S SPECIAL FUNDING SOURCES, OBLIGATIONS, AND BENEFIT PACKAGES

NORMAN A. COHEN, MD

Many anesthesia practices receive payments from facilities to provide specific clinical services or complete administrative tasks. In a 2004 American Society of Anesthesiologists (ASA) survey, 57% of practices received stipends of one sort or another, and 91% of academic practices received institutional support. Almost 10% of the stipends exceeded $3 million/year!

Clinical service stipends frequently address provision of obstetric or trauma anesthesia coverage, because the income potential compared to the cost of providing these services is not favorable. Cardiac anesthesia is another area that may receive support, because such a large percentage of patients are covered by the poor-paying Medicare program.

One of the most frequent types of stipends, although one of the lowest-paying, is for medical director services. Medical director responsibilities may include departmental scheduling, addressing operating room operational issues, and quality and cost improvement initiatives. Paying an anesthesiologist to fulfill these responsibilities is often seen as money well spent by facilities.

EXCLUSIVE CONTRACTS

A substantial number of hospitals and other surgical facilities have entered into exclusive relationships with anesthesia groups to provide specified anesthesia services.

Advantages and Disadvantages. For the hospital, an exclusive agreement usually provides guaranteed anesthesia coverage for the operating rooms, obstetric suite, and sometimes the intensive care unit (ICU). The hospital often has the ability to bypass medical staff due-process rules to quickly address perceived issues of quality. If the group does not meet its contractual obligations, the hospital frequently has the option to terminate the agreement, with automatic relinquishment of medical staff privileges. When this option is present, the hospital has significant power and influence over the group.

Hospitals cannot enter into exclusive arrangements lightly, particularly if they control a substantial part of the local health care market. Displaced physicians can and often do sue. Although legal decisions in federal courts

© 2006 Mayo Foundation for Medical Education and Research

have allowed hospitals to enter into exclusives with reasonable cause, such as exhausting other attempts at providing necessary services or addressing disruptive behavior, in at least one state, a displaced physician was able to use his state's "right to work" law to earn a substantial settlement.

For the group, being able to control staffing can lead to more efficient and thus more profitable delivery of care. In addition, exclusives are often associated with stipends to make up for income shortfalls from new service obligations, such as trauma calls or dedicated obstetric anesthesia coverage. Being in control of hiring allows the group to select new members with a work ethic and focus that is consistent with the group's goals.

An exclusive arrangement also exposes a group to multiple risks. Groups sometimes use their monopoly at the hospital to increase fees. If the fees rise above average market rates without reasonable justification, this may indicate predatory pricing and subject the group to possible antitrust litigation.

The group is also usually responsible for providing a guaranteed level of staffing. If illness, departure of employees, or other factors lead to a shortfall, the group may need to pay expensive *locum tenens* rates to meet coverage requirements; otherwise, it risks potential loss of the contract. The hospital may use its power over the group to influence contracting decisions with payers. If these requests are honored, the group may suffer disastrous drops in payment rates from key insurers.

Pass-Through Requirements. In an exclusive contract with a group, the terms of the agreement with the hospital often require that particular conditions be repeated in each employment agreement. These "pass-through" requirements may include automatic surrendering of privileges upon termination of the group's contract, waiving of certain medical staff due-process rights, and possible restrictions on providing care at facilities that compete with the hospital. Although state law may prevent some of these terms from being enforced—noncompete agreements being a notable example—these conditions are often seen in employment agreements, and the group views these items as non-negotiable.

VACATIONS AND BENEFITS

Depending on the method by which pay is determined, you may receive either paid or unpaid vacation. Typically the group will allow a maximum number of weeks away from the practice. Groups often have a vacation lottery to assure a fair distribution of vacation time while still assuring adequate numbers to meet clinical obligations. Vacation may or may not be negotiable, but, at the very least, you need to understand the system and determine the number of weeks allowed.

As an employee, the group may offer health insurance, disability insurance, and professional liability insurance. You may be responsible for paying some or all of the premiums out of your gross income. You have the right to request and receive a summary of the benefits offered, with an estimate of the cost and source of the funding. You may be able to participate in the group's retirement plan. Sometimes the plan precludes participation until you have worked for a defined period, such as 1 year.

203

ALWAYS AVOID THE BAD JOBS—KNOW WHAT TO EXPECT IN CONTRACTS

NORMAN A. COHEN, MD

As a new physician joining a group or as a *locum tenens* physician working with a staffing agency or directly with a group, you are almost certain to enter into legal contracts that define the obligations of each party and the manner in which you will receive compensation for the services you provide. At some point you may have the opportunity to acquire an ownership interest in the group, and this ownership will also be bound by a contract. This review of the types of agreements is greatly simplified from a legal point of view, but it should give you a basic understanding to guide you when you start encountering these documents.

EMPLOYMENT

A physician employment agreement defines the relationship between you and the group that will be employing you. It usually defines the term during which it will be in effect, options for renewing the agreement, methods for terminating the relationship, responsibilities of the two parties, "hold harmless" or indemnification clauses, and requirements for maintaining records. In the body of the agreement or as an attachment, the contract will include the method by which your pay will be calculated and the frequency of payments.

The employer will be responsible for paying certain taxes and withholding federal, state, Social Security (FICA) and Medicare taxes. As mentioned in Chapter 202 on exclusive contracts, pass-through requirements may also be found in this agreement. The employer has a right to control the employee with regard to shifts worked, vacation granted, clinical assignments made, and even establishing policies that relate to the delivery of medical care. In return, the employer bears responsibility for supervising your performance and acting to correct any deficiencies.

INDEPENDENT CONTRACTOR

An independent contractor is a person or entity such as a limited-liability company (LLC) or corporation that enters into an agreement to provide specific services but is not subject to the control of the other party as to the manner in which the service is delivered. *Locum tenens* physicians often enter into independent-contractor agreements to provide a specific service, such

© 2006 Mayo Foundation for Medical Education and Research

as anesthesia care, for a limited time frame. The group hiring the *locum* has no control over the manner or type of medical care delivered; however, the agreement requires the *locum* to obtain privileges at the health care facility and comply with all medical staff requirements.

For a group, the advantage of an independent-contractor agreement is having no responsibility for taxes and benefits and not being subject to certain employment laws. The Internal Revenue Service (IRS) has specific requirements that must be met to receive independent-contractor tax treatment. If the group violates these requirements, most notably that of control, the IRS may disallow the independent-contractor agreement, subjecting the group to back taxes and penalties.

You should note that when a group has an agreement with a health care facility, that contract is an independent-contractor agreement. The facility and the group each has defined responsibilities, but the details, manner, and means of accomplishing the tasks are left to each party.

SHAREHOLDER OR LLC MEMBERSHIP

If you are offered ownership interest in a corporation, you will be required to sign a shareholder's agreement and will be issued a stock certificate after paying a defined sum. The agreement will include some definitions of terms; any restrictions on the purchase, transfer, or sale of stock; election of the board of directors; and rules on voting for corporate business decisions.

A membership agreement for an LLC is known as an "operating agreement." It is essentially a combination of by-laws and a shareholder's agreement, and it defines the governing rules for the company and the responsibilities of the members, with particular attention to contribution of additional capital, distribution of profits, and allocation of tax obligations, because these are passed through to the owners. Responsibility for management, regular meeting requirements, dissolution of the LLC, and limitations on the transfer of a particular LLC member's ownership interest to an outside party are also frequently included in the agreement.

NEGOTIATIONS

You have every right to negotiate with the group to change aspects of the agreement that you (and, hopefully, your lawyer) find particularly troubling. Some requests, including vacation amount, pay, or call requirements, may be granted, often depending on how desirable the group finds you.

As mentioned, some elements may be non-negotiable because of requirements in other agreements that the group is bound to honor. In the same way, some contractual items may be "make or break" for you. If the group does not honor your request on those matters, then you may have to make the difficult decision to look for another opportunity.

TERMINATION

Most employment contracts include two methods for termination—with and without cause.

Termination with Cause. If you or the group fails to meet defined obligations, then one of the parties may be in "breach" of the contract's terms. If, after notification of the problem, the offending party fails to fix the matter or "remedy the breach" consistent with the terms of the agreement, the contract can be terminated. The time frame for termination is usually either immediate or after a very short term. For example, if the group is obligated to maintain your professional liability insurance but fails to do so and fails to fix the problem, then you may have the right to terminate immediately. The contract may also define damages that the party in breach must pay to the other. It is fairly rare for an employer to terminate a physician for cause, because the facts may not be clear-cut and thus may be subject to subsequent legal entanglements; however, if there is a clear danger to the safety of patients or others in the workplace, the group may have no choice but to exercise for-cause termination, as the financial risk of not proceeding immediately may be considered too great.

Termination without Cause. Almost all agreements include a "termination without cause" section. It typically gives either party the right to terminate the agreement without a specific reason, provided the required notification is given in the specified manner. Typical notification time frames are 60 or 90 days in a physician employment agreement, and written notification is almost always required.

This section works for both parties, as it allows the employee to end the relationship without waiting an unreasonable period of time to change jobs, and it allows the group to terminate an employee who is not meeting the group's expectations. It is important to note that although an agreement may have a term of 1 or 2 years (or some other period), the effective length of the contract is only as long as the termination-without-cause notification period. If you have a 90-day without-cause termination clause, you effectively have a contract with a 90-day term.

INDEMNIFICATION

Many contracts include indemnification agreements. Indemnification is the payment of a sum of money in compensation for a loss or injury. A group may require you to pay for any loss created by your medical negligence for which the group was also found financially responsible. On the other hand, if you acted in good faith and coded an anesthetic procedure correctly, but the group's agents changed that code before submitting the charge, you would want to be financially compensated for any loss you suffer as a consequence of a subsequent compliance claim. With regard to the issue of medical negligence, your professional liability insurance will cover any damages assigned to you (up to the limits of the policy) but will typically not cover any party you have agreed to indemnify. If you choose to sign an agreement like this, you should make sure that the group is also listed as a covered entity or "additionally named insured" on your liability insurance agreement.

CONTRACT REVIEW

Although I have read hundreds of contracts and worked with many attorneys over the years on contract matters, I am by no stretch of the imagination an attorney or any sort of expert on contracts. I have tried to provide you with my observations of some of the basic concepts and pitfalls found in agreements that you might come across during your attempt to find a good job.

It is absolutely essential that you seek competent legal advice before entering into any agreement of this level of importance. This does not excuse you from doing your best to understand the key terms and conditions of the agreement before you sign. You should find an attorney familiar with health care contracts, licensed in your state, with no relationship with the group with which you will be contracting. The state medical association or anesthesiology component may be able to provide a list of attorneys who qualify. It is well worth the money and could save you the high cost of disentangling yourself from a bad relationship.

CODING AND PAYMENT—MAKE SURE YOU GET PAID

204

UNDERSTANDING MEDICAL CODING AND THE HEALTH CARE PAYMENT SYSTEM

NORMAN A. COHEN, MD

INTRODUCTION TO MEDICAL CODING

When we give anesthesia, one of our most important jobs is to communicate effectively with our patient, surgeon, operating room (OR) staff, and postanesthesia care unit (PACU) nurse. To get paid for our work, we also have to communicate effectively with another audience—the payer. This process of formally communicating our work to those who will pay us is known as *medical coding.*

Diagnostic and procedure codes are the *lingua franca,* the descriptive taxonomy, that allows us to classify both the diagnoses justifying our work as well as the procedures that describe the work performed. A payment system associates a value with each covered procedure. *Covered procedures* are medical services for which insurers have agreed to provide compensation. The payment-system value may list an arbitrary dollar amount or a *relative value unit* (RVU) for each covered service. A relative value system defines a value relationship among all procedures on the payer's fee schedule. Payers convert an RVU into a payment amount by multiplying the RVU by a *conversion factor,* which defines the monetary value of each RVU. The list of payment amounts or RVUs for all covered services is known as a *fee schedule.*

In the following chapters, we will discuss the basics of coding for all sorts of medical services commonly performed by anesthesiologists, including the anesthetic service, line placements, pain management, critical care, and evaluation and management. We will also learn about the resources available to code correctly, the elements of the Medicare payment system, and a brief overview of Medicaid and third-party insurance payment systems.

We will spend a fair bit of time examining specific payment rules and policies of the Medicare system. Medicare is a dominant player in the health care system. Because Medicare's system for developing payment policies is open to public scrutiny and comment, Medicare's influence on other payers is significant, making understanding of these rules quite important. As the old saying goes, "He who has the gold makes the rules."

Before diving into this material, I need to provide a disclaimer. At the time of this writing, I serve as the chairman of the American Society of Anesthesiologists (ASA) Committee on Economics as well as the ASA's representative to the American Medical Association (AMA) Relative Value System

ⓒ 2006 Mayo Foundation for Medical Education and Research

Update Committee (RUC); however, the coding guidance, interpretations, and advice presented in the following chapters represent my opinions only. This information does not, in any way, represent the official positions of either the AMA or the ASA. Also, any errors in the information that follows are mine alone.

Best coding practices change over time. I have made every effort to provide accurate information as of the late fall of 2006, the time when I submitted this material for publication. It is essential that you review the latest coding information from the AMA, ASA, Medicare, private payers, and your local billing experts when investigating any medical coding question; however, the foundation that you will create from reading the following chapters will help you formulate the right questions to ask and efficiently guide you to the correct source to obtain the answers you need to get paid correctly and completely for the work you do.

In the discussion of procedural coding, I will be using code examples from the American Medical Association's *Current Procedural Terminology* (CPT). Fair use of that material requires the following statement: Current Procedural Terminology (CPT) is copyright 2006 American Medical Association. All Rights Reserved. No fee schedules, basic units, relative values, or related listings are included in CPT. The AMA assumes no liability for the data contained herein. Applicable FARS/DFARS restrictions apply to government use.

CONCLUDING COMMENTS

In the following chapters we cover a great deal of material. We will learn about diagnosis and procedure codes, both their use and the process that creates them. We will explore specific coding areas of importance to anesthesiologists. We will learn about the coding resources available to help you get paid for your work. And finally, we will cover specific but important issues pertaining to public and private health insurers. Believe it or not, this material, while seemingly quite detailed, only scratches the surface of medical coding and payment policy. My goals in presenting this information is to help you both recognize what you don't know and know enough to ask the right questions at the right time. The final and most important goal is to help you get paid fairly while avoiding expensive mistakes.

The AMA and ASA kindly provided me permission to cite specific information from their publications. I would not have been able to produce the text that follows without the guidance and counsel of the outstanding physicians and staff at both the AMA and the ASA. In particular, I would like to thank Marie Mindeman at the CPT, Sherry Smith at the RUC, and Sharon Merrick and Karin Bierstein at the ASA. I value their friendship and their willingness to teach me as I learned the intricacies of the code development and valuation process over the past decade. I am also indebted to my physician mentors at the ASA, including Chuck Novak, Alex Hannenberg, Jimmy McMichael, and Stan Stead, who both helped me learn the intricacies of this complex material and gave me the opportunity to put this knowledge to use for our profession.

Lastly, I would like to give my greatest thanks to my wife and best friend Michelle and my daughter Allie, both for allowing me the time away from the family to pursue my interests in this area as well as the encouragement to share this information with you.

205

THE STRUCTURE OF MEDICAL CODES

NORMAN A. COHEN, MD

For the most part, payment for medical services in the United States in 2006 is tightly connected to the procedure or procedures performed. In addition, those who pay for the bulk of medical services, insurers such as Medicare, Medicaid, United Healthcare, Aetna, and others, require that the patient has a medical condition that justifies performing the procedure. To meet these medical necessity requirements, physicians must not only tell the payer what was done by reporting a procedure code but must also provide the reason by reporting a diagnosis code. In a later chapter we will discuss medical necessity policies, but first let us explore the structure of medical codes.

Medical codes consist of two elements, a unique identifier and a text descriptor. The identifier is a unique but arbitrary sequence of characters, which may be limited in length (e.g., five characters) and character composition (e.g., digits in the first four characters and digits or capital letters in the last character). The text descriptor provides an unambiguous and discrete exposition of the characteristics covered by the code. For purposes of submitting claims, the identifier is exactly equivalent to the text descriptor; therefore, your billing office or billing service only needs to submit the code identifier(s) to get the payment process started. The text descriptor, which is often very long, can remain happily in your computer or coding reference book and not waste bandwidth or paper.

As an example, the procedure code defined in the American Medical Association's Current Procedural Terminology (CPT);[1] procedure coding system that describes a single-shot epidural steroid injection at L3–4 is

Code: 62311

Descriptor: Injection, single (not via indwelling catheter), not including neurolytic substances, with or without contrast (for either localization or epidurography), of diagnostic or therapeutic substance(s) (including anesthetic, antispasmodic, opioid, steroid, other solution), epidural or subarachnoid; lumbar, sacral (caudal)

Let's spend a few moments considering all the key elements of this code and descriptor. Note that the identifying code is five characters long. All

---

[1]Current Procedural Terminology © 2006 American Medical Association.® All Rights Reserved. Applies to all CPT code references in this chapter.

© 2006 Mayo Foundation for Medical Education and Research

current CPT codes are exactly five characters in length and all mainstream, widely used, and nonexperimental codes consist of five digits. The descriptor clarifies that the procedure refers to an injection excluding an indwelling catheter (the what), not including neurolytics (other codes describe neurolytic injections) regardless of whether contrast is used. This code can be used for injecting either diagnostic or therapeutic substances. Some procedures may have different codes depending on whether the purpose of the procedure is to diagnose or treat. 62311 is applicable for epidural or subarachnoid injections in the lumbar, sacral, or caudal region (the where). In fact, a different code, 62310, describes similar injections in the cervical or thoracic area. When procedure codes are very similar but differ in anatomic location or target, they frequently have identifying codes in close sequence. These are sometimes referred to as a family of codes. 62310 and 62311 comprise a small family of codes.

Now that we have a basic understanding of the building blocks for medical coding, let's get into some of the nitty-gritty of coding and provide a historical context.

206

A detailed look at describing diagnoses using the International Classification of Diseases

Norman A. Cohen, MD

Describing medical services for billing purposes involves selecting a procedure code and a supporting diagnosis code. The International Classification of Diseases (ICD) is far and away the most prevalent system for reporting diagnoses and the American Medical Association (AMA) Current Procedural Terminology (CPT) (*Current Procedural Terminology* © 2006 American Medical Association.®All Rights Reserved. Applies to all CPT code references in this chapter) publication is the primary way to report the services of physicians and many allied health professionals. In some situations, physicians may need to use Medicare's Health Care Procedural Coding System (HCPCS) when reporting procedural services. In addition, hospitals use a section of the ICD to report inpatient procedural services. In the next few years, hospitals will transition to a new edition of ICD, many years in the making, known as ICD-10.

Diagnosis Coding

In the United States, the system for reporting medical diagnoses is the International Classification of Diseases Ninth Revision—Clinical Modification, or ICD-9-CM. The World Health Organization (WHO) developed the ICD system. The National Center for Health Statistics (NCHS) and the Centers for Medicare and Medicaid Services (CMS) maintain the ICD-9-CM, which has been modified from the WHO's ICD-9 to address specific requirements of the U.S. health system. ICD-9-CM is "the official system of assigning codes to diagnosis and procedures in the United States." Agencies that categorize mortality data from death certificates use the unmodified ICD-9 system. The WHO first published ICD-9 in 1979, and the U.S. government published ICD-9-CM at about the same time. As we will discuss when considering procedural coding, the diagnosis and procedural coding systems will see major changes when the next version of ICD, the tenth revision, becomes the standard in just a few years.

ICD-9-CM has three volumes. Volume 1 lists all disease code numbers and descriptors in the form of a very long table. Volume 2 has an alphabetical index to the disease entries. And Volume 3 contains an alphabetical index and

© 2006 Mayo Foundation for Medical Education and Research

a tabular list of the procedural coding system used by hospitals for describing surgical, diagnostic, and therapeutic interventions. In this section, we will discuss the codes found in Volumes 1 and 2, and address Volume 3 in the chapter on procedural coding.

The ICD-9-CM divides diseases into 17 broad categories. Examples include "diseases of the nervous system and sense organs," "diseases of the digestive system," and "congenital anomalies." In addition, a supplementary classification system, known colloquially as "V-codes," describes situations when conditions other than current disease or injury are applicable. One would report a past history of a now-inactive condition or a family history of a disease state with a V-code rather than a primary diagnosis code. For example, a family history of a malignant neoplasm in the gastrointestinal tract (V16.0) could support a screening colonoscopy at a younger age than is currently recommended for the general population. Think V-codes for risk factors and diagnosis codes for known patient conditions.

Insurers, both public and private, also use these supplementary classifications to help define medical necessity requirements in payment policies. Recently, insurers have grappled with coverage for bariatric surgery. In 2006, the CMS introduced a series of new V-codes into the ICD-9-CM to define ranges of body mass index (BMI) between 30 and 39 (V85.30 to V85.39), as well as 40 and over (V85.4) in the adult population. Some payers may provide coverage for bariatric surgery at a BMI >35 only if the patient has other conditions such as diabetes or hypertension, or for all patients with a BMI >40. These new codes allow for reporting the patient characteristic known as body mass index, which is neither a disease nor an injury, but most certainly a risk factor!

The disease/injury diagnosis codes consist of up to five digits, with a decimal point separating the first three digits from the last two. The codes range from 001 to 999.9. The digits to the left of the decimal point provide the primary diagnosis, while the digits to the right provide significant qualifications to the diagnosis. For example, ICD-9 code 401 describes essential hypertension. 401.0 is essential hypertension, malignant, 401.1 is essential hypertension, benign and 401.9 is essential hypertension, unspecified.

The ICD-9-CM does not provide a simple code-number breakdown between sections. So, rather than having all diagnoses for diseases of the circulation in an easily remembered range such as 300 to 399, the actual range is 390 to 459.9. For this reason, those without a photographic memory will need either a printed or an electronic version of ICD-9 handy for diagnosis coding. In addition, payers require diagnosis codes to be submitted to the most specific level possible in order to support the procedure performed. This means that you must code to the last digit possible. With rare exceptions, a code without numbers after the decimal place, sometimes called a *truncated* code, is not an acceptable diagnosis code for submission; therefore, almost all the codes submitted will be four or five characters in length (excluding the decimal point). To illustrate, a patient undergoes a heart transplant for an idiopathic cardiomyopathy. The anesthesiologist should report diagnosis code 425.4—"other primary cardiomyopathies" rather than the less specific truncated code 425—"cardiomyopathy" when submitting a claim for anesthesia for heart transplant (CPT procedure code 00580).

Multiple diagnoses and diagnosis codes may apply. An anesthesiologist may need to report a diagnosis or diagnoses to support the surgical procedure as well as different diagnoses to support invasive monitoring or provision of acute pain procedures.

Let's look at an example to help put these concepts into practice. Suppose that you provide anesthesia for a thoracotomy to remove a lung tumor in the right lower lobe. Previous needle biopsy identified this tumor as a squamous cell carcinoma. You also inserted an arterial line for perioperative monitoring as well as a thoracic epidural for postoperative pain management at the request of the surgeon. With great trepidation, you search for supporting diagnoses in the ICD-9-CM. You are relieved to find a section on neoplasms (Section 2) that lists primary neoplasms by specific sites. Code 162 describes malignant neoplasms of the trachea, bronchus, and lung, and code 162.5 qualifies 162 by location—lower lobe, bronchus, or lung. Bingo! We have a diagnosis to support the anesthetic procedure.

The primary surgical diagnosis code will likely support the use of an arterial line. Other diagnosis codes that would also support this ancillary procedure include V10.1—personal history of malignant neoplasm, trachea, bronchus, or lung, as well as 799.02—hypoxemia. To find the codes that support placement of an epidural for acute pain, one should look in Volume 2 of the ICD-9-CM, the alphabetical listing of code descriptors. If one searches for "pain," Volume 2 refers you to the codes for pain, organized by the site of the pain. With the 2007 edition of ICD-9-CM, effective for use in October 2006, CMS has published a series of new acute pain codes in the range 338.1 to 338.19. We find that 338.12 describes our situation perfectly, as its descriptor is "acute postthoracotomy pain NOS" (where NOS indicates "not otherwise specified").

Previously, many payers requested that V58.49, "other specified aftercare following surgery," be used as the indication for acute postoperative pain procedures; however, the 2007 ICD-9-CM has appended, "change or removal of drains" to this code, making its use for this purpose no longer correct. For those interested in following the updates to ICD-9-CM, the CMS has a web page dedicated to this purpose. You can find it at www.cms.hhs.gov/ICD9ProviderDiagnosticCodes/07_summarytables. asp#TopOfPage.

Whether you will need to provide specific diagnosis codes for each procedure you perform depends on your local situation. In my experience, I have never had to submit specific ICD-9 codes to my billing staff; however, I have had to submit narrative descriptions of all applicable diagnoses, which my practice's coding professionals then use to determine the specific supporting diagnosis code or codes. Even though you may not need to identify the diagnosis codes by number, possessing familiarity with the coding system will allow you and your billing staff to report your services more promptly and accurately. The likely result will be more timely payment. Understanding that a common reason for an insurer to delay or deny payments is a mismatch between the diagnosis and procedure codes gives one a great incentive to get diagnosis and procedure coding right the first time!

207

A DETAILED LOOK AT PROCEDURE CODING—CURRENT PROCEDURAL TERMINOLOGY, HCPCS AND ICD

NORMAN A. COHEN, MD

The dominant procedure coding system to report physician services, including anesthesia care, is the American Medical Association (AMA) Current Procedural Terminology, Fourth Edition (CPT-4).[1] (*Current Procedural Terminology* © 2006 American Medical Association.® All Rights Reserved. Applies to all CPT code references in this chapter). Other procedural coding systems include the Healthcare Common Procedure Coding System (HCPCS), ICD-9-CM (Volume 3), and the soon to be implemented ICD-10 PCS.

CPT

First released in 1966, the American Medical Association has annually updated and published Current Procedural Terminology (CPT), now in its fourth edition. As mentioned in previous chapters, CPT is a systematic listing of procedural services performed by physicians and other health care workers, organized into distinct categories such as evaluation and management, anesthesia, surgery, and radiology. CPT includes three "categories" of codes, designated by roman numerals I through III. Category I codes describe commonly performed and medically accepted procedures and services. Technology encompassed within the procedure must have already received U.S. Food and Drug Administration (FDA) approval and be in widespread use across different types of practice settings. Category II codes are supplemental tracking codes used for performance measures, which are becoming increasingly important as "pay for performance" initiatives gain traction. These tracking code numbers are currently four digits followed by the letter "F." Category III codes represent emerging technology and help facilitate data collection about the medical efficacy of new and perhaps experimental services. Category III codes are temporary and automatically "sunset" after 5 years, unless interested parties submit a request for renewal. These codes have four digits followed by the letter "T."

---

[1]Current Procedural Terminology © 2006 American Medical Association.® All Rights Reserved. Applies to all CPT code references in this chapter.

© 2006 Mayo Foundation for Medical Education and Research

Originally, CPT had a distinct surgical focus. In those simpler times, only four digits were necessary to identify all the services described. In 1970, the AMA expanded CPT to include diagnostic and therapeutic procedures across specialties and simultaneously expanded the code range to five digits to accommodate the significantly increased number of services listed.

The 1980s saw the U.S. government adopt CPT for reporting Medicare Part B (physician) services, Medicaid services, and outpatient surgical procedures. CPT also became the dominant method to report physician services to private payers. The passage of the Health Insurance Portability and Accountability Act of 1996 (HIPAA) cemented CPT's dominance, as the government selected it as the required system for reporting physician services electronically.

All decisions regarding code selection for CPT rests with its Editorial Panel. The AMA Board of Trustees receives nominations from organized medicine and the health care industry, both public and private, for physician representation on the Panel. The Board of Trustees is solely responsible for the selection of all Panel members. In addition to 11 AMA-nominated members, the Blue Cross/Blue Shield Association, the Health Insurance Association of America (HIAA), the American Hospital Association (AHA), and the Centers for Medicare and Medicaid Services (CMS) each nominate one physician representative. The Health Care Professionals Advisory Committee (HCPAC), representing the interests of allied health professionals, nominates two nonphysician health professionals to the Panel. Of the 11 AMA-nominated seats, seven are termed "regular" and four are "rotating." Those with regular seats may serve up to two 4-year terms, while rotating seats are limited to a single 4-year term. The Panel also has an executive committee consisting of a chairman, vice-chairman, and three elected members of the Panel, one of whom represents the private-payer community.

The CPT Advisory Committee advises the Editorial Panel on all code submissions brought forward for consideration. Each of the 107 specialty societies and military service groups with membership in the AMA House of Delegates has a designated representative to the Advisory Committee. The advisors are responsible for reviewing every code submission and offering comments on whether the code and its descriptor meet criteria for acceptance into CPT. Although the CPT process is open, meaning that anyone can submit a code proposal (with medical specialty societies and industry representatives being the most common participants), the Editorial Panel will only consider a code if at least one advisor has indicated support for the proposal. In addition to reviewing code proposals, advisors also assist in the refinement of CPT, prepare technical educational materials, and promote CPT to their specialty organizations and physicians in general.

The CPT Panel meets three times a year. Any new or substantially revised Category I code approved by the CPT Panel is sent to the joint

AMA–Specialty Society Relative Value System Update Committee (RUC) for establishment of work, practice expense, and liability relative value units. We will discuss the role of the RUC in more detail elsewhere. After the RUC achieves consensus on valuation, the codes and values are submitted to CMS for inclusion in the Resource Based Relative Value System (RBRVS). CMS maintains the RBRVS and updates it annually.

Code development is a time-consuming process! Let's follow the process for successfully developing and valuing a new code by assuming that the American Society of Anesthesiologists (ASA) submitted a code proposal for consideration at the February 2006 CPT meeting. The ASA submitted a *code change request* in November 2005. In December, CPT Advisors had the opportunity to comment and indicate support or opposition. The CPT Panel considered the code proposal and Advisor comments at its February 2006 meeting. The Editorial Panel approved the code; therefore, CPT staff forwarded the new code and final descriptor to the RUC for consideration at the RUC's April 2006 meeting. Between February and April, the ASA and any other specialty societies interested in the new code conducted a RUC survey to help the RUC determine the work value. After presentation and debate, the RUC accepted the ASA's recommended base unit value for this service. In early May, the RUC forwarded its annual list of recommendations to CMS, including the new ASA code. In August 2006, CMS published a Notice of Proposed Rule Making (NPRM) for the 2007 Physician Fee Schedule in which the agency accepted the new CPT codes into the RBRVS including acceptance of the RUC's recommendation. After the required public comment period, the agency published the Physician Fee Schedule final rule, in early November 2006. The new service, with the CMS-approved value, was recognized by Medicare as a payable service beginning January 1, 2007. All in all, it takes between 14 and 21 months to take a code proposal from conception to birth.

The author adapted much of the information in this section from the description of the CPT-RUC code development process found at the AMA web site and in various AMA publications. In particular, I refer the reader to this AMA web page describing how a code becomes a code: www.ama-assn.org/ama/pub/category/3882.html.

In the introductory comments to this section, we described the structure of a typical CPT code. After completing our survey of the various procedure coding systems, we will turn our attention to the procedure codes commonly reported by anesthesiologists, pain physicians, and intensivists.

HCPCS

CMS updates the Healthcare Common Procedure Coding System every year. It consists of two sections or "Levels." Level I is the current year's AMA Current Procedural Terminology list of codes and descriptors just described.

Level II describes products, supplies, and services not included in CPT but commonly used to provide medical care. Examples include ambulance services, certain drugs, and durable medical equipment. For anesthesiologists practicing pain medicine, an understanding of HCPCS Level II codes is necessary for correct payment for a number of services. For example, many Medicare carriers require submission of "J-codes" in order to receive payment for implanted drug pump refills. "J-codes" describe drugs that are administered other than via the oral route.

Temporary codes, describing procedures or professional services not yet in CPT, may be listed in the section for G-codes. Medicare may assign payments in the physician fee schedule to these codes. G-codes derive their name from their code number format, that being the letter "G" followed by four digits. If CMS determines that it will pay for the G-code service and the service requires anesthesia, then the anesthesia care is typically paid as well. CMS has also been using G-codes to describe new performance measures, similar to CPT Category II codes. CMS is currently using some G-codes in its Physician Voluntary Reporting Program (PVRP).

ICD-9-CM, VOLUME 3

In the late 1970s the U.S. government developed a procedural coding system designed for inpatient hospital services. This system became Volume 3 of the ICD-9-CM and is used to this day to describe procedures performed in the hospital. From the inception of the Medicare program in 1966 through 1982, Medicare paid hospitals retrospectively based on the charges submitted. In 1983, the U.S. Congress mandated that hospital inpatient services be paid prospectively, based on the anticipated cost of providing care for a patient with a specific diagnosis. These *diagnosis-related groups* (DRG) blend a diagnosis with the typical procedures, tests, and other services necessary to care for the typical patient. Medicare adopted the ICD-9-CM, Volumes 1 and 2, for diagnoses and Volume 3 for procedural coding in the development of the DRG system.

Procedure codes in ICD-9-CM have four digits, and Volume 3 has fewer than 4,000 codes total. This compares to around 8,600 codes in CPT. The ICD system allows only 10 codes in a family of procedures; once the family is full, either CMS combines codes or finds a different place in the book for the additional codes. Separating similar codes into distant areas can hamper efforts to code accurately and efficiently. One issue that is particularly relevant to anesthesiologists is that Volume 3 of ICD-9-CM does not address anesthesia services at all.

As an example of an ICD-9, Volume 3, procedure code family, code 34.5 has a descriptor of "pleurectomy." Code 34.51 represents decortication of lung and code 34.59 describes other excision of pleura, excluding biopsy of pleura (34.24) and pleural fistulectomy (34.73). The astute reader, and that's anyone reading this book, certainly recognized that both 34.51 and 34.59 are subtypes of pleurectomy.

Volume 3 of ICD-9-CM has two parts, a tabular listing of procedures by body system with 16 categories in all, and an alphabetic index to procedures. This organization is very similar to that for Volumes 1 and 2. It is also a fairly straightforward process to crosswalk an ICD-9-CM procedure code to the comparable CPT procedure code. As will be seen in the next section, this relationship does not hold in the next iteration of the ICD system, ICD-10 PCS.

ICD-10 PCS

As the ICD-9-CM ages and medical technology advances, CMS has become increasingly aware of deficiencies in its system for diagnostic and procedural coding. The World Health Organization (WHO) released ICD-10 for diagnoses in 1993. Beginning in 1990, CMS began developing a replacement for the procedural coding element, ICD-9 CM, Volume 3, which would become part of the U.S. version of ICD-10. The name for this replacement is ICD-10-PCS, where PCS stands for *procedural coding system*. Initially, CMS considered replacing CPT with ICD-10-PCS for reporting medical services; however, the agency received significant resistance from the physician community. Organized medicine objected to using ICD-10-PCS for reporting physician services for a number of reasons. These reasons included the cost of modifying business processes and likely delay in payments during a transition from CPT, the complexity of the new system, substantial organizational differences from CPT, and the use of terminology foreign to most physicians and physician coders. Its creators designed ICD-10-PCS, like ICD-9-CM Volume 3 before it, for procedure coding for hospitalized patients. This focus has led to a number of weaknesses in reporting physician services performed in the office or other outpatient settings.

ICD-10-PCS uses a seven-character alphanumeric system for reporting procedures. Each character has a specific meaning within the chapter or section of the code set. The first character defines the section, and the second character usually, but not always, indicates the body system. Assigning meaning to the actual code characters is a significant departure from previous procedural coding systems. One should note that the 31 body system characters are not consistent with nomenclature for body systems typically used by physicians.

As an example of some of the problems with ICD-10-PCS, let us look at just one aspect of describing endotracheal intubation with this system. PCS requires determining whether the target organ is the "trachea" or the "tracheobronchial tree," because one of the seven characters requires this specification. Like intubation, many other services are not easily coded with PCS. Examples include multiple trauma, which would require seven-character codes for each body system suffering trauma, or a Whipple procedure, which has multiple elements (pancreatectomy, choledochojejunostomy, etc.), each of which would have to be separately coded. This code-building exercise, while having the advantage of being easily extensible to new procedures and services and better suited for computerized data analysis, is not terribly user-friendly to physicians and office staff familiar with the current CPT system.

To give you a flavor of an ICD-10-PCS code, let's consider the code for a laparoscopic appendectomy (CPT code 44970). The PCS equivalent would be 0DTJ4ZZ:

0: Section = Medical and surgical
D: Body System = Gastrointestinal system
T: Root Operation = Resection
J: Body Part = Appendix
4: Approach = Using a percutaneous endoscopic approach
Z: Device = None
Z: Qualifier = None

Now "0DTJ4ZZ" really rolls off the tongue, doesn't it?

The diagnostic piece of ICD-10 is very similar to ICD-9. The significant changes are an increase in the number of digits from five to seven and the capability to designate laterality of condition, where appropriate. These changes lead to a dramatically larger code space, which will allow for anticipated growth in the number of medical diagnoses and conditions. By allowing for laterality, coders can accurately match the surgical target to the diagnosis, such as right-sided shoulder pain after surgery supporting a right-sided interscalene block. One might anticipate fewer delays in payments with these changes. The United States adopted ICD-10 (the version published by the World Health Organization) for reporting mortality data in 1999. At the time of this writing, ICD-10-CM and PCS will likely be implemented around 2010; however, CPT will remain the selected code set for reporting physician services in and out of the hospital.

208

SPECIFIC CODING ISSUES

NORMAN A. COHEN, MD

CODING ANESTHESIA PROCEDURES

No matter the specialty, physicians need to be familiar with the coding conventions for reporting the services they commonly perform. Anesthesiology is no exception. In this chapter we briefly discuss the history of the anesthesia coding system and cover the codes that describe anesthesia care. In Chapter 209 we will learn about the unique anesthesia payment system.

Before the 1960s, the anesthesiology profession, like medicine as a whole, had no "system" for reporting its services. Physicians billed their patients directly for the services rendered. Each physician or group established its own fees using individual determinations of the value of the care provided. A senior member of my former group recalls that in the early days of her practice, she charged a fixed percentage of the surgical fee. Although this system was elegant in its simplicity, those who provide anesthesia know that the relationship between surgical effort and anesthesia effort is highly variable.

The explosive growth of third-party payers in the late 1950s and 1960s created a need for better ways to both describe and define the value of anesthesia care. In the early 1960s, trailblazers in California developed the California Relative Value Guide, a systematic listing of anesthesia services and recommended values for each service. Only a few years later, the American Society of Anesthesiologists (ASA) adopted much of the California guide and began publishing the *ASA Relative Value Guide* (RVG) in 1962. The ASA, through its Committee on Economics, continues to publish an annual update to this document. As a member of that committee since 1997 and currently its chair, this author has been actively involved in the preparation of this guide for a number of years.

The RVG evolved fairly rapidly, but the ASA received a legal challenge from the U.S. Federal Trade Commission, which claimed that the publication of relative values promoted illegal price fixing. The ASA prevailed in court in 1979. Ironically, the 1989 *Relative Value Guide* became the basis for Medicare's anesthesia payment system, which we will discuss in a later chapter.

The *ASA Newsletter* published a brief but excellent history of the *Relative Value Guide* in 2004. You can download it from www.asahq.org/Newsletters/2004/09_04/ogunnaike.html.

© 2006 Mayo Foundation for Medical Education and Research

ANESTHESIA PROCEDURE CODES

The American Medical Association Current Procedural Terminology (CPT)[1] (*Current Procedural Terminology* © 2006 American Medical Association.® All Rights Reserved. Applies to all CPT code references in this chapter) organizes the codes describing anesthesia care primarily by body region, with each code encompassing one or more surgical procedures. Some anesthesia services are not easily categorized by body system, leading to special sections for radiologic, burn, obstetric, and miscellaneous other services.

In some cases a single anesthesia code can cover hundreds of surgical procedures. When we discuss coding resources later on, you will learn about the ASA Crosswalk publication, which provides a systematic association between every diagnostic or therapeutic CPT procedure that may require anesthesia and one or more anesthesia services.

Each anesthesia code has an associated base unit value. CPT does not publish the relative values; however, the ASA *Relative Value Guide* does. An underlying principle of the anesthesia relative value system is that all procedures having the same base value and anesthesia time are equivalent in work. For example, anesthesia for an open reduction and internal fixation of a proximal femur fracture taking 90 minutes is equivalent to anesthesia for hysterectomy also lasting 90 minutes, because both anesthesia services have 6 base units assigned. We will discuss methods for calculating anesthesia payments in Chapter 209.

Anesthesia services have their own section in CPT, and the range of anesthesia code numbers is 00100 to 01999. CPT lists approximately 270 anesthesia services. As one progresses through each anesthesia section, the hundreds digits is incremented by one. For example, the code family for spine and spinal cord anesthesia procedures fall in the code range 00600 to 00699. The next section in CPT, "upper abdomen," covers the codes 00700 to 00799. Not every code number in the anesthesia section has a code assigned, allowing room for future growth in the code set.

Here are a few examples of anesthesia codes:

00326—Anesthesia for all procedures on the larynx and trachea in children <1 year of age

00541—Anesthesia for thoracotomy procedures involving lungs, pleura, diaphragm, and mediastinum (including surgical thoracoscopy); utilizing one-lung ventilation

01402—Anesthesia for open or surgical arthroscopic procedures on knee joint; total knee arthroplasty

---

[1]*Current Procedural Terminology* © 2006 American Medical Association. ® All Rights Reserved. Applies to all CPT code references in this chapter.

As you may have noticed, the codes have a specific structure as described in this meta-description:

> Anesthesia for <[specific surgical procedure] OR procedures on [body region] OR [body region] procedures>; <subcategory>

Although most anesthesia codes stand alone, CPT does include a few "add-on" codes that are reported with other services. For example, the procedure codes describing burns include add-on codes to describe large-surface-area burns. Also, when a caesarean section is done after placement of a labor epidural, one would report CPT code 01967, describing neuraxial analgesia for labor, as well as add-on code 01968, describing caesarean section following neuraxial labor analgesia.

A key point for any procedural coding, including anesthesia services, is that the code selected must be the one that most specifically describes the service. To learn more about finding the best fit between the surgical procedure and the anesthesia service, see the discussion of the ASA Crosswalk in Chapter 211.

The following sections will investigate major coding issues that anesthesiologists commonly face. These areas include evaluation and management services, acute and chronic pain procedures, and invasive line and monitoring procedures. During this review, I will try to provide enough background information and specific guidance to help you code correctly. In some cases, I will refer you to primary sources for additional information for topics that are sufficiently complex to preclude an accurate and succinct presentation in this book.

CODING OTHER COMMONLY PERFORMED SERVICES—EVALUATION AND MANAGEMENT

Evaluation and management (E/M) services are the most frequently reported type of medical service, comprising more than 40% of all Medicare physician payments. Office visits, consults, critical care management, emergency medicine evaluations, and numerous other services are all part of the larger evaluation and management family. Although the anesthesiologist who works primarily in the operating room does not perform nearly as many reportable E/M encounters as does his medical and surgical colleagues, understanding E/M is still very important. In 2004, about 7% (~$114 million) of all Medicare payments to anesthesiologists were for E/M services. For two anesthesiology subspecialty areas, pain and critical care medicine, E/M comprises a significantly larger share of total revenue.

This section discusses visits, consults, and critical care services. I will not discuss other E/M services, which are rarely performed by anesthesiologists, such as nursing home visits, preventive medicine services, and care plan oversight.

Visits and consults have various levels of service. These levels reflect the time and work involved in caring for the patient. The key service elements involved in E/M include the history, physical examination, and medical decision making. In some situations, counseling and coordination of care may dominate. In these cases, the total time spent in counseling and coordination determine the appropriate E/M code to report. Other characteristics that help determine which E/M codes to report include the site of service (office or facility) and whether the patient is new to the practice or previously seen. Both site of care and prior patient contact often affect payment level.

As with many elements of the payment system, a seemingly simple question such as "Is this a new patient?" has a nuanced and complex answer. According to CPT, a new patient is "one who has not received any professional services from the physician, or another physician of the same specialty who belongs to the same group practice, within the past 3 years." Medicare, for once, has a slightly less restrictive approach. For Medicare patients, the CPT definition applies except that Medicare limits the definition of "professional services" only to E/M services.

This difference is important to anesthesiologists. For example, a surgeon sends a Medicare patient to your pain clinic for evaluation and treatment of radicular pain affecting the back and left leg. Assume that one of your partners provided anesthesia to this patient for a cholecystectomy 12 months earlier, and further assume that both you and your partner have listed your specialty with Medicare as "anesthesiologist." Because this is a Medicare patient, the previous anesthesia care, not being an E/M service, would make the pain management evaluation a new patient service; conversely, by the CPT definition applied by most other payers, this hypothetical E/M service would be for an established patient. Also, if your specialty designator is "pain medicine" or "interventional pain medicine" and your partner's is "anesthesiologist," then by either definition, you practice a different specialty than your partner, making this a new patient encounter no matter the payer (but please note the important change in CPT definition beginning in 2007 described below). One final point to make the answer to this "simple" question complete: The requirement for being in the same "group practice" is that if the practice bills for both you and your partner using the same Federal tax ID number, then you are in a group practice with the other physician. My former employer has practice sites throughout Oregon, all operating under the same tax ID number. So if I performed an E/M service on a patient in Corvallis, Oregon, that another anesthesiologist in the group cared for 90 miles away in Portland within the previous 3 years, then CPT would consider this patient to be an established patient. It is important to note that as of 2007, CPT changed the definition of new versus established patient to indicate that "same specialty" means "same specialty or same sub-specialty," provided the tax ID number for both providers is the same. I do not know whether the Medicare definition will change to match the CPT definition.

The level of service within a family of E/M codes can depend either on the complexity of the key service elements or, when counseling and coordination of care are the dominant activities, on the total time spent with the patient. Because determining the correct level of service has proven somewhat difficult and Medicare and other payers were suspicious of "up-coding" of services, CMS has published documentation guidelines to help assure that physicians code E/M services correctly. These guidelines, last updated in 1997, are available at www.cms.hhs.gov/MLNEdWebGuide/25_EMDOC.asp.

Correctly determining a level of service using these documentation guidelines is fairly complex. The guidelines categorize each element and subelement of service into a hierarchy that, taken as a whole, allows for determining the correct level of service. Rather than repeating these verbatim or alternatively oversimplifying the guidelines so much that the reader may, by using the simplified description, determine the level of service incorrectly, I urge every anesthesiologist to read the guidelines and have them available as a resource when coding evaluation and management encounters. Another excellent source of general information and overview of all the E/M services is the introduction to the E/M section in each year's CPT publication. I also strongly encourage you to consult with a certified medical coder with recent experience in E/M coding periodically, to confirm that your assignment of level matches both current best practices and the information in the medical record. E/M services are an ongoing area of review by government investigators and private insurers, as these services are both high in volume and have the potential for fraudulent or abusive billing. *Caveat venditor*—"Let the seller beware."

A number of useful articles written by Karin Bierstein, J.D., M.P.H., who serves as the ASA's Associate Director of Professional Affairs, pertain to the use of E/M codes by anesthesiologists. These are available at the ASA web site:

www.asahq.org/Newsletters/1999/02_99/PractMgmt_0299.html
www.asahq.org/Newsletters/2001/04_01/pm0401.htm
www.asahq.org/Newsletters/2002/2_02/pm202.htm

Visits. CPT lists visit codes for both office/outpatient and inpatient encounters. The office/outpatient codes differentiate between new (codes 99201 to 99205) and established patients (99211 to 99215). One reports the office codes when the patient is seen in the office, an outpatient clinic or any other ambulatory facility.

Anesthesiologists may use the outpatient visit codes in a number of circumstances. As an example, a neurosurgeon sends a patient to the pain clinic for the first in a planned series of epidural steroid injections. The pain physician/anesthesiologist performs a history and physical examination, reviews the neurosurgeon's office records and any relevant laboratory or imaging studies before determining that the patient is an acceptable candidate for an epidural steroid trial. The physician documents these findings in the medical record. Because the surgeon made a specific request for treatment before the anesthesiologist saw the patient, this evaluation does not meet the criteria of a consultation. If the patient meets the criteria for a new patient, then the anesthesiologist should report one of the new-patient visit codes; otherwise, the established-patient codes apply. For subsequent epidural steroid injections, the review of intervening history usually is encompassed within the epidural procedure payment itself; however, if the patient develops a new condition requiring evaluation, the evaluation may warrant reporting a subsequent care E/M service.

As another example, an elderly male patient reportedly in good health comes to your ambulatory surgery center for a shoulder arthroscopy. You perform your usual preoperative anesthetic evaluation and discover that the patient has a previously unrecognized harsh systolic murmur radiating to the neck. Further questioning reveals increasing frequency of chest pain and near-syncopal episodes that the patient "didn't want to worry the doctor about." You determine that the patient requires a visit to the cardiologist and an echocardiogram before proceeding with an elective surgical procedure. Because you cancelled the case and the intention of the surgeon was for you to treat the patient by administering an anesthetic (keeping you from reporting a consult), you document your findings and report an office/outpatient visit code of the appropriate level. The choice of new or established patient depends on the criteria as previously described. By the way, you hear from the surgeon a week later that the patient had critical aortic stenosis with 95% stenoses of the LAD and circumflex coronary arteries. You then dislocate your shoulder patting yourself on the back for your clinical acumen, leading the surgeon to schedule you for *your* shoulder arthroscopy!

CPT lists inpatient visit codes for the initial visit by the *admitting physician* (codes 99221 to 99223) and subsequent hospital visit codes that may be reported by any physician providing care in the hospital (codes 99231 to 99233). The admitting physician may report the initial hospital care codes whether or not the patient is new to that physician's practice. Unless a physician other than the admitting physician meets the specific requirements for performing a consultation (see "Consults" below), that physician would most likely report codes 99231 to 99233 for a hospital E/M service.

Anesthesiologists rarely admit patients to the hospital; however, if you are the admitting physician, then these codes 99221 to 99223 are probably the codes you need to report for the admission.

While we rarely admit patients, we do report subsequent hospital care codes with some frequency. For example, your trauma surgeon has admitted a patient who suffered a nondisplaced distal radius fracture in a motor vehicle accident. The orthopedic surgeon has placed a splint and does not believe that surgical management will be necessary; however, the patient suffers from a pre-existing complex regional pain syndrome, so you have been asked to place a continuous brachial plexus block for acute pain management. The patient is new to you and your practice, so you review the medical record including laboratory studies, perform a focused history and physical examination, and determine that the patient is an acceptable candidate for the suggested treatment. You document your findings in the medical record and may report a subsequent-care hospital code (99231 to 99233) for the evaluation as well as the continuous block code (code 64416), assuming you place the continuous catheter. We will discuss many of the important principles for acute and chronic pain procedure reporting, as well as the CPT modifiers that may apply, in the section on coding other commonly performed services—acute and chronic pain coding.

Anesthesiologists need to be aware that the anesthesia base units include payment for the usual preanesthesia evaluation and postanesthesia care. In fact, Medicare and most private insurers have claims-processing software that automatically rejects any claims for an evaluation and management service other than critical care performed on the same date as an anesthetic.

Following this line of thought, the careful reader may wonder whether one may bill separately for the preoperative visit when the patient comes to the anesthesia pre-op clinic. For the typical patient, the answer is "no," these services are typically not separately payable. When the service either significantly exceeds the usual evaluation for the scheduled surgical procedure or when the surgeon specifically requests a consultation from an anesthesiologist, then the service may qualify as an E/M service, subject to separate payment. For the formal consult situation, please see the "Consults" discussion that immediately follows this paragraph. When the preoperative visit substantially exceeds the norm, one may report a visit code of the appropriate level and site of service. As always, the documentation needs to meet the E/M guidelines for the level of service chosen; additionally, the record entry should clearly reflect the evaluation and medical decision making over and above that seen in a normal preanesthesia evaluation.

Consults. In a consult, one physician requests that another physician evaluate a patient and provide written recommendations or opinions as to managing an aspect of that patient's condition. With consults, the key points to remember include:

- The referring physician is not transferring care to the consultant.
- This is a physician-to-physician request.
- The medical record of the referring physician documents the request for consultation.
- The consultant must provide a written report of his or her findings with recommendations to the referring physician.

A patient cannot request a consultation independently. A consultant can order additional testing and may see the patient on more than one occasion to complete the evaluation; however, the consultant would report the subsequent patient encounters with visit codes.

The consult codes apply to both new and established patients, but the codes do differentiate between inpatient and outpatient settings. Given the increased complexity of both the medical decision making and time necessary to evaluate the patient appropriately, the consult codes carry a significantly higher valuation in the RBRVS than do visit codes.

Most frequently, anesthesiologists receive consult requests to evaluate exceptionally complex cases and to provide recommendations on preparing these patients for surgery. Another common reason for an anesthesiology consult is to get recommendations on managing acute and chronic pain problems. To bill for a consult, the anesthesiologist must satisfy the requirements described above. One of the key differences between a consult and a visit code is the expectation of the referring party. With a request for a consult, the expectation is that the anesthesiologist will provide written recommendations to the referring physician regarding patient management and that the responsibility for care remains with the referring physician. With a referral for a visit, the expectation is that the anesthesiologist will both evaluate *and* treat an already-diagnosed condition.

Preoperative Clinics. We have just spent some time learning about consults and visits performed by anesthesiologists. Many anesthesia groups offer preanesthesia clinics. Are these clinics self-financing from clinical revenue? The short answer in most cases is "no" regarding self-financing; however, the overall benefits to the practice may make staffing a clinic worthwhile. These benefits, as we will see below, may include improved goodwill and enhanced operating room efficiency.

When is a visit to a clinic separately reportable for payment? In addition to a request for an anesthesia consult, certain clinic visits may also be compensable if they exceed the usual preoperative evaluation included in the anesthesia base units.

As a rule of thumb, if the evaluation in the clinic identifies the need for increased evaluation, optimization of medical status, or additional diagnostic testing as a prerequisite for proceeding with the anesthetic, then the clinic visit may meet the criteria for a reportable E/M service. An example may be useful. Let's say a male college basketball player presents to the clinic for a preoperative evaluation for an anterior cruciate ligament repair. During physical examination, notable findings include a faint diastolic murmur, exceptionally long fingers and hands, and some joint laxity. The patient's family history is remarkable for sudden death at an early age in an uncle and grandfather. The patient has never been evaluated for Marfan syndrome. You contact the orthopedic surgeon and recommend echocardiography before surgery to evaluate for possible aortic root or valve pathology. Your evaluation in the clinic clearly exceeds the typical preanesthesia evaluation for a sports-medicine surgical procedure, and I believe that if it is appropriately documented, this service would justify separate payment as an outpatient visit service.

Because an anesthesia practice can submit E/M claims for only a small subset of patients seen in a preoperative clinic, the obvious question is how one makes such an endeavor financially viable. To answer this question, one must determine who benefits most from these clinics. While patients benefit through assurance that they are in medically optimal condition before surgery and from reducing the rate of cancellations the day of surgery, patients assume that this is part of our obligation to them and that they should not have to pay a premium for this benefit. Both the surgeon and the anesthesiologist benefit through improved productivity and reduced complications; however, neither the surgeon nor the anesthesiologist typically sees enough direct gain to justify the additional cost. The facility, which garners the lion's share of the perioperative health care payment, definitely benefits the most from an efficient operating room. Surprise delays and cancellations are exceptionally costly to the hospital because of nonproductive staff, unused equipment, and wasted supplies. Given all these considerations and recognizing that the surgeon is unlikely to contribute significant funds, pursuing facility financing often makes the most sense.

If your practice is seeing a high rate of delays and cancellations on the day of surgery related to patient preparation, "gain sharing" with the facility to jointly create and staff a clinic may be a business decision that will pay great dividends for both parties going forward. In addition to improved patient and surgeon satisfaction ("goodwill"), increased anesthesiologist productivity can reduce overall personnel requirements. With increased income, the practice has more options to invest in the business. Likewise, the facility can use an efficient operating suite as a marketing tool to attract surgeons and patients, can pay adequately to retain staff, and can invest in equipment and personnel to maintain the facility's competitive position.

Critical Care. Anesthesiologists participated actively in the creation of the medical specialty now known as critical care medicine. Fittingly, many anesthesiologists still provide nonanesthesia medical services to the critically ill of all ages. In the following paragraphs we will review the key requirements for coding these services, as well as some important caveats.

CPT provides an excellent overview of the components of critical care in the CPT Evaluation and Management Section of each year's CPT publication. Some of the key points listed include the following:

- Critical care involves the delivery of medical care to patients who have potentially life-threatening illnesses or injuries that threaten one or more organ systems.
- Medical decision making in critical care is of high complexity, involving assessment, manipulation, and support of key or "vital" organ systems so as to both prevent further patient deterioration and help induce recovery.
- Examples of vital organ system failure include circulatory failure, shock, central nervous system failure, hepatic failure, and respiratory failure.
- Although application of advanced technology and interpretation of multiple physiologic parameters is often a part of critical care, a critical care service does not require these elements, most notably in life-threatening circumstances that develop suddenly.
- A physician may provide critical care over multiple days, whether or not the physician makes changes in the therapeutic plan, as long as the patient's condition qualifies, the medical decision making is of sufficient complexity, and the time involved in direct patient care is sufficient to qualify.
- Although critical care is most typically delivered in a critical care unit, a physician may deliver critical care outside of that setting.
- Conversely, not all patients lodged in a critical care unit meet the requirements for reporting of a critical care service.
- If neither the patient condition nor the medical care delivered meet the criteria for critical care, the physician should report an appropriate E/M service, such as a visit code.

CPT includes a number of critical care service codes, which cover the adult (CPT codes 99291 to 99292), pediatric (99293 to 99294), and neonatal (99295 to 99296) populations. By definition, adult critical care applies to patients >24 months of age, pediatric to patients from 29 days through 24 months of age, and neonatal to patients 28 days old or less. CPT limits the neonatal and pediatric codes to the inpatient setting; however, one can report the adult codes in either the inpatient or outpatient setting. Outpatient settings may include an emergency department or the office. The neonatal and pediatric codes include all work done during the initial *day* of critical care or each subsequent day. The adult codes include the work done during the initial 30 to 74 *minutes* (99291) or each subsequent 30 minutes (99292). For outpatient neonatal or pediatric critical care, CPT instructs the physician to use the adult critical care codes.

When a physician attends a critically ill patient during transport, that physician should report the adult critical care codes for those patients >24 months old or the specific pediatric transport service codes 99289 and 99290 when the patient is 24 months or less in age.

As noted above, the adult critical care codes reflect the actual time spent in delivering critical care. This time can be discontinuous and the codes reported should reflect the sum of all discontinuous time for a given day. The time should include both face-to-face time and other time spent on the floor or unit in reviewing records, interpreting tests, communicating with family or other care givers, and documenting findings. Critical care time must bear directly on the management of the specific patient; administrative meetings or educational sessions in the ICU do not count toward critical care time. Critical care time for an individual patient should not include any time spent managing other patients in the critical care unit or other locations, nor should it include time spent off the floor or unit. The medical record entry should include documentation of the time spent caring for the patient.

Discussions with family or care givers count as critical care only to the extent that these discussions bear directly on patient management. For example, critically ill patients are often unable to provide a history or provide informed consent. Obtaining a patient history or consent for a procedure from the family would count as reportable time in these circumstances; however, time spent updating the family on the patient's status unrelated to obtaining consent or history would not count.

If the total time spent caring for the adult patient is <30 minutes, then the physician reports an appropriate E/M service. For critical care lasting between 30 and 74 minutes, the physician would report 99291 (Critical care, evaluation and management of the critically ill or critically injured patient; first 30 to 74 minutes). And for each 30-minute block after 74 minutes (i.e., 75 to 104 minutes, 105 to 134 minutes, etc.), the physician would additionally report one or more codes 99292 (each additional 30 minutes [list separately in addition to code for primary service]). As an example, let's assume that you have spent 130 minutes of reportable face-to-face and floor time on a given calendar day caring for a postsurgical critically ill patient, who is suffering from shock and respiratory failure. When submitting this service for payment, you should report a 99291 for the first 74 minutes and two 99292s for the additional 56 minutes.

As mentioned, the neonatal and pediatric critical care service codes differ both in duration and site of service requirements from the adult critical care codes. The definition of critical care does not vary with age; however, the need to account for every minute spent with the patient is not necessary for neonates and infants requiring critical care services. CPT does allow separate reporting of delivery services and newborn resuscitation, including endotracheal intubation performed as part of the resuscitation, with the initial-day neonatal critical care code (99295). For neonates <5 kg in weight who are not critically ill but do require intensive observation and frequent interventions, CPT provides a family of "continuing intensive care services." For neonates weighing >5 kg, physicians should use the subsequent hospital care visit codes (99231 to 99233).

CPT lists several services as being inclusive within the critical care service and thus not separately reportable. These services include interpreting cardiac output measurements, chest radiographs, pulse oximetry, blood gases, and other data stored in computers (e.g., electrocardiogram tracings, hemodynamic data, etc.). Other bundled services include gastric intubation, temporary transcutaneous pacing, ventilator management, and certain vascular access procedures (i.e., peripheral intravenous or needle placement, venipuncture and venous blood collection, blood collection from an implantable venous access device, and arterial blood draw). Any other service may be separately reported. Common examples include central venous pressure (CVP) catheter or arterial line placement, endotracheal intubation, and echocardiography. When performing these separately reportable services, you should not include the time spent doing so in your critical care time.

The National Correct Coding Initiative (NCCI) is Medicare's way of linking codes that should not be reported at the same time. We will address NCCI in more detail in a later chapter; however, one of the exclusions important to anesthesiologists is Medicare's decision to deny payment for E/M services on the same day as an anesthetic. Critical care is a notable exception to this rule. So if you provide critical care services and anesthesia care on the same day to the same patient and you meet the reporting requirements for critical care, you may be paid for both services.

CODING OTHER COMMONLY PERFORMED SERVICES—ACUTE AND CHRONIC PAIN CODING

As experts in all aspects of pain management, our physician colleagues frequently request that we evaluate and manage acute and chronic pain conditions. Management options range from prescribing medications to physical therapy or other noninvasive modalities to personally performing peripheral or neuraxial nerve blocks or even placing neuraxial catheters or stimulators.

In this section we focus on the coding of acute pain management services as well as a few commonly performed chronic pain procedures. We will also discuss certain guidelines to help prevent you from running afoul of payer rules involving these services.

General Guidelines, Caveats, and "Medical Necessity." Anesthesiologists often perform neuraxial blocks, plexus injections, and peripheral nerve blocks in their efforts to reduce acute pain associated with surgery or trauma. Because physicians other than the anesthesiologist also have responsibilities for pain management, payers have established certain prerequisites before compensating for these services. For surgical procedures, payments to the surgeon cover managing typical postoperative pain. Medicare rules prohibit separate payment for pain management procedures to the surgeon. In addition, payment for patient-controlled intravenous analgesia (IV PCA) is inclusive in the global surgical payment. Many private payers also follow Medicare's payment rules, so this decision applies more broadly than just to Medicare.

Because payers already compensate the operating physician for routine pain management services, these payers often require that the surgeon specifically delegate to the anesthesiologist responsibility for perioperative pain management. This request may take the form of a written order, a note in the medical record, or a verbal request to the anesthesiologist. If the surgeon's request is verbal, the anesthesiologist should make a written note of this request on the anesthesia record, in the progress notes, or in the procedure note itself.

When a nerve block is the primary means for delivering surgical anesthesia, the ASA, CPT, and most payers consider payment for that block to be included in the payment for the anesthesia service. If the block's purpose is to provide postoperative pain relief, a different anesthetic technique is primary, and the block only "incidentally" contributes to the anesthetic, then the block may be separately payable. From a payment perspective (but not necessarily that of patient safety), the anesthesiologist may place the nerve block before, during, or after the anesthetic and still receive separate payment. For example, let's say an elderly woman presents for a shoulder hemiarthroplasty and this patient has a general anesthetic. If you place an interscalene block at the beginning of the case before anesthesia induction, then you can charge separately for the brachial plexus block, because the primary anesthetic technique was general.

Because one can place blocks during the anesthetic itself, I have often been asked whether placing a block influences reporting of anesthesia time. My (admittedly conservative) advice is that if one places the block before induction of anesthesia, then the anesthesia time does not start until after one has completed block placement. If one chooses to place the block sometime between anesthesia induction and the time that the patient can be safely transferred to the care of the PACU nurse, then placement of the block does not affect reporting of anesthesia time, because your responsibilities toward managing the anesthetic are in no way diminished while placing the block.

In the final scenario, one may place the block in the PACU or on the floor. In this situation, one should end anesthesia time before block placement. In this definition, "induction of anesthesia" would also apply to a combination of neuraxial block for anesthesia and peripheral or plexus block for postoperative pain control. One often sees the situation of two regional anesthetic techniques in total knee arthroplasties, in which the primary anesthetic is a spinal or epidural, but the surgeon often also requests a single-shot or continuous femoral nerve block for more prolonged postoperative pain relief.

Although most physicians recognize the many benefits of pain control, pain management interventions can be expensive and do expose the patient to additional risks. For these reasons as well as the fear (well founded or not) that anesthesiologists, driven by greed, perform unnecessary pain procedures, many payers have established "medical necessity" policies for pain management services. Although every anesthesiologist should be familiar with such payer policies, it is incumbent upon each of us to make the medical judgment to provide a pain management intervention ethically, based on patient condition, surgical intervention, and the balancing of risk and benefit to the patient. If we cannot reasonably justify the proposed intervention, then we shouldn't perform the procedure. It's that simple! Although most of us do the right thing, I often hear about some in our profession who, for whatever reason, perform pain management interventions that don't pass this simple "smell test." I fear that we will be faced with increasingly onerous payer policies that work to limit our autonomy in medical decision making, as long as we have colleagues who deliberately push the limits of propriety and professionalism.

In June 2006, the ASA's leadership issued a general statement on medical necessity for anesthesia care in response to the growing number of private payers trying to limit payments for anesthesia for gastrointestinal endoscopy. Previously, the AMA had published a definition of medical necessity. Although it should be obvious to you that medical necessity requirements extend beyond just pain management services, the attention of payers to the medical necessity for and coverage of pain management services made this a reasonable place to introduce this concept. For further information, I refer you to a number of documents for a better understanding of how our professional organizations view medical necessity:

www.asahq.org/Washington/ASA   PositionStatementonMedicalNecessity060406.pdf

www.asahq.org/Washington/GuidryWeb.pdf

www.ama-assn.org/ama1/pub/upload/mm/368/mmcc_4th_suppl_1.pdf

For those who still doubt that interventional pain services are the subject of intense payer scrutiny, I note that among the fastest-growing "minor" procedures in the Medicare population are spinal injections. Payers definitely notice areas of rapid growth! The Office of the Inspector General (OIG), Medicare's enforcement arm, publishes the results of its enforcement actions. Several recent cases involve incorrect billing for pain management services: http://oig.hhs.gov/fraud/enforcement/administrative/cmp/cmpitems.html.

Specific Procedures. Acute pain management procedures for surgical and trauma pain most commonly involve the diagnostic or therapeutic nerve block injection series (CPT 64400 to 64450) or neuraxial injections (62310 to 62319). Anesthesiologists who practice chronic pain management also often diagnose and manage spinal pain with transforaminal epidural and facet injections (64470 to 64484), treat sympathomimetic pain syndromes (64505 to 64530), introduce neurolytic substances (64600 to 64681), manage neuraxial (63650 to 63688) and peripheral (64550 to 64573) nerve stimulators, and place (62350 to 62362) and refill (95990 to 95991) neuraxial pumps.

Some CPT codes differentiate between single and continuous techniques. Neuraxial blocks (spinal or epidural) have single-injection versions that differentiate between cervical/thoracic (62310) and lumbar/sacral (62311) placement, along with similar continuous versions (62318 and 62319, respectively). Several of the peripheral plexus and nerve blocks also have continuous versions, notably those targeting the femoral and sciatic nerves and the lumbar and brachial plexuses. One should note that currently CPT lists only a continuous lumbar plexus block, and not the single variant. There is currently significant interest in the regional anesthesia community to develop a code for the single-injection version.

For most payers, all of these pain management procedures fall under the general payment rules for RBRVS services. The ASA's *Relative Value Guide* lists anesthesia unit equivalents for most of these procedures; however, only a handful of payers recognize these ASA values. For those payers that follow Medicare rules or RBRVS, it is important to note the global period for these services. For example, all the continuous nerve block procedures, with the exception of the continuous neuraxial blocks, have a 10-day global. That means that any visits associated with managing the continuous block that occur within 10 days of placement are included in the procedure payment and not separately billable. For the continuous neuraxial blocks (62318 and 62319), the global period is 0 days.

The method for reporting ongoing management of continuous spinals and epidurals is different from that for the continuous peripheral and plexus blocks. The anesthesiologist reports subsequent management of a *continuous neuraxial infusion* performed *in the hospital* with the anesthesia code 01996, which is worth 3 anesthesia base units. If epidural management occurs in the outpatient setting or if the patient receives only bolus injections through the catheter, then the anesthesiologist should report the appropriate hospital or outpatient E/M visit codes. The reason for this seemingly bizarre approach is that the descriptor for 01996 specifically applies only to inpatients and only to management of continuous neuraxial infusions. One of the frequently asked questions that we receive at the ASA's Committee on Economics is whether one can report 01996 for a long-acting spinal or epidural narcotic injection with drugs such as preservative-free or liposomal-encapsulated morphine. Although there is additional physician work and risk involved in managing these injections, we recommend that when anesthesiologists evaluate and manage patients consistent with the E/M guidelines, they should document interventions and report a visit code on the day after the injection. Because these are not continuous infusions, ongoing management does not qualify as a 01996 procedure. This care is typically at the level of a low-acuity visit (e.g., CPT 99231), but, on occasion, the total work performed may justify a higher-level visit.

CPT Modifiers. In the following paragraphs we will discuss the CPT modifiers that frequently apply in coding acute and chronic pain management encounters. Many payers require the reporting of modifiers to demonstrate that the procedure code being submitted is not included in the payment for other services. For the actual descriptors for these modifiers and specific CPT instructions, see Appendix A of the current-year CPT publication.

When an anesthesiologist performs an acute pain management procedure on the same day as an anesthetic service, he or she should append modifier 59 to the pain management procedure code. This modifier indicates to the payer that the pain management procedure is a "distinct procedural service," and that the pain management procedure was not the primary anesthetic for the surgical procedure.

We previously discussed the situation in which a physician refers a patient to a pain management clinic. On that first visit, the work involved in evaluating and examining the patient, reviewing records and test results, and determining that the patient is an appropriate candidate for an interventional procedure may qualify as a separately reportable E/M service. If the E/M service and the interventional procedure occur on the same day, CPT advises the use of modifier 25, which is a "Significant, separately identifiable evaluation and management service by the same physician on the same day of the procedure or other service."

On occasion, the physician may perform multiple procedures on the same visit, or she may perform the same procedure bilaterally. For multiple procedures, CPT requires reporting modifier 51 for most codes, and for bilateral procedures (e.g., bilateral femoral nerve blocks), the second procedure should include modifier 50. Some codes, such as add-on codes (ZZZ globals in RBRVS), or those listed in Appendix E of CPT, do not require reporting modifier 51 when performed with other procedures. Because many payers reduce payments for second and subsequent procedures, the physician should append modifier 51 to the lesser-valued service. For most bilateral procedures, the second side also receives reduced payments; however, some CPT descriptors note that the procedure code applies to both unilateral and bilateral interventions. For these codes, it would be inappropriate to report modifier 50.

When one uses image guidance, the appropriate imaging service should have modifier 26 appended. This indicates that the payer should compensate only for the professional component of the service. Please see the next chapter's discussion of transesophageal echocardiogram (TEE) reporting for a complete description of modifier 26.

When the patient needs to have the procedure repeated on the same day or some other day during the global period, CPT provides modifier 76 for a return on the same day or modifier 78 for a return to the operating room during the postoperative period. Sometimes, a patient requires an unrelated intervention during the global period for another procedure. Once again, CPT comes to the rescue with modifier 79.

Considering all these modifiers makes me glad that I am an anesthesiologist and do not have to deal very frequently with many of these matters.

CODING OTHER COMMONLY PERFORMED SERVICES—LINES, TEE, EMERGENCY INTUBATION, AND VENTILATOR MANAGEMENT

In addition to pain management and E/M, anesthesiologists commonly perform several other services, such as invasive lines, transesophageal echocardiography, emergency intubation, and ventilator management. In the following sections I review many of the key issues with reporting these services and some of the pitfalls that anesthesiologists should avoid.

Invasive Lines. Anesthesiologists commonly place arterial, central venous (CVP), and pulmonary artery (PA) catheters for many reasons. While *monitoring* the data arising from these lines is part of routine anesthetic care, the value of an anesthetic service never includes bundled payment for *placing* invasive monitoring lines. The ASA even has published a formal statement on this issue, which can be found at www.asahq.org/publicationsAndServices/standards/Intravascular.pdf. This statement has and will likely continue to be of value to anesthesia groups facing payer denials for line placement services.

In the section on modifiers, we discussed that payers often reduce the payment of second and subsequent procedures when a physician performs multiple procedures in the same setting. We also noted that CPT maintains a list of "modifier 51–exempt" codes that are not subject to this payment reduction. When one performs an invasive line procedure along with an anesthetic, the invasive line procedure is not subject to payment reduction. Currently, both arterial lines and PA catheters are on the multiple procedure exempt list. This means that when one places both an arterial line or a PA catheter along with another nonanesthesia procedure, the physician receives full payment for the lines.

A few years ago, CPT substantially modified the codes for CVP placement. Because central access can include tunneled and nontunneled catheters with and without subcutaneous access ports, and because the work of placing these catheters can vary dramatically by age, the CVP code set tries to cover all these eventualities. In practice, CPT has two central line codes of interest to the typical anesthesiologist. These codes describe nontunneled centrally inserted catheters for patients 5 years of age or older (36556) and for those younger than 5 years of age (36555).

Over the past few years, physicians have increasingly used ultrasound guidance for vascular access. CPT code 76937 describes this modality. When used in the facility and when the physician does not own the ultrasound machine, the physician should append modifier 26 to the service on the claim. In 2004, Medicare received >200,000 claims for this service, compared to about 600,000 for nontunneled central access in adults. Radiologists performed 85% of the ultrasound procedures, while anesthesiologists were barely a blip on the screen at under 1%. To report the ultrasound code, the physician must accomplish all of the following tasks:

Scan potential access sites.

Check for vessel patency.

Visualize the needle actually entering the target vessel.

Maintain a permanent record of the images (electronic or print).

Formally document the findings in the CVP procedure note or a separate report.

Practices that charge for ultrasound guidance in 100% of their line placements may run a risk of being audited. Diagnostic imaging is one of the fastest-growing families of procedures, and the payers have noticed. Even though ultrasound may be helpful in a number of circumstances, no one has proven that it is medically necessary to use ultrasound in every case. I strongly encourage anyone using ultrasound guidance not only to meet *all* the criteria listed above but also to include the reasons (diagnoses) justifying its use in each and every case. Some common reasons that would support the use of ultrasound include morbid obesity, coagulopathy, history of difficult central access, or history of intravenous drug abuse. Others may apply as well. Use your medical knowledge in determining whether ultrasonic guidance is beneficial to the patient. Your convenience alone is unlikely to justify the additional expense to either your patient or your patient's insurer.

Transesophageal Echocardiography. Given its proven utility in the management of patients with cardiovascular disease, it should be no surprise that the use of TEE has grown rapidly since its introduction in the 1980s. Over the 10-year period from 1994 to 2004, Medicare volume for TEE nearly tripled. Anesthesiology is second only to cardiology in the number of services performed. CPT includes seven procedures that one can use to report TEE services. Medicare has assigned an XXX global period to all the TEE codes, meaning that the surgical global concept does not apply. XXX global procedures are not subject to reporting of modifier 51, and thus payers pay the fee schedule value without any multiple procedure reduction.

As with most imaging services in the RBRVS, the TEE codes have a global payment amount as well as a professional and technical component. When a physician owns the equipment, employs the technical staff, and performs the service, he gets paid the global payment; however, if someone else owns the equipment and employs the technical staff, the physician gets paid the professional component (PC) and the other party gets paid the technical component (TC). The PC includes payment for the physician's work, physician-related practice expenses, and physician liability, while the technical component includes no payment for work but does include practice expenses associated with the use of the equipment and liability of the technical staff. The sum of the PC and TC for a service equals the global payment. When a physician submits a charge for the professional component of a service, she appends the modifier 26 to the code. The owner of the equipment and employer of the staff uses the TC modifier.

Three TEE codes address standard diagnostic TEE (93312 to 93314), three codes address TEE for congenital anomalies (93315 to 93317), and the final TEE code addresses the use of TEE for perioperative monitoring (93318). CPT has defined four components of a TEE service: Probe placement, image acquisition (with permanent recording), interpretation, and report preparation. CPT has also grouped these services into bundles: The full service comprising all four elements; the probe placement service only; and the image acquisition, interpretation, and report services without probe placement.

TEE codes 93312 and 93315 are the full-service codes. To report this service, the physician must perform all four elements, including preparation of a written report. The physician should not just restate calculated values such as ejection fraction, aortic valve area, or jet velocity; he should also demonstrate his acumen by interpreting these values and making medical judgments regarding significance. Use of adjectives such as "severe," "moderate," or "mild" help demonstrate the interpretation element of the service.

In the OR, it is common for an anesthesiologist to place the probe and the cardiologist to acquire and interpret the images. In this situation, the anesthesiologist would submit either 93313 or 93316 for the probe placement, and the cardiologist would submit 93314 or 93317 for the image acquisition, interpretation, and report. The RBRVS value for 93313 + 93314 is the same as 93312; likewise, 93316 + 93317 is the same value as 93315.

I know from personal experience that some cardiologists ask the anesthesiologist or even the echocardiography technician to acquire the images during the procedure. Because the anesthesiologist (or the technician, for that matter) does not perform the interpretation or prepare the report, the anesthesiologist should report only the probe placement code. Because the cardiologist has not acquired the image, she has not completed all the required elements of code 93314 or 93317. In my opinion, the cardiologist should append modifier 52, indicating a reduced service; however, I doubt that this occurs with any frequency.

The TEE code for perioperative monitoring, 93318, includes probe placement, real-time image acquisition, and interpretation of dynamically changing cardiac function, often resulting in therapeutic interventions. Early in my tenure on the ASA Committee on Economics, I served on a work group that developed this code. We believed that in most cases, intraoperative TEE was a distinctly different service from diagnostic TEE, involving frequent assessment of cardiac function under dynamically changing conditions. Although we succeeded in both having CPT approve a code that described these activities and getting a fair value recommended by the RUC, CMS determined that Medicare would not pay for "monitoring," making code 93318 an uncovered service. Unfortunately, many other payers followed Medicare's lead. Given this situation, physicians code almost all intraoperative TEEs as diagnostic TEEs, or, less commonly, as TEEs for congenital anomalies. Keep in mind, though, that to report a diagnostic TEE, you need to perform the elements of the examination described above.

An interesting factoid is that, despite CMS not paying for the intraoperative monitoring code, physicians, 50% of whom were cardiologists, reported 2,500 cases of 93318 to Medicare in 2004. It pays to know what Medicare actually covers!

Emergency Intubation. As experts in airway management, anesthesiologists often urgently or emergently perform endotracheal intubations. CPT code 31500 describes this service. Anesthesiologists should not report 31500 for endotracheal intubation that occurs as part of a general anesthetic. The base + time units for the anesthesia service include the work of endotracheal intubation; however, if a patient requires urgent/emergency reintubation in the PACU or elsewhere after the end of reportable anesthesia time, the anesthesiologist can report 31500, and should include a 59 modifier to indicate that this reintubation was a distinct procedural service. Given that CCI and other "edit" software may initially disallow payment for 31500 on the same day as an anesthetic service, including a copy of the procedure note for the intubation along with the claim may help reduce a delay in payment.

Critical care is another area where payment rules may not allow reporting of 31500 on the same day. The critical care services include emergency intubation when performed. The August 2004 CPT Assistant did identify one situation involving critical care when one may report both emergency intubation and a critical care service on the same day. If a newborn requires intubation as part of the initial neonatal resuscitation in the delivery room, the intubation is not performed as a convenience before transport to the neonatal intensive care unit (NICU), and the documentation supports the necessity for intubation in the delivery room, then the physician can report and be paid for 31500 in addition to neonatal critical care.

CPT lists emergency intubation on the modifier 51 exempt list. This status means that if one performs emergency intubation along with another service (e.g., arterial line, central venous line, etc.), payers should pay both services without the multiple procedure payment reduction.

Ventilator Management. CPT recently made a number of changes to the ventilator management codes that took effect in 2007. For anesthesiologists, the key codes to know are 94002 for the first day of ventilator management and 94003 to be reported on each subsequent day of management.

The elements included in ventilator management include establishing initial settings, periodic assessment of both clinical and laboratory findings relevant to ventilator care, establishing the clinical goals, adjustment of settings as indicated, interventions to treat the underlying causative condition for or complications related to the respiratory failure, and defining the weaning protocol for use when the respiratory failure resolves. Given the extent and number of tasks included in ventilator management, anesthesiologists should not expect to be paid for this service merely by providing initial ventilator settings and doing nothing further; however, if the anesthesiologist does provide initial settings, manages weaning from the ventilator, directs the extubation, and documents those activities, then reporting ventilator management in most cases is appropriate.

If the anesthesiologist reports an evaluation and management service, including critical care, on the same day that the physician also performed inpatient ventilator management, the anesthesiologist should report only the E/M code. The physician should consider the time and work involved in ventilator management along with all other evaluation and management services in determining the appropriate level and type of E/M. Risking the restatement of the obvious, ventilator management is an inclusive component of critical care and should not be separately reported the same day as critical care.

As is true for E/M services, Medicare does not allow reporting of initial ventilator management on the same day as an anesthetic service. This may also be true for other payers that follow Medicare payment policies and guidelines. If ventilator care does continue onto subsequent days and the anesthesiologist provides ventilator care, he can report the subsequent ventilator care code each day he performs the service, beginning the day after the anesthetic.

209

GETTING PAID FOR ANESTHESIA SERVICES

NORMAN A. COHEN, MD

This chapter discusses the anesthesia relative value system as well as the dominant payment system for most other physician services, the Resource-Based Relative Value System (RBRVS). Anesthesiologists need to be familiar with both, as the methods by which insurers calculate payments for our services often involve both systems.

ANESTHESIA PAYMENT SYSTEM

The anesthesia payment system dates back to the early 1960s, when the California Medical Association published an anesthesia relative value guide. This was one of the first examples of a relative value system, in which one valued a physician's service in comparison to all other physician services. The American Society of Anesthesiologists (ASA) adopted this system in the mid-1960s and has published a relative value guide annually for many years.

This payment system consists of several elements: Base units, time units, and modifier units. Each unit is equal in value.

Base Units. In the ASA *Relative Value Guide* (RVG), every anesthetic service has a base unit value assigned. Currently, the base units range from 3 units to 30 units, and the base units reflect the amount of work involved in the pre-anesthetic evaluation, the postanesthetic management, the administration of fluids and blood, intraoperative monitoring, and the overall complexity and intensity of the anesthetic service. *Table 209.1* provides examples of base unit values for various anesthetics.

Time Units. The creators of the anesthesia relative value system understood that the time involved in providing anesthesia care was not in the control of the anesthesiologist. They also understood that time could be highly variable between surgical procedures that were otherwise identical in anesthetic complexity. Therefore, the anesthesia relative value system explicitly identifies time as part of the payment formula. Each time unit represents a defined period of anesthesia care, most typically 15 minutes. According to the ASA, anesthesia time begins when the anesthesiologist begins to prepare the patient for anesthesia in the operating room or equivalent area and ends when the patient is safely placed under postanesthesia care. One can think of this as "hands on to hand-off."

© 2006 Mayo Foundation for Medical Education and Research

TABLE 209.1	EXAMPLES OF BASE UNIT VALUES FOR VARIOUS ANESTHETICS	
CODE	**DESCRIPTOR**	**BASE UNIT**
	Surgical Procedure Example	
01810	Anesthesia for all procedures on nerves, muscles, tendons, fascia, and bursae of forearm, wrist, and hand	3
	Carpal Tunnel Release	
00790	Anesthesia for intraperitoneal procedures in upper abdomen including laparoscopy; not otherwise specified	7
	Laparoscopic Cholecystectomy	
01173	Anesthesia for open repair of fracture disruption of pelvis or column fracture involving acetabulum	11
	Open Repair of Acetabular Fracture	
00562	Anesthesia for procedures on heart, pericardial sac, and great vessels of chest; with pump oxygenator	20
	Aortic Valve Replacement	
00796	Anesthesia for intraperitoneal procedures in upper abdomen including laparoscopy; liver transplant (recipient)	30
	Liver Transplant	

Most private payers allow rounding to the next higher anesthesia unit after a certain number of minutes. For example, assume that the practice reports time in 15-minute increments. A particular anesthesia case lasts 66 minutes. The practice may have established a policy to round to the next time unit after 5 minutes. In that situation, the example case would be worth 5 time units. The Medicare program, many Medicaid programs, and some private payers round to the nearest minute. In that case, the example case would be worth $66/15 = 4.4$ time units.

Although 15-minute time units are common, some regions have historically reported time in 10- or 12-minute time units. Some practices may also increase the number of units charged per hour after a procedure exceeds a certain duration.

A common error in billing for anesthesia services is to charge for anesthesia time for parts of the service that should not be included in reportable anesthesia time. Some anesthesiologists mistakenly "start the clock" during the preoperative interview immediately before the scheduled surgical procedure. The preoperative interview is included in the base unit payment for the service and is outside of reportable time. Another example of incorrect time reporting is to include time spent in the recovery room with the patient after care has been turned over to the postanesthesia care unit (PACU) nurse. Again, this is part of the base units and is not separately reportable. A gray area exists around charging anesthesia time for placement of epidurals or nerve blocks used exclusively for postoperative pain relief. Because insurers pay separately for these services, I do not start the anesthesia clock until after placing the block when that placement occurs before anesthesia induction. If the block is the primary means of anesthesia for the surgery, then insurers do not allow separate payment, so in these circumstances, I do start anesthesia time before placing the block.

Anesthesia time reporting can be a compliance nightmare, so be sure to check whether your practice has specific rules or guidelines with regard to time reporting. If the group does not, strongly encourage it to do so. Most well-run practices with an up-to-date compliance plan do have time reporting policies. Having a well-reasoned compliance plan in place and following that plan can be a great help if you are ever unfortunate enough to have to face an investigation of your billing practices.

Reporting time for labor analgesia is highly variable, partly because the anesthesiologist is not in personal attendance throughout the procedure in most cases, partly because the anesthesiologist may be managing multiple labor analgesia procedures at the same time, and partly because the total charge for a prolonged labor case, if billed as is typical for an operating room case, can be very large, possibly exceeding the entire fee charged by the obstetrician for 9 months of care! As one might imagine, neither patients nor our obstetrical colleagues are very happy when this occurs.

The RVG provides guidance on the underlying principles that one should use in developing a charge system for labor analgesia care. It also lists four methods consistent with these principles. These methods include usual anesthesia time subject to a cap, 1 unit per hour plus actual face-to-face time, incremental time-based fees (0 to <2 hours, 2 to 6 hours, >6 hours), and a flat fee regardless of total time. In surveys of anesthesia practices, ASA has found that most use one of these four variants, with no particular method being particularly dominant.

Modifiers and Qualifying Circumstances. Anesthesia coding modifiers identify specific circumstances that increase the complexity, intensity, or risk of performing an anesthetic service. The RVG and the American Medical Association (AMA) *Current Procedural Terminology* (CPT) list a number of modifiers that may be reported. The most commonly reported modifiers are those for physical status, extremes of age, and emergencies. Other modifiers describe special procedures that affect the anesthetic, such as controlled hypotension and induced total-body hypothermia.

The RVG recommends specific values for some of these modifiers. For example, the RVG values physical status 1–2 (P1, P2) at 0 units, but awards P3 1 unit, P4 2 units, and P5 3 units.

Some modifiers have highly variable differences in work, and the RVG notes that the value should be determined by "individual consideration" or "I.C." The RVG defines Modifier 22, "Unusual Procedural Services," as "When the service(s) provided are greater than that usually required for the listed procedure, it may be identified by adding modifier '22' to the usual procedure number. A report may also be appropriate. I.C."

Let's assume that you perform an anesthetic for a laparoscopic cholecystectomy. You give the neuromuscular reversal agents and the patient develops profound hypotension and bradycardia, requiring cardiopulmonary resuscitation (which is successful). You could report modifier 22 along with your code for the primary procedure (00790), provide a report documenting the additional and exceptional work, and request additional payment accordingly. This additional payment is the "individual consideration" noted in the RVG. Realistically, many payers refuse to make that additional payment, and even if they do, the claim is often initially denied and paid only on appeal.

Medicare, many Medicaid, and some private payers do not pay for physical status, emergency, extremes of age, or other modifiers listed in the "Qualifying Circumstances" and "Modifiers" sections of the RVG. Be sure to check with your local billing staff to determine payer policies in your area. For payers that do not accept modifiers or qualifying circumstances, the anesthesiologist sees about a 10% lower payment on average. This is an important contractual point to address when negotiating with payers.

So why does the ASA relative value system allow recognition of the anesthesia modifiers and the Medicare system does not? This is a very reasonable and often-asked question. The answer lies in a fundamental difference in philosophy about valuation of physician services. The ASA system historically did not consider patient condition in the determination of base unit values. Physical status and qualifying circumstances were the mechanism to address additional work related to patient condition.

When Medicare implemented the RBRVS in the early 1990s, an underlying principle was that the value for physician work would be based on the "typical patient" undergoing the procedure. With this approach, patient condition was integral to the valuation of the service. At the same time, Medicare, after much pressure from organized anesthesia and with some legislative direction from Congress, implemented the anesthesia payment system alongside RBRVS, basing it on the 1989 ASA *Relative Value Guide*. The ASA saved the "base + time" methodology; however, Medicare disallowed reporting of qualifying circumstances for anesthesia care, using the "typical patient" methodology of the RBRVS as a justification. If surgeons, internists, radiologists, and other physicians could not have their payments adjusted based on medical condition, then neither would the anesthesiologists.

When Medicare implemented the RBRVS and the anesthesia payment system, the anesthesia conversion factor decreased from $20.01 in 1990 to $13.94 in 1992, a 30% drop. This was due to Medicare's attempts to "align" the value of anesthesia services on the same scale as the rest of the RBRVS system. The method used to make that alignment has been lost in the fog of history. What rarely gets mentioned is the cost of the loss of modifiers to anesthesiologists. This may have added an additional 15% or more to the cuts incurred, because elderly patients are more likely to have higher physical status scores and to meet the criteria for extremes of age than the average patient.

MULTIPLE SURGICAL PROCEDURES

When multiple surgical services are performed during a single anesthetic event and no single anesthesia code adequately describes all these services, the anesthesiologist should choose the one anesthetic service from all that apply that has the highest base unit value. Medicare also requires appending the CPT modifier 51 to the anesthesia code to indicate that the anesthesiologist provided anesthesia care for multiple surgical procedures, according to the Medicare Claims Processing Manual, Chapter 12, Section 50 (www.cms.hhs.gov/manuals/downloads/ clm104c12.pdf).

As an example, consider the case of a trauma procedure in which the surgical team performs a craniotomy for subdural hematoma and an exploratory laparotomy with splenectomy. Both the anesthesia code for intracranial procedures (00210) and the code for upper-abdominal intraperitoneal procedures (00790) apply. Because the craniotomy anesthetic has a higher base unit value (11 units) than the intraperitoneal procedure (7 units), the anesthesiologist should report code 00210-51. In addition, the anesthesiologist should also submit the combined anesthetic time for both procedures.

Sometimes the anesthesiologist performs both an anesthetic and one or more other procedures at the same setting. These other procedures may include such things as invasive lines, nerve blocks for postoperative analgesia, or a transesophageal echocardiography study. We have already described the correct methods to report these services in an earlier chapter.

CONVERSION FACTOR

Each anesthesiologist or anesthesia group establishes the dollar value of each unit. The sum of base, time, and modifier units, multiplied by a "conversion factor," produces the amount charged for the anesthetic service.

The anesthesiologist or his group frequently enters into contracts with public and private payers. These contracts usually stipulate a conversion factor that will be used to calculate payments for anesthesia services, and the value of this conversion factor is usually different from and less than the practice's published conversion factor.

Insurance contracts may also list a conversion factor or fee schedule for nonanesthesia services. If the contract includes a second conversion factor, it is typically a conversion factor for the RBRVS payment system described in the next chapter. In a recent AMA survey, >75% of private payers use the

RBRVS system in one or more of their contracts. In my work with the ASA's Committee on Economics, I have learned that a small number of practices have successfully negotiated the use of the ASA assigned base units associated with nonanesthesia services. In these contracts, the base unit values for evaluation and management visits, line placements, pain blocks, etc., are multiplied by the contracted anesthesia conversion factor to determine payments for these services.

210

MEDICARE ISSUES

NORMAN A. COHEN, MD

This chapter reviews the origins and payment methodology of the dominant payment system for most physicians, the Resource-Based Relative Value System or RBRVS. In addition to Medicare and most Medicaid programs, >75% of private payers use the RBRVS in determining payments to physicians. We also consider the steps taken by Congress to control growth in the RBRVS program and the difficult choices faced by anesthesiologists regarding participation in Medicare's payment system for physicians.

HISTORY OF MEDICARE—HOW WE GOT TO THE RBRVS

President Lyndon Johnson signed the legislation creating the Medicare program into law in 1965. In its initial form, the Medicare program included two distinct areas of responsibility: Payment for inpatient hospital care and certain long-term nursing services through Part A, and payment for physician and outpatient services through Part B. The law stipulates separate funding and eligibility requirements for Part A and Part B. Those who individually or through their spouse have contributed more than 40 quarters to FICA (Social Security and Medicare tax) do not pay separately for Part A coverage. Part B, on the other hand, is an optional benefit that requires payment of a monthly premium. In addition to Part A and Part B, Congress more recently created Part C to encompass Medicare managed care ("Medicare Advantage") plans and Part D to provide prescription drug insurance coverage.

From the inception of the Medicare program in 1965 until the early 1990s, the government paid physicians for services to Medicare beneficiaries based on "usual and customary" charges. Then, beginning in the mid-1970s, physician charges began increasing faster than anticipated, leading to the first of many steps to control growth in the program. In 1975 Congress limited increases in physician charges to growth in the Medicare Economic Index (MEI), a calculated value, similar to the Consumer Price Index, that measures growth in the operating expenses facing physicians. The index also includes an offsetting adjustment for economy-wide productivity growth. During the period from 1984 to 1991, Congress determined the maximum allowable growth in charges annually.

During the 1980s, rapid growth in the cost of medical services led to a review of the Medicare payment system. What was abundantly clear to

© 2006 Mayo Foundation for Medical Education and Research

health care policy analysts at the time was that market forces and the use of historical prices had proven ineffective in producing a rational pricing system for physician services. These analysts noted wide geographic variability in the charges for the same services and seemingly no discernible relationship among the time, effort, risk, and incurred costs in providing care and the charges requested for that care.

Several other factors contributed to the sense of urgency that something needed to be done. With improved access to health care for the elderly along with the development of expensive new drugs and technologies, our seniors were beginning to live longer and use more resources than government actuaries had originally estimated. It was also becoming abundantly clear that the "baby boomer" demographic tidal wave was going to create substantial stress on the system. Then, as now, policy pundits, supported by the self-interest of certain segments of the medical community, beat the drum about inadequate payments for primary care as well as the perverse incentives in the payment system that promoted *intervention* rather than *prevention*.

During the 1980s, a team of Harvard researchers led by William C. Hsiao analyzed the components of physician work, making realistic comparisons across all physician services possible for the first time. Hsiao defined physician work as being dependent on the time involved, the mental effort and judgment expended, the physical effort and technical skill required, and the psychologic stress that occurs when an adverse outcome has serious consequences. Through physician surveys, Hsiao determined relative work values and times for a broad array of physician services. Once these key services had values, the researchers then used a number of techniques to assign values to the remaining services, thus creating a comprehensive relative value scale for physician services. In 1988 Hsiao submitted this work to the Health Care Financing Administration (renamed in the early 2000s the Centers for Medicare and Medicaid Services [CMS]). Then, in 1989, Congress passed the Omnibus Reconciliation Act (OBRA89), mandating the transition of Medicare physician payments from the previous charge-based system to Hsiao's resource-based relative value system (RBRVS). The provisions of this law took effect in January 1992, and the RBRVS was born. Along with instituting the RBRVS, OBRA89 also provided for a system to control the growth in Medicare spending, known as Medicare Volume Performance Standards, and limited the ability of a participating physician to bill the patient for the difference between Medicare's payment and the normal physician charge.

HOW RBRVS DETERMINES PAYMENTS AND UNDERSTANDING GLOBAL PERIODS

Medicare assigns each RBRVS service separate relative value units (RVU) for work, practice expense, and professional liability insurance. The Center for Medicare and Medicaid Services (CMS) updates these values annually. Each geographic region has a geographic adjustment factor to correct for variations in local costs from the national average. The sum of the geographically adjusted RVUs, multiplied by the national RBRVS conversion factor, produces the allowed Medicare payment. Medicare beneficiaries are also responsible for a defined percentage of the charge as well as an annual deductible amount that the beneficiary must satisfy before Medicare begins paying. Hsaio's work at Harvard established the spectrum for work RVUs. Initially, Medicare determined practice expense and professional liability RVUs based on historical charges. Later on, both these parts of the RBRVS triad became resource-based.

The RBRVS system classifies procedures into a number of "global periods." Within the global period, the Medicare payment for the service reflects *all* usual services related to the procedure. The global period begins either the day before the procedure for major procedures or the day of the procedure for minor procedures. The global period continues from the day of the procedure and ends after the number of days assigned.

Major procedures have a global period of 90 days (090 global period). Minor procedures have a global period of either 0 (000 global period) or 10 (010 global period) days. For some procedures, the global period does not apply; thus the payment covers only the procedure itself, and the physician can report and have Medicare pay for other services without reduction in payment for multiple procedures or the need to report modifiers to justify these other services. These services have a global period of XXX assigned. For some services, Medicare has determined that they are always reported with another service, and associated services are included in the global payment for the other service. These "add-on" codes have a ZZZ global period. Finally, for a number of services, Medicare does not assign a global period, delegating this responsibility to the regional Medicare carriers. These services have a global period of YYY, and are typically unlisted surgical procedures. *Table 210.1* lists some examples of procedures known to anesthesiologists and the Medicare-assigned global period.

So what does the RBRVS consider to be included in procedures with a global period? Here's the answer:

Preoperative visits—Preoperative visits after the decision is made to operate, beginning with the day before the day of surgery for major procedures and the day of surgery for minor procedures

Intraoperative services—Intraoperative services that are normally a usual and necessary part of a surgical procedure

Complications following surgery—All additional medical or surgical services required of the surgeon during the postoperative period of the surgery because of complications that do not require additional trips to the operating room

TABLE 210.1	EXAMPLES OF PROCEDURES KNOWN TO ANESTHESIOLOGISTS AND THE MEDICARE-ASSIGNED GLOBAL PERIOD	
CODE	**DESCRIPTOR**	**GLOBAL**
47562	Laparoscopic cholecystectomy	090
64416	Brachial plexus block, continuous	010
36620	Arterial line	000
93312	Transesophageal echocardiography, with probe placement, image acquisition, and interpretation	XXX
64484	Trans-foraminal epidural, additional level	ZZZ
27599	Unlisted procedure femur or knee	YYY

Current Procedural Terminology © 2006 American Medical Association.® All Rights Reserved. Applies to all CPT code references in this chapter.

Postoperative visits—Follow-up visits within the postoperative period of the surgery that are related to recovery from the surgery

Postsurgical pain management—By the surgeon

Supplies and miscellaneous services—Items such as dressing changes; local incisional care; removal of operative pack, removal of cutaneous sutures and staples, lines, wires, tubes, drains, casts, and splints; insertion, irrigation, and removal of urinary catheters, routine peripheral intravenous lines, nasogastric and rectal tubes; and changes and removal of tracheostomy tubes.

The anesthesia services, CPT codes 00100 to 001999, function effectively as XXX codes; however, CPT, the ASA, and Medicare have published specific reporting rules that address the elements included in the anesthesia service, reporting of time, and handling of multiple procedures, among other things, as described in other chapters in this section.

HOW THE GOVERNMENT HAS TRIED TO CONTROL MEDICARE GROWTH WHILE PLACATING PHYSICIANS WHEN NECESSARY

The RBRVS has seen several substantial changes since its inception. These include institution of resource-based payments for practice expense in the mid-1990s and resource-based payments for professional liability insurance in the early 2000s. Other changes included moving from separate conversion factors for surgical, medical, and other services to a single conversion factor in 1999, as well as replacement of the Medicare Volume Performance Standards (MVPS) with the Sustainable Growth Rate (SGR) formula in 1998. The MVPS created huge annual swings from negative to positive and back again, making the annual updates highly unpredictable. As mentioned above, the SGR formula replaced the MVPS in 1998. The SGR formula, which ties payment updates to a combination of growth in the national economy and comparison of Medicare expenditures to defined allowable targets, initially produced positive updates during the economic boom of the late 1990s; however, the slowing of the economy and other factors described below have produced negative updates since the early 2000s. Congress has acted several times to stay the pain by giving physicians positive updates for a year or two at a time, but the cumulative SGR tab has continued to grow. At the end of 2006 that deficit was approximately $140 billion, and the Medicare program as a whole was looking at cuts in the conversion factor of -5%/year until 2015 and beyond. Despite calls from many organizations, including the AMA, specialty societies, and even MedPAC (the independent commission that advises Congress about Medicare payment adequacy), the ever-increasing budgetary cost of fixing the SGR formula has resulted in Congressional inaction in dealing with the core of the problem.

Ironically, the growth in Medicare spending that is leading to the negative SGR annual updates has little to do with increases in anesthesia or surgical care volume. Most of the growth has occurred in pharmaceuticals administered in the physician's office (primarily chemotherapy drugs), imaging services, level and volume of evaluation and management services, and the transfer of services previously provided in the hospital and now provided in the outpatient setting or the office. Believe it or not, facility fees for ambulatory surgery centers and hospital outpatient departments come from the Medicare Part B "physician" pool. Also, physicians, both radiologists and others, have opened office-based imaging facilities with magnetic resonance imaging, computed tomography, and other expensive services now being paid out of Part B funds. In combination, all these factors have led to explosive growth in Medicare Part B expenditures that automatically result in SGR cuts. In a stereotypical "Catch-22," the specialties having the least to do with growth in the SGR are paying the greatest cost in terms of reduced payments from Medicare.

MEDICARE PAYMENTS ARE TERRIBLE. MUST I PARTICIPATE IN MEDICARE?

In my role as chair of the ASA Committee on Economics, ASA members frequently ask me the following questions:

> "Will Medicare fix our payments only if there is an access problem to anesthesia services?"
>
> "Can I drop out of Medicare?"
>
> "What are the repercussions of doing so?"

Although the questions I receive usually focus on anesthesiologists' participation in Medicare, the answers to these questions apply to all physicians and health care professionals who are paid under Part B of the Medicare program. The answer to the first question is most definitely "yes"; however, as we will soon see, getting to a critical-access problem is particularly difficult for our specialty. Defining access adequacy is challenging. To demonstrate payment inadequacy, the question that government analysts must answer is whether payment rates are so low that Medicare beneficiaries are less likely than other insured patients to get elective or urgent services in a timely fashion. To answer this question, these analysts look at a number of factors, including the rate of provider participation, whether physicians are accepting new Medicare patients, and whether Medicare patients have the same ready accessibility to certain key services as does the general public. Although there has been much talk about an "access crisis" every time Medicare threatens to cut physician payments, the reality has been that beneficiary access has not suffered so far, at least using the measures just described.

To answer the last two questions, one must understand what contracting with Medicare means. Essentially, a contracting physician has three options: Be a participating provider, be a nonparticipating provider, and "opt out" of the program entirely. I will describe the definitions of these terms and some of the implications of choosing one designation or another. Once one has this background, then one can make the personal and often challenging choice regarding Medicare contracting status.

In agreeing to be "participating providers" in the Medicare program, physicians must limit their charge to the Medicare-allowed amount. In return, Medicare agrees to pay the physician directly for Medicare's share of the service, and the allowed payment is 5% more than that provided for a nonparticipating physician. Nonparticipating physicians have the option to charge slightly more than the Medicare-allowed amount; however, those nonparticipating physicians need to collect their full payment from the patient, because Medicare pays the patient directly when the provider is nonparticipating.

The choice to throw in the towel completely and "opt out" of the Medicare program is exceptionally difficult. Once physicians make this choice, Medicare requires the physicians to enter into private payment contracts with their Medicare-eligible patients; however, these physicians must notify Medicare when they first enter into such a contract, and the Agency prohibits the physicians from billing Medicare for **any** Medicare services performed for a period of 2 years from the initiation of that first contract. To be crystal clear, if one opts out of Medicare and provides any Medicare-covered service to a Medicare beneficiary, then one *must* enter into a private-payer contract. Medicare does make an exception for emergency treatment of a patient who does not have a private contract with the physician. By opting out of Medicare, the physician also agrees not to participate in Medicare Advantage plans in addition to fee-for-service Part B

Medicare. Full details of the provisions for an "opt-out" can be found at www.cms.hhs.gov/manuals/downloads/bp102c15.pdf.

For hospital-based physicians such as anesthesiologists, the "opt-out" option is particularly onerous for several reasons. The lack of an ongoing doctor–patient relationship makes the patient very unlikely to enter into a private payment agreement with an anesthesiologist. Thus, receiving any payment at all for the care provided becomes extremely unlikely for members of our specialty. Imagine the process of requiring every Medicare patient to sign a private contract with you before surgery. Your entreaties will probably be met with confusion, disbelief, and possibly outright anger. Rightly or wrongly, these patients believe that they are *entitled* to receive your care and that you are *obligated* to participate in Medicare. Also, anesthesiologists who work at hospitals often do so under a contractual arrangement. In these situations, hospitals typically mandate in the contract that the anesthesiologist be enrolled in the Medicare program.

So, unlike our primary care colleagues, who can set up boutique, non-Medicare practices, the opt-out "option" is, for most anesthesiologists, not an option at all. And because opt-out is not a realistic option for our specialty, critical access shortages for anesthesia services are unlikely to occur. Access levels for medical and surgical services will likely become critical long before that occurs for anesthesia care.

211

WHAT ARE THE CODING RESOURCES TO HELP ME CODE CORRECTLY?

NORMAN A. COHEN, MD

Because correct coding leads to proper payment, and incorrect coding can be *very* expensive, a plethora of coding resources from many sources are available to physicians. This chapter describes the basic resources that I think every anesthesiologist should have available to code correctly:

- Current-year Current Procedural Terminology (CPT) Standard Edition
- Current-year American Society of Anesthesiologists (ASA) Relative Value Guide
- Current-year ASA Crosswalk

In addition, I also describe a few other resources that can be very helpful in addressing more complex coding needs.

AMA CURRENT PROCEDURAL TERMINOLOGY (CPT)*

The American Medical Association (AMA) publishes two versions of the annual CPT manual, a standard edition and a more detailed professional edition. In addition, the AMA also publishes a number of periodicals to provide correct coding advice *(CPT Assistant)* and updates on changes in the CPT *(CPT Changes)*. The AMA also offers electronic versions of CPT and its family of publications, including the excellent *Code Manager*. I refer any reader interested in procedural coding (and most anesthesiologists should be) to the AMA website (www.ama-assn.org/ama/pub/category/3113.html) for information on purchasing AMA coding resources.

At a minimum, I believe that every anesthesiologist should have a copy of the *CPT Standard Edition* for the current year. Personally, I prefer the *CPT Professional Edition*, as it includes a number of additional features, such as anatomic and procedural illustrations, and coding rules and guidelines. The cost for either is fairly reasonable, and with an AMA membership, the purchaser receives a substantial discount. You are a member of the AMA, aren't you?

CPT undergoes many changes every year, so using an out-of-date copy can easily lead to coding errors. *Always use coding products that are up to date!*

---

*Current Procedural Terminology © 2006 American Medical Association.® All Rights Reserved. Applies to all CPT code references in this chapter.

© 2006 Mayo Foundation for Medical Education and Research

For those who want to go beyond the basics, I strongly recommend *Code Manager,* an electronic resource that includes CPT, International Classification of Diseases (ICD)-9, Medicare Diagnosis Related Groups (DRG's), Healthcare Common Procedure Coding System (HCPCS) codes, and more. A subscription to *CPT Assistant* is invaluable. An archive of previous *CPT Assistant* articles is also available for purchase in electronic form, and this archive can be referenced from *Code Manager* or as a stand-alone product. The *CPT Professional Edition* includes all references to *CPT Assistant* articles for every code. All of these products and more are available from the web address cited above.

THE ASA RELATIVE VALUE GUIDE

The chapters on procedure coding and the anesthesia payment system made mention of the American Society of Anesthesiologists (ASA) *Relative Value Guide* or RVG. The RVG is a product of the ASA's Committee on Economics. Having served on this committee for 10 years both as a member and currently as its chair, I can vouch for the substantial efforts made by the committee and ASA staff to assure that the RVG is both a valuable resource and as accurate as humanly possible.

The ASA publishes the RVG annually in both printed and electronic forms. The RVG includes a definition of terms, a listing of the CPT anesthesia codes, and the ASA's recommended base unit values, a number of nonanesthesia CPT codes for procedures commonly performed by anesthesiologists with anesthesia base unit value recommendations, a number of ASA-approved position and guideline statements, and a summary of ICD-9 headers for assistance in diagnosis coding. The RVG also provides some additional coding guidance that supplements that available from CPT.

The printed version of the RVG is a bargain, currently priced at $15 for ASA members and $25 for nonmembers. Although I strongly recommend that anesthesiologists have a copy of CPT as well, many anesthesiologists use the RVG as their sole coding resource. You can order a copy of the RVG directly from the ASA through the "Publications and Services" link at the ASA website (http://asahq.org).

Like CPT, the RVG changes every year. We add new codes, revise existing codes and even delete codes. Our coding comments also change over time, as does the ASA's positions and guidelines included in the RVG. For these reasons, using the current-year RVG is a necessary requirement for correct coding of anesthesia services.

ASA CROSSWALK

First published in 1995 and updated annually thereafter, the *ASA Crosswalk* has become *the* standard in associating surgical CPT codes to the most correct anesthesia code or codes. The brainchild of Stanley Stead, M.D., M.B.A., the Crosswalk systematically lists a primary anesthesia code as well as possible alternative codes that best describe the anesthesia care for each diagnostic or therapeutic procedure that may have an associated anesthetic. Dr. Stead has served as the Crosswalk's editor since its inception. Each year, he convenes the Crosswalk Editorial Panel, who, together, create anesthesia crosses for new codes, review and alter as necessary the crosses for revised codes, review suggestions referred to the ASA from users of the Crosswalk, and periodically review all CPT codes for Crosswalk accuracy. I have had the pleasure of serving on the Editorial Panel with Dr. Stead for several years. Although the work of reviewing thousands of codes is exceptionally tedious, mind-numbing, and time-consuming, the end product is an exceptionally valuable resource to the specialty, making the effort most worthwhile.

To get an understanding of the value of the Crosswalk, let's consider an example. Your surgeon has performed a thoracotomy and left lower lobe resection. The anesthetic care involved one-lung ventilation. Your question is, "What's the most accurate code to describe the anesthesia service?"

The surgical CPT code for this procedure is 32480. Looking up 32480 in the 2007 Crosswalk reveals that anesthesia code 00541 is the primary cross and 00540 and 00548 are the alternative crosses. Code 00541 (15 base units) describes anesthesia for intrathoracic procedures utilizing one-lung ventilation, code 00540 (12 base units) describes the same thing without one-lung ventilation, and code 00548 (17 base units) describes anesthesia for procedures on the trachea and bronchi (excluding reconstruction). The Crosswalk also lists two coding comments. The first reminds the user to take into account whether the anesthetic utilized one-lung ventilation, and the second notes that the physician should report code 00548 only when the surgeon reports CPT add-on code 32501. This add-on code indicates performance of a bronchoplasty. For this case, the anesthesiologist should report code 00541, because the surgeon did not perform a bronchoplasty and the patient received one-lung ventilation as part of the anesthetic. Repeat this process for over 6,000 codes, and you get a flavor of the Crosswalk's value.

Although the Crosswalk is a terrific reference, it is not a stand-alone product, the ASA intends for the Crosswalk to be used hand-in-hand with both the RVG and CPT. Because the Crosswalk includes material from both CPT and the RVG, both of which change annually, the Crosswalk changes significantly every year as well. Again, use of the most current version of any of these publications is essential. As with the RVG, one may order the Crosswalk in either electronic or book form directly from the ASA (http://asahq.org).

212

NAVIGATING A HAZARDOUS ROAD

NORMAN A. COHEN, MD

GETTING PAID FOR ANESTHESIA CARE BY MEDICARE

In previous chapters I mentioned a number of ways in which the Medicare program handles anesthesia differently from many other payers. For example, Medicare does not allow for payment of anesthesia modifiers, such as physical status or extremes of age. Medicare insures a substantial percentage of patients for most anesthesia practices, usually between 25% and 50%; therefore, understanding this payer well is essential to good practice management.

In the following discussion, we will look more deeply into Medicare payments for anesthesia care under the Resource-Based Relative Value System (RBRVS), the Correct Coding Initiative edit process, and a number of important Medicare payment policies.

PAYMENT FOR ANESTHESIA

Medicare pays for anesthesia services under the American Medical Association (AMA) *Current Procedural Terminology* (CPT)* codes 00100 to 01999, using a version of the anesthesia base + time system described previously. Medicare maintains a list of base unit values for each anesthesia service. This list is similar but not identical to the American Society of Anesthesiologists (ASA) listing of base unit values. To determine time units, Medicare uses the actual anesthesia time to the nearest minute divided by 15 minutes per unit. Medicare adds base and the calculated time units together and multiplies the total by the conversion factor to determine the allowed payment amount.

For example, a Medicare beneficiary undergoes a total hip replacement (CPT 01214, 8 base units) lasting 124 minutes. This makes the time units equal to 124/15 = 8.3 and the total units for the case 8 + 8.3 = 16.3. The allowed payment for the service is then $17.77 × 16.3 = $289.65 (in 2006).

Medicare publishes a national conversion factor, but federal law mandates that the agency adjust payments geographically for all Part B services (not just anesthesia) to reflect the regional cost variation for payroll, equipment, supplies, etc. Medicare calculates geographic practice cost indices (GPCI) for work, practice expense, and professional liability

---

Current Procedural Terminology © 2006 American Medical Association.® All Rights Reserved. Applies to all CPT code references in this chapter.

© 2006 Mayo Foundation for Medical Education and Research

insurance for each defined region. Medicare listed 91 specific geographic regions in 2006, and 93 in 2007. For example, in Oregon, where I practice, Medicare lists two regions—Portland, and the rest of Oregon. So Portland ($17.07/unit) ends up having a different anesthesia conversion factor than the rest of the state ($16.73), because the two areas have different GPCI values. Each year, the ASA posts the GPCI-adjusted conversion factors on the ASA website. For 2006, one can find the posting at www.asahq.org/Washington/2006AnesCFREVISED.pdf.

ANESTHESIA CONVERSION FACTOR

Each year since the inception of the RBRVS, Medicare has updated both the anesthesia and the RBRVS conversion factors. When setting the initial conversion factor, Medicare used some of the Harvard RBRVS research data (see previous chapter) to link the work of anesthesia work to the work of other medical services. The Centers for Medicare and Medicaid Services (CMS) also used historical charge data to set the value of the practice expense and professional liability insurance (PLI) components for anesthesia payments. The ASA has long disagreed with Medicare's initial method of setting the anesthesia work relationship, and was successful in getting a large update with the first and a very small update in the second Five Year Review of physician work. The ASA is still fighting this battle at the time of this writing.

A number of factors have played a role in influencing the annual updates. We have previously learned about the tools Congress has mandated to rein in growth in the Medicare program. Unless Congress stipulates otherwise, Medicare must apply the sustainable growth rate formula (SGR) as part of the annual update. For the past several years, the SGR update would have reduced the conversion factor by >4% a year; however, Congress has acted several times to delay those cuts. Unfortunately, Congress has not yet acted to replace the SGR with something better.

Other factors that have affected the conversion factor updates are required budget neutrality adjustments and significant changes in the practice expense and professional liability insurance methodologies. With only a few exceptions, whenever a change in payment for services exceeds $20 million, Medicare must apply a budget neutrality adjustment. The Five Year Reviews of physician work and some changes in new and revised codes have exceeded this threshold, resulting in budget neutrality adjustments. After the first Five Year Review, the budget neutrality adjustment led to >5% decrease in the conversion factors. For all intents and purposes, the Part B payment pool is of fixed size, so changes in work, practice expense (PE) and Professional Liability Insurance (PLI) values lead just to a redistribution of the pool, not any overall increase.

Because some updates apply only to a single component of the RBRVS (work, PE, and PLI) and because an anesthesia service handles these components through the conversion factor and not through procedure-specific values, Medicare has applied these sorts of updates to the relevant "share" of the conversion factor. The next section describes this share concept in greater detail.

WORK, PRACTICE EXPENSE, AND PROFESSIONAL LIABILITY INSURANCE SHARES

In the section on RBRVS, we learned that each (nonanesthesia) service in that payment system has values assigned for work, PE, and PLI. The RBRVS codes also may have different values depending on where the physician performs the service.

The Medicare anesthesia payment system does not use fixed procedure-specific values; however, the law requires Medicare to consider the values for these three components in physician payments. To address this requirement, Medicare allocates anesthesia work, PE, and PLI through "shares" of the conversion factor. In 2006, the national average Medicare anesthesia conversion factor was $17.77/unit, and work comprised 78%, PE 13%, and PLI 9% of each anesthesia relative value unit. In dollar terms, that means that, in the Medicare program, each anesthesia unit equals $13.86 for work, $2.31 for PE, and $1.60 for PLI.

In the RBRVS, payments often differ depending on where the service takes place. Medicare has the option to assign different PE values for a service performed in the hospital and the office. Unfortunately, in anesthesia care, payments are the same for hospital and office-based anesthesia care, and that value is always at the hospital (facility) rate. Because the anesthesia payment system uses a global expression of practice expense through the PE share of the conversion factor, there is no simple way for Medicare to allocate the expenses of office-based anesthesia care accurately. So Medicare doesn't! At the time of this writing, ASA has begun to explore methods to fix this problem and hopefully will have a solution in place in the next year or two.

CMS RESOURCES

The CMS maintains a comprehensive website that provides a great deal of information about the Medicare program. The CMS also hosts an anesthesia-specific page with links to very useful information: www.cms.hhs.gov/center/anesth.asp. This page also includes links to the Medicare Learning Network, a repository of articles explaining many aspects of the program, and to local carrier websites. Medicare also hosts a number of email subscription lists that provide periodic updates documenting program changes.

The Medicare contractors that process Medicare claims for various regions within the United States also host websites to provide carrier-specific information. These are the places to go to learn about Local Carrier Determinations (LCD), which are policies describing coverage requirements. We will talk more about LCDs later.

For physicians who are new to practice, I highly recommend requesting a copy of the *Medicare Physician Guide: A Resource for Residents, Practicing Physicians, and Other Health Care Professionals.* You can order this from the Medicare site (http://cms.meridianksi.com/kc/main/kc_frame.asp?kc_ident=kc0001&loc=5) in either a printed or CD-ROM form. Medicare does not charge for this document. You should receive a copy within a few weeks after ordering it.

GETTING PAID BY MEDICARE FOR RBRVS SERVICES

When anesthesiologists perform any covered nonanesthesia service for a Medicare beneficiary, the agency makes most payments using the RBRVS system. The formula requires knowing the national RBRVS conversion factor; your regional work, PE, and PLI GPCIs; and the work, PE, and PLI RVUs for the service. The formula is

$$CF \times (RVUw \times GPCIw + RVUpe \times GPCIpe + RVUpli \times GPCIpli)$$

where

CF = national CF

RVUw, RVUpe, RVUpli = work, practice expense, and pli RVUs for the specific service

GPCIw, GPCIpe, GPCIpli = the locale-specific geographic practice cost indices

Medicare publishes these values each year and provides an online tool to look up the relevant information at www.cms.hhs.gov/apps/pfslookup/step1.asp.

Beginning in 2007, the CMS, over the objection of almost all physicians, decided to address the budget neutrality changes from the third Five Year Review through a "budget neutrality adjustor" applied to the work component only, rather than making an adjustment to the RBRVS conversion factor; therefore the formula listed above has changed slightly, to

$$CF \times (RVUw \times GPCIw \times BNA + RVUpe \times GPCIpe + RVUpli \times GPCIpli)$$

where BNA is the budget neutrality adjustor.

For 2007, the BNA will be 0.8994 based on published information available in the 2007 fee schedule final rule (www.cms.hhs.gov/apps/ama/license.asp?file=/physicianfeesched/downloads/1321-fc.pdf), published in November 2006. I can guarantee that reading Medicare proposed and final rule publications will make you a more rested person, because these publications are terrific soporifics.

UNDERSTANDING THE NATIONAL CORRECT CODING INITIATIVE

Quoting Medicare's description of the National Correct Coding Initiative (hereafter referred to as CCI), the purpose of the CCI program is to "promote national correct coding methodologies and to control improper coding leading to inappropriate payment in Part B claims." Furthermore, "the purpose of the CCI edits is to ensure the most comprehensive groups of codes are billed rather than the component parts. Additionally, CCI edits check for mutually exclusive code pairs. These edits were implemented to ensure that only appropriate codes are grouped and priced" (www.cms.hhs.gov/NationalCorrectCodInitEd).

We have already discussed the concept of the global period for RBRVS services. The global concept implies that a given service may encompass a combination of other services. For example, the full diagnostic transesophageal echocardiography (TEE) service code 93312, which we discussed previously, includes the services in code 93313 (probe placement) and code 93314 (image acquisition, interpretation, and report). CCI edits prevent the same physician from reporting code 93312 with either code 93313 or 93314 on the same day.

Medicare considers a number of CPT services to be integral to the anesthesia care. Examples include but are not limited to placement of an intravenous catheter (36000), venipuncture (36410), and intravenous infusion/injection (90760 to 90768, 90774 to 90775). In the rare circumstance that the anesthesiologist performs these services on the same day, but not as part of the anesthetic, he or she can report these services with modifier 59, indicating a "distinct procedural service." For example, you care for a patient with a history of drug abuse and poor vascular access. After the patient returns to the floor from the PACU, you get a call that the patient's intravenous (IV) catheter has infiltrated and your expertise is needed to restart the IV. You do so and report the service (36000) with modifier 59. You should document in the medical record the placement of the catheter, with date and time of placement, which will support that the service occurred after the conclusion of the anesthetic.

On occasion, a physician may perform two or more services that in combination are subject to a CCI edit. If relevant CPT modifiers apply, then the physician may report the service with the appropriate modifier in order to justify separate payment. Let's consider an example relevant to anesthesiologists. Suppose that you receive a request to consult on a trauma patient for pain management. You perform, document, and prepare a report for an inpatient consultation, making recommendations on options available to the trauma team. Later that day, the patient presents for emergency surgery, you are the anesthesiologist on the hook, and you perform the anesthetic. Normally, CCI edits prevent the same physician from reporting an evaluation-and-management (E/M) service, with the exception of critical care services, on the same day as an anesthetic. The reason for this edit is to prevent reporting of the routine preoperative anesthesia assessment as an E/M visit. However, in this example, the E/M visit bore no relationship to the anesthesia care. To indicate that CMS should pay for the E/M service and override the standard edit, the anesthesiologist can append modifier 25 to the E/M service, which indicates a "significant, separately identifiable evaluation and management service by the same physician on the same day of the procedure or other service." Because the documentation supports that the consultation was not a preoperative assessment, CMS should pay for both the anesthesia care and the E/M visit.

For more information on the National Correct Coding Initiative, see the NCCI manual, available at www.cms.hhs.gov/NationalCorrectCodInitEd/Downloads/manual.zip. This series of documents provides the same exceptionally detailed information available to Medicare carriers regarding use of CCI edits. The ASA currently has a representative who helps advise the NCCI contractor on code edits of interest to anesthesiologists. Before Medicare opened this process to medical specialty and public comment, carriers used "black box" edits without publishing the actual logic employed. Unsurprisingly, these edits were often clinically incomprehensible to those in practice, with most physicians considering the whole affair to be an example of "big brother" government at its worst. After extensive efforts by organized medicine, the CMS developed the current process. With the move to a more transparent system, the level of public furor over the use of edits has diminished dramatically.

UNDERSTANDING MEDICARE CLAIMS MODIFIERS

Medicare has established a number of policies that directly affect the delivery of anesthesia care to patients. Although the following discussion is in no way comprehensive, it will introduce you to a number of important Medicare reporting requirements. We will discuss medical direction, medical supervision, the anesthesia teaching rule, an overview of Medicare local and national medical necessity policies, and upcoming changes in Medicare carrier contracting.

Medicare and Anesthesia Delivery. Anesthesiologists can provide anesthesia care in a number of ways. An anesthesiologist can either personally perform the entire anesthetic, work as part of an anesthesia care team with nurse anesthetists or anesthesiology assistants, or teach anesthesiology residents. Nurse anesthetists may either work under the medical supervision of another physician, usually a surgeon, or in some states can practice independently without physician oversight. Let's take a look at some Medicare requirements for these modes of practice. For complete and detailed information, refer to Chapter 12, Section 50, of the *Medicare Claims Processing Manual* (MCPM) (www.cms.hhs.gov/manuals/downloads/clm104c12.pdf). Medicare has a number of specific claims modifiers that one reports, depending on the mode of anesthesia delivery:

AA—Anesthesia services performed personally by the anesthesiologist

AD—Medical supervision by a physician; more than four concurrent anesthesia procedures

G8—Monitored anesthesia care (MAC) for deep, complex, complicated, or markedly invasive surgical procedures

G9—Monitored anesthesia care for a patient who has a history of a severe cardiopulmonary condition

QK—Medical direction of two, three, or four concurrent anesthesia procedures involving qualified individuals

QS—Monitored anesthesia care service

QX—Certified Registered Nurse Anesthetist (CRNA) service; with medical direction by a physician

QY—Medical direction of one CRNS by an anesthesiologist

QZ—CRNA service: without medical direction by a physician

Personally Performed Anesthesia. When an anesthesiologist personally delivers an anesthetic, reporting of the service to Medicare is fairly straightforward. The physician reports the appropriate anesthesia code and includes the Medicare claims modifier "AA," which indicates that the anesthesiologist personally performed the anesthetic.

Besides personal administration of an anesthetic, an anesthetic service can qualify as personally performed when the physician is teaching a single resident, is involved in no other case concurrently, and qualifies as a *teaching physician* (as defined in Chapter 12, Section 100, of the *Medicare Claims Processing Manual*). A similar policy applies when the anesthesiologist is continuously involved in a single case with a student nurse anesthetist.

On rare occasions, the services of both an anesthesiologist and a CRNA or anesthesiology assistant (AA) may be medically necessary, provided that no other concurrent care for other patients occurs. A trauma patient suffering hemorrhagic shock and requiring massive transfusion is an example of a situation when two sets of anesthesia hands are medically necessary. In this situation, both the anesthesiologist and the CRNA or AA would submit claims. The anesthesiologist would report the anesthesia code with the AA modifier and the anesthetist would report the code with the QZ modifier. Medicare requires that both providers submit supporting documentation with the claim. For all other situations involving a single case with both an anesthesiologist and a CRNA or AA, see the medical direction rules below.

Medical Direction. Anesthesia medical direction refers to concurrent care when an anesthesiologist directs two, three, or four qualified personnel (CRNA or AA) and performs certain mandated activities:

Performs a preanesthetic examination and evaluation

Prescribes the anesthesia plan

Personally participates in the most demanding procedures in the anesthesia plan, including induction and emergence

Ensures that any procedures in the anesthesia plan that he or she does not perform are performed by a qualified anesthetist

Monitors the course of anesthesia administration at frequent intervals

Remains physically present and available for immediate diagnosis and treatment of emergencies

Provides indicated postanesthesia care

According to the MCPM, the medically directing anesthesiologist:

> Must participate only in the most demanding procedures of the anesthesia plan, including, if applicable, induction and emergence. Also for medical direction services furnished on or after January 1, 1999, the physician must document in the medical record that he or she performed the pre-anesthetic examination and evaluation. Physicians must also document that they provided indicated postanesthesia care, were present during some portion of the anesthesia monitoring, and were present during the most demanding procedures, including induction and emergence, where indicated.

Medicare has stipulated that the medically directing anesthesiologist can provide several services while still qualifying for medical direction. These include attending to an emergency of short duration in the immediate area, administering labor analgesia, periodic but not continuous monitoring of a labor patient, receive a patient in preoperative holding, attend to or discharge patients from the PACU, or handle scheduling matters. Some Medicare carriers have also provided further clarification of allowable activities that can occur during medical direction. In 1999, Georgia's carrier published a series of "Questions and Answers," available at www.cahabagba.com/part_b/education_and_outreach/newsletters/georgia/ 1999/nov99/nov99pg12.htm, about medical direction, which other carriers have since adopted. In the discussion of Medicare medical necessity policies, we will discuss ways to determine your carrier's policies on this and other issues.

Regarding pre- and postanesthesia visits, the CMS has clarified that a different physician in the same group can perform the preanesthesia visit. Also, any qualified anesthesia provider (CRNA, AA, resident, or anesthesiologist) in the group can perform the postoperative visit.

Concurrency is an important issue that anesthesiologists must understand if they are involved in medical direction. We previously covered the definition of anesthesia time, when we discussed the base-plus-time payment system for anesthesia services. If two cases overlap by even a minute in reportable anesthesia time, then the concurrency for medical direction purposes is 2. In fact, if the end time of one case and the beginning of the next are exactly the same time, Medicare considers these cases to overlap, making the concurrency 2. For any specific case, the maximum number of overlapping cases determines the concurrency. So, if at some point during the case you had medical direction responsibilities for four cases total, even if only for a minute or two, your concurrency is 4. One calculates concurrency independently for each case, with the maximum number of cases directed during that case determining the total concurrency. Also, one does not consider the insurance status of the patients in calculating concurrency.

Money, as is true with so many things, is the reason that concurrency is so important. For medically directed cases, Medicare pays the physician 50% of the allowable fee and the nurse anesthetist/AA 50% of the fee. The total payment is the same as if the anesthesiologist personally performed the case. If, at any point while medically directing, the concurrency level reaches five or more cases, then all overlapping cases at that point become *medically supervised* cases, with payment to the anesthesiologist at the much lower supervised rate as discussed below. This dramatically reduces payments to the physician in situations in which the anesthesiologist does not bill for the anesthetists, such as occurs when the hospital employs the CRNA or AA. For groups that commonly direct four anesthetists at the same time, errors in reporting start and end times can lead to a concurrency level >4. Even worse, if the times on the anesthesia record demonstrate concurrency >4, the times on the billing slip do not, and the billing clerks did not catch the error, then the group may have filed incorrect claims for medical direction, when medical supervision was the service provided. If caught on an audit, this can turn into a costly event, as Medicare may consider this a fraudulent or abusive claim. Such a finding may have civil or criminal penalties.

When you medically direct two, three, or four concurrent cases, you report the appropriate anesthesia code with the QK claims modifier and each anesthetist reports his or her services with the anesthesia code and the QX modifier. In the event you medically direct one anesthetist, you report your service with the QK modifier and the anesthetist reports his or her service with the QY modifier.

If you do not meet the criteria for medical direction, you should report your service as *medical supervision*, using the AD modifier for the physician service and the QZ modifier for the anesthetist's services.

Medical Supervision. When concurrency exceeds four cases or the anesthesiologist does not accomplish the required elements of medical direction, the anesthesiologist must report his or her role in the case as medical supervision, using the "AD" claim modifier. Nurse anesthetists report the case with the QZ modifier.

In terms of payment, the nurse anesthetist is eligible to receive 100% of the allowed charge (less any co-pay or deductible). The anesthesiologist can receive payment equal to 3 units, plus one additional time unit if the documentation supports the anesthesiologist's presence at induction.

Independent and Medically Supervised Anesthetists. If a physician supervises a nurse anesthetist or, in states allowing independent practice of anesthesia by nurses, a nurse anesthetist works unsupervised, the nurse anesthetist reports the QZ modifier with the anesthesia claim. A number of states allow anesthesia assistants to provide anesthesia care; however, unlike nurse anesthetists, no states allow an anesthesia assistant to work without supervision by a physician. In cases in which the supervising physician does not meet medical direction criteria, the AA reports the claim with a QZ modifier and the physician reports the AD modifier.

Monitored Anesthesia Care. Once upon a time, in the dark ages of anesthesia (around the time I began training), there was an anesthesia service known as "local standby." In these cases, the anesthesiologist provided monitoring and sedation services for minimally invasive procedures, while being prepared to convert to general anesthesia. The Healthcare Financing Administration (HCFA), the predecessor of the CMS, decided in the 1980s that it would pay for anesthesia standby services; however, many other payers created barriers to payment for local standby care. In 1986 the ASA introduced the term "monitored anesthesia care," usually referred to as MAC, to help differentiate other physician standby services from an anesthesia service not associated with a general or regional anesthetic. For more information on the history and current status of MAC, see the 2004 article in the *ASA Newsletter* that I co-authored with my predecessor as chair of the Committee on Economics, Dr. James McMichaels, available at www.asahq.org/Newsletters/2004/06_04/whatsNew06_04.html.

Although Medicare will pay for a *medically necessary* MAC service, the agency does require that those providing MAC report claims modifier QS with the anesthesia code. Because Medicare pays only for medically necessary services, whether performed by an anesthesiologist or not, and because the agency and its carrier contractors have concern that not all MAC services are, in fact, necessary, many carriers have published *local carrier determinations*

(LCDs), which define combinations of services and patient conditions (often expressed as a list of ICD-9-CM codes) that support medical necessity for MAC. In fact, Medicare has published two claims modifiers that a number of carriers use in their LCDs to support the need for MAC anesthesia:

G8—Monitored anesthesia care (MAC) for deep, complex, complicated, or markedly invasive surgical procedures

G9—Monitored anesthesia care for a patient who has a history of a severe cardiopulmonary condition

Since each carrier that has issued an LCD on MAC differs significantly in the details of the policy's implementation, you can search at the CMS website (www.cms.hhs.gov/mcd/search.asp?clickon=search&) for policies that are currently in effect. If you need to contact your carrier directly, you can download a list of contact numbers and websites as a Microsoft Excel file from www.cms.hhs.gov/MLNProducts/downloads/CallCenterTollNumDirectory.zip.

As an example of a MAC LCD, the interested reader can view the Noridian MAC policy. Noridian covers about 12 Western states. The Noridian MAC policy for my state, Oregon, can be found here at www.cms.hhs.gov/mcd/viewlcd.asp?lcd_id=14947&lcd_version=14&basket=lcd%3A14947%3A14%3AMonitored+Anesthesia+Care+%28MAC%29%3ACarrier%3ANoridian+Administrative+Services%7C%7C+LLC+%2800821%29.

Anesthesia Teaching Rule. The federal government has identified the need to financially support medical education as a societal goal. Through direct and indirect graduate medical education payments, institutions that provide training of physicians in residency programs receive compensation for the expenses incurred. Physicians involved in teaching residents must meet certain requirements; however, in return, Medicare often allows the teaching physician to care for more than one patient at a time, while still receiving full payment for each service. For example, surgeons may participate in two overlapping cases, provided that the surgeon is available for the *key and critical portions* of each procedure, *as determined by the teaching surgeon.* For E/M visits, a single physician can teach up to four residents concurrently, provided that the teaching physician is present for and documents involvement in the self-defined *key and critical portions* of the service. In certain circumstances, when a primary care facility has received an exception from the CMS, residents can perform certain low-level procedures (CPT codes 99201 to 99203 and 99211 to 99213) and the teaching physician can submit claims for those services without even being present!

Unfortunately for anesthesia training programs, Medicare has singled out teaching anesthesiologists for special treatment since 1994, and this has not been a good thing for the specialty. Unlike surgeons or medical specialists, who receive full payment for concurrent care, teaching anesthesiologists receive full payment only if they teach one-on-one and have no overlapping case responsibilities. If an anesthesiologist oversees two concurrent cases, with either or both being resident cases, Medicare instructs the teaching physician to treat both cases as medically directed; however, unlike for CRNAs or AAs, Medicare pays only 50% of the allowed charge for the teaching physician and pays nothing for the resident for concurrent teaching cases.

Given that teaching hospitals often care for a disproportionate share of Medicare beneficiaries, this payment policy has created a significant and increasing financial hardship. The situation has become worse because of both Medicare's very low anesthesia payment rates and the failure of those rates to keep pace with inflation. Surveys of academic anesthesia departments demonstrate that the teaching payment policy alone costs the average department >$400,000 a year, and costs some programs as much as $1 million/year. The ASA has fought this Medicare policy both with the CMS and most recently before Congress itself. Although this effort has not yet been successful yet, fixing the teaching rule is currently the number-one legislative priority for the ASA.

UNDERSTANDING THE DIFFERENCE BETWEEN NATIONAL AND CARRIER POLICIES

The law covering Medicare gives the CMS Administrator fairly broad discretion to implement Congressional action through the regulatory process. The Administrator can authorize a National Coverage Determination (NCD), which can alter national Medicare policy. All Medicare carriers need to follow these NCDs. As an example of an NCD, Congress authorized the CMS to develop a screening benefit for abdominal aortic aneurysm as part of the Deficit Reduction Act of 2005. In August 2006, Dr. Mark McClellan, the CMS Administrator at the time, announced implementation of this new benefit effective in 2007. As part of the administrator's power to interpret legislation through regulation, Dr. McClellan limited coverage to at-risk individuals (positive family history, men 65 to 75 years old with a history of smoking, or other patients with risk factors determined by an independent agency). Congressional legislation instructed the CMS to provide this benefit; the CMS determined how to implement this legislation through a National Coverage Determination.

In actual practice, the CMS rarely introduces NCDs, deferring to the carriers to make policy determinations that make sense for local circumstances. Such a carrier policy is known as a *local coverage determination* or LCD. This practice has both good and bad points. On the good side, these policies affect only a part of the country. If the carrier implements a bad policy, then only a small region of the country suffers. On the other hand, if the policy is fair and reasonable, physicians in other areas can use the policy as a model for their carriers to follow. Having the potential for inconsistent policies in neighboring states does make billing more complicated, however!

Most Medicare medical necessity policies affecting anesthesiologists are actually LCDs. Carriers have introduced LCDs for MAC, pain management, TEE, and many other services. Many policies arise from claims data suggesting overuse, misuse, or abuse of certain procedures. The search page at the CMS website will allow you to research the NCDs and LCDs that may affect your practice (www.cms.hhs.gov/mcd/search.asp?clickon=search&).

Because both LCDs and NCDs implement Medicare law through regulation, both the CMS and the carriers must publish these proposals and allow public comment before implementation. Practicing physicians can provide valuable input into policy development, helping to assure that limitations are clinically sound, necessary care will not be unreasonably restricted, and that the policy does not create excessive administrative hassles. At the CMS, the Medicare Coverage Advisory Committee (MCAC) advises the Administrator on national coverage policy development (www.cms.hhs.gov/FACA/02_MCAC.asp). And at the carrier level, each contractor has a Carrier Advisory Committee (CAC) for each state. For larger states, in which more than one carrier may have responsibility for coverage, that state may have more than one CAC. Virtually every state has an anesthesiologist sitting on its carrier's CAC, and the ASA recently successfully nominated an anesthesiologist to serve on the MCAC.

Because the local carriers have significant power in affecting anesthesia practice, the ASA has fostered communications among anesthesiologists who serve on the CACs. The ASA Committee on Economics serves as a resource for our CAC members, as does our excellent staff in Washington, D.C., and Park Ridge, Illinois. Truly, these anesthesiologists who serve the specialty and medicine as a whole are unsung heroes. For those of you who find this process interesting and who might want to serve your specialty in this role, I strongly encourage you to contact your state anesthesia society or the ASA Washington Office. We'll do all that we can to mentor you in this pursuit.

MEDICARE CONTRACTING REFORM

In 2003, Congress passed the Medicare Prescription Drug, Improvement and Modernization Act (MMA). One of the provisions of this law instructed the CMS to significantly change the administration of Part A and Part B to make the process more dynamic, efficient, and responsive to the needs of beneficiaries and providers. In response, the CMS will be replacing the current fiscal intermediaries (Part A) and carriers (Part B) with 15 regional Medicare Administrative Contractors (another MAC) that will serve both Part A and Part B. The CMS will also create four additional MACs to handle durable medical equipment and home health/hospice claims processing.

In July 2006, the CMS awarded the first A/B MAC contract, which covered Arizona, Montana, North Dakota, South Dakota, Utah, and Wyoming. The CMS will determine the rest of the contractors by September 2008. For details on the program, see the CMS web page on Medicare Contracting Reform at www.cms.hhs.gov/MedicareContractingReform/01_Overview.asp#TopOfPage.

One interesting outgrowth of this process has been the requirement for the MACs to consolidate existing LCD policies within the new coverage regions. Thus far, the contractors have chosen to implement the least restrictive requirements of overlapping policies. If this trend continues, some of the more onerous local medical policies may be replaced with something better.

A BRIEF LOOK AT MEDICAID AND ANESTHESIA

NORMAN A. COHEN, MD

Medicaid, created at the same time as the Medicare program, is a welfare program that provides medical benefits and long-term care assistance to certain groups. The program is funded jointly by the states and the federal government, but each state administers the program independently, consistent with federal guidelines. The program is voluntary; however, every state has participated since 1982. Each state determines eligibility requirements, but, in general, poor children, pregnant women, the blind, disabled, and impoverished elderly are the groups most likely to receive Medicaid assistance. Medicaid provides both medical assistance and long-term care coverage for those who qualify. In 2001, >46 million Americans received Medicaid coverage, at a cost of $278 billion in 2003.

Dr. Marc Leib serves as a medical director for the Arizona managed-care Medicaid program and was a recent appointee to the American Society of Anesthesiologists (ASA) Committee on Economics. I once heard Dr. Leib answer a question about Medicaid programs by saying, "If you've seen one Medicaid program, you've seen one Medicaid program." Because each state administers its program, determines eligibility, and defines payments for physician services independently, I can provide little advice about Medicaid here that is broadly applicable.

In the late 1990s, I worked with ASA staff to conduct a survey of Medicaid payment policies and rates across the country. The results of this exercise matched Dr. Leib's experience. I could demonstrate little commonality in payment methodology, rates, or extent of coverage for anesthesia care. More recently, the ASA again conducted a focused survey to determine Medicaid payment rates. The only "good" news is that for states that use the base-plus-time payment system for anesthesia services, the average conversion factor is slightly higher than Medicare's. For most specialties, Medicaid payments are lower than Medicare's. You shouldn't believe for a moment that Medicaid gives preferential treatment to anesthesiologists. It's just that Medicare pays for anesthesia care at an exceptionally low rate.

To learn the specific requirements of your state's Medicaid program that are applicable to your practice, you should consult with your practice manager or billing staff, review the Medicaid pages at the Centers for Medicare and Medicaid Services (CMS) website, www.cms.hhs.gov/home/medicaid.asp, and contact your state Medicaid administrative agency.

© 2006 Mayo Foundation for Medical Education and Research

A BRIEF LOOK AT OTHER PAYERS

NORMAN A. COHEN, MD

After Medicare and Medicaid, the balance of income from professional services comes from private third-party health insurers, state and private worker's compensation programs, military health plans (Champus), the Veterans Administration, automobile insurers, and the patients themselves. You or your group may have contracts with one or more of these entities that tie your payments to an agreed-upon conversion factor, or, less commonly, to a *capitated rate*.

In a capitated agreement, the physician or group agrees to accept a guaranteed payment for each member of the health plan each month. In return, the physician must provide services for the plan's patients when indicated. Unlike fee-for-service medicine, under which the physician's income depends on performing visits and procedural services, capitated payments completely change the incentives, such that doing less maximizes your income. After a brief flurry of interest in capitation as a way to control the growth in health care expenditures, beneficiaries began fighting back, demonstrating that in some cases health plans and physicians were withholding needed services.

Other than capitation, insurers offer a number of payment mechanisms in their contracts to compensate anesthesiologists for their services. Most use the anesthesia base, time, and modifier system. Recently, some payers have started using incentive payments to reward quality. Reducing unnecessary testing, minimizing cancellations, and administering antibiotics in a timely fashion are all things by which anesthesiologists can help reduce direct and indirect costs of care. To the extent that practices can quantify these accomplishments, they have an opportunity to earn these incentive payments.

Other insurers guarantee to contracting physicians access to their patients but insist that the contracting physicians share some in the financial risk of insuring these patients. These plans often share risk by withholding a defined percentage of the agreed-upon payment, with the withheld amount being payable only at some future date if certain financial and other contractual goals are met. If your contract includes withholds, make your financial plans based on never seeing the withheld money. If you do get something, it truly qualifies as a bonus!

© 2006 Mayo Foundation for Medical Education and Research

For most anesthesiologists, patients with traditional third-party insurance still comprise the most lucrative sector of their business. With conversion factors on average over threefold higher than Medicare's rates, the value to the practice is clear. Looking forward, the future is not as rosy. With the "baby boomer" generation approaching Medicare eligibility age, with private health premiums increasing at double-digit rates, with large employers restricting health benefits or moving jobs oversees, and small employers unlikely to provide health benefits at all, the opportunity to maintain income through cost shifting to these payers is likely to shrink or vanish in the coming years. Whether the current fragmented health care financing "system" will actually survive in anything like its current form is considered unlikely by most health care economists and prognosticators; therefore, the likelihood of the status quo remaining stable is exceptionally small.

Private insurers are beginning to respond by consolidating through mergers to gain market power and by trying to cut costs. Health insurers can control costs by reducing payment rates, using risk-adjusting premiums, limiting coverage to a subset of all procedures, or establishing medical necessity guidelines for expensive and/or high-volume services. Until recently, major private insurers had few medical policies that affected anesthesiologists directly. Recently, though, several large payers, including Aetna, Wellpoint, Health Net, and others, have identified rapid growth in the use of anesthesia care for gastrointestinal endoscopies. Like Medicare with their MAC policies, these and other payers have started to establish medical necessity criteria for receiving anesthesia care associated with endoscopy. I would not be at all surprised to see similar policies produced for acute pain management and other elective services if volumes for those services increase more rapidly than desired by the insurers; furthermore, I believe that physician practices will face increasing difficulties in negotiating rate increases, because consolidation of insurers has reduced competition and increased the insurers negotiating leverage.

This is the second time in my career that I have seen the pendulum swing toward increased power for insurers while simultaneously hearing increasing cries about a looming health care crisis. Although I am not certain how all of this will evolve, I do know that we will likely have an interesting ride!

215

RESPECT IN THE OPERATING ROOM: BE GOOD ... NO, BE GREAT

GRACE L. CHIEN, MD AND TAMMILY R. CARPENTER, MD

What makes a good anesthesiologist? What makes a great one? We believe that in considering these questions, anesthesia providers can adopt principles established in successful businesses. Treacy and Wiersema suggest four keys to great success, all of which must be met: (i) excelling in one value discipline (product leadership, operational excellence, customer service); (ii) maintaining threshold standards of performance in the other value disciplines; (iii) improving value year after year; and (iv) building a well-tuned operating model focused on delivering unmatched value. The first two keys represent a framework for what is needed for success. The latter two speak to enduring success.

Product leadership involves delivery of an innovative or especially high-quality product. In anesthesiology, product leadership may result from subspecialty expertise or facility with newer techniques or technology such as transesophageal echocardiography, regional nerve block catheters, or difficult-airway management devices. Anesthesia providers with these skills may have an initial edge, but maintaining this advantage over time may be challenging. Even in the absence of unique subspecialty or technical expertise, focus on the delivery of exceptional quality to create product leadership. The ability to apply current knowledge is key. Recognize, critically interpret, and implement significant medical or surgical (not only anesthesiology) outcomes literature. For example, surgical-site infection-prevention initiatives in the Institute for Healthcare Improvement's 100K Lives Campaign are based on outcomes data reported in cardiac surgical and general medical journals. Simultaneously, understand details of the case at hand (e.g., How long will the procedure likely last? Is the aorta going to be clamped above or below the renal arteries? How long until the aortic clamp is to be removed?); understand how your choices will affect outcomes. Actively seek information you need to know to make good decisions for the patient and for others in the room with whom you share responsibility.

Operational excellence means being timely, time-efficient, cost-effective, and consistent. Be prepared and organized for your cases. Prepare for subsequent cases so that you minimize the need to return to the room before bringing the next patient back. Shape your practice to minimize the

© 2006 Mayo Foundation for Medical Education and Research

duration, but more important, the variability, of your procedural and emergence times through recognition of key factors, creation of a thoughtful plan, and efficient movement from one plan to a suitable alternative if needed (e.g., develop your own equivalent of the American Society of Anesthesiologists' difficult airway algorithm for neuraxial blocks, arterial cannulation, central venous catheters, etc.). One fundamental manufacturing principle is that understanding and minimizing variability through process control is critical to making gains in quality. Be consistent and predictable, yet look actively for opportunities to improve your routine practices.

Customer intimacy involves meeting your customers' needs or concerns. Learn your customer's preferred name and put it to use. Make your customers feel that they are important, heard, attended to with a range of services, and that their unique needs are met in a timely manner. Who are your customers? Patients are obviously customers, but so are your anesthesiology colleagues, surgeons, operating room nurses and technicians, pre- and postoperative nurses, anesthesia technicians, biomedical engineers, housekeepers, administrators, and any others who contribute to the overall success of an operating team. Consider the important role of housekeeping staff, whose job includes cleaning all surfaces and devices in an operating room in the same short turnover time that you have. When you keep your area relatively clean and tidy on a regular basis and communicate focused special needs early (e.g., spatter on a particular cable, a nearly empty hand hygiene dispenser), you further infection control measures, you respect the work of the housekeeper, and you gain reciprocal respect. Treat your peers with respect and, perhaps more important, adopt an egalitarian approach. People notice if you mistreat or disrespect any individual, particularly behind his or her back, and then they will wonder what you say about them behind their backs.

What are your customers' needs? Your understanding of your customers' critical factors for success and their preferences, and how you meet them, is contingent on good communication. Good communication is dependent on recognition and appreciation of the idea that different people have inherently different preferred ways of dealing with the world. Several personality inventories (e.g., the Myers-Briggs Type Indicator, Keirsey Temperament Sorter, and many others) illustrate this concept. Know your own preferred style. Couple it with understanding those of your customers and you will minimize misunderstandings.

Communicate at a time that is comfortable for all parties. As annoying as it is to you to be asked something in the midst of performing an anesthetic induction and intubation, so will it be annoying if you ask a team member something when he or she is focused on a critical task. When possible, discuss plans ahead of time to "get on the same page" and to avoid conflict in pressured situations. Respect the surgeon with focused brevity; concentrate on his or her concerns about a given case, likely challenges, options you might be considering to address everyone's concerns, and your recommendations and rationale. Sometimes a strategy of providing limited options, as in parenting, allows others to participate in the decision while ensuring that you are also happy with the result.

Conflict in the OR often represents divergent goals of different members of the care team. Don't fuel a fire; instead, defuse it. The Thomas-Kilmann Conflict Mode Instrument is an example of a simple instrument to learn about your and others' different preferred styles of handling conflict. Use any one of the five different modes (avoiding, accommodating, compromising, competing, and collaborating) as appropriate and effective. At times, you may be an effective "team player" by being cooperative ("don't sweat the small stuff"), but when something is important or urgent, balance cooperativeness with assertiveness lest the team miss a critical piece of information or perspective.

In conflict situations, focus on each party's goals rather than proposed actions. Pause to clarify what you want and why. Reflect on facts rather than emotion. Intuition may be important but must be recognized for what it is. What is the actionable benefit of your plan? If a given case is being postponed, how will the results of a cardiology consultation change your management? What is the risk of your plan? Is the required duration of antiplatelet therapy after percutaneous coronary intervention (or risk of continuing antiplatelet therapy perioperatively) appropriate relative to the risk of progression of underlying disease during postponement of surgery? Reflect also on positions the other party is likely to take and why.

Discuss contentious matters in private whenever possible. If the issue can be deferred, consider making an office appointment to meet with the other party. Always leave the other party a graceful exit, especially in the circumstance of an unavoidably public encounter. When you share your concerns, remind everyone that your mutual goal is a good patient outcome. Listen actively; a party who has been heard is more likely to acquiesce to a plan other than his or her own. Negotiate, rather than demand; consider alternatives or compromises that would be acceptable to both parties.

Once you understand what is needed, how do you deliver the product? Deming is widely credited with improving production in postwar Japan (e.g., Toyota automotives, Sony electronics). His principles have been applied across many disciplines, and many can be applied directly to managing an effective and efficient OR. In addition to emphasizing quality and process control principles, Deming also advocated: (a) creating an atmosphere of purposefulness in which all members of the team are focused on patient care and safety; (b) breaking down barriers between departments and adopting a win–win approach to patient care, thus ensuring that all team members are working toward the same goal; (c) recognizing and utilizing the fact that team members have different abilities, capabilities, and aspirations; (d) driving out fear and building trust so that everyone can work more effectively; (e) setting appropriate expectations (perfection is unachievable, and threats of punishment only create adversarial relationships, further lowering chances for success); and (f) removing barriers that rob people of joy in their work. We recommend modeling these behaviors. Set the tone for a favorable climate in which each team member performs to the best of his or her ability, thereby furthering quality patient care. Maintain an upbeat attitude and keep working on improvements.

In summary, understand the breadth and depth of effort it takes to excel as an anesthesia provider. A threshold-level performance is required in each of product leadership, operational excellence, *and* customer intimacy. Acknowledge and address your weak areas, develop as many strengths as possible, and work toward continual improvement. Learn about yourself; communication and people skills are not merely "touchy-feely" intangibles but are based in successful business principles.

- Be a jack of all trades. . .
  - Know your stuff, *and*
  - Deliver it well, *and*
  - Be respectful of others
- . . . and master of one:
  - Master yourself.
- Be great. Respect will follow.

SUGGESTED READINGS

Deming WE. *Out of the Crisis.* Cambridge, MA: MIT Press; 1982.

Deming WE. *The New Economics for Industry, Government, Education.* 2nd ed. Cambridge, MA: MIT Press; 2000.

Goleman D. *Emotional Intelligence: Why It Can Matter More Than IQ.* New York: Bantam Books; 1995.

Institute for Healthcare Improvement, 100K Lives Campaign, Prevention of Surgical Site Infection, www.ihi.org/ihi/programs/campaign, November 2006.

Keirsey D. *Please Understand Me II: Temperament, Character, Intelligence.* Del Mar, CA: Prometheus Nemesis; 1998.

Thomas KW, Kilmann RH. *Thomas-Kilmann Conflict Mode Instrument.* Mountain View, CA: Consulting Psychologists Press; 1974.

Treacy M, Wiersema F. *The Discipline of Market Leaders: Choose Your Customers, Narrow Your Focus, Dominate Your Market.* New York: Perseus; 1995.

INDEX

Note: Page numbers followed by *f* indicate figures; page numbers followed by *t* indicate tables.